Surgery of the

Liver, Pancreas and Biliary Tract

Edited by

JOHN S. NAJARIAN, M.D.
JOHN P. DELANEY, M.D.

Surgery of the

Liver, Pancreas and Biliary Tract

Edited by

JOHN S. NAJARIAN, M.D.
JOHN P. DELANEY, M.D.

Selected papers and discussion from the Annual Continuation Course in Surgery, "Surgery of the Liver, Pancreas and Biliary Tract," University of Minnesota, Department of Surgery, Minneapolis, Minnesota.

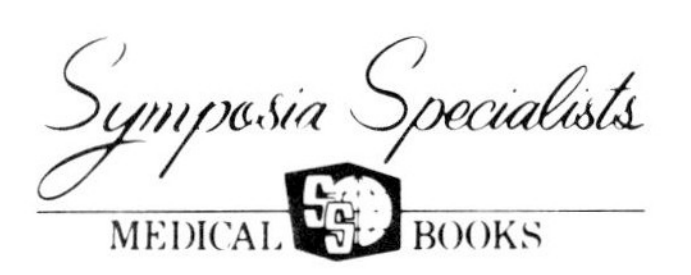

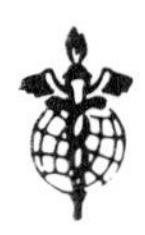

STRATTON INTERCONTINENTAL MEDICAL BOOK CORPORATION
381 Park Avenue South, New York, New York 10016 and London

Library of Congress Catalog
Card No. 74-27862

ISBN 0-88372-025-6

Symposia Specialists

MIAMI, FLORIDA, 33161

Printed in the U.S.A.

Contents

Preface

A long-standing tradition for the University of Minnesota Department of Surgery has been to present an annual Continuation Course. In the past few years the enrollment has increased markedly. More than 700 surgeons were registered at the Course from which this book originated. The growing popularity is attributable, in part, to generally increased interest in continuing education but more, we think, to the excellence of the speakers and the quality of the presentations. In organizing the program, a simple criterion was used to invite the visiting professors, namely, who is the leading expert on the topic. Participants from the United States and abroad were supplemented by members of the faculty of the University of Minnesota Medical School Departments of Surgery, Medicine, Pediatrics and Anesthesiology.

The book is planned to span a broad area of general surgery. In this context, surgery is viewed as including certain basic science topics which provide the intellectual basis for surgical practice. This book is not intended as a comprehensive coverage of surgery of the liver, pancreas and biliary tract. It is not conceived of as a substitute for standard textbooks nor for journals. Rather, the topics chosen emphasize the controversial and relatively new developments.

The book is divided into five sections. The first two articles deal with the technique of splenectomy and the hematologic indications for its performance. The second section covers selected topics in physiology and surgery of the biliary tract. Particularly noteworthy are the chapters on the new areas, dissolution of gallstones, nonoperative instrumentation of the bile ducts, and retrograde cholangiography. The third section deals with surgery of the pancreas. Topics of special current interest in this group of papers are those of resection for acute pancreatitis and the concept of peritoneal lavage for treatment of this entity, as outlined in "Acute Pancreatitis: The Toxic Effects." The fourth section of the book concentrates on surgery of the liver. In fact, at least half of the section is medical in orientation, dealing with such topics as hepatitis B antigen, differential diagnosis of jaundice, chronic active hepatitis, alcoholic hepatitis and cholestasis. The editors make no apology for this medical orientation. When dealing with the complex problems that arise in caring for the jaundiced patient, the surgeon indeed must be an "internist who operates." The final section of the text reviews the various surgical interventions for complications of portal hypertension.

We were very pleased with the Continuation Course and trust that the reader will find this book, the proceedings of the course, stimulating, provocative and informative.

John S. Najarian, M.D.
John P. Delaney, M.D.

I

Spleen

The Technique of Splenectomy

Robert M. Zollinger, M.D.

Introduction

Splenectomy is commonly performed in association with operations on the upper abdomen. During the last 25 years, almost 2,000 splenectomies have been performed at The Ohio State University Hospitals. A great majority of these were carried out for either primary or secondary hypersplenism. The special interest of our medical colleagues in hematologic disorders has been responsible for the large number of patients operated upon for hypersplenism. The incidence of hypersplenism appeared to peak in 1964, but has since declined. The number associated with trauma has steadily increased. Incidental splenectomy has also been a more and more common indication. This group includes those patients who had splenectomy during such extensive operations as total gastrectomy, pancreatectomy or procedures for malignancy of the left colon. In addition, there seemed to be an increase in splenectomies incidental to operations for benign gastrointestinal disease which clearly indicated the need for review of the technique being carried out.

Preoperative Evaluation

Before carrying out a splenectomy, the surgeon must be familiar with the indications other than trauma, since the various indications for splenectomy sometime present different pre- and postoperative problems. It is helpful to know whether the hypersplenism is primary or secondary, since the primary group is a much better surgical risk. Patients with secondary hypersplenism have a severe primary disease such as lymphoma. Furthermore, approximately one half of the patients will have had steroid therapy, and it is important to take this into consideration in the immediate preoperative period with replacement of steroids, doubling the

---

Robert M. Zollinger, M.D., Department of Surgery, The Ohio State University College of Medicine, Columbus.

dosage of steroids on the day after surgery, and the continuation of steroid therapy during the postoperative period. Failure to do so may precipitate acute adrenal insufficiency in the early postoperative period. Other factors to be considered include whether chemotherapy has been given as well as the status of the bone marrow. In our cases, a hematologist with wide experience in bone marrow evaluation has carried out this procedure. If there is no activity within the bone marrow, splenectomy has usually been contraindicated. The various newer procedures for portal hypertension make splenectomy a less frequent operation than in former years. Finally, the age and general condition of the patient are, of course, very important. The older the patient and the more serious the primary disease, the higher the risk. Since the most common indication for elective splenectomy tends to be thrombocytopenic purpura, it is important to have platelet transfusions and whole blood available. Blood should not be given, however, in patients with hereditary spherocytosis because of the possibility of inducing hemolytic crisis.

Surgical Considerations

Although some prefer the subcostal incision, we have used either the left paramedian or a midline incision. The midline incision is especially important in patients having a staging procedure for Hodgkin's disease, since dissection of the aortic lymph nodes may be necessary.

In the presence of a low platelet count, every individual vessel should be ligated. It is advantageous to take time to ligate all of these bleeding points except when the platelet count is quite low. Under those circumstances, the clamps may be left in place and the abdomen opened in the hope of reversing the bleeding by ligation of the splenic artery and removal of the spleen. As soon as the abdomen is opened, it is important to search for accessory spleens, before hemorrhage in the surrounding tissues masks the smaller ones. If this is delayed, pseudoaccessory spleens may develop due to hemorrhage beneath the subserosa around the hilus of the spleen, the gastrocolic ligament or even posterior to the spleen itself. When one accessory spleen is found, additional ones should be sought. It has been our experience that the incidence of accessory spleens averages about 12% but the range varies from 7% with incidental or traumatic splenectomy, when no effort is made to find them, to 15% in hypersplenism and 22% in staging procedures for Hodgkin's disease. When the operation is carried out for hypersplenism, the end result will be compromised unless all splenic tissue is removed. The importance, therefore, of removing the accessory spleens cannot be overemphasized.

Fabri et al [1] in a recent review found that incidental splenectomy had emerged as the most common type of splenic surgery. Such increase was largely the result of radical operations on the stomach, pancreas or colon, renal transplantation, hepatic disease and splenectomy for staging Hodgkin's disease. There were many cases in this group where the splenic capsule was torn during an operation on the upper abdomen, and it was believed safer to remove the spleen than to attempt repair of the capsule. Unfortunately, it was found that the addition of splenectomy to major surgical procedures was accompanied by increased rates of morbidity and mortality. In a group of 136 patients who had operations on the stomach, pancreas and colon without splenectomy, the surgical mortality was 5% and 32% had postoperative complications. Patients who underwent gastrointestinal surgery with splenectomy had a mortality of 28% and a considerably higher incidence of subphrenic abscess (8.8%) and hemorrhage (2.2%) than in surgery for hypersplenism. In other words, the incidental removal of the spleen during an elective procedure is not as harmless as was formerly believed.

Surgical Technique

The technical aspects of splenectomy are not particularly challenging if the surgeon is familiar with the various anatomic relations of the spleen. Years ago Dunphy [2] described the spleen as part of an anatomical sandwich. The gastrosplenic ligament is the bread while the pancreas itself is perhaps the meat and the splenorenal ligament might be compared to the posterior layer of the sandwich.

In the presence of a traumatic rupture of the spleen, bleeding must be controlled as quickly as possible; and for that reason, mass ligation of the pedicle may be indicated. However, it is safer for the patient if a meticulous and anatomic approach is carried out. The initial step is to divide the gastrosplenic ligament and individually ligate the short gastric vessels. The gastrosplenic ligament is usually divided in order to open the lesser sac preliminary to ligating the splenic artery. The gastrosplenic vessels are separated by several centimeters, permitting individual clamping and ligation. It is important to transfix the vessels on the gastric side to the gastric wall in order to avoid hemorrhage should postoperative gastric distention occur. A small bite in the gastric wall is included in the suture, preliminary to ligation of the contents of the clamp. As soon as three or four of these vessels have been ligated, it is possible to get a clear view of the pancreas and to identify the tortuous course of the splenic artery. The splenic artery may vary in size, but usually it can readily be seen beneath the peritoneum unless it is hidden by multiple, enlarged lymph nodes. The location of the splenic artery can also be identified by palpation if the patient is obese. A long right-angle clamp is then used to isolate the splenic artery and surrounding structures preliminary to ligating it with 00 silk. At this point, whole blood transfusions may be started in patients with low blood levels regardless of the cause. Ligation of the splenic artery also tends to decrease the size of the spleen, at least temporarily, and makes it easier to manipulate without tearing the capsule. In previous years, some had recommended injection of adrenalin directly into the spleen to effect this same shrinking response.

One of the difficult portions of splenectomy involves separating the fundus of the stomach from the very tip of the spleen. If this is not done carefully and under direct vision, two complications may result: injury to the fundus with a high-output fistula which tends to be quite serious; or, second, the surgeon may forget the double blood supply to the fundus in this area. After ligation of the superficial layer of gastrosplenic vessels, it is important to remember that there is a sizable gastric vessel about 2 cm from the curvature itself. If this vessel is overlooked, massive hemorrhage is liable to occur, particularly in the presence of portal hypertension. When all the splenic vessels have been divided, along with the splenic artery, any adhesions between the spleen and parietes are lysed. Some have suggested that even the peritoneum should be excised along with the spleen when adhesions are severe, but we have not found this to be necessary. When applying traction to the spleen, the surgeon should avoid tearing the splenic capsule since seeding of splenic tissue may occur, with the development of splenosis.

It is worthwhile to pull down on the contracted spleen with the right hand and with the left hand incise the peritoneum over the left adrenal gland and continue as far posteriorly as possible. The hands can then be changed, with the left hand maintaining upward traction, and the splenorenal ligament can immediately be divided. When there are sizable vessels in this structure, clamps may be applied on the lateral side to adequately control all bleeding points. Likewise, the colon may on occasion be adherently attached to the inferior surface of the spleen. Usually, the spleen and the tail of the pancreas can be easily mobilized toward the midline and outside the peritoneal cavity. Packs are applied in the left upper quadrant after active bleeding points have been clamped and tied. In the management of the pedicle, it is important to avoid injury to the tail of the pancreas, which sometimes is almost confluent with the splenic tissue.

Difficulties with postoperative bleeding are more likely to result from failure to control bleeding points in the tail of the pancreas than elsewhere. The splenic artery should be separately identified along with the splenic vein, which tends to remain hidden beneath the artery and in the pancreatic tissue. The tail of the pancreas is gently separated from the hilus of the spleen and all bleeding points tied.

If it is important to conserve blood, the splenic artery has sometimes been divided, leaving only the splenic vein attached. At this time, the spleen is compressed in order to provide an autotransfusion to the patient. Finally, only the splenic vein remains to be doubly clamped and tied. The major vessels to the pedicle should be ligated first and then transfixed distally. Fatal hemorrhages have occurred when the needle has been blindly passed through the pedicle with a resultant tearing of the splenic vein.

After the spleen has been removed, the tail of the pancreas is again carefully inspected for evidence of hemorrhage, and likewise the area of the splenocolic ligament and the omentum are searched for accessory spleens. Sometimes it is possible to peritonealize the splenic bed. A long right-angle clamp is used to stabilize the peritoneal margins, thus facilitating placement of these sutures. Following this, it is essential to biopsy the lymph nodes above the pancreas and from the retroperitoneal tissue as well as from the mesentery of the small bowel. We have done this routinely, particularly in patients having splenectomy for hypersplenism. In addition, a wedge biopsy of the liver is taken. We usually use a transfixing suture of silk on either side in order to provide a biopsy of the margin of the liver several centimeters wide. Additional sutures are taken in order to make certain that there is no chance of postoperative bleeding. A strip of Gelfoam is sometimes applied over the wound. Pathologic examination of these biopsies may well convert the diagnosis of primary hypersplenism to secondary hypersplenism.

Staging for Hodgkin's Disease

A recent indication for splenectomy has been as a staging procedure for Hodgkin's disease [3] (Fig. 1). Not only must the spleen and all the accessory spleens be removed, but also biopsy of the liver and the retroperitoneal lymph nodes, including any enlarged lymph nodes that may have been shown up by lymphangiography, should be done. It may be necessary to open the lesser sac to mobilize the left side of the pancreas to gain access to the enlarged lymph nodes, especially on the left side of the

HODGKIN'S DISEASE

SPLENECTOMY•

Secondary Hypersplenism•

? Abdominal Involvement•

Biopsy Liver & Periaortic Nodes

Excision Periaortic Nodes T_{12} L_3

Open Marrow Biopsy - Iliac Crest

Final Staging - Definitive Therapy

FIG. 1. A recent, important indication for splenectomy has been as a staging procedure for Hodgkin's disease.

aorta, or in the tissues adjacent to the aorta, or gently separate it with excision, with sufficient biopsies to determine if they are involved with Hodgkin's disease. In the presence of Hodgkin's disease, not only should the vessels of the tail of the pancreas be identified with silver clips, but also the site of any lymph node biopsy as well as obvious tumors within the liver or at the site of liver biopsy. These markers are used in subsequent irradiation therapy to indicate whether they are being distorted by recurrent disease.

Conclusions

The technical considerations which are extremely important include making certain that all accessory spleens are identified early (Fig. 2). When one is found, there may be others. Approximately 15%-20% should be recovered. The short gastric vessels should be transfixed to avoid hemorrhage in the presence of postoperative gastric distention. Except in the presence of massive hemorrhage with a ruptured spleen, individual ligation of all bleeding points with preliminary opening of the lesser sac and ligation of the splenic artery is believed to be the best surgical approach. The surgeon should avoid injury to the fundus of the stomach, particularly keeping in mind that it may be confluent with the uppermost portion of the hilus of the spleen. Furthermore, he should not forget the secondary blood supply to the fundus of the stomach, particularly in the

TECHNICAL CONSIDERATIONS

Identify accessory spleens (early)
Transfix short gastric vessels
Preliminary ligation of splenic artery
Avoid injury · Fundus
Tail of Pancreas
Splenic Capsule
Peritonealize splenic bed ?
Delay closure · Observe bleeding

FIG. 2. Familiarity with the anatomical relationships of the spleen combined with meticulous operative technic will ensure satisfactory morbidity and mortality rates associated with splenectomy.

presence of a very large spleen or portal hypertension. The tail of the pancreas should be protected from injury and the surgeon should identify the relationship between the tail of the pancreas and the hilus of the spleen as early as possible. All bleeding points in the tail of the pancreas should be carefully ligated. Tear of the splenic capsule should be avoided because of the danger of splenosis. When possible, the splenic bed should be peritonealized, but this is not absolutely necessary.

Summary

Familiarity with the anatomical relationships of the spleen combined with meticulous operative technic will ensure satisfactory morbidity and mortality rates associated with splenectomy. Biopsy of the liver as well as the retroperitoneal lymph nodes should often be considered essential in the majority of elective splenectomies.

References

1. Fabri, P. J., Metz, E. N., Nick, W. V. et al: A quarter century with splenectomy. Changing concepts. Arch. Surg., 108:569, 1974.
2. Dunphy, J. E.: Splenectomy for trauma: Practical points in surgical technique. Amer. J. Surg., 71:450, 1946.
3. Hellman, S.: Current studies in Hodgkin's disease. New Eng. J. Med., 290:894, 1974.

Splenectomy for Hematologic Disease

Seymour I. Schwartz, M.D.

Over the past decade, as a consequence of a dialogue with enlightened hematologists, we have had personal experience with well over 250 patients in whom splenectomy was performed for hematologic disorders. We collated the first 200 sequential cases, all of whom have had follow-up (Fig. 1). The largest group had idiopathic thrombocytopenic purpura (ITP) and there is a significant number of patients with hereditary spherocytosis and what we shall term, and describe later as malignant hemopathy.

It is appropriate to begin with a consideration of the hemolytic anemias. They are generally classified as congenital or acquired. The congenital types are due to an intrinsic abnormality of the erythrocytes, while the acquired anemia is related to an extracorpuscular factor, acting on an intrinsically normal cell. The most common congenital anemia for which splenectomy is performed is hereditary spherocytosis in which the red cells are smaller than normal, unusually thick and almost spherical in shape. A defective cell membrane is responsible for an increased osmotic fragility, ie, (Fig. 2) the cells disrupt in a saline concentration of 0.75 gm% in contrast to the normal of 0.5%. Both the spherical shape and intrinsic changes in the membrane cause these cells to be more rigid and less deformable than normal cells; this factor seems to be responsible for the difficulty encountered by the cells in passing through the splenic pulp, since following splenectomy, the half-life of the red cells becomes normal and clinical cure occurs. Hereditary spherocytosis is certainly regarded as a surgeon's delight. The spleen is usually enlarged. The salient features of the disease are anemia and jaundice in addition to splenomegaly. It is unusual for the anemia to be severe. Because cholelithiasis is reported in 30%-60% of cases, with gallstones of the pigment variety, all patients should have a cholecystogram preoperatively. Chronic leg ulcers, without varicose veins, represent an unusual complication of the disease and will not heal unless

Seymour I. Schwartz, M.D., Professor, Department of Surgery, University of Rochester School of Medicine, N.Y.

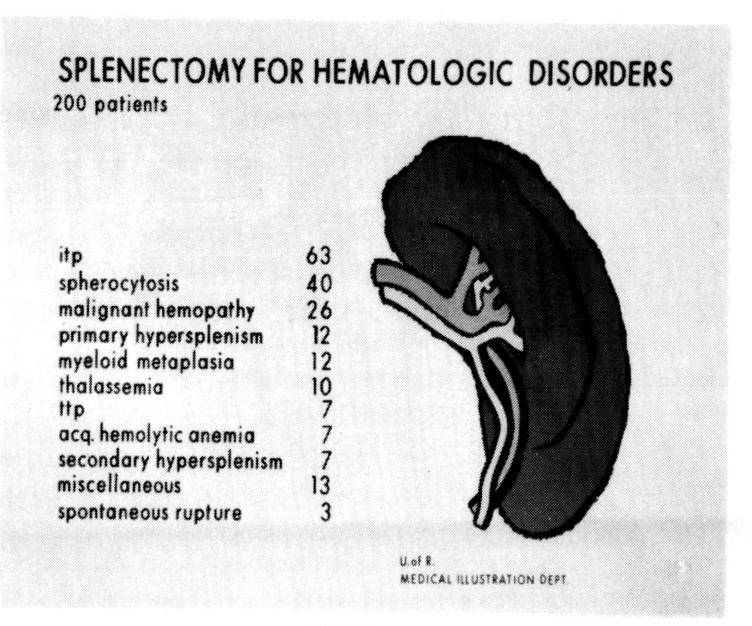

FIGURE 1.

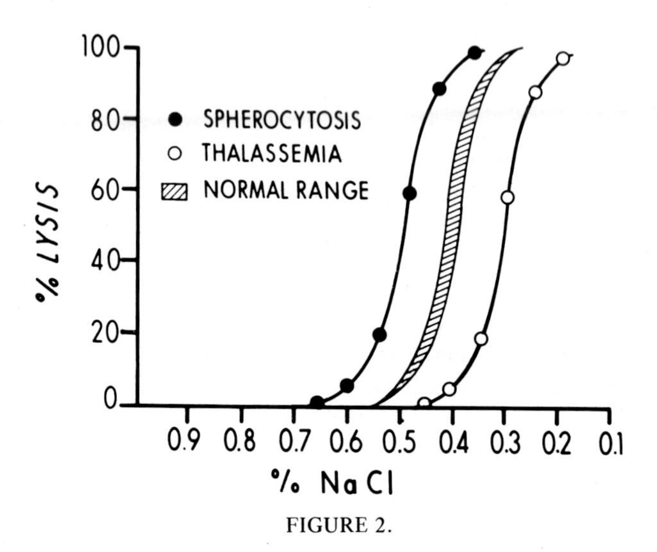

FIGURE 2.

splenectomy is performed. Splenectomy constitutes the sole therapy and results of removal of the spleen are generally excellent. In our experience with 40 patients, all had excellent results, and there were no deaths (Fig. 3). Within a few days following removal of the spleen, the erythrocytes achieve a normal life span, jaundice is reduced and there is gradual improvement of the anemia. Interestingly, the erythrocyte morphology and membrane abnormality are not altered, and the increased osmotic fragility perisists. The gallbladder is always explored at the operative procedure and concomitant cholecystectomy is performed if stones are present. Because of the theoretical risk of increased infection, we now generally recommend that the operation be delayed until the third or fourth year of life, and give antibiotic therapy postoperatively.

Another hereditary abnormality, elliptocytosis (Fig. 4), is quite rare, usually exists as a harmless trait, but may cause hemolytic anemia. In these patients, over 90% of the red cells are involved in the elliptical process; the disease is thought to occur in about 0.04% of the population. Symptoms and manifestations are similar to those of hereditary spherocytosis, and splenectomy is indicated in all symptomatic cases. Removal of the organ is almost always followed by lasting decrease in hemolysis and corrected

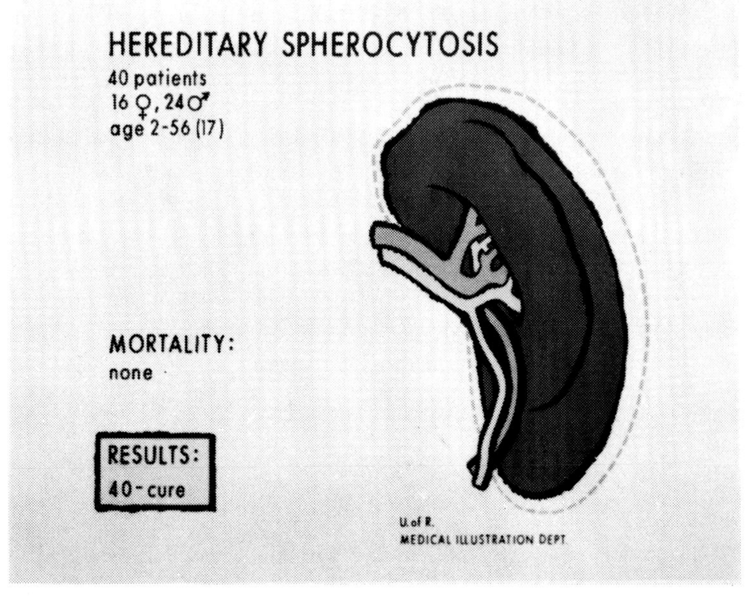

FIGURE 3.

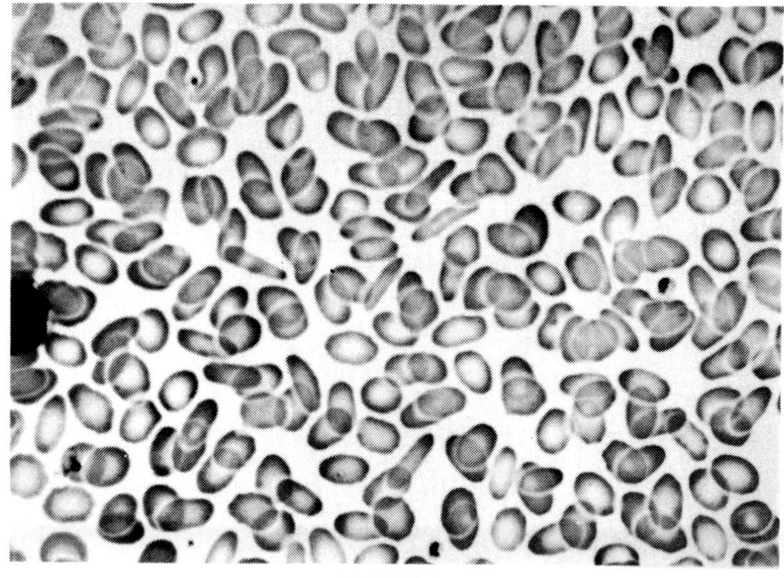

FIGURE 4.

anemia, while the morphologic abnormality of the red cell remains unchanged.

Thalassemia, or Mediterranean anemia, is a congenital anemia, due primarily to a defect in hemoglobin synthesis. It exists in two degrees of severity: thalassemia major, or Cooley's anemia, which is a serious disorder, often fatal in childhood, and thalassemia minor which is comparatively mild in adolescents and adults. Gradations between the two have been called thalassemia intermedia. The disease is transmitted by either parent as a dominant trait, with thalassemia major representing the homozygous state. Thalassemia intermedia is usually either an unusually severe variant of thalassemia minor, or thalassemia minor coupled with another inherited defect in the hemoglobin or red cell metabolism. The hemoglobin deficient cells are thin and misshapen, appearing in many bizarre forms, including target cells and cell fragments (Fig. 5). Because of their low hemoglobin content, they are able to absorb more fluid than normal without bursting, resulting in increased red cell resistance to hypotonic saline.

We have had a reasonable experience with thalassemia in view of the high percentage of Italians in our population. In fact, the disease was named by Drs. Whipple and Bradford in our auditorium at a pediatric grand rounds. Surgically we are concerned only with patients who present

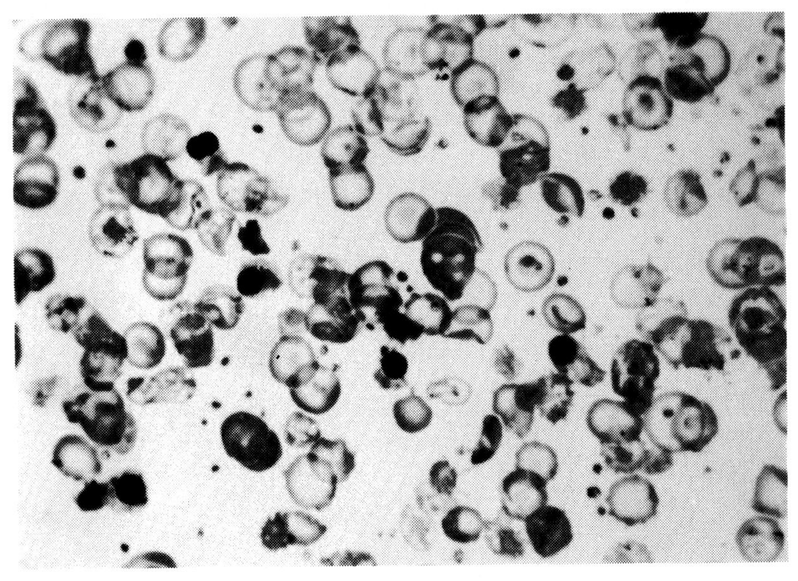

FIGURE 5.

with manifestations of anemia of significant proportions, jaundice and splenomegaly. Recurrent infections occur frequently in these cases, often leading to the death of the more severely involved patient. Gallstones were reported in about 25% of these patients. Transfusions are required at regular intervals, but since most children accommodate to a lowered hemoglobin level, it is better to maintain a hemoglobin of about 10 gm rather than continually transfuse. In the experience with ten cases, there was one death four years after surgery. Transfusion needs were reduced in all nine survivors (Fig. 6). In general, the best results associated with splenectomy were obtained in older children and in young adults with large spleens in whom excessive splenic sequestration could be demonstrated.

To complete the consideration of hemolytic anemias for which surgical intervention may be required, we come to the acquired type known as idiopathic autoimmune hemolytic anemia, the distinguishing feature of which is a direct or indirect Coomb's Test positivity for an antibody in the patient's red cell or in the serum. These patients are generally managed medically with steroid therapy. Splenectomy is indicated if steroids are ineffective, or if excessive doses of steroids are required, or perhaps if steroids are contraindicated. In these patients sequestration studies using 51-Chromium tagged red cells are particularly pertinent. One measures the

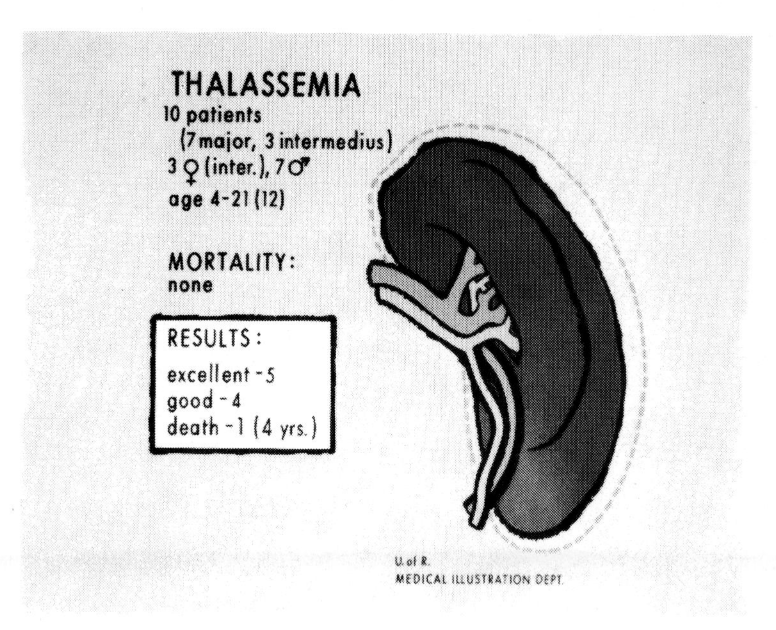

FIGURE 6.

spleen to liver index, which normally is 1 to 1; if the index is greater than 2 to 1, then one can anticipate effective results subsequent to splenectomy.

We have operated on seven patients who were refractory to medical therapy. Six of the seven have had excellent responses. There were no operative deaths. Two patients did require short-term steroid therapy (Fig. 7).

Idiopathic thrombocytopenic purpura heads the list of diseases requiring splenectomy in our series. It is of interest that in 1916, Kaznelson, who was a fourth year medical student, suggested that the procedure could induce an increase in circulating platelets. For many years therapeutic reliance was placed on splenectomy. However with the availability of steroid therapy in the 1950s, there was an impetus for reevaluating the therapeutic results. Much of the confusion regarding the efficacy of therapy stems from the inclusion of a variety of disorders in the nomenclature of ITP. The term should be reserved for ecchymotic and petechicial disorders characterized by a subnormal platelet count in the presence of a marrow containing normal or increased megakariocytes, in the absence of any systemic disease or history of drug ingestion. The platelet count in these patients is generally 50,000 or less. The bleeding

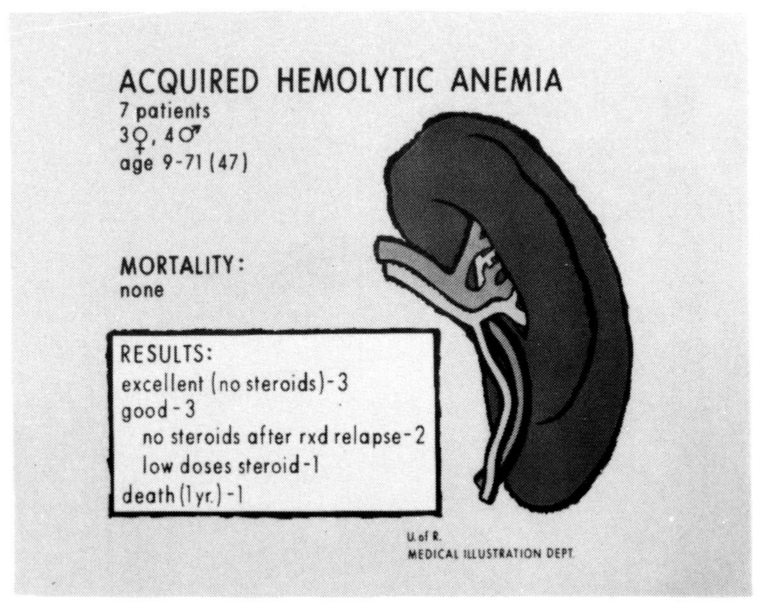

FIGURE 7.

time is prolonged, and platelet survival following transfusion is shortened. Examination of the bone marrow reveals megakariocytes to be normal or increased in number; qualitatively they demonstrate degranulation of the cytoplasm, pseudopodia and vacuolization (Fig. 8).

The argument concerning the relative value and disadvantages of steroid therapy relates largely to the evangelical pleas for steroid therapy by Dr. Dameshek, who reported that the platelets increased to normal levels in 90% of acute cases and 60% of chronic cases (Fig. 9). Most of these patients continued to receive steroid therapy and became Cushionoid.

Other experiences did not substantiate the data presented by Dameshek. In contrast, the results achieved by splenectomy are much more impressive with a success rate of between 60% and 90% (Fig. 10). If we consider those series in which comparative response to steroids and splenectomy was evaluated, there is no question that splenectomy produced a more favorable response. Failures with steroid therapy did not affect subsequent success with splenectomy (Fig. 11).

In our personal experience with 63 patients, 51 of 56 available for follow-up had permanent remission. There were three temporary relapses requiring steroids for short periods of time (Fig. 12).

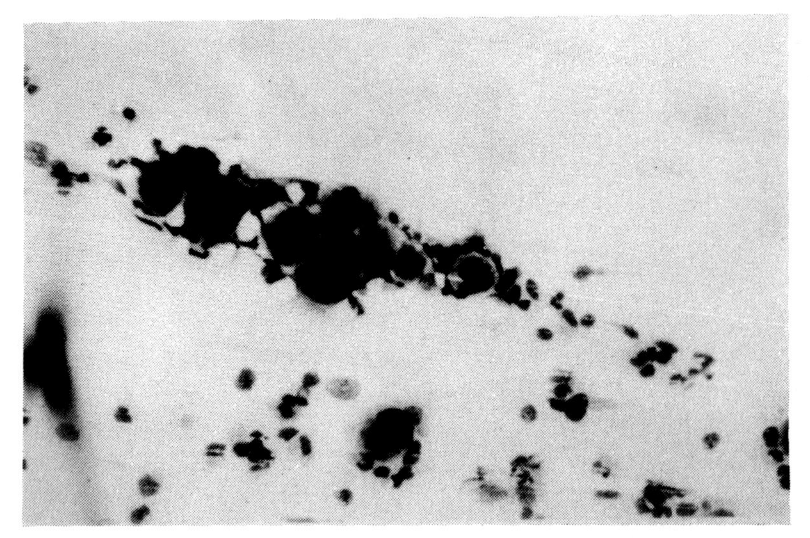

FIGURE 8.

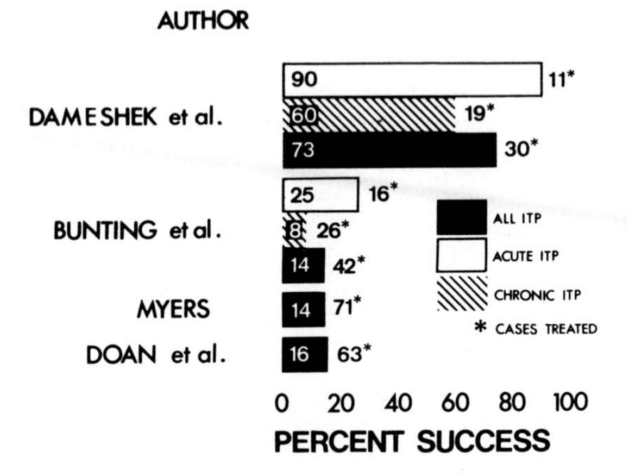

FIGURE 9.

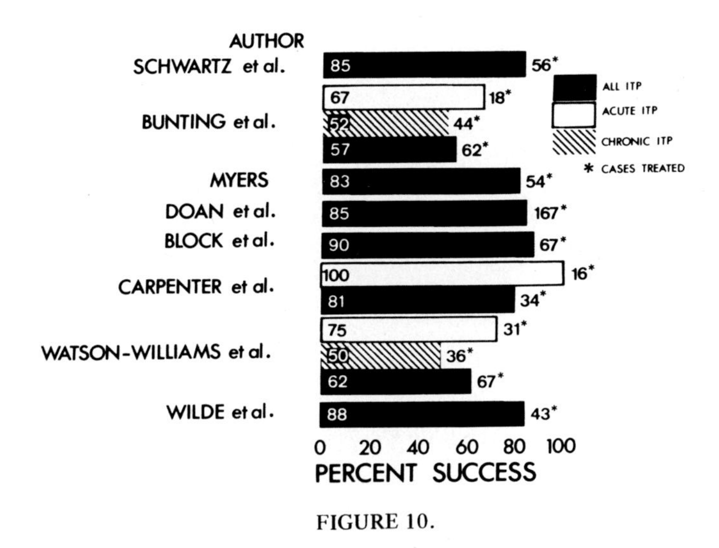

FIGURE 10.

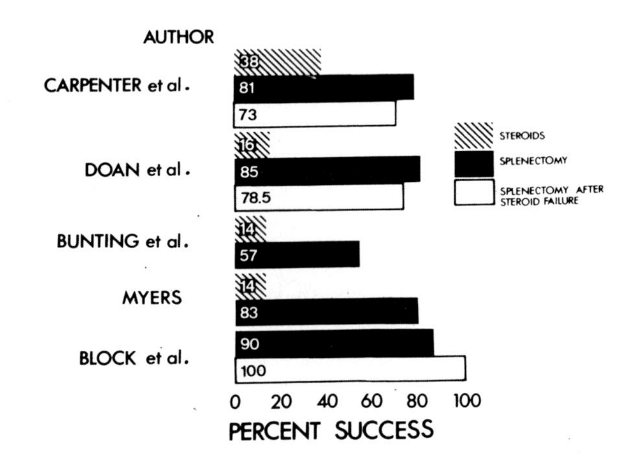

FIGURE 11.

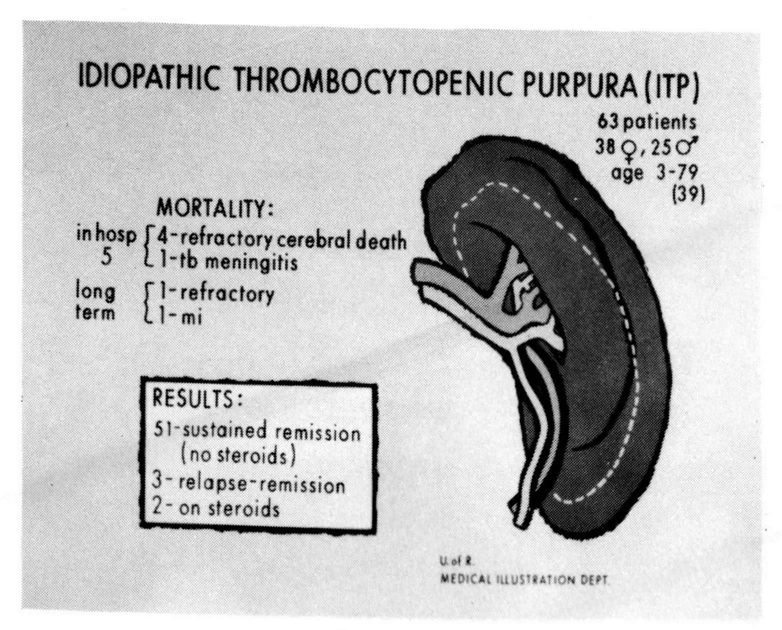

FIGURE 12.

In our experience, four postoperative deaths related to the surgical procedure occurred only in patients who had splenectomy for emergency reasons, ie, fulminant disease with uncontrollable hemorrhage or intracranial bleeding. During the same period, we had two patients with ITP admitted for elective splenectomy, who developed manifestations of intracranial bleeding in the course of the preoperative preparation and died. Thus, we feel that any manifestation of possible intracranial bleeding is preemptive to emergency surgery. One of the concerns regarding splenectomy was the idea that disseminated lupus developed with increased frequency after operation. This is not true in our series, or in the experience of others. It is now believed that many of the patients classified as ITP in the Dameshek series, in fact, had systemic lupus prior to surgery. This diagnosis can be made by histologic evaluation of the spleen.

Thrombotic thrombocytopenic purpura is a disease of the arterioles and capillaries in which the hematologic alteration in response to splenectomy is such that it merits inclusion in this discussion. The role of the spleen has been hard to define. We have had experience with seven patients (Fig. 13) who had the classic clinical symptoms: fever, purpura, hemolytic anemia, neurologic manifestations and signs of renal disease. In the majority of cases, the disease follows a rapid downhill course. Our

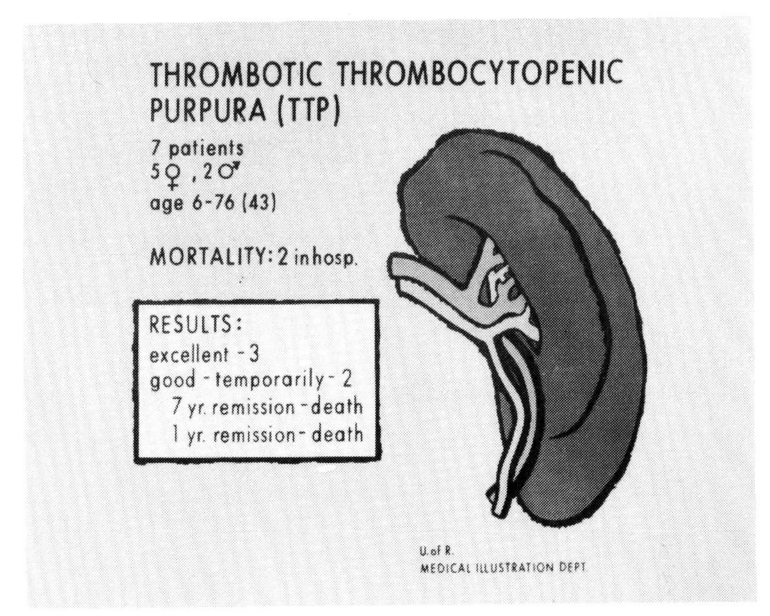

FIGURE 13.

experience with seven patients suggests an aggressive approach in that three patients had an excellent and sustained response, while two were temporarily improved after splenectomy. Collating the data (Fig. 14) about 300 cases have been reported with an overall survival of 8.6%. For nonsplenectomized cases the rate was 5.4%, whereas 40% of all splenectomized cases, 50% of those who were reasonable risks, survived. More important is the fact that of the 26 reported survivors, 17, or 65%, had been splenectomized. Our regimen, therefore, includes massive doses of steroids and emergency splenectomy in these patients.

In 1939, Wiseman and Doan described a disease consisting of splenomegaly and neutropenia in which splenectomy was curative. A few years later they enlarged the concept to include patients who were pancytopenic. The etiology is unknown. The patients have a hyperplastic marrow and corticosteroids rarely affect the process. Once the diagnosis is made, splenectomy is indicated in view of the excellent results (Fig. 15). We are somewhat concerned with the diagnosis in that over half of the patients whom we have cared for following splenectomy have subsequently developed a lymphomatous process or reticulum cell sarcoma. This parallels the experience of others leading to the question of whether this disease actually exists as a separate entity.

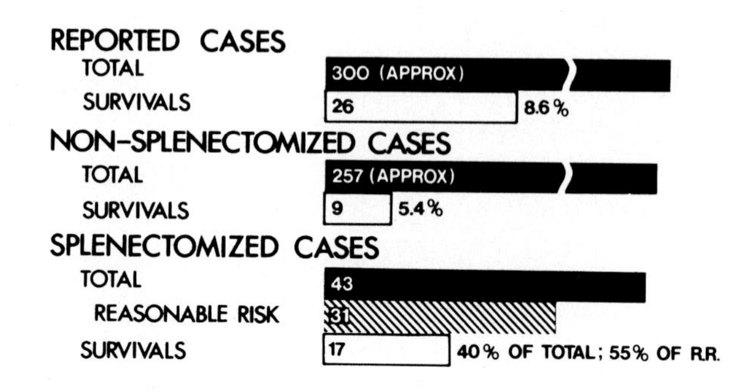

FIGURE 14.

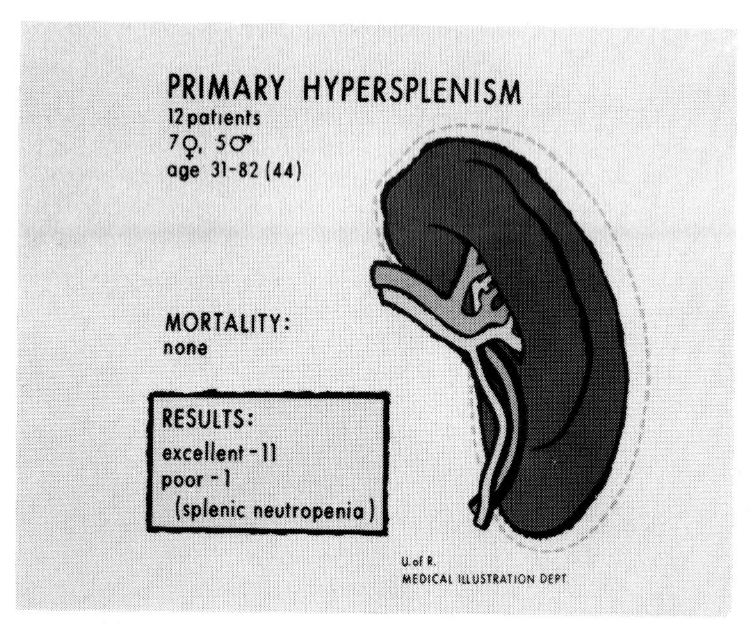

FIGURE 15.

Among the hematologic diseases for which splenectomy is advised, the most demanding is myeloid metaplasia, a panproliferative process manifested by increased proliferation of marrow elements in liver, spleen and lymph nodes. It is now recognized that the old concept that removal of the spleen has an adverse effect on the hematologic picture has no support. Splenectomy, in fact, has a position in the armamentarium for patients with symptomatic splenomegaly, multiple painful infarcts and hypersplenism requiring increasing transfusion. The first line of defense in these patients includes transfusion therapy, hormone therapy, alkylating agents. Splenectomy is indicated only if these fail. Adhering to these indications, we have operated on 12 such patients. Seven had an excellent response. We have seen no deleterious effects on the hematologic picture. Three patients progressed to myelogenous leukemia, as would be anticipated (Fig. 16).

Splenectomy is indicated in a variety of malignant diseases, for palliation and reduction of the hypersplenism (Fig. 17). Once again, the demonstration of increased uptake of radioactive labeled cells is associated with a more predictable response. Although it does not alter the course of the disease, it does improve patients with Hodgkin's disease and other

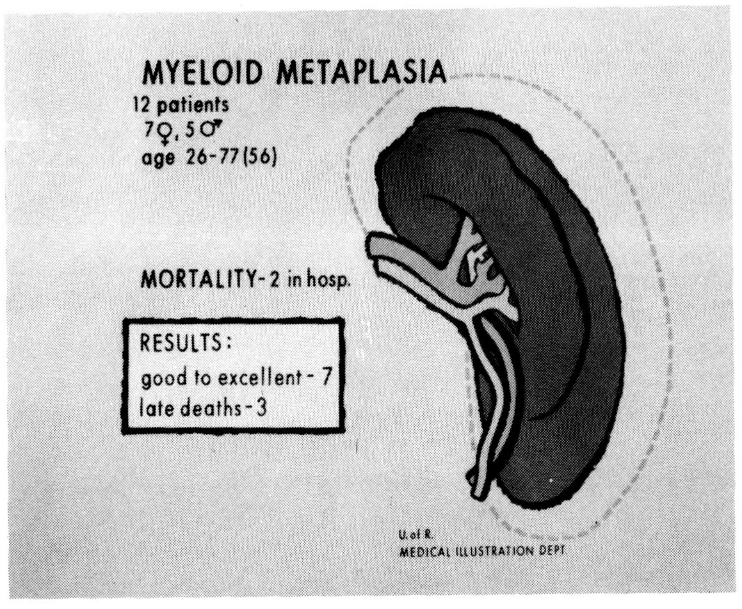

FIGURE 16.

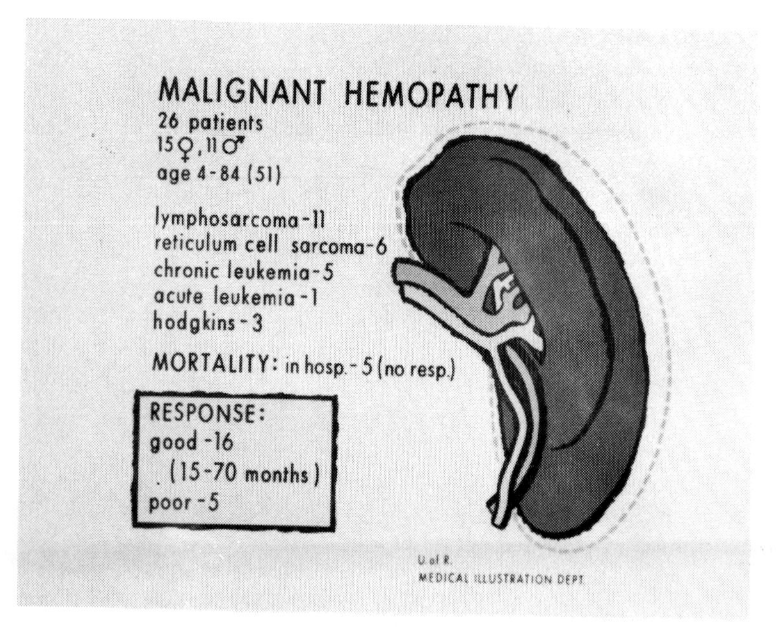

FIGURE 17.

malignancies and, to a greater extent, patients with lymphosarcoma. In these diseases, a plea is made for early splenectomy, ie, once the hypersplenic phenomenon is diagnosed. The yield is a reduction in subsequent infections and a possible extension of the use of radiation therapy and chemotherapy without associated reduction in circulating cells.

Recently the great explosion with regard to Hodgkin's disease has been the application of staging, which includes liver biopsy, splenectomy, and retroperitoneal node biopsy performed to provide a more precise definition of intra-abdominal disease. Time permits just an abbreviated synopsis of the present state of the art. The findings at laparotomy and histologic evaluation of these organs have been correlated with the patients' symptoms, physical findings, liver function tests and radiographic findings. As far as splenic involvement is concerned, the percentage of errors for patients thought to have splenic involvement was 38%, while operative evidence of splenic involvement was determined in 36% of patients whose spleens were judged to be normal. The liver is suspected of being infiltrated with Hodgkin's disease if there is evidence of hepatomegaly or if liver function tests are abnormal. Although uncommon, liver involvement indicates a poor prognosis and generally dictates a therapeutic regimen based on chemotherapy. Preoperative suspicion of Hodgkin's disease involving the liver was incorrect in 45% of patients, whereas the percentage of errors in those livers which were judged to be normal was only 4%. In this regard, we have had personal experience with two patients, judged to be Stage IA, with no suggestion of abdominal involvement. At operative staging the livers were involved, converting them from a therapeutic regimen based on radiation to chemotherapy. With reference to lymphangiography, in those cases where the nodes were thought to be normal, operative staging demonstrated involvement in about 50%. Conversely, when the nodes were thought to be abnormal, only 20% were demonstrated as abnormal by surgery. This is a hard figure to dissect, since perhaps the surgeon had not biopsied a representative node. Collating all cases in regard to a change in stage, we can see that in 27% of the cases, the stage was increased by operative procedure, whereas in 15%, the stage was decreased.

Where do we stand at present regarding the heated argument concerning the applicability of operative staging? All authors agree that the procedure is indicated for patients with diagnosed Hodgkin's disease who present with evidence or suggestion of disease in the upper abdomen, providing that the patient does not have significant icterus or major hepatic dysfunction. Disagreement regarding the applicability of staging of Hodgkin's disease centers around Stage IA and IIA patients. We feel that the safety of the procedure and the opportunity to increase our knowledge of pathogenesis, and the possibility of facilitating treatment justify routine surgical staging of patients as an integral part of the therapeutic regimen. As a part of staging, the enlarged spleen is removed before the disease becomes advanced. At this time splenectomy can be carried out with a reduced risk. Radiation to the left kidney and left lower lobe of the lung is obviated, thus reducing the incidence of nephritis and pneumonitis. Splenectomy is also prophylactic in regard to the hypersplenism which may limit either radiation or chemotherapy. In reference to the operation itself, the nodal biopsy should be extended to include the mesenteric nodes and the nodes in the hepatoduodenal ligament, in addition to the retroperitoneal nodes since isolated involvement of each of these groups of nodes has been demonstrated. The miscellaneous categories (Fig. 18) include Felty's disease, in which the anemia is corrected, but the arthritis is not altered, Gaucher's disease in which the patients are improved symptomatically, and sarcoid disease generally for a significant splenomegaly. We had three spontaneous ruptures of the spleen in patients with hematologic disorders and surgery was carried out with good immediate results.

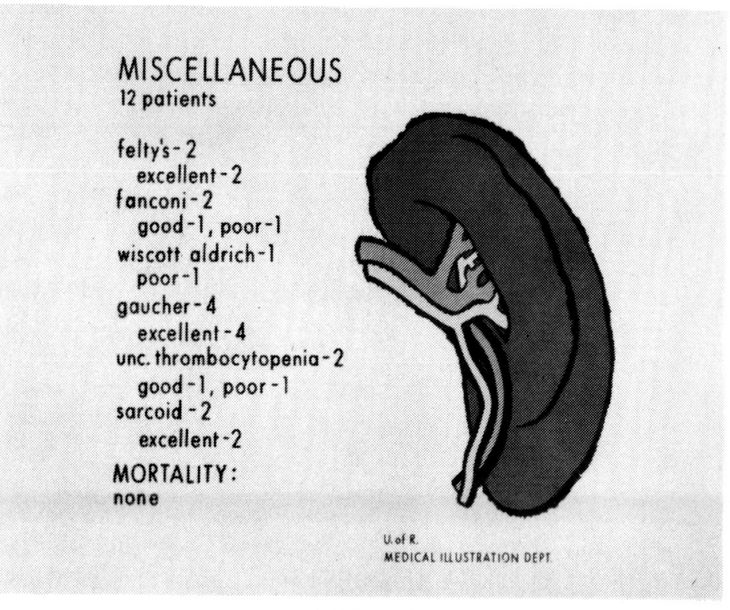

FIGURE 18.

It is appropriate to conclude with a series of general preoperative and postoperative considerations. Platelet packs are generally not administered preoperatively to patients who are thrombocytopenic, due to hematologic disorder, since they are rapidly destroyed by the spleen and therefore not effective. In such patients we perform rapid splenectomy, and if bleeding continues, platelets are administered after the spleen is removed. Patients with malignant lymphoma and leukemia may have cryoglobulinemia and blood should therefore be administered at room temperature. For patients with thalassemia and, more particularly, those with acquired hemolytic anemia, typing and crossmatching may be extremely difficult, and sufficient time should be alloted preoperatively to accumulate the blood which may be required during operation. A point which I would like to make regarding surgery is the need to search for accessory spleens in all of these patients. The locations of accessory spleens were most commonly in the hilum of the spleen extending to the ovary and even to the testis (Fig. 19). The incidence is reported to be between 14% and 30% in patients with hematologic disorders.

Overall mortality in our series was 7% (Fig. 20) but all deaths were related to the basic disease and, in general, occurred in critically ill or moribund patients. In good risk patients, there were no deaths, and a

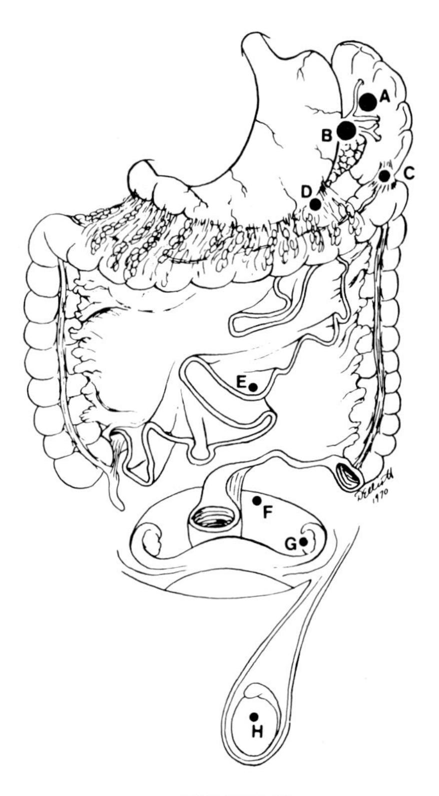

FIGURE 19.

similar experience has been noted in most large series. Complications are appreciable, occurring in 18% of cases. Most frequent is that of left lower lobe atelectasis. Wound complications, septicemia and subphrenic hematoma occur almost exclusively in patients with myeloproliferative disorders and malignant hemopathy, which yields significant bleeding from the splenic bed. An excessive elevation in platelet count with increased platelet adhesiveness, particularly in patients with myeloid metaplasia, has been reported. These factors have been implicated in the greater incidence of thrombophlebitis and pulmonary embolism following splenectomy; however, there is no good correlation between the incidence of these complications and the platelet count. Of our four patients with postoperative venous thrombosis, only one had a significant elevation of the platelet count. We do not use anticoagulants in the postoperative period, since they do not alter platelet adhesiveness. Our long-term follow-up of splenectomized patients has revealed no increased incidence of infection,

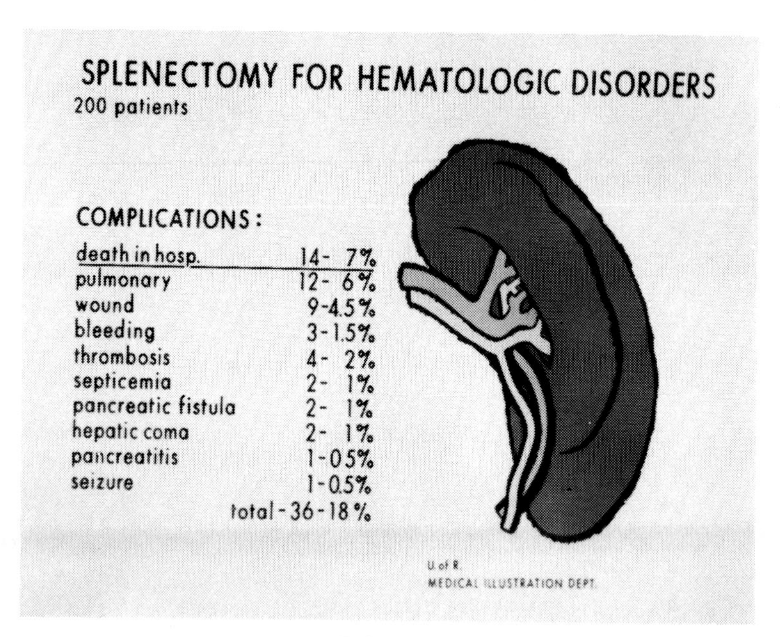

FIGURE 20.

but most feel that splenectomy for hematologic disorders should be delayed, if at all possible, until the age of 2, based on the demonstration that the spleen does participate in the formation of macroglobulinemic bacterial antibodies during the first two years of life. Recently, there have been alarming reports of disseminated viral, pneumonococcal and hemophilus infections following splenectomy, but more data are required. The spleen had been originally described by Galen as the organ of mystery. The mystery still persists, but a continued dialogue between physicians and surgeons might provide some of the answers.

Bibliography

Eraklis, A. J., Kevy, S. V., Diamond, L. K. et al: Hazards of overwhelming infections after splenectomy in childhood. New Eng. J. Med. 276:1225, 1967.

Schwartz, S. I., Adams, J. T., and Bauman, A. W.: Splenectomy for Hemotologic Disorders. Current Problems of Surgery, May, 1971.

Schwartz, S. I. and Cooper, R. A., Jr.: Surgery in the diagnosis and treatment of Hodgkin's disease. Advances in Surgery, Ch. 5, Vol. 6, 1972.

II

Biliary Tract

Medical Therapy for Stones in the Biliary Tract

Alan F. Hofmann, M.D.

Introduction

In the last five years there has been an exciting growth in our understanding about why people get gallstones. I think the reason that this did not occur sooner was because cholecystectomy has been such a safe and effective operation. I would like to review for you where we stand with respect to medical dissolution of gallstones. I am going to say that chenodeoxycholic acid, a primary bile acid in man (which I shall term chenic acid), when given orally in doses of about 1 gm/day will dissolve radiolucent gallstones present in radiologically visualizing gallbladders in one to three years in relatively asymptomatic patients about half the time. When the medicine is discontinued, stones will recur in some patients. Most radiopaque gallstones will not respond. I also want to mention briefly our attempts to dissolve common duct stones in patients who have previously had cholecystectomies. Finally, I want to review the current status of dissolution of common duct stones by T-tube infusions of bile acid solutions. All of the clinical work has been carried out in collaboration with Dr. Johnson L. Thistle, who, in fact, is entirely responsible for the clinical aspects of the studies to be discussed.

Gallstone Formation and Dissolution

The majority of gallstones are mostly cholesterol. Cholesterol is a white, waxy substance, totally insoluble in water [1]. It is soluble in bile where it is present in aggregates of bile acid and lecithin molecules which are called micelles (micelle means a little cluster of molecules). The

Alan F. Hofmann, M.D., Professor of Medicine and Physiology, Mayo Medical School; Associate Director, Gastroenterology Unit, Division of Gastroenterology, Mayo Clinic and Mayo Foundation, Rochester, Minn.

cholesterol sits inside of the micelle like the hole in the doughnut. In patients with cholesterol gallstones, bile is obviously saturated with cholesterol. This was clearly shown by the late Charles Johnston, a surgeon in Detroit [2]. Johnston and others, such as Andrew Ivy, also showed that if a gallstone were placed in the gallbladder of the dog, which is known to have extremely unsaturated bile, it would dissolve rapidly, confirming an observation made before the turn of the century by Naunyn and his associates.

There must be multiple steps in gallstone formation. Obviously, the first step is the occurrence of supersaturated bile in the gallbladder. Then, nucleation must occur with the formation of cholesterol crystals. The crystals clump together and enlarge by continuing deposition of crystals. As the stone enlarges, it may damage the mucosa; and this may initiate a vicious circle, in that the damaged mucosa may be more permeable to bile acids, and loss of bile acids through the mucosa may increase the saturation of bile. But clearly we cannot initiate stone formation or have continuing stone growth without supersaturated bile being in the gallbladder. That is why it is reasonable to attack the problem here.

What do we mean by supersaturated bile? Let me discuss the uncommon manner in which bile composition is frequently depicted. If one has three substances that add up to 100%, one can plot the relative proportions of each in two dimensions by using triangular coordinates. Some examples of three variables which add up to 100% might conveniently be shown in this manner. What are the constituents of a martini? Gin, vermouth and water. What is the composition of your diet? Fat, carbohydrate and protein. What is the source of your income? Medical school, outside consulting fees, private practice.

Between 1963 and 1966, Dr. Donald Small, now Professor of Medicine at Boston University, working in Paris studied the behavior of mixtures of cholesterol, lecithin and bile acid simulating the composition of bile. The chemicals were mixed in small bottles, allowed to reach equilibrium and then scrutinized by polarizing microscopy. His results [3] defined the solubility of cholesterol in this system, and they are most conveniently presented using triangular coordinates. Figure 1 shows his results. The line defines the limits of the micellar zone, and for samples whose composition lies below it, a clear micellar solution, just like water, will obtain. Above the line, cholesterol crystals will form at equilibrium. If the sample is not at equilibrium, a clear micellar but supersaturated solution will be present.

When Dr. Small came back to Boston he was joined by Dr. William Admirand, now at the University of California in San Francisco. They

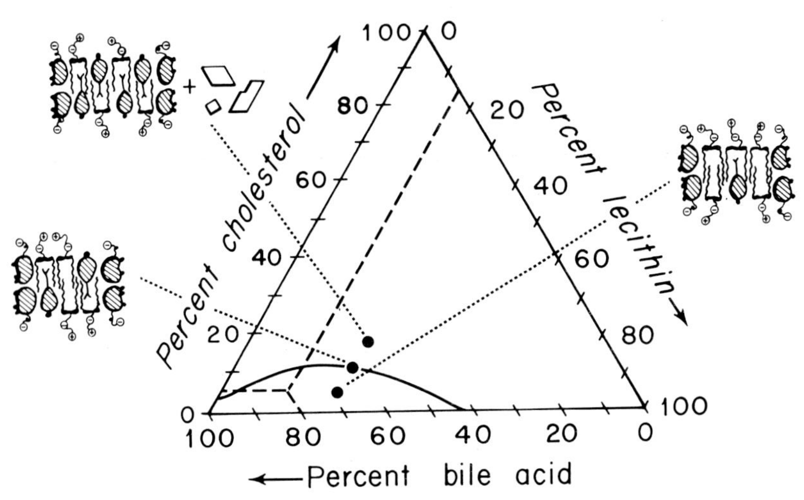

FIG. 1. Phase equilibria present in a model system simulating bile. Model system contains four components – bile acids, lecithin, cholesterol and water. Diagram shows physical state of the constituents in relation to concentration. Since there are four components in the system, there are three degrees of freedom. One should show the phase equilibria present using a tetrahedron. However, since bile contains 5%-15% solids, it is 85%-95% water, and one can show the phase equilibria present at a fixed water concentration, for example, 90% by a triangle, which in fact is a plane through the tetrahedron. Now one has only two degrees of freedom and any composition can be represented by a triangle in which each axis is the percentage either molar or by weight of one of the components.

Here, the base of the triangle is bile acid composition in moles percent. Any point on a line parallel to the base opposite the 100% bile acid apex (*lower right*) defines samples with constant bile acid composition. Similarly, any point on a line parallel to the base defines samples with constant cholesterol composition. Dash lines intersect at a point representing the following composition: bile acids, 80%; lecithin, 15%; cholesterol, 5%. Curved, solid line represents the limits of the micellar zone as defined by Admirand and Small. Any point lying on or below the line is a clear micellar solution. Points lying above the line indicate a supersaturated solution or a saturated solution containing crystalline cholesterol.

It is now recognized that the solubility line at true equilibrium is somewhat lower than that originally described by Admirand and Small.

acquired bile at surgery from patients undergoing cholecystectomy as well as healthy controls. They found, as would be predicted, that patients with gallstones in general had bile which was saturated or supersaturated whereas, patients without gallstones generally had bile which was unsaturated [4] (Fig. 2). A priori this should be true. But Dr. Admirand and Small showed it experimentally.

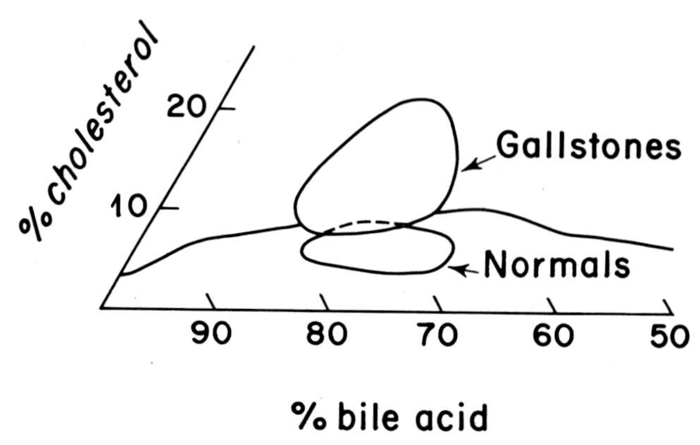

FIG. 2. Approximate range of lipid composition of fasting-state gallbladder bile, as shown on triangular coordinates, when obtained from patients with gallstones in healthy subjects. In patients with gallstones, bile is supersaturated or contains cholesterol crystals. In some instances it can be transiently unsaturated, but continuous unsaturation of bile in cholesterol gallstone patients is probably only observed during chenic acid administration. Normal subjects usually have unsaturated bile. The presence of supersaturated bile should be associated with increased risk for development of cholesterol gallstones.

How can we make bile unsaturated? Let me begin by reading a quotation from Dr. Charles Johnston, who was the Professor of Surgery at Wayne [2]. Dr. Johnston wrote: "We should have some means of removing the stones by metabolic means. The bile we have been using is cholic acid. When we give this to patients, a strange thing happens, more cholesterol comes out together with bile salt and lecithin. I have some hope that there will be other substances which will not cause this great increase in cholesterol excretion." He went on to write: "We are now studying some of the bile acids, such as chenic acid, which are found in human bile in smaller quantities. They are hard to come by, so we have to synthesize them ourselves. It really should be a matter of trying one substance or another until we find one which will not increase cholesterol (secretion) and cause saturation of human bile. This should be possible, because in animals, bile is unsaturated." This statement made some 17 years ago was quite prophetic. About five years ago, Drs. Thistle and Schoenfield working in our group at the Mayo Clinic showed, in women with gallstones, that chenic acid (which, as Dr. Johnston said, is made synthetically) made bile unsaturated in cholesterol whereas cholic acid or placebo did not [5] (Fig. 3). This study was carried out over four months. No definite changes in gallstones were detected by cholecystogram, but it showed that the defect in bile composition in patients with gallstones could be corrected.

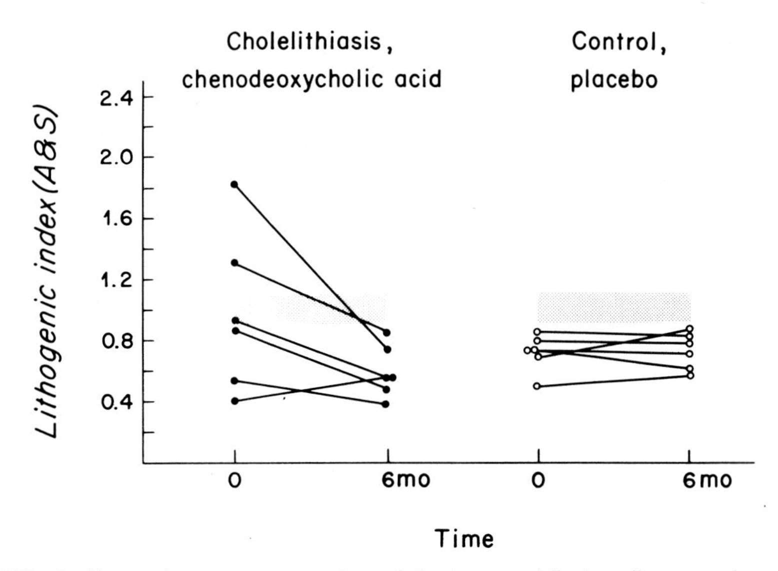

FIG. 3. Change in percent saturation of fasting-state bile in gallstone patients receiving chenic acid (*left*) or healthy subjects receiving placebo (*right*). Percent saturation is defined as [(cholesterol concentration in sample/cholesterol solubility at saturation in sample) × 100] using the phase diagram shown in Figure 1 to estimate cholesterol solubility at saturation. The initials A and S refer to Admirand and Small.

On the basis of that historic experiment, Dr. John Thistle and I, about three years ago, began a randomized trial. We took men and women with relatively asymptomatic radiolucent gallstones in radiologically visualizing gallbladders.

We gave patients chenic acid or cholic acid or placebo in doses averaging 20 mg/kg body weight per day. There were approximately 17 patients in each group. We did x-rays, bile composition, various metabolic studies and also toxicity studies. In brief, cholic acid did not work and, as expected, gallstones did not dissolve in the patients receiving placebo. The only efficacious substance was chenic acid [6].

Where do we stand then at 18 months? In our 18 patients, we have five whose stones have disappeared, six whose stones are getting smaller, six whose stones have not changed; and one patient has developed a nonfunctioning gallbladder. If the six patients whose gallstones are diminishing in size will eventually achieve complete dissolution, and we think that they will, this will be a response of 11 out of 18, or slightly greater than 50%. My guess is that this is going to be the experience of the majority of Western countries, that is, slightly more than half of radiolucent gallstones are going to respond to chenic acid.

Why didn't stones dissolve in all patients? In all probability the resistant radiolucent stones contained a surface of calcium bilirubinate or other noncholesterol materials, and of course some of the stones were probably pure bilirubin stones. We cannot predict stone composition from the x-ray appearance.

What about radiopaque stones? These are difficult to define. We might include stones with sufficient calcium so that they may be seen by a flat plate or radiolucent stones containing an inner calcium core visualized during routine cholecystography. If the stones get smaller during chenic acid therapy, it is only the lucent component which dissolves in our experience. We believe that most radiopaque gallstones will not respond. Figure 4 shows stones dissolving during chenic therapy.

What about toxicity? In our hands we have not seen any significant elevation of alkaline phosphatase; abnormal BSP retention has not occurred. No patient has become jaundiced. We did observe SGOT elevations about 1½ times normal in five of 27 patients, but these were transient in virtually all instances (Fig. 5). Altogether, in this country and in Europe there have been about 60 liver biopsies; no significant abnormalities have been discovered. However, the drug is unequivocally hepatotoxic in the Rhesus monkey where it causes portal tract inflammation. It is because of the animal toxicity that all clinical trials in this country have been frozen by the Food and Drug Administration, until additional animal toxicity studies are completed. I might note that the hepatotoxicity in the Rhesus monkey is signaled by striking elevations in transaminase and leucine amino peptidase, appears to be dose related and rapidly disappears when therapy is stopped.

What about serum lipids? Serum cholesterol levels do not change. Serum triglyceride levels actually diminish by about 20% in people taking chenic acid. We have done cholesterol pool size measurements by isotope dilution and there is no change in the size of the exchangeable cholesterol pools [7].

So, at the moment, on the basis of the animal studies, if there is toxicity in man, it is likely to be hepatic, is likely to be manifested by changes in the usual liver function tests and should be reversible; but it has not been observed as yet. Any patient who receives chenic acid must have his serum transaminase monitored regularly.

Chenic acid causes a profound change in the bile acid metabolism of the patient. The majority of patients with gallstones have small bile acid pools when this is measured by isotope dilution. Chenic acid enlarges the bile acid pool and biliary bile acids become predominantly chenic acid [8].

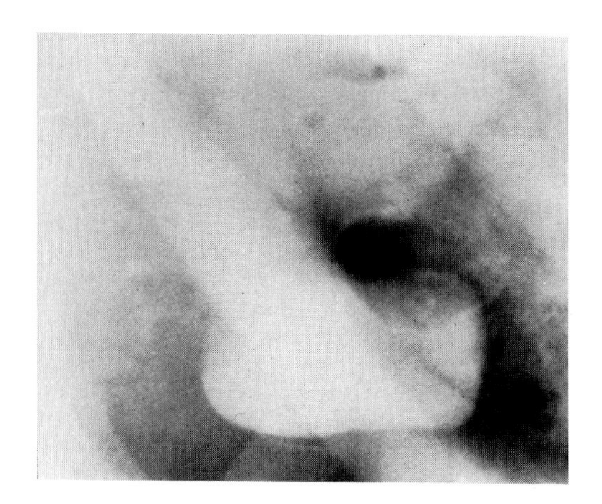

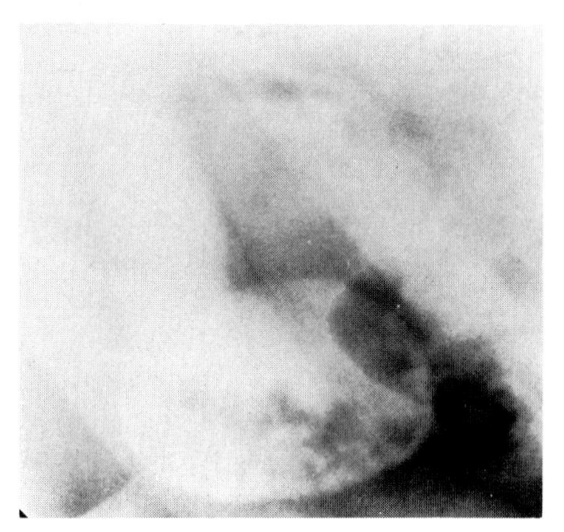

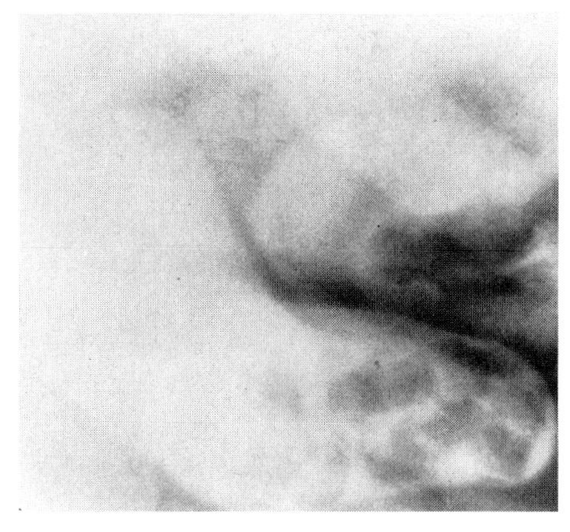

FIG. 4. Radiolucent gallstones before (*top*), after six months (*center*), and 12 months (*bottom*) of chenic acid therapy. Multiple radiolucent gallstones respond most rapidly to drug therapy. Recurrence may be observed when the drug is stopped.

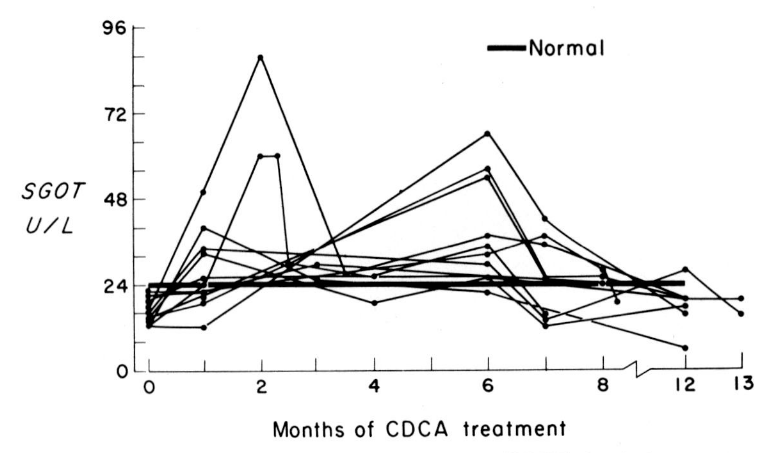

FIG. 5. Serum glutamic oxaloacetic transaminase (SGOT) levels in a group of gallstone patients receiving chenic acid for gallstone dissolution. The elevation is transient and modest, and not exhibited by the majority of patients ingesting chenic acid. The solid horizontal line represents the upper limits of normal values at the Mayo Clinic.

The mechanism of action, however, does not appear to be expansion of the bile acid pool but rather a specific decrease in cholesterol secretion in bile [9]. When this is measured by a duodenal perfusion technique, chenic acid decreases the amount of cholesterol secreted, and this is the major effect. Thus, the mechanism of action of chenic acid therapy is totally different than T-tube infusion, which I will discuss in a moment.

When treatment with chenic acid is stopped, bile rapidly becomes supersaturated again [10]. If bad bile is the villain, and the gallbladder once again contains supersaturated bile, stones should recur, if there is nucleation.

We have now followed five patients for 12 to 18 months following stone disappearance; recurrence by x-ray has occurred in two. Perhaps this demonstration that chenic acid therapy may only be temporarily successful in some patients may please the surgeons, since it suggests that medical therapy may be only palliative whereas cholecystectomy is curative. However, it seems likely that we may develop new approaches to maintaining bile in an unsaturated state following gallstone dissolution.

Finally, I want to mention briefly that Dr. Thistle is also carrying out an uncontrolled trial of chenic acid therapy for patients with common duct stones. No patient is admitted to this trial until such treatment has been judged to be in the patient's best interest by an independent medical-surgical team. So far, only one of 11 patients has shown complete disappearance; obviously, we cannot be certain that dissolution was induced by chenic acid therapy.

T-Tube Infusions With Bile Acid Solutions for Retained Common Duct Stones

Elimination of duct stones by T-tube infusion with sodium cholate the sodium salt of cholic acid, the other primary bile acids in man, is based on two different principles, in my judgment. First, we have dissolution of the stones by the micellar solution of sodium cholate; perhaps stone disintegration also occurs and if so we may have simultaneous litholysis and lithoclasis. Second, there is probably enhanced passage of duct stones by infusion of fluid per se into a T-tube.

The rationale of this treatment is that there should be fairly rapid micellar solubilization of cholesterol under sink conditions, that is, when there is no cholesterol in the system. In solutions of sodium cholate, stones dissolve much more rapidly than if lecithin is present, even though the addition of lecithin increases the total solvent capacity of cholate solutions at equilibrium [11].

The alternative to sodium cholate infusion is extraction with the Dormia basket [12]. To use this technique one must remove the T-tube first. If the basket extraction attempt is unsuccessful, one may pass a Robinson catheter into the tract and then into the common duct (using fluoroscopic guidance) and then perfuse the retained stones through this catheter.

At the Mayo Clinic in Rochester, Dr. Nicholas LaRusso and Dr. John Thistle have been carrying out a controlled study on patients with nonobstructing stones in the common duct distal to the T-tube. Patients are not studied until two weeks after biliary surgery to allow spontaneous passage, and eligible patients require evidence of good liver cell function with minimal or no elevation of transaminase, bilirubin or alkaline phosphatase. We ask approval for entering patients into this study by an uninvolved physician and surgeon. I believe it is desirable to clear any such studies with the Food and Drug Administration, but this is a personal judgment. The Food and Drug Administration has not issued a judgment as to what legal requirements pertain to this particular mode of treatment.

The general approach is as follows. Prepare a solution of sodium cholate and use an overflow manometer to keep the pressure not greater than 20 cm. A nasojejunal tube may be passed so that the infused cholate can be aspirated, or cholestyramine may be infused at about 2 gm/hr to prevent diarrhea. We have been using probanthine to relax the sphincter, but others have not. Informed consent is obtained. We infuse the cholate (75 mM in half strength saline), obtain bilirubin and alkaline phosphatase at regular intervals and then monitor the stone size by T-tube cholangiograms.

For the infusion, one attaches the infusion line to a manometer which should have an overflow arrangement. In patients with duct obstruction, Dr. Way and his associates [13] have used a catheter through which the cholate is infused and around which it regurgitates back out of the T-tube. With this arrangement, the nasojejunal tube is not necessary. Sodium cholate, 75 mM or 100 mM, has been used and is considered to be safe. I don't believe that one should use deoxycholate and there is no rationale for using chenodeoxycholate (chenic acid). A paper has recently been published showing a certain enhancing effect on dissolution rate of quaternary ammonium detergents [14]. (This idea was first advanced by Higuchi and his co-workers on the basis of in vitro studies on dissolution kinetics [15].) Quaternary ammonium surfactants are quite toxic in man, and I believe that they should not go into patients without a great deal of animal study. Heparin has been claimed to be of value in uncontrolled studies [16], but I believe that it will be of no value by itself. Conceivably, its addition to sodium cholate infusions may enhance the dissolution rate [14], but there is little hard evidence that this is true.

The efficacy of this mode of therapy appears to be diminishing with time when compared to the original data published by Admirand et al [17]. They reported success in 12 of 22 patients, with response generally occurring in three days. Recently, Kern's group in another uncontrolled study reported success in five of six patients within five days of beginning sodium cholate infusions [18]. In this study, the rate of infusion was 30 ml/hr of a 100 mM solution. Our own results are quite disappointing. We used saline for four days or 75 mM cholate for four days in randomized order. As yet, we have seen no unequivocal stone dissolution, although one stone has certainly passed during the trial. It is difficult for me to believe that our poor results can be explained by the use of 75 mM sodium cholate rather than a 100 mM solution.

In summary, this is an experimental procedure. It works slowly and in only some patients. The rationale is unclear, and certainly some stones are passing just because of the infusion per se. Severe diarrhea has been reported, but this can be controlled by nasojejunal aspiration or cholestyramine infusion. Pancreatitis has been reported, and I have heard third-hand about the development of cholangitis. In my judgment, only sodium cholate has been shown to be safe, and no other bile acid should be used. The status of heparin is unclear, and quaternary amines should not be added until additional animal studies are done.

Summary

There has been real progress in developing new pharmacological approaches to gallstones and common duct stones. My associate, Dr. John Thistle, who has been in charge of our therapeutic studies with chenic and cholic acid is continuing to expand our experience with biliary stones and we will continue to pursue some of the unsolved problems. In my judgment, oral chenic acid will eventually be important as a valuable alternative to surgery in patients with radiolucent gallstones in functioning gallbladders, especially those with greater risks for cholecystectomy. We need new agents which will rapidly dissolve recurrent stones in patients with T-tubes, and we must develop a rational, effective approach to sludge.

References

1. Carey, M. C. and Small, D. M.: Micelle formation of bile salts. Arch. Intern. Med., 130:506-527, 1972.
2. Johnston, C. G. and Nakayama, F.: Solubility of cholesterol and gallstones in metabolic material. Arch. Surg., 75:436-442, 1957.
3. Bourges, M., Small, D. M. and Dervichian, D. G.: Biophysics of lipid associations. III. The quaternary systems lecithin-bile salt cholesterol-water. Biochim. Biophys. Acta, 114:189-201, 1967.
4. Admirand, W. H. and Small, D. M.: The physicochemical basis of cholesterol gallstone formation in man. J. Clin. Invest., 47:1043-1052, 1968.
5. Thistle, J. L. and Schoenfield, L. J.: Induced alterations of persons having cholelithiasis. Gastroenterology, 61:488-496, 1971.
6. Thistle, J. L. and Hofmann, A. F.: Efficacy and specificity of chenodeoxycholic acid therapy for dissolving gallstones. New Eng. J. Med., 289:655-659, 1973.
7. Hoffman, N. E., Hofmann, A. F. and Thistle, J. L.: Effect of bile acid feeding on cholesterol metabolism in gallstone patients. Mayo Clin. Proc., 49:236-239, 1974.
8. Danzinger, R. G., Hofmann, A. F., Schoenfield, L. J. et al: Effect of oral chenodeoxycholic acid on bile acid kinetics and biliary lipid composition in women with cholelithiasis. J. Clin. Invest., 52:2809-2821, 1973.
9. Northfield, T. C., LaRusso, N. F., Thistle, J. L. et al: Effect of chenodeoxycholic acid therapy on biliary lipid secretion in gallstone patients, abstracted. Gastroenterology, 64:780, 1973.
10. Thistle, J. L., Yu, P. Y. S., Hofmann, A. F. et al: Prompt return of bile to supersaturated state followed by gallstone recurrence after discontinuance of chenodeoxycholic acid therapy, abstracted. Gastroenterology, 66:789, 1974.
11. Higuchi, W. I., Prakongpan, S., Surpuriya, V. et al: Cholesterol dissolution rate in micellar bile acid solutions: Retarding effect of added lecithin. Science, 178:633-634, 1972.

12. Mazzariello, R.: Review of 220 cases of residual biliary tract calculi treated without reoperation: An eight-year study. Surgery, 73:299-306, 1973.
13. Way, L. W., Admirand, W. H. and Dunphy, J. E.: Management of choledocholithiasis. Ann. Surg., 176:347-359, 1972.
14. Lahana, D. A., Bonorris, G. G. and Schoenfield, L. J.: Gallstone dissolution in vitro by bile acids, heparin and quaternary amines. Surg., Gynec. Obstet., 138:683-685, 1974.
15. Higuchi, W. I., Prakongpan, S. and Young, F.: Dissolution rates of cholesterol monohydrate crystals and human gallstones in bile acid lecithin solutions; Enhancing effect of added quarternary ammonium salts. J. Pharm. Sci., 67:1207, 1973.
16. Gardner, B.: Experiences with the use of intracholedochal heparinized saline for the treatment of retained common duct stones. Ann. Surg., 177:240-244, 1971.
17. Admirand, W. H. and Way, L. W.: Medical treatment of retained gallstones. Trans. Ass. Amer. Physicians, 85:382-387, 1972.
18. Lansford, C., Mehta, S. and Kern, F., Jr.: The treatment of retained stones in the common bile duct with sodium cholate infusion. Gut, 15:48-51, 1974.

Research described in this paper was supported by NIH grants AM-16770 and AM-15887, as well as grants-in-aid from the Mead Johnson Company, the Lilly Research Foundation and Weddel Pharmaceuticals.

Manometry and Physiology of the Bile Ducts

Thomas Taylor White, M.D.

From a practical point of view the main causes of symptoms requiring reoperation on the biliary tree are residual or retained stones and stenosis of the sphincter of Oddi. The majority will present with recurrent symptoms of partial biliary tract obstruction within one year of the initial operation. Since these patients make up from 4% to 6% of all patients undergoing cholecystectomy in the United States, studies of the intraductal biliary pressure are of some clinical importance.

The normal intraductal biliary pressure is regulated by the secretory pressure of the liver, the distensibility of the gallbladder and the resistance of the choledochal and ampullary sphincters. The normal resting pressure in the common bile duct is higher than that of the gallbladder to insure filling of the latter. The opening pressure of the sphincter is from 5 to 50 mm of water higher than the resting pressure. Pain in the right upper abdomen occurs only when the common bile duct pressure is 20 cm or more above the passage pressure. The gallbladder pressure increases above the bile duct pressure during contraction, at which time the sphincters at the distal end of the bile duct relax. Naturally this reciprocal effect disappears when the gallbladder and ducts are chronically inflamed and filled with stones.

There are three main sphincters at the lower end of the bile duct – the ampullary, the inferior choledochal and the superior choledochal (Fig. 1). The distance between the lowest and the top of the highest sphincter may be as much as 25 mm, explaining why a sphincterotomy does not significantly alter intrabiliary pressure as measured via the T-tube during the postoperative period [1, 2]. Only complete division of all three sphincters will reduce the pressure. In the patient with intact sphincters, it

---

Thomas Taylor White, M.D., Clinical Professor of Surgery, University of Washington School of Medicine; Active Staff, Swedish and University Hospitals, Seattle, Wash.

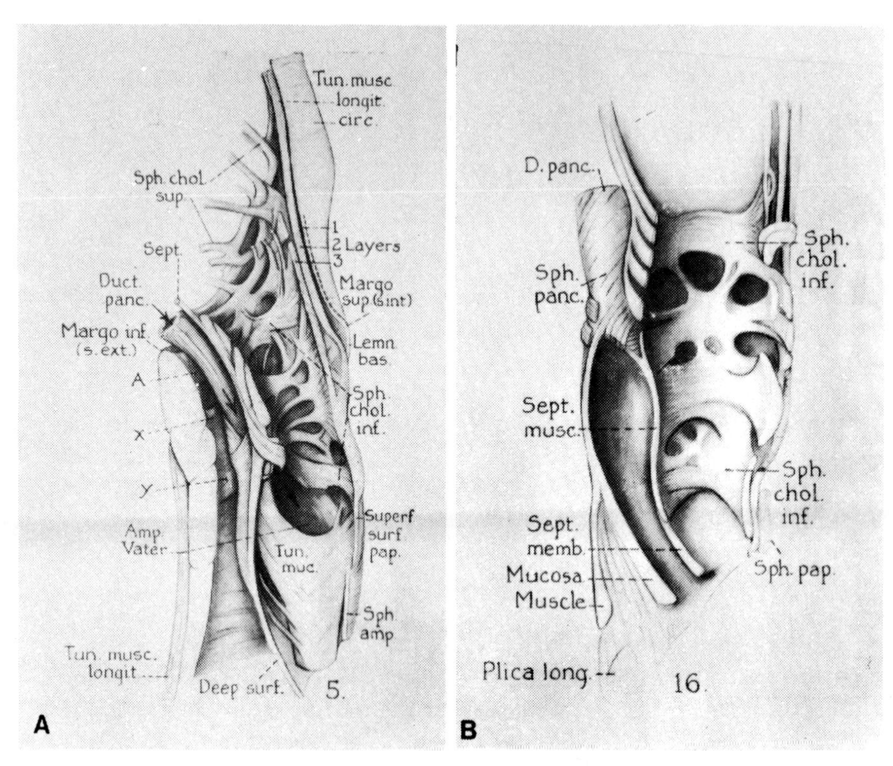

FIG. 1. (A) Dissection of the ampullary area. From Boyden, 1957. The pancreatic duct is shown by three arrows. The sphincter of the ampulla (sph. amp.), inferior choledochal (sph. chol. inf.) and superior choledochal sphincters (sph. chol. sup.) can be seen. (B) Second dissection from Boyden, 1957, showing pancreatic inferior choledochal and papillary sphincters.

appears that the predominant factor in determining biliary pressure in a patient who has had cholecystectomy is the choledochal sphincter tone, and that electrical activity must be present in the sphincter before flow can take place. In spite of statements by Burnett and Shields to the contrary, more recent studies have shown that there is no peristalsis in the common bile duct, only a milking action of the several sphincter muscles at its distal end [3, 4]. Relaxation is produced by cholecystokinin, pituitrin, probanthine and amyl nitrite. The contraction produced by morphine and opium derivatives lasts for 15 to 30 minutes, and demerol, for a shorter time. As a rule the sphincter does not significantly relax with papavarine or epinephrine. Atropine does reduce the spasm produced by morphine, but does not relax the sphincter by itself [4-7]. The vagus nerves probably do not affect the sphincter of Oddi, but may be involved in the maintenance of its tone as they are in the maintenance of gallbladder tone [4, 7, 8]. We know that the gallbladder does enlarge after vagotomy, but is not otherwise affected [9, 10].

It is obvious that stones in the distal bile duct, mechanical irritation of the sphincter muscles with resulting spasm and/or scarring, the presence of congenital abnormalities of the sphincter, or a tumor of the papilla will increase the intrabiliary pressure. Thus, in order to reduce the pressure, one must remove the stones and rid the patient of his ductal obstruction, whatever be the basis for it. Operative cholangiograms are especially useful in finding large stones within large ducts and demonstrating complete obstruction at the lower end of the bile duct. They are notoriously weak in showing more stones within a small duct, particularly those less than 3 mm in diameter. This patient had ten stones in her common bile duct, nine of which could not be seen in x-rays even in retrospect (Fig. 2). None of

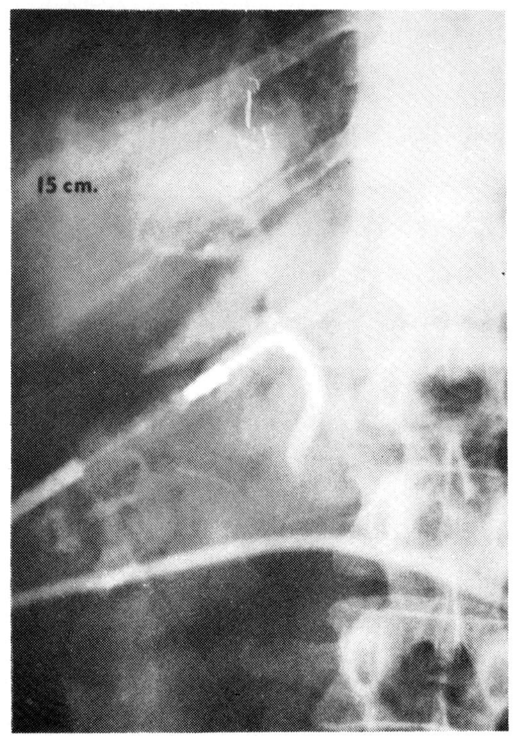

FIG. 2. Stones cannot be seen in the distal duct in this picture, nor has dye entered the duodenum at this pressure. Several small stones were present.

these stones were over 2 mm in diameter. We were only able to discover these stones because the passage pressure of the sphincter was elevated well over the normal pressure of 16 cm of water. One can argue that stones of this size would pass anyway and that their removal is meddlesome. Yet the high instance of residual or recurrent stones and of spasm of and/or stricture of the sphincter of Oddi suggests that this pathology must be at least partially on this basis.

On the continent of Europe and in South America, biliary surgery has been profoundly influenced by the addition of manometry and flow rates to cholangiography [6]. Stenosing processes at the sphincter or papilla which cannot be seen on routine x-rays and stones under 4 mm in diameter are not usually visualized by cholangiograms, but they can be revealed through the use of manometry and flow rates. One patient had had a prior cholecystectomy and numerous normal intravenous cholangiograms. When the catheter was inserted into the residual cystic duct, the bile climbed up into the catheter to a level of 35 cm above the duct. It was on this basis alone that the sphincteroplasty was carried out, with fibrosis found.

We have purchased and used both the manometric cholangiographic apparatus proposed by Prof. Hess [6-8, 11, 12] and that developed by

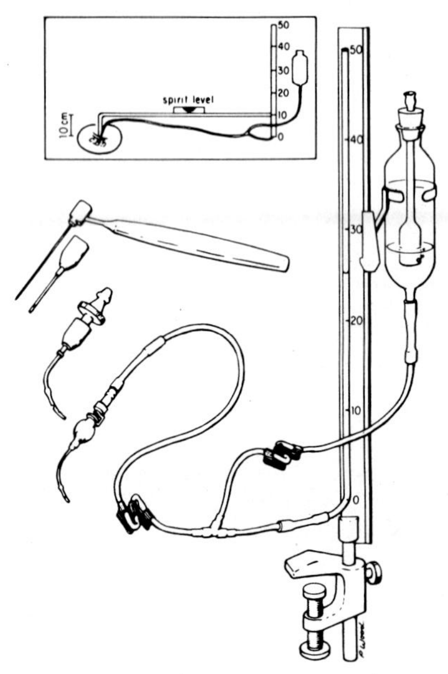

FIG. 3. Caroli-Fourès manometer with cannulas.

Professors Caroli and Fourès. We have used the latter device in 100 patients (Fig. 3). Without going into all the details, you can see in Figure 4 that the intrabiliary pressures in the patients with dilated common bile ducts were considerably higher than those with the normal ducts (6). This graph (Fig. 4) shows the relationship between pressure and diameter in the ducts. As you can see, obstructed or stone-containing bile ducts vary from 6 mm to 25 mm in diameter, with virtually all of the abnormally large ducts having a high pressure. While it did the job, we found this apparatus cumbersome and have abandoned it.

We are now using a simpler apparatus (Fig. 5) with a cannula having a minimum internal diameter of 1 mm which will allow the passage of at least 10 ml of saline per minute into the duodenum (Fig. 6). It also includes some intravenous tubing and a 50 ml syringe into the top of which has been placed a cork with a small glass pipe passing down to the 10 cc mark so that we can have constant pressure. This apparatus is held

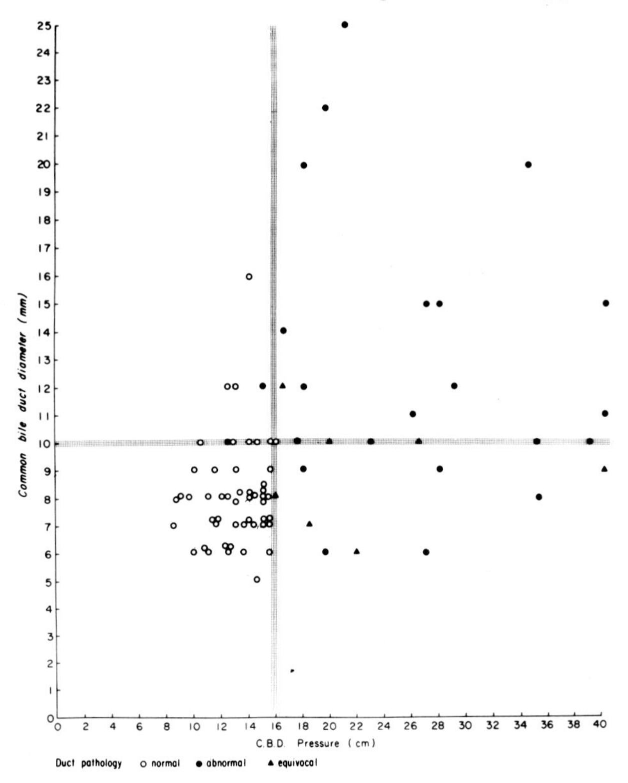

FIG. 4. Relationship between size of the duct and opening pressure.

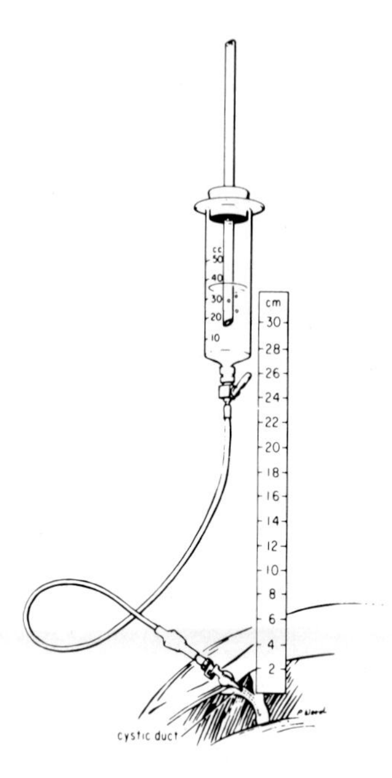

FIG. 5. Flow and pressure apparatus.

30 cm above the common bile duct. If 10 ml of saline or more passes out of the syringe into the duodenum in one minute, the duct is considered to be normal (Fig. 7). After this is done, the cholangiogram is taken. When that is completed, a residual pressure is taken. The results of our first 300 patients with this technique are shown here (Table 1). We feel that this is not only a simpler, but also a somewhat more sensitive test than the one proposed by Caroli, since it combines flow, pressure and cholangiograms [5, 13]. While we do all three as a routine, since we are using this as an experimental procedure, at the moment we are evaluating the patients

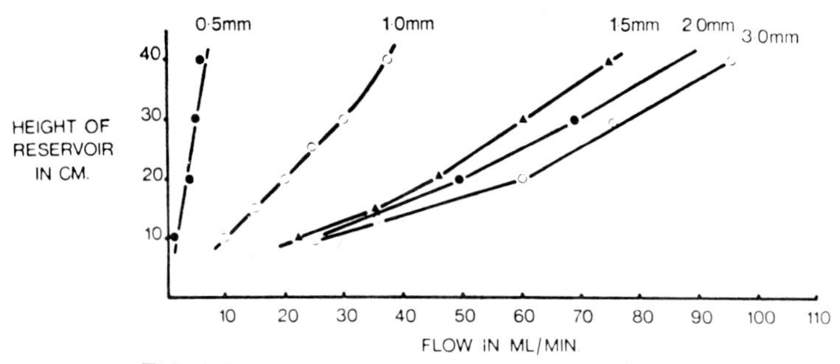

FIG. 6. Relationship of flow to outflow tract diameter.

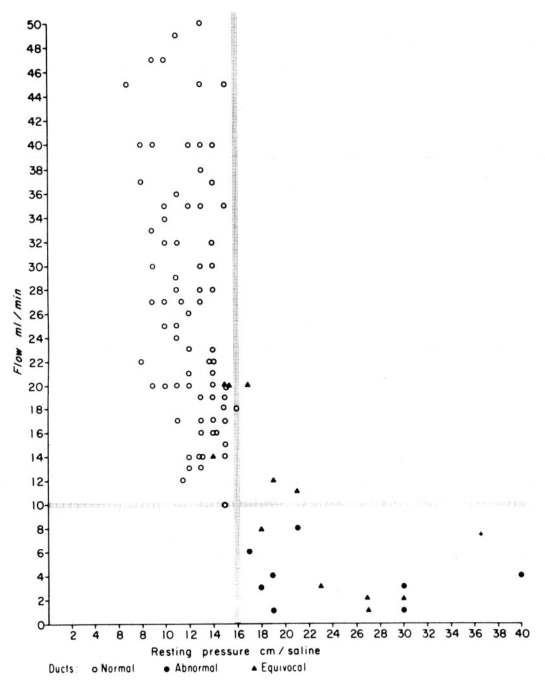

FIG. 7. Relationship between pressure and flow and normality.

Table 1. Comparison of Accuracy of Cholangiography, Flow Rates and Resting Pressures Alone or in Combination

	False Negative		*False Positive*		*Total*	*Accuracy Rate*
Cholangiography	16/281	(5.7%)	6/281	(2.1%)	22/281	92.2%
Flow	6/193	(3.1%)	4/193	(2.1%)	10/193	94.8%
Resting pressure	9/281	(3.2%)	18/281	(6.4%)	27/281	90.4%
Flow and resting pressure	5/193	(2.6%)	3/193	(1.6%)	8/193	95.9%
Flow and cholangiography	0/193	(0%)	1/193	(0.5%)	1/193	99.5%
Pressure and cholangiography	5/281	(1.9%)	6/281	(2.1%)	11/281	96.1%

on which these two approaches were used five years ago. We think that in the final analysis, the flow and pressure measurements alone could be used as a screening technique for common duct pathology in patients undergoing routine cholecystectomy.

In summary, we have found that with cholangiography alone there are at best approximately 6% false negatives and 2.5% false positive findings. Combining this technique with pressure and flow measurement reduces the false negatives and positives to under 1%. Measurement of flow alone produced 95.5% accuracy, pressure alone 92% accuracy and pressures and flows together 99.1% accuracy. All in all, we have found about 7% more pathology using these techniques than by the usual techniques of palpation, cholangiography and clinical judgment.

References

1. Boyden, E. A.: Anatomy of the choledochoduodenal junction in man. Surg. Gynec. Obstet., 104:641, 1957.
2. White, T. T. and Harrison, R. C.: Reoperative gastrointestinal surgery. Boston:Little Brown and Co., 1973.
3. Burnett, W. and Shields, R.: Movements of the common bile duct in man: Studies with image intensifier. Lancet, 2:387, 1958.
4. Hand, B. H.: Anatomy and function of the exhepatic biliary system. Clinics in Gastroenterology, 2:3, 1973.
5. Daniel, O.: The value of radiomanometry in bile duct surgery. Ann. Roy. Coll Surg. Eng., 51:357, 1972.
6. Hess, W.: Surgery of the biliary passages and the pancreas. New York:Van Nostrand, 1965.
7. Hopton, D. and White, T. T.: An evaluation of manometric operative cholangiography in 100 patients with biliary disease. Surg. Gynec. Obstet., 133:949, 1971.
8. Schein, C. J. and Beneventano, T. C.: Biliary manometry: Its role in clinical surgery. Surgery, 67:255, 1970.
9. Johnson, F. E. and Boyden, E. A.: Effect of double vagotomy on motor activity of the human gallbladder. Surgery, 32:591, 1952.
10. Rudick, J. and Hutchinson, J. S. F.: Evaluation of vagotomy and biliary function by combined oral cholecystography and intravenous cholangiography. Amer. Surg., 162:234, 1965.
11. Hopton, D. and White, T. T.: Effect of hepatic and celiac vagal stimulation on common duct pressure. Amer. J. Dig. Dis., 16:1095, 1971.
12. McCarthy, J. D.: Radiomanometry during biliary operations. Arch. Surg., 100:424, 1970.
13. White, T. T. et al: Radiomanometry, flow rates and cholangiography in the evaluation of common bile duct disease. Amer. J. Surg., 123:73, 1972.

Partially supported by NIH Grant CA-AM 14380 and American Cancer Society Grant CI 82.

Endoscopic Retrograde Cholangiography

Robert L. Goodale, Jr., M.D.

The correct preoperative diagnosis of extrahepatic biliary tract disease can be extremely difficult and challenging. Better diagnostic techniques have long been sought, especially when serum bilirubin levels of 3 mg% or greater make oral or intravenous cholangiography worthless. The advent of the side-viewing fiberoptic duodenoscope as developed by the Japanese has brought a major advance in the diagnosis of biliary tract disease. The ampulla is now visualized and cannulated under direct endoscopic vision. Radiopaque solution is instilled into the biliary tract and the pancreatic duct, with an overall success rate of visualization approaching 89%, as the experience of the endoscopist increases with time. This method appears to be a practical, low-risk technique. The major advantage is that by noninvasive means, we can delineate the ductal system in the presence of jaundice. The method was first introduced by Oi [1], Takagi [2] and Ogoshi [3] in Japan, independently, in 1970.

Vennes and Silvis [4], from the Minneapolis Veterans Administration Hospital, reported the first successful series of cases in this country in 1972. Since that time, the technique has gained in acceptance and popularity worldwide. The low but definite morbidity, the amount of time required to master the technique and the expense will probably always restrict this to an in-hospital procedure, to be done only on selected cases, after the more routine diagnostic tests have failed. Endoscopic cholangiography and pancreatography are the most difficult endoscopic procedures presently done. Figure 1 shows the cannulation of an ampulla of Vater with a 1.7 mm teflon catheter inserted in the orifice. The tube has been guided there by the duodenoscope.

The indications for endoscopic retrograde cholangiography in patients with jaundice due to possible extrahepatic obstruction include patients with recurrent jaundice or jaundice following biliary tract surgery, or

---

Robert L. Goodale, Jr., M.D., Associate Professor, Department of Surgery, University of Minnesota Medical School, Minneapolis.

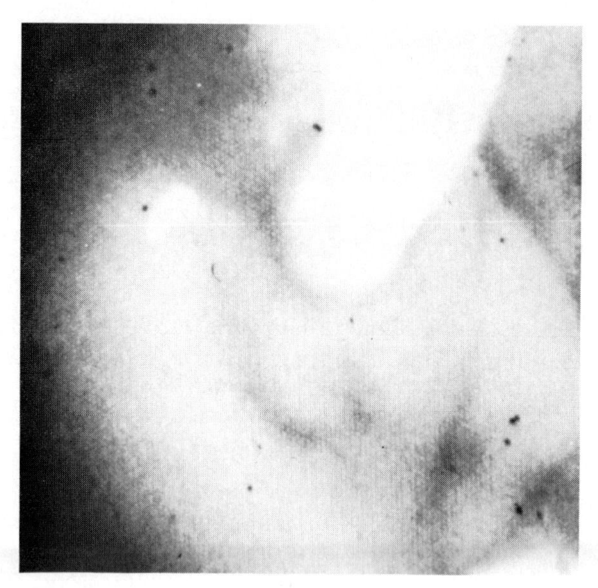

FIGURE 1.

patients with known primary liver disease who develop cholangitis. Patients who have received any possible hepatotoxic drugs within the last six months are also candidates.

The contraindications include the unavailability of a surgical team prepared to operate within 24 hours, should biliary obstruction be found. We have learned that cholangitis can flare up immediately following the endoscopic procedure. If a surgeon is not available or the patient is not in condition for operation, this procedure should not be done. Pyloric obstruction and duodenal obstruction are relative contraindications, but where the narrowing is not too severe the study can be undertaken. Uncooperative or comatose patients can ruin an expensive fiberoptic instrument and thus cause a lot of financial grief. Involuntary biting of the fiberoptic shaft may greatly damage the scope. Infection with Hepatitis B viremia is another contraindication. These instruments cannot be autoclaved and there is a risk of viral transmission despite cleansing with soap and alcohol solutions.

The results of endoscopic cholangiography in 38 patients with jaundice of uncertain etiology at the University of Minnesota Hospital are shown in Figure 2. With very few exceptions, prior intravenous cholangiography was nondiagnostic. There were 28 patients (71%) in whom successful visualiza-

PATIENTS WITH JAUNDICE OF UNCERTAIN ETIOLOGY

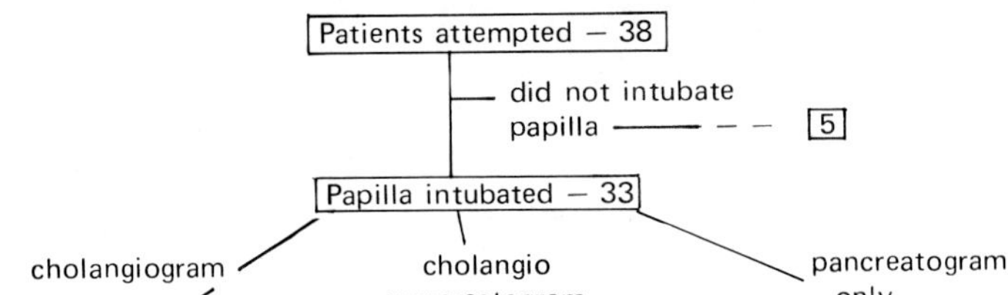

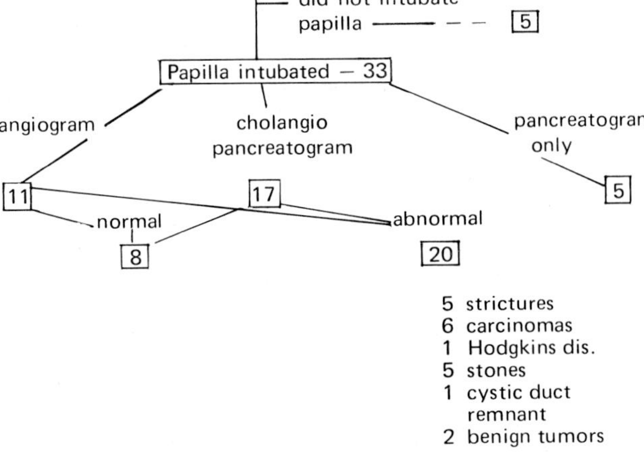

FIGURE 2.

tions of the common duct and biliary system were obtained. A cholangiogram alone was obtained in 11 and cholangiopancreatograms obtained in 17. In five patients only a pancreatogram was obtained. It was not that we did not try to obtain cholangiography; however, for technical reasons, only the pancreatic duct was visualized.

Twenty cholangiograms were abnormal. Strictures and stones were the most common findings. Seven of the nine tumors were malignant, one of them being a bile duct carcinoma and five pancreatic duct carcinomas. There was one case of extrahepatic obstruction due to Hodgkin's disease with nodal compression.

There were five instances of unsuccessful cannulation attempts. Some failures were associated with our early inexperience with the technique. A few difficulties resulted from pyloric narrowing or an abnormally located ampulla. There are always going to be some anatomic variations, which will preclude a 100% success rate in cannulation.

Some cases will illustrate the value of endoscopic cholangiography. A 79-year-old man entered the hospital with painless jaundice and a 15 pound weight loss. The presumptive diagnosis was of a malignancy. However, as shown by Figure 3, a dilated common duct with multiple stones was demonstrated by the retrograde cholangiogram. Several stones

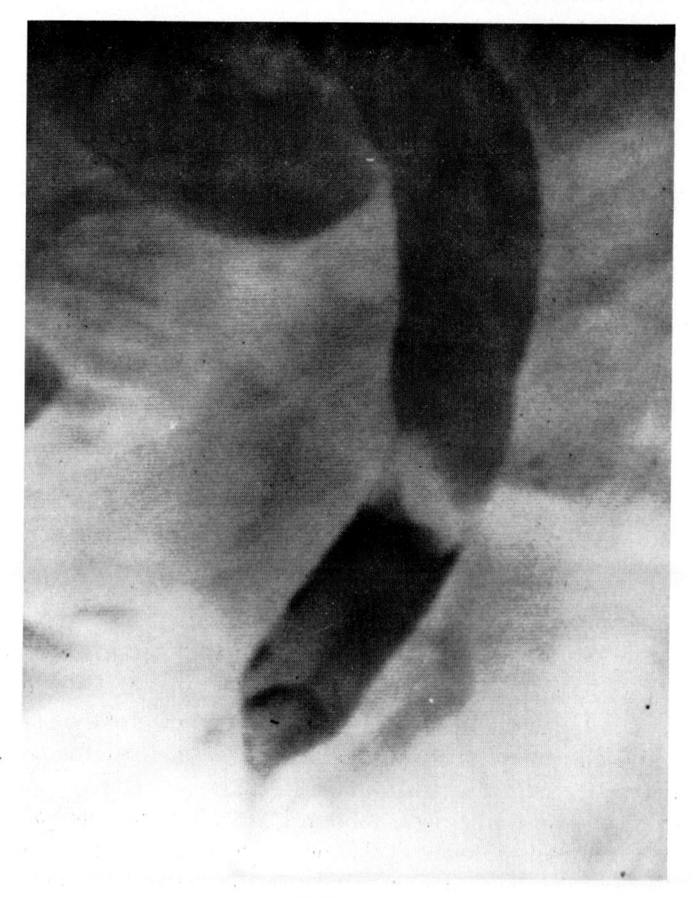

FIGURE 3.

were impacted in the distal end of the duct. The stones were removed uneventfully at the time of surgery.

A second case is that of a 69-year-old lady who entered the hospital with epigastric pain, fever and chills. A cholecystectomy had been performed ten years previously. An incidental endoscopic finding, at the time of cholangiography, was a benign gastric ulcer that had not been demonstrated by the upper gastrointestinal x-ray examination. The retrograde study shows a dilated common duct and intrahepatic radicals. One rounded common duct stone is clearly visible (Fig. 4) and a second is just evident.

A 53-year-old man with hyperthyroidism had been treated by propylthiouracil. He noted the insidious onset of jaundice with bilirubin

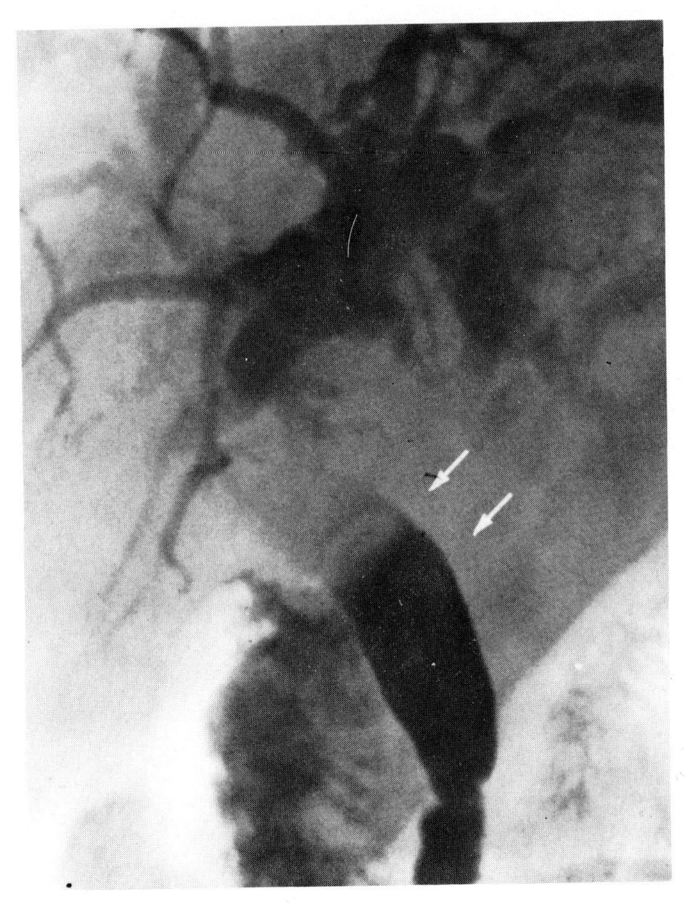

FIGURE 4.

rising to 10 mg%. There was a strong suspicion that he might have a malignancy. Actually, however, a normal caliber common duct, a normal gallbladder and normal intrahepatic radicals were demonstrated by endoscopic cholangiography. A percutaneous needle biopsy showed a chronic hepatitis probably secondary to the thyroid medication (Fig. 5). The jaundice subsided with discontinuance of the medication.

The next cholangiogram is that of a 52-year-old lady who entered with weight loss and nausea, which had been treated for months with Compazine®. Then she developed painless jaundice. Endoscopic cholangiography showed a normal common bile duct faintly outlined (Fig. 6) and a normal gallbladder. However, the intrahepatic ducts could not be filled and a high complete intrahepatic obstruction was suspected. At the time

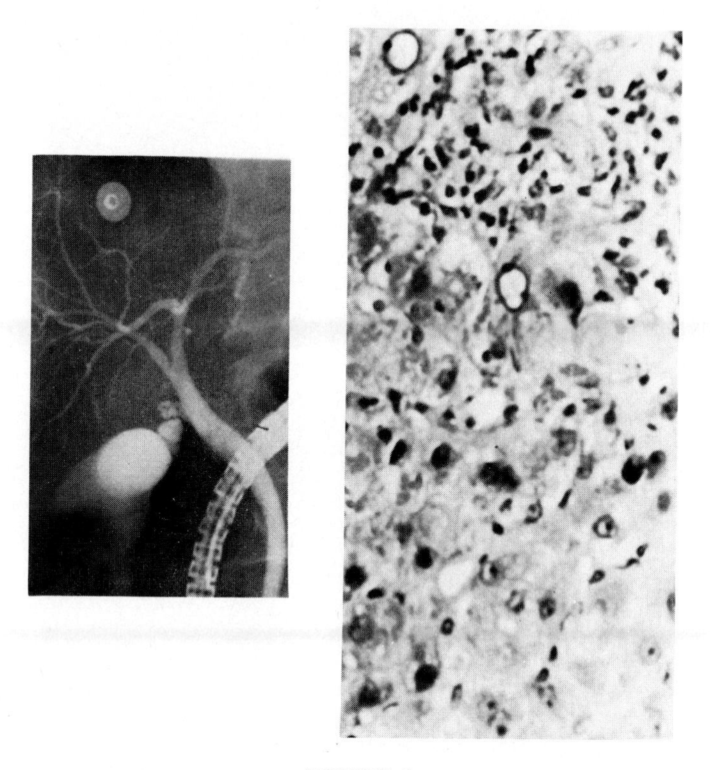

FIGURE 5.

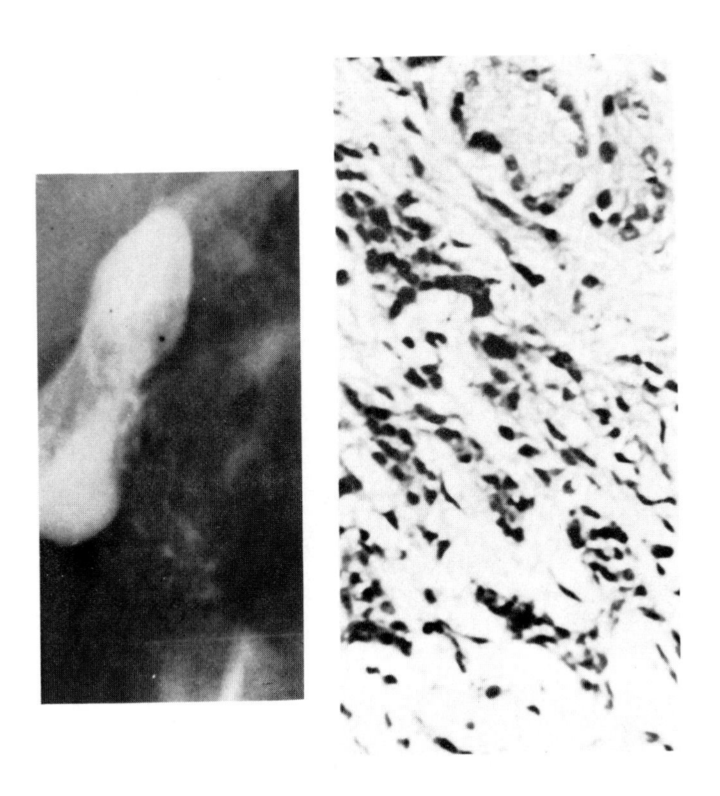

FIGURE 6.

of surgery, a bile duct carcinoma was found (Fig. 6) which completely obstructed the intrahepatic ducts.

A 65-year-old man developed liver function studies suggesting obstruction. Upper GI series showed a polypoid lesion in the second portion of the duodenum in the area of the ampulla. Endoscopic biopsies showed a benign adenoma of the ampulla. Because of evidence of pancreatic and biliary ductal dilation as shown on the cholangiogram, a resection of the adenoma was carried out (Fig. 7).

A 53-year-old man underwent a kidney transplant. He did well for six months and then developed fever, chills, jaundice and right upper quadrant pain. Endoscopic cholangiography revealed a normal sized common duct,

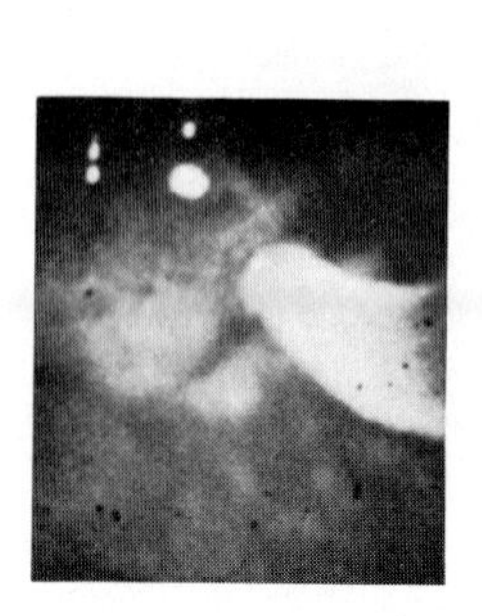

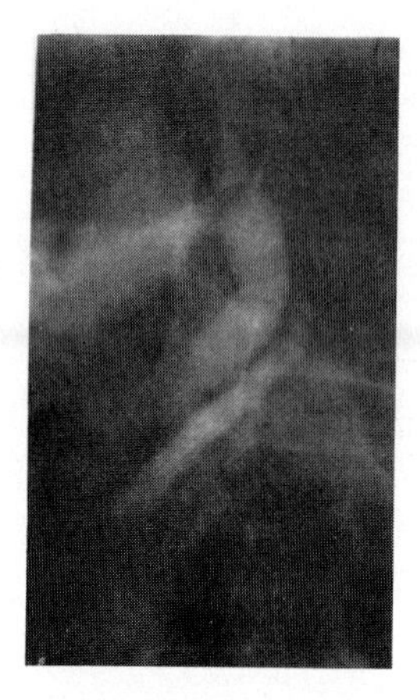

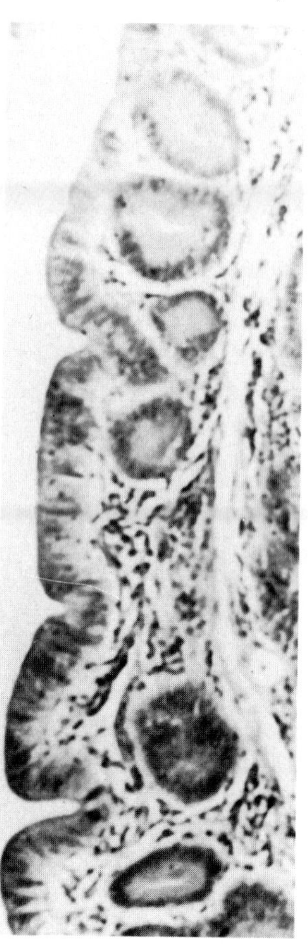

FIGURE 7.

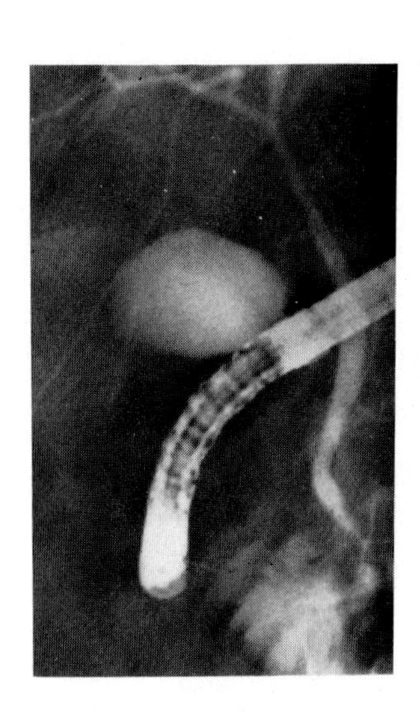

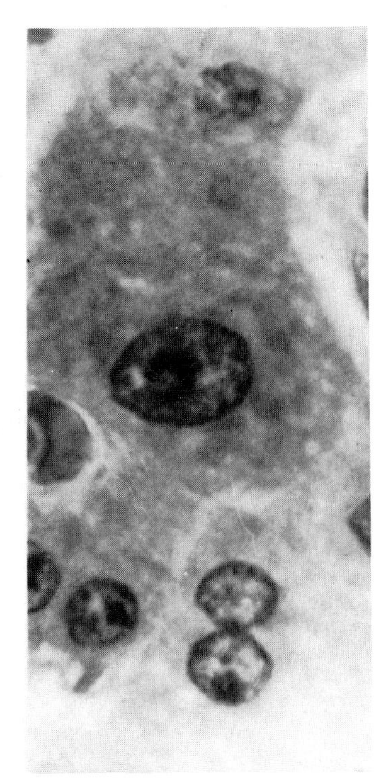

FIGURE 8.

gallbladder and intrahepatic radicals. No operation was performed. At autopsy, it was found that he had cytomegalic inclusion bodies (Fig. 8) in many organs, including the liver. The jaundice was clearly hepatocellular.

A final case is that of a 19-year-old girl who underwent cholecystectomy, then developed painless jaundice. An endoscopic cholangiogram shows dilated intrahepatic ducts, with a lobulated filling defect just above the cystic duct remnant (Fig. 9). At surgery, there was a cystadenoma of the liver, arising in the left lobe and impinging on the right and left hepatic ducts. The endoscopic cholangiogram clearly favored a diagnosis of tumor rather than stone.

Three complications occurred and are ones that we would hope to avoid in the future. Two cases of cholangitis occurred: one quite severe due to the fact of a three day delay before surgical correction of an obstructed biliary duct. If obstruction is found, we now administer antibiotics, such as gentamycin or Keflin. The experience of others indicates the use of gentamycin has reduced the overall incidence of

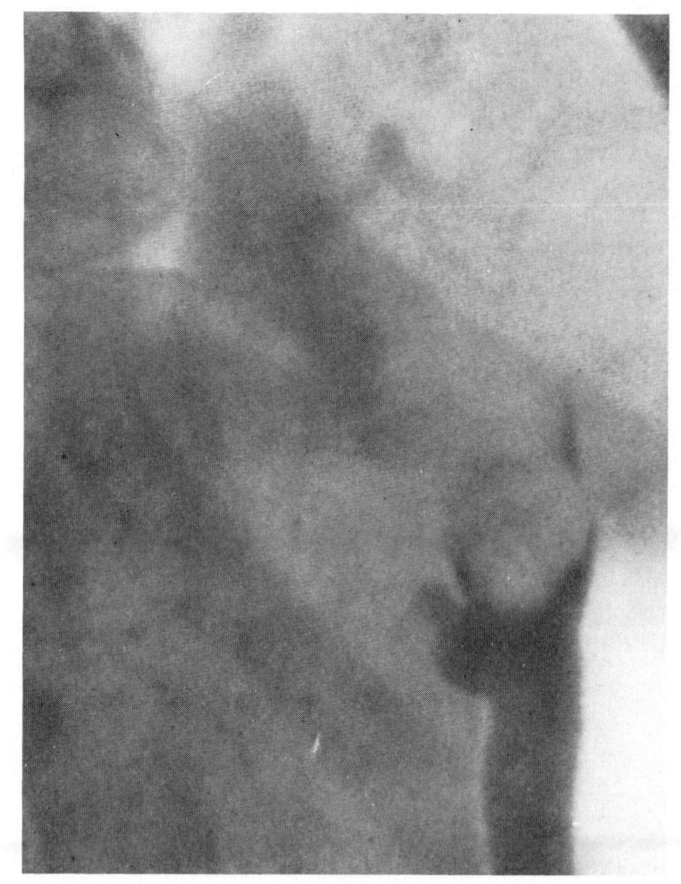

FIGURE 9.

cholangitis from 1.5% to 0.2%. Our own incidence of cholangitis is 5.3%. There has been one death in our experience. Endoscopic cholangiography was undertaken in a patient in septicemic shock with bile peritonitis and we would now regard cannulation to be contraindicated in all patients not in condition to undergo surgery.

In conclusion, endoscopic retrograde cholangiography is proving to be a practical and valuable noninvasive diagnostic procedure which can help the surgeon dealing with biliary tract disease. One of its greatest uses is in identifying clearly those patients with primary cholestatic or hepatocellular jaundice and thereby saving them the risk, expense and discomfort of an unnecessary operation.

References

1. Oi, I.: Fiberduodenoscopy and endoscopic pancreatocholangiography. Gastroint. Endosc., 17:59-62, 1970.
2. Takagi, K. et al: Retrograde pancreatography and cholangiography by fiber duodenoscope. Gastroenterology, 59:445-452, 1970.
3. Ogoshi, K., Tobita, Y. and Hara, Y.: Endoscopic observations of the duodenum and pancreato-choledochography using duodenal fiberscope under direct vision. Gastroint. Endosc. (Tokyo), 12:83-96, 1970.
4. Vennes, J. A. and Silvis, S. D.: Endoscopic visualization of bile and pancreatic ducts. Gastroint. Endosc., 18:149-152, 1972.

Should Silent Gallstones Be Treated by Cholecystectomy?

Henry Sosin, M.D.

The incidence of gallstones in the United States is of major proportion. It is estimated that approximately 7% of the total population have cholelithiasis. In several autopsy studies, the incidence of cholelithiasis approximates 11%. In Table 1, it can be seen from extensive autopsy series that females have more cholelithiasis than males, and that whites have significantly more gallstone disease than blacks. Although not represented in the table, it is also known that the Indian populations have an even higher incidence of cholelithiasis. Also, one can note that there is an increased incidence of gallstone disease with age. The incidence of silent biliary stone disease is much more difficult to assess. In necropsy studies, this percentage has varied between 16% and 77%. This incidence seems extremely high. However, one would have expected most patients with symptoms to have been operated upon, possibly raising the incidence of "asymptomatic" stones. In addition, modest symptoms from calculus disease probably were not reported on premortem records (Table 2). The prevalence of silent biliary calculi in the normal population is the figure which is most meaningful. Several authors have attempted to assess this problem (Table 3). Most of the papers listed really dealt with nonoperated patients who were relatively asymptomatic. However, these patients were discovered most frequently because of prior symptoms. Only the report by Wilbur of 1,233 patients was truly a survey of asymptomatic patients. Seven and one-half percent of all of these gentlemen, who were over the age of 40, had biliary calculi and only 4.8% were truly asymptomatic. When one considers that the incidence of stones in any age group for females is approximately double that of males, one could surmise that the true incidence of silent stones in an asymptomatic population over the age of 40 would approximate 7½% to 10%.

Henry Sosin, M.D., Associate Professor, Department of Surgery, University of Minnesota School of Medicine, Minneapolis.

Table 1. Autopsy Frequency of Gallstones (Newman)

Age	*White Males*	*White Females*	*Negro Males*	*Negro Females*
0-19	0.1%	0.1%	0.01%	0.01%
20-29	1.0%	5.0%	0.2 %	2.0 %
30-39	2.0%	9.0%	1.0 %	5.0 %
40-49	6.0%	15.0%	2.0 %	10.0 %
50-59	9.0%	24.0%	5.0 %	11.0 %
60-69	13.0%	30.0%	7.0 %	17.0 %
70-79	18.0%	34.0%	8.0 %	18.0 %
> 79	22.0%	38.0%	10.0 %	23.0 %

Table 2. Prevalence of Silent Biliary Calculi – Necropsy

Author	*Patients*	*%Asymptomatic*
Newman	5,375	77.0%
Robertson	1,027	61.0%
Kozoll	1,874	33.8%
Stewart	6,000	16.4%
Crump	1,000	32.2%

Table 3. Prevalence of Silent Calculi – Real Population

Author	*Patients*	*Stones*	*Silent*
Truesdell	500	50 – 10.0%	2 – 1.0%
Comfort		998	112 11.0%
Lund		526	34 6.3%
Ralston		116	14 12.0%
Colcock		3246	134 4.0%
Wilbur	1,233	92 – 7.5%	59 4.8%

Table 4. Development of Symptoms, Complications and Mortality

	Patients	*Symptoms*	*Complications*	*Mortality*
Comfort	112	51 – 46%	24 – 21%	3 – 2.7%
Lund	526	50%	25%	14 – 2.7%
	34	33%	7 – 20%	
Ralston	116		51%	3 – 2.6%
Wenckert	781	254 – 33%	35%	13 – 1.7%
Bolt	7	12 – 15%	16 – 71%	

The question proposed here is how best to handle a patient with truly unsuspected or silent biliary calculi. In order to decide the best course to follow, one must balance the risk of disease vs. the risk of surgical removal. Therefore, one must attempt to ascertain the incidence of the development of symptoms, the incidence of further complications, the frequency of associated disease and the mortality from biliary tract disease itself if left untreated. On the other hand, one must know the surgical mortality, morbidity of elective cholecystectomy and the possibility of other nonoperative therapy. Table 4 details the development of symptoms in those patients reported as having relatively nonsymptomatic stones. The incidence of subsequent symptoms approximates 35%-40% and the incidence of complications of biliary disease is approximately 25%. The mortality associated with biliary calculi alone is approximately 2.5%. In the study reported by Lund (Table 5), the mortality from untreated biliary tract disease increases with age to a high of 7.2% in patients over age 65. This figure is important in order to make comparisons with increased operative mortality with age.

The incidence of or association of carcinoma of the gallbladder with biliary stone disease has traditionally been used as an argument for elective cholecystectomy. The necropsy series by Newman (Table 6) does document that there is an increased incidence of carcinoma in patients with biliary calculi and that the increased incidence of carcinoma follows

Table 5. Mortality of Gallbladder Disease (Lund)

Age	*Mortality*	*%*
< 46 yrs	0 – 150	0
46 – 55 yrs	1 – 123	0.8%
56 – 65 Yrs	4 – 128	3.1%
> 65 yrs	0 – 125	7.2%
	14 – 526	2.7%

Table 6. Gallbladder, Carcinoma and Calculi at Autopsy (Newman)

Age	*Males With Stones*	*Males Without Stones*	*Females With Stones*	*Females Without Stones*
20-29	0/4	0/54	0/5	0/44
30-39	0/6	0/83	3/17	0/75
40-49	0/22	0/159	1/44	0/127
50-59	1/42	1/278	10/78	0/159
60-69	3/83	0/370	4/112	1/178
70-79	2/50	0/163	4/55	1/179
> 79	0/9	0/28	3/16	0/16
	2.7%	0.09%	7.6%	10.13%

Table 7. Cancer of Gallbladder

	Patients	*Number*
Lund	526	3 – 0.6%
Ralston	116	2 – 1.7%
Wenckert	1402	5 – .4%

Table 8. Mortality from Cholecystectomy With Age

	<60 Years		*>60 Years*	
	Patients	*Mortality*	*Patients*	*Mortality*
Wenckert	3079	.13%	518	.8%
Hoff		1.0 %		5.0%
Iback 1962-66	275	.7 %	151	4.0%
Seltzer 1963-67	712	.6 %	378	3.4%
Meyer 1958-64	921	.5 %	340	7.6%

Table 9. Surgical Mortality With Age (Wenckert)

	Patients	*Mortality*	*Patients*	*Mortality*
Uncomplicated	355	0	151	0
Complicated	203	.99%	72	11 – 15.3%
	558	2 – .4%	223	11 – 5%

in time the incidence of biliary calculi. The incidence of carcinoma of the gallbladder increases approximately 70-fold over the normal population if the patient does have gallstones. However, the total incidence remains quite small. This has been estimated to be 0.5%-1.0% of patients (Table 7) with gallstones. Although the increased incidence of cancer is real, and as we will see it does approximate the operative mortality for elective cholecystectomy, the fear of cancer cannot be used as a strong argument in favor of elective cholecystectomy. It does remain, obviously, a factor.

On the other side of the balance, one must consider the operative mortality from cholecystectomy. For elective cholecystectomy under the age of 60 years, the operative mortality approximates 0.5% (Table 8). In addition, one can see that the operative mortality in patients over 60 increases in one series to a figure of 7.6%, which equals the mortality from biliary lithiasis in patients not having undergone elective cholecystectomy. In a series reported by Wenckert, the operative mortality also increased in the presence of complications from biliary tract disease (Table 9). There was no reported mortality in patients even over the age of 60 if the disease was uncomplicated. However, when complications arose, a mortality of 1% occurred in the age group under age 60, but the age group over age 60 experienced a 15% operative mortality rate. Waiting for asymptomatic patients to develop complications of biliary tract disease requiring urgent surgery seems to be an unwise course to follow. If one selects mortality rates associated with only elective cholecystectomy, the figures are even better. In several series the mortality rate for elective cholecystectomy averaged 0.5% (Table 10).

These figures indicate that approximately 50% of patients with asymptomatic biliary calculi will develop symptoms at a future date. Moreover, 25% will develop complications of biliary tract disease. In general, we have seen that the mortality of biliary tract disease alone approximates 2.5% and that in the age group over age 65 the mortality from biliary tract disease is 7.2%. In addition, an incidence of 0.5% to 1% malignant change may be expected. On the other hand, we have seen that

Table 10. Surgical Mortality in Elective Cholecystectomy

	Cases	*%Mortality*
Method	565	.35
Glenn	1444	.3
Wenckert	557	.18
Hoff	589	2.0
Seltzer	1090	1.6
Holm	1467	.9
Meyer	680	.9

Table 11. Silent Gallstones

Disease Risk		*Surgical Risk*
Symptoms	50.0%	Operative mortality elective 0.5%
Complications	25.0%	
Mortality from disease	2.7%	With complications,
> 65 years	7.2%	With age,
Cancer	0.5-1.0%	Other treatment ?

the operative mortality for elective cholecystectomy is 0.5%. Table 11 summarizes these data. We know that mortality of operative intervention will increase with age and with the occurrence of complications of biliary tract disease. Although we are aware that physiologic manipulation by the use of chenodeoxycholic acid is now under experimental trial, we have learned that this method is at present relatively ineffective and still under research control. The conclusion that is logically reached is that all patients with known biliary calculi, in the absence of very strong contraindications to surgery, should undergo elective cholecystectomy and other appropriate biliary tract operations when required.

Bibliography

Berk, J. E.: Treatment of silent gallstones. Mod. Treatm., 5:2, 505, 1968.

Carey, J. B.: Natural history of gallstone disease. Mod. Treatm., 5:497-499, 1968.

Colcock, B., Killen, R. B. and Leach, N. G.: The asymptomatic patient with gallstones. Amer. J. Surg., 113:44-48, 1967.

Comfort, M. W., Gray, H. K. and Wilson, J. M.: The silent gallstone; A ten to twenty year follow up study of 112 cases. Ann. Surg., 128:931, 1948.

Glenn, F. and Grafe, W. R.: Historical events in biliary tract surgery. Arch. Surg., 93:848, 1966.

Lund, J.: Surgical indications in cholelithiasis: Prophylactic cholecystectomy elucidated on the basis of long term follow up in 526 nonoperated cases. Ann. Surg., 151:2, 153, 1960.

Method, H., Mehn, W. H. and Frable, W. J.: "Silent" gallstones. Arch. Surg., 85:138, 1962.

Meyer, K. A., Capos, N. and Mittelpunkt, A.: Personal experiences with 1,261 cases of acute and chronic cholecystitis and cholelithiasis. Surgery, 61:5, 661, 1967.

Newman, H., Northup, J., Rosenblum, M. et al: Complications of cholelithiasis. Amer. J. Gastroent., 50:476, 1968.

Ralston, D. E. and Smith, L.: The natural history of cholelithiasis. Minn. Med., 48:327, 1965.

Truesdell, E. D.: The frequency and future of gallstones believed to be quiescent or symptomless. Ann. Surg., 119:1, 232, 1944.

Wilbur, R. and Bolt, R.: Incidence of gall bladder disease in "normal" men. Gastroenterology, 36:251, 1959.

Wenckert, A. and Robertson, B.: The natural course of gallstone disease. Gastroenterology, 50:3:376, 1966.

Choledochal Sphincteroplasty or Choledochoduodenostomy

Thomas Taylor White, M.D.

There has always been a great deal of discussion as to which treatment is best for benign obstruction of the lower portion of the common bile duct [1-11]. A number of surgeons [2, 3, 5, 7] feel that choledochoduodenostomy is always the best procedure for this purpose. On the other hand, Jones [4] has advocated the use of sphincteroplasty in virtually all such situations. Only recently has there been a discussion as to the relative merits of the two procedures, with the idea that sphincteroplasty would be better used in some circumstances and choledochoduodenostomy in others. On the basis of such comparisons, Hoerr feels that choledochoduodenostomy is a much better procedure, while others [7, 8, 10, 11] feel that the underlying pathological features are more important in determining both the choice and the morbidity of the procedure used. We prefer to do sphincteroplasty if there is a choice, because there will be no stasis in the distal blind loop remaining after the latero-lateral anastomosis which we usually use. We tend to use choledochoduodenostomy in older, sicker patients and sphincteroplasty in younger, healthier patients.

Specific Indications for Sphincteroplasty as Opposed to Choledochoduodenostomy

Where the patient is found at operative cholangiography to have not only a stricture of the ampulla, reflux of nearly all the dye into the pancreas, and a diffusely hard pancreas which is not constricting the intrapancreatic portion of the bile duct, sphincteroplasty with a special effort to surgically divide the pancreatic duct sphincter is preferred (Fig. 1). We do this because stricture of the pancreatic duct can occur alone or in combination with a stricture of the sphincter of Oddi, and both

---

Thomas Taylor White, M.D., Clinical Professor of Surgery, University of Washington School of Medicine; Active Staff, Swedish and University Hospitals, Seattle, Wash.

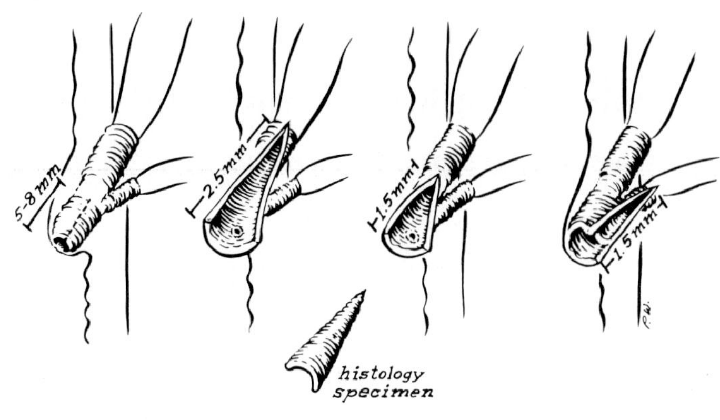

FIGURE 1.

problems can be solved at the same time. In both instances, the principal cause of the stricture and/or spasm is prior passage of a common bile duct stone. Stricture of either/or both sphincters can occur without any history of jaundice or common bile duct stones, probably due to the passage of stones from the cystic into the common bile duct without this situation being clinically detectable. For this reason, we feel that in dealing with distal bile duct obstruction, where repeated attacks of pancreatitis have occurred, therapeutic disobstruction of both ducts should be carried out.

Narrowing of the Intrapancreatic Bile Duct

If the patient has a significant narrowing of the intrapancreatic bile duct, it is obvious that sphincteroplasty would be of no value because of persistent obstruction above this point (Fig. 2). A choledochoduodenostomy is the procedure of choice in this instance because of the relative simplicity of suturing the bile duct to the adjacent duodenum.

Where the Duodenum Must Be Explored

The duodenum must be explored whenever there is uncertainty as to whether or not there is an ampullary or other intraduodenal tumor and where there is a stone impacted in the ampulla which cannot be removed from above. Under these circumstances, sphincteroplasty is preferable as a method of decompression of the distal bile duct, because the single incision which is used for duodenal exploration can also be used for performance of a sphincteroplasty without making a secondary, higher incision for the performance of a choledochoduodenostomy.

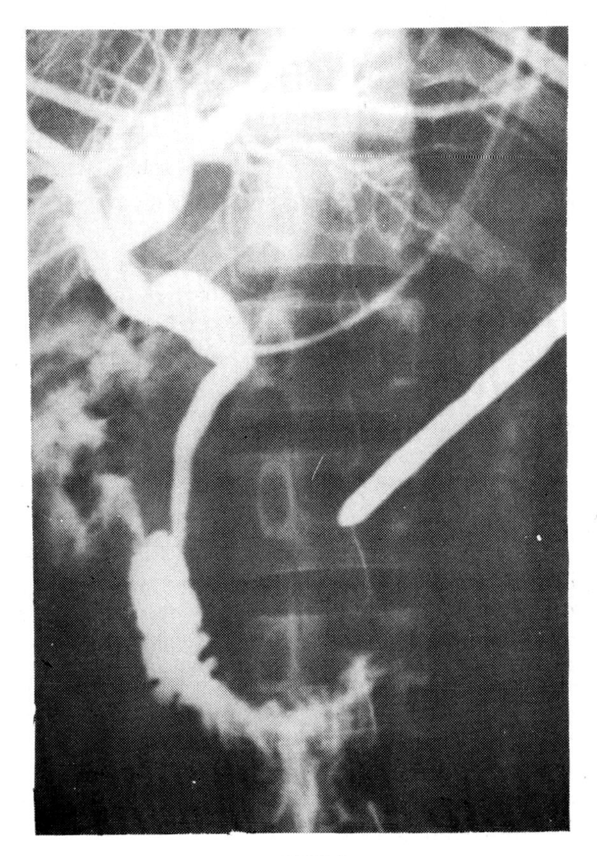

FIGURE 2.

Where There Are Recurrent or Retained Stones

If the problem is thought to be due to biliary mud, bilirubin stones or sludge (with or without the presence of a compacted stone made of this material), it probably is on the basis of chronic ductal obstruction, usually ampullary stenosis. Under these circumstances, we feel that sphinctero-plasty is best if the duct is less than 15 mm in diameter; either a choledochoduodenostomy or a sphincteroplasty if it is between 16 and 25 mm in diameter; and a choledochoduodenostomy if it is over 26 mm in diameter. We do not have the bias in favor of choledochoduodenostomy which Dr. Hoerr has [7, 10, 11].

Aside from the above considerations, duodenotomy is still a hazardous procedure, and it is for this reason that it is recommended that the average surgeon use the method more familiar to him. On the other hand, the morbidity of the two procedures is about the same. The underlying pathology is more important in determining morbidity [8, 10].

Out of my 136 sphincteroplasties and 32 choledochoduodenostomies, I have had three postoperative deaths following sphincteroplasty and two following choledochoduodenostomy. A postoperative abscess or fistula developed in five and three died during the postoperative period after sphincteroplasty. One of the deaths was due to acute gastrointestinal bleeding secondary to a stress ulcer of the stomach, one from breakdown of an accompanying cystogastrostomy and a third from liver failure. The mean diameter of the bile ducts in the patients who underwent sphincteroplasty was 10.0±1.3 cm and that for choledochoduodenostomy was 22.5±13.3 cm.

Technical Aspects

In doing either procedure, we use a generous exposure which will identify all the duodenal and ductal areas. The operative cholangiogram should be made prior to any manipulation of the ampulla to avoid spasm of the ampulla which will falsely give the impression of obstruction because of the manipulation. The sphincter of Oddi has three sphincters: one at the papilla, one at the junction of the pancreatic and distal bile duct and one at the bile duct sphincter. A cut of approximately 2.5 mm in length is required to cut all three sphincters (Fig. 1). In effect, one is producing a transduodenal choledochoduodenostomy. We always prefer to open the duodenum only after doing a thorough Kocher maneuver by cutting the peritoneum along the reflection of the duodenum on the posterior abdominal wall. It is much easier to locate the distal end of the common bile duct and bring the duodenum into an anterior position for duodenotomy if such a dissection has been carried out. This maneuver is helpful in doing either a sphincteroplasty or a choledochoduodenostomy.

Sphincteroplasty

When I do a sphincteroplasty, I use a high duodenal incision (Fig. 3) either with a probe in the common bile duct or after having found the end of the bile duct after mobilization of the pancreas and duodenum. We cut the seromuscular layers first, push them back and then cut the mucosa, so that we can later longitudinally close the duodenum in two layers, the mucosa first and then the seromuscular layer. We use a high incision to avoid a difficult postoperative problem if a fistula does occur. If a large enough probe is passed so that it stops at the duodenal wall, it can be

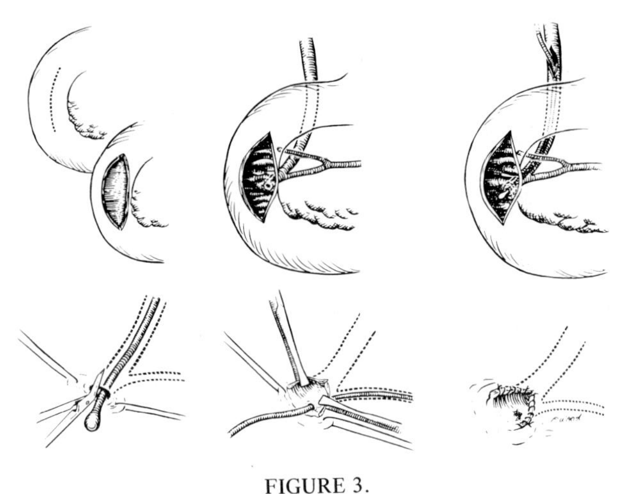

FIGURE 3.

clearly seen through the duodenal mucosa by its metallic color. We then place a mucosal suture on either side of the probe to hold the area taut. An iris, a sharp-pointed dura or a Potts scissors can be used to open the sphincter. Once this is done we place a suture through the mucosa and the sphincter mechanism along this side using 4-0 chromic catgut. Once this has been carried 25 mm to the top of the incision, a wedge is cut loose from the medial side and the suture is carried down on this side. Before the mucosal sutures are placed, a probe or a catheter should be inserted into the pancreatic duct to avoid oversewing its opening with resultant postoperative pancreatitis (Fig. 4).

Choledochoduodenostomy

Mechanically, this is the most straight-forward approach to an area which is easy to get at at either a primary or secondary procedure. On the other hand, after many secondary operations on the bile duct, mobilization of the ducts is difficult enough to warrant making the anastomosis to the jejunum instead. The duct must be at least 15 mm in diameter before a choledochoduodenostomy is undertaken. Smaller ducts are difficult to anastomose. The main approaches are latero-lateral (Figs. 5 and 6) and end-to-side. As to the pros and cons of the two procedures, the latero-lateral is easier and can be carried out much more rapidly than the end-to-side. While we consider the latter a better procedure because one can ligate the distal duct and prevent accumulation of material in the blind distal loop, there is considerable difference of opinion as to which type of

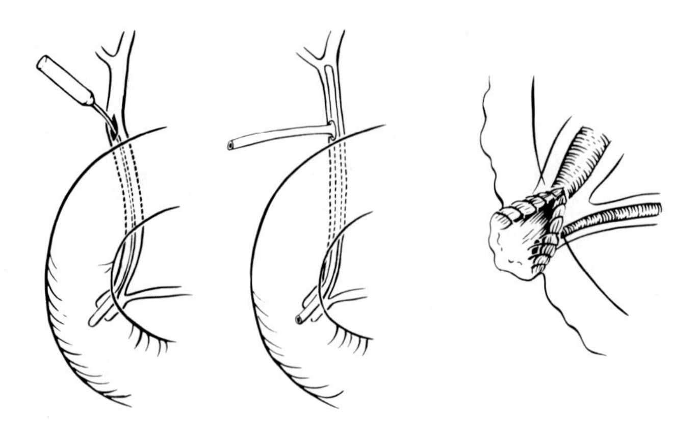

FIGURE 4.

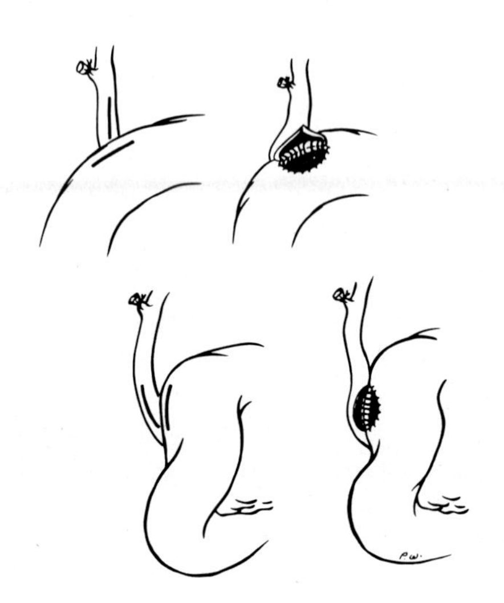

FIGURE 5.

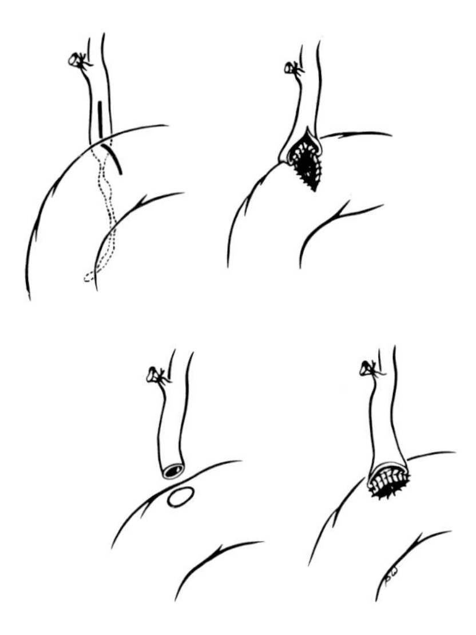

FIGURE 6.

anastomosis works better. The latero-lateral procedure allows the surgeon to make a larger opening (20-25 mm), which seems preferable generally speaking, but an end-to-side anastomosis with a 15 mm or greater opening is certainly large enough. Since one procedure allows as much reflux as the other, there is no basis for choice in this regard. As a matter of fact, there is just as much reflux into the biliary tree following a sphincteroplasty as in any type of decompressive procedure. Further, the latero-lateral anastomosis does not require dissection of the duct below the point of anastomosis and through areas of scarring, infection, bile debris, cholangitis and pancreatitis. There has been a great deal of heated discussion about this, particularly from those who fear stasis of the lower end of the duct. Still, cholangitis is a real problem only when there is partial rather than total obstruction of any type of anastomosis.

Thus, I recommend a good wide sphincteroplasty or choledochoduodenostomy through uninflamed tissue above unobstructed intestine. In the latter instance a Roux-y choledochojejunostomy is preferable.

References

1. Acosta, J. M. and Nardi, G. L.: Papillitis: Inflammatory disease of the ampulla of Vater. Arch. Surg., 92:354, 1966.

2. Capper, W. M.: External choledochoduodenostomy: An evaluation of 125 cases. Brit. J. Surg., 49:292, 1961.
3. Degenshein, G. A. and Hurwitz, A.: The techniques of side-to-side choledochoduodenostomy. Surgery, 61:972, 1967.
4. Jones, S. A., Steedman, R. A., Keller, T. B. et al: Transduodenal sphincteroplasty (not sphincterotomy) for biliary and pancreatic disease: Indications, contraindications, and results. Amer. J. Surg., 118:292, 1969.
5. Madden, J. L., Chun, J. Y., Kandalaft, S. et al: Choledochoduodenostomy, an unjustly maligned surgical procedure. Amer. J. Surg., 119:45, 1970.
6. Shingleton, W. W. and Gamburg, D.: Stenosis of the sphincter of Oddi. Amer. J. Surg., 119:35, 1970.
7. Stuart, M. and Hoerr, S. O.: Late results of side-to-side choledochoduodenostomy and of transduodenal sphincterotomy for benign disorders. A twenty-year comparative study. Amer. J. Surg., 123:67, 1972.
8. Thomas, C. G., Jr., Nicholson, C. P. and Owen, J.: Effectiveness of choledochoduodenostomy and transduodenal sphincterotomy in the treatment of benign obstruction of the common duct. Ann. Surg., 173:845, 1971.
9. Way, L. W., Admirand, W. H., and Dunphy, J. E.: Management of choledocholithiasis. Ann. Surg., 176:347, 1972.
10. White, T. T.: Indications for sphincteroplasty as opposed to choledochoduodenostomy. Amer. J. Surg., 126:165, 1973.
11. White, T. T. and Harrison, R. C.: Reoperative gastrointestinal surgery. Boston:Little Brown Co., 1973.

Figures 1, 3-6 from White and Harrison [11].

Partially supported by NIH Grant CA-AM 14380 and American Cancer Society Grant CI82.

Panel Discussion

Moderator: H. Sosin, M.D.

Panelists: A. Hofmann, M.D. R. L. Goodale, M.D.
S. Schwartz, M.D. T. T. White, M.D.
R. M. Zollinger, M.D.

Dr. Sosin: Most of the questions received involve the incidence of pancreatitis. Since the artery to the spleen is ligated, presumably at some point proximal to the tail of the pancreas, how often is pancreatitis seen, and are serum and urine amylase determinations done to find chemical pancreatitis?

Dr. Zollinger: The pancreas has a very adequate blood supply. We have never feared pancreatitis from the ligation of the splenic artery above the pancreas and we will do it at any place that it comes easy. This was demonstrated by Frank Leahy years ago, with many procedures on the pancreas. We routinely do the amylase determinations at night, not because we fear it so much but just as a check, particularly if the patient has distention, or a lot of back pain. I don't see pancreatitis very frequently and don't fear pancreatitis from ligation of the artery.

Dr. Sosin: Do you measure urine amylases on your patients, postoperatively, routinely?

Dr. Zollinger: Yes, pretty much so. In most upper abdominal surgery, we have been doing that. Maybe it is a bad habit, but we do it after biliary surgery, gastric surgery, splenic surgery. The more you look, the more you find and the more you are aggravated by it; maybe we had better stop it.

Dr. Sosin: Dr. Schwartz, would you like to comment on the incidence of pancreatitis?

Dr. Schwartz: I guess that we do not see pancreatitis, because we don't do amylase determinations after splenectomy. The only two complications that we recorded, as I indicated, were fistulas and they both closed spontaneously. But we do not do an amylase study after routine splenectomy.

Dr. White: These complications do occur, as indicated by the fact that I have two patients in the hospital with pancreatic cysts following splenectomy, right at the present time. I am happy to say that I was not the original surgeon. It does occur. The real need is one of being aware that they can occur.

Dr. Zollinger: What did they do, a mass ligation in the middle of the pancreas when they took the spleen out?

Dr. White: Vascular surgeons did the operations.

Dr. Zollinger: Vascular surgeons?

Dr. White: Yes, vascular surgeons.

Dr. Zollinger: They are not safe to do splenectomies.

Dr. Sosin: Dr. Schwartz, could you please mention contraindications to splenectomy, especially in cases of splenomegaly?

Dr. Zollinger: This I want to hear!

Dr. Schwartz: I am trying to formulate an answer. The present thesis is that presented a patient with splenomegaly, after the internists go through a variety of studies, and cannot establish a diagnosis, we will operate on these patients. And, more often than not, we have provided a diagnosis of either lymphoma, or some sort of a sarcomatous process. Splenomegaly, alone, is becoming more and more an indication, in the absence of portal hypertension, for splenectomy. If I were to answer the direct question, I would say that splenectomy, alone, is not indicated in the patient with portal hypertension, secondary to hepatic disease, because it does not alter portal pressure. The only circumstance in which splenectomy, alone, may be important in a patient with portal hypertension would be the circumstance of increased afferent flow, which is described rarely in tropical splenomegaly. We have seen it twice, in patients with myeloproliferative disorders. In these very large spleens, with myeloidmetaplasia, removing the spleen did alter portal hypertension. So my answer would be, just in secondary hypersplenism; otherwise, splenomegaly, in general, is an indication for surgical extirpation.

Panelist: I think the question is directed toward the problem of whether the spleen is a myeloproliferative organ in myelometaplasia. I tried to make the point that it is not. There is an extraordinarily inappropriate paper in the literature, as recent as 1972, in the *Journal of Surgery*, in which, for some reason, a surgeon and a hematologist got together and, for another reason which I don't understand, the journal accepted the paper. Nevertheless, it indicates that they had a patient with myeloid metaplasia and they were disturbed as to whether the spleen was bad or good, so they removed one half of it. I think that they are to be complimented in getting away with the patient alive and covering the surfaces of the spleen. In myeloproliferative disorders there is no danger in removing the spleen, as far as the hematologic picture is concerned.

Dr. White: I think that there is one other thing which hasn't been mentioned. In patients who have islet cell tumors to the left of the aorta, and even more, in patients with chronic pancreatitis, there is no point in taking the left side of the pancreas out without taking the spleen out. One of the problems that you get into, if you do take the pancreas out without taking out the spleen, is that you may get splenic vein thrombosis and, later, a big, football-sized spleen which is painful and which gives later difficulty. So I would suggest that you take it out when you are going to do a left pancreatectomy. Do you agree, Dr. Zollinger?

Dr. Zollinger: Yes; I didn't know that there was any other way, actually. I think that it is pretty tedious to dissect the pancreas off of the splenic vessels.

Dr. White: There are people who do that.

Dr. Zollinger: Do they?

Dr. White: Oh, yes!

Dr. Zollinger: Well, they ought to be in a cage if they try it.

Dr. White: I am glad that Dr. Zollinger agrees with me.

Dr. Sosin: This question is directed to any member of the panel who would care to attempt to answer it. It concerns the preparation of a patient with a hematologic disorder prior to splenectomy.

Dr. Schwartz: There are several points to be made. First, it depends upon the patient. Rarely can you bring a patient in one day and operate on him on the next day. This is particularly applicable to patients with acquired hemolytic anemia and who are very difficult to type and to cross-match, patients with Hodgkin's disease and reticulum cell sarcoma who have a cryoglobulinemia and then you have to consider the fact that you don't want to give the blood cold. The main evangelical point about the preparation of patients and the biggest error that is made is giving the patient platelets preoperatively, when the patient is extremely thrombocytopenic, with a platelet count approaching zero, whether he has I.T.P., or secondary hypersplenism. I think that there is no point in this. Our approach is very similar to the one that Dr. Zollinger alluded to: get in rapidly, leave the clamps on, get the spleen out. Almost invariably, the bleeding will stop before the platelets come up. They are being consumed and, therefore, you don't see it in the peripheral smear. If the bleeding continues, then you give platelets after the spleen is removed. If you are going to give platelets, then you have to give them appropriately and, to me, that means about 15 or 20 platelet packs and no less. I think the point to take home, as far as preparation, is not to give the patients platelets preoperatively. Do you agree, Dr. Zollinger?

Dr. Zollinger: Yes, I agree to that. I think that it takes maybe one to two weeks to get patients ready until the hematologist is absolutely convinced that the bone marrow activity is adequate. They may want to survey the activity of the spleen and liver with survival studies. I would be very hesitant to remove a spleen unless a competent hematologist had surveyed the bone marrow. I am a little worried when pathologists evaluate the bone marrow. I think that the hematologists who are used to doing this can give you a much truer picture. You can get into trouble by taking out the spleen, on occasion. But I think, as Dr. Schwartz has said, that this is becoming less and less frequent. I don't know about platelets. I remember one of our junior colleagues once measured blood volume, Dr. Schwartz, in patients with purpura and he found quite a deficiency. We used to laugh when they slipped our patients whole blood on the basis of replacing their blood volume and not worry so much about platelets. We thought that they bled into their tissues perhaps more than had been realized. But we wouldn't admit that in the presence of our colleagues because we want to stay pretty clubby with them. But this did impress us.

Dr. White: Our hematologists are inclined to have the platelets given immediately as the splenic pedicle is clamped. We don't wait around to see whether they are going to rise. It is done as we go along.

Dr. Schwartz: I would think that we give no platelets in well over 75% of the patients of I.T.P. It gives us a better method of evaluating postoperatively. In reference to the point that Dr. Zollinger made about blood volume, interestingly enough, some new studies have just come from Denmark. All patients with significant splenomegaly have a marked increase, about a 100% increase, in their blood volume. Nobody knows exactly why. This appeared in *Acta Chirurgica Scandinavica* about three months ago. They have extraordinary increases in their blood volume, which has not been defined as to its reason; so I would not be worried about a reduced blood volume in any patient with splenomegaly.

Dr. Zollinger: But, in purpura, you said the spleen was small.

Dr. Schwartz: Yes, that is correct.

Dr. Zollinger: You read too much, Dr. Schwartz.

Dr. Schwartz: I am sorry to hear that, because I usually read your articles.

Dr. Zollinger: I can write trash, just the same as you. I have to defend myself.

Dr. Sosin: You have no comment about Dr. Schwartz being the editor? Let me ask Dr. Hofmann this question: The members of the audience would like to know, with respect to chenodeoxycholic acid treatment, what the cost is, what the patient intolerance is to the drug and would you comment about the toxicity, not only of chenodeoxycholic acid, but of lithocholic acid, which is the secondary acid?

Dr. Hofmann: The cost for the national study will be about 40 cents per day for a dose somewhere between 500 mg and 1 gm per day. Chenodeoxycholic acid is a white powder which is given in gelatin capsules. No one knows what the ultimate cost will be. The drug is probably not patentable. A number of pharmaceutical companies are trying to decide how involved to become. Chenodeoxycholic acid is usually prepared by chemical synthesis from cholic acid, which is obtained from ox bile. This is why most of the companies engaged in its production have ready access to meat packing facilities. These are large companies, such as Canada Packers and Weddell Pharmaceuticals (U.K.), both in the meat packing business.

The side effects, as far as patients are concerned, are essentially none. I think that they have been amplified unnecessarily and perhaps unwisely in the literature. In the initial Mayo Clinic studies, patients were given increasing doses until they had diarrhea and then the dose was cut back. To my knowledge, no patient has ever been reported, and I have not heard about any anecdotally, who could not achieve satisfactory bowel patterns on a therapeutic dose. The converse is also true, however. A number of patients who, reportedly, had constipation have had this problem solved by taking chenodeoxycholic acid. These studies are not controlled, in that the observer was aware that the patient was on chenodeoxycholic acid and there may have been observer-patient interaction.

In the national study, which is being funded by a $7 million NIH contract, if the toxicity studies, which are now being carried out in Matawan, Michigan, give results, which suggest to the Steering Committee of the National Cooperative Gallstones Study that they can proceed, then, this autumn, 1,000 patients with asymptomatic gallstones will be enrolled in a completely double-blind trial featuring high-dose, low-dose and placebo. That probably will be the best source of information as to whether patients really do feel better taking chenodeoxycholic acid.

When patients take chenodeoxycholic acid, colon bacteria remove a 7-hydroxy group and make a new bile acid called lithocholic acid. As people take more chenodeoxycholic acid, they make more lithocholic acid. You and I absorb very little of this from the colon. When it goes to the liver it is sulfated and we rapidly excrete it. There are not good data but we think the same thing is happening in patients who take chenodeoxycholic acid. They absorb a little bit more lithocholic acid from the colon, they sulfate it and lose it. In our laboratory, we have just worked out decent methods for measuring lithocholate in blood and bile. We'll find out whether these mild transaminase elevations are related to lithocholic acid. At the moment it is not known. One species – the rabbit – rapidly converts chenodeoxycholic acid to lithocholic acid and gets cirrhosis very soon after taking chenodeoxycholic acid. If there are some people who are just like rabbits, they are going to have trouble. But, so far, we haven't seen it.

Dr. Sosin: Isn't there also hepatoma reported in either mouse or rat with high doses of lithocholic acid?

Dr. Hofmann: I think that Dr. Palmer had an abstract on high doses of lithocholic acid. I don't think that it was chenodeoxycholic acid. The animals got peliosis hepatis, which is the occurrence of blood-filled sinuses in the liver; I believe that one of those animals got a hepatoma. But the bile acid metabolism is very different in small animals and this pathology was observed only after very high doses and a very long time. I don't think that the data are relevant to man. Perhaps I am seeing it in my own way. But I don't think so. If there is a lithocholic acid effect, it is clearly reversible from the animal work. You can stop the drug and it will go away. So, at the moment, we don't think that there should be any problem of permanent liver disease. There is unequivocal toxicity in the monkey, and this is why things are moving so slowly. The scenario that seems reasonable, to me, is we should first begin with the patient who has a retained common duct stone, then proceed to the patient that is at high risk for surgery, say, one who has had three coronaries. It will be a very long time before we can have any certainty that our drug is as good as the mortality figures which you showed for the elective cholecystectomy in the relatively asymptomatic patient.

Dr. Goodale: Do you think that there is going to be some difficulty when the chenodeoxycholic acid starts to dissolve the stones if they get small enough to get into common duct and cause acute jaundice and cholangitis?

Dr. Hofmann: The only thing which is predictable about "chenotherapy" is that I will be asked that question. All I can say is that we haven't seen it in our 70 patients. So far it has not been reported. Every stone which is large was once smaller and had the opportunity then to pass into the common duct. There will only be a limited time when this can happen. But I can say that we are worried about it.

Dr. Sosin: I am going to read this question verbatim and thereby remove myself from any editorial comment: "What has become of the best treatment for retained common duct calculi, that is, a flush of the common duct through the T-tube with chloroform and ether?" I open that up to the panel for discussion.

Dr. Zollinger: That is before my time. I don't know. I think that that was the old pre-Bomb stuff, wasn't it? You put it in there and then left the room while the patient boiled? I have heard about it for a long time, but I have never used it. I don't think that it has been used for a long, long time.

Dr. White: I would say, never. We had several patients in which this was attempted at Swedish Hospital within the last two or three years and they were all failures. I had never really seen this done before. One of our other staff members decided that he would try it, but it didn't work. What we have done, however, is what Dr. Hofmann discussed earlier, running cholic acid into the common bile duct, with a pump, somewhat as he showed. We treated about 12 patients so far with something around 75% of the stones having disappeared by one means or another. The assumption is that they have either passed or dissolved. Some of them got smaller. It takes quite a while. It may take as long as a week to ten days. Since Dr. Burhenne has come along with his steerable basket, we have been more inclined to remove single stones with this approach.

Dr. Schwartz: I saw that treatment once as a house officer and decided then never to use it. It is nice that it was used in the Swedish Hospital because I regard it as a sort of internal sauna bath, with the patient heating up all over. But, as far as the cholic acid infusion, I am a little concerned about the efficacy and how one will double-blind the cholic acid as Doctors Way and Dunphy have done. There are several papers that indicate that stones have been flushed through with just Ringer's lactate and saline. So I am not sure how you can equate this with the chemical dissolution, other than the mechanical alteration. I think that we are reaching a point with Dr. Burhenne's contributions, that this is going to become a radiologic exercise rather than a chemical one.

Dr. Zollinger: I am surprised that Dr. Dunphy didn't use Irish whiskey. He always has.

Dr. Schwartz: He didn't want to waste it.

Dr. Sosin: I was going to ask you whether he was going to take it himself or whether he was going to give it to the patient?

Dr. Zollinger: I would agree. I think that simple saline irrigation alone is about as useful as anything else.

Dr. White: I would like to say one thing. I am not in the position of defending cholate. We thought that it should be studied under controlled conditions and are doing just that. Our results aren't very good. Certainly, there is an effect of the fluid per se, but the cholate may cause the stones to fragment. It may release some of the glue holding them together. One difference, it seems to me, is that if you elect to use the basket, you must remove the T-tube, and then have to do the infusion through a catheter which is put into place. I would like to find an infusion that will work or not work in 48 hours. If that doesn't work, you pull out the tube and try the basket. It seems to me that if we can find a fast, rapid agent, there should be a use for it.

Dr. Sosin: Dr. Hofmann, in your presentation, you very quickly discharged the idea of the use of heparin. Would you care to comment upon any biochemical or physical-chemical properties of that substance that make you feel that it is not efficacious?

Dr. Hofmann: I don't ever like to be skeptical about anything that I haven't worked on with my own hands. Dr. Gardner showed that it changed the zeta potential of cholesterol particles and I accept his electrophoresis experiments. However, there is no reason why it should dissolve cholesterol. Conceivably, it could have an effect on the mucopolysaccharides. To my knowledge, the only people who have looked at in vitro are Dr. Schoenfeld, who has a paper which shows a statistical effect, but an effect of negligible magnitude (*Surgery, Gynecology and Obstetrics,* 138:683, 1974). Dr. Higuchi, a physical chemist, in Michigan, found no effect. A number of people have come up to me at meetings and have told me anecdotally that heparin alone had no effect. I don't understand how it should work. It is my experience that if somebody publishes a favorable report, and somebody does two or three experiments and gets a negative result, they usually don't bother to publish their results. To my knowledge, we haven't had anything confirming Dr. Gardner's report. At the moment, I am skeptical about it, but I don't like to rule it out completely.

Dr. Sosin: Why not use atropine or Valium or some sphincter-relaxing agent along with an infusion of cholic acid?

Dr. Hofmann: As I said, Dr. John Thistle suggested that we use probanthine, and we have done so, but then you have about three variables at once that you want to study.

Dr. Sosin: Dr. White, there are several questions regarding your measurement of common duct pressure. In patients with an abnormal pressure, that is, greater than 16 cm and flow less than 10 ml, do you always open the common duct? How do you know what the pathology is, whether it is a stricture or a spasm related to the operative manipulation at the time? Do you also use drugs as relaxing agents prior to the time that you do your infusion studies? How do you tell the difference between resting and opening pressure?

Dr. White: During our study period on the first 300 patients, which we are now following up at five years, if there was a high pressure and a low flow, and the pressure was not reduced or the flow was not increased by giving nitroglycerin, or amyl nitrite, we opened the common bile duct. In all but one patient we found pathology. Do I use drugs? Yes, I do. We give amyl nitrite or nitroglycerin. How do we measure the opening versus the resting pressure? It is not possible to do it, unless you use the Caroli apparatus to get the opening pressure when you get continuous bubbling. We don't use that apparatus or measure the opening pressure at the present time. We simply measure the residual pressure, that is, the pressure after a flow study and then let the fluid run down in the pipe. Does this increase the morbidity? No, it does not. Does it increase the number of common ducts explored? The answer is both yes and no. We have done something different from what we would have done to begin with. We didn't explore in about 7% of the patients where we would have on the basis of clinical findings. In others, we did explore, where we would not have done so, on the basis of clinical impression and x-rays. The length of time to do these studies and x-rays, using the original Caroli apparatus, averaged out seven minutes, with the anesthetist using a stop watch. It took five minutes for the flow and pressure study plus x-rays.

Dr. Sosin: Dr. Goodale, how do you exclude infectious hepatitis from your series of jaundiced patients? Do you examine for Australia antigen before your retrograde cholangiography? Second, what is the incidence of cholangitis following retrograde study? Has this been a problem?

Dr. Goodale: Usually, these patients are pretty well worked up before we get to the step of recommending retrograde endoscopic cholangiography. If there is a suspicion of infectious hepatitis, Australia antigen studies are done. At the present time, we would not perform the study in the case where there is a positive Australia antigen and the patient has active hepatitis at the time. If the patient does not show evidence of an active hepatitis and there is a suspicion of an extrahepatic block, we go ahead and do the study. Our incidence of cholangitis is 5.2%, two cases out of 38 who were studied. This is a little higher than the reported series of others, which is about 1.5% cholangitis as a result of the endoscopic retrograde cholangiography. I didn't mention, but I should have done so, that when you do find a blocked duct, with dilatation and obvious obstruction, if the patient hasn't been placed on antibiotics, you should do so immediately – either Keflin or gentamicin. A number of them will develop acute cholangitis following the study. Some people have mixed dye with antibiotic, gentamicin placed right into the radiopaque medium and have cut the incidence of acute cholangitis down to approximately 0.2%.

Dr. Zollinger: What do you do if you were so unfortunate as to carry this out on a patient who proved to have hepatitis? What do you do with the instrument? You can't sterilize it. Do you put it in a museum? Do you put it out in the hall? What do you do with it? Can you wait so many months and then the hepatitis will go away?

Dr. Goodale: First, we cleanse our instrument, just mechanically, with betadine solution.

Dr. Sosin: Will betadine kill virus?

Dr. Goodale: It won't kill the virus.

Dr. Zollinger: It will make them hungry.

Dr. Goodale: We have, from time to time, gas-sterilized the instrument.

Dr. Zollinger: Does your insurance company like that idea?

Dr. Goodale: I think that this is the best that we can do at the present time.

Dr. Zollinger: But if you did the study on a hepatitis patient, you would gas it?

Dr. Goodale: We gas-sterilize the instrument after washing it out.

Dr. Zollinger: But you would use the instrument again?

Dr. Goodale: We will use it again. We have to!

Dr. White: This instrument costs $5,000, so after paying that much money for it, you can't just let it lie there. American Cystoscope Makers Institute has been very upset about this. They are afraid that they are going to get sued sometime and they actually did devise a special rapid gassing apparatus, with the idea that perhaps they would no longer be eligible for a lawsuit.

Dr. Sosin: Dr. Goodale, this question regards a comparison between the use of transduodenal retrograde cholangiography versus percutaneous cholangiography. Would you care to comment about the merits of both? Percutaneous cholangiography versus retrograde cannulation?

Dr. Goodale: This is a very important question. I would suggest that if you demonstrate complete block high up in the biliary system, by retrograde cholangiography, you know nothing about the state of the proximal architecture. In this case, depending upon the eagerness of the surgeon, how badly he wants to have the information about the intrahepatic ducts, which sometimes is very critical, I would recommend a transhepatic or a percutaneous cholangiogram.

Dr. White: You wouldn't just push and push and push and push, until you got dye through?

Dr. Goodale: There is no way that you can do that. You are working with small Teflon tubes that just don't have a great deal of pushing ability.

Dr. Sosin: Are any other panel members using percutaneous cholangiography?

Dr. Zollinger: Yes, I use it and like it. I have a colleague in the x-ray department, Dr. Molnar, who has carried this out in many cases.

Dr. White: We use it regularly.

Dr. Sosin: Dr. White, with reference to your presentation, you mentioned the ampulla, and the question is: If the sphincter is so long, and if such a great incision is required, how frequently do you find yourself outside the posterior wall of the duodenum? And, if so, then what do you do?

Dr. White: With a sphincterotomy, you could just make a split, where you were down at the distal end within the duodenum and just stop the bleeders. We always do this, as we expect such an opening to occur in a large proportion of our patients. I oversew the lateral side of the cut first, without going down the medial side. The reason for doing this is that the pancreatic duct is on the medial side. Usually we go right up to the top of the incision, and only after that is done do we take a specimen and then come down on the medial side with the catheter in place. That really makes it a transduodenal choledochoduodenostomy.

Dr. Zollinger: Dr. White, when should I do a sphincteroplasty? I only do one about once every decade. I have an open mind on the subject, as you can tell. You like to do it and you enjoy doing it. I can appreciate that.

Dr. White: Everybody gets brought up differently. I got brought up to do sphincterplasties first and so we didn't have a great many complications. I think that you need to do sphincteroplasties in patients who have had acute pancreatitis in the recent past, where you think that there is a stricture or obstruction at the duodenum. You also should do them in instances, I believe, where there are small stones down at the distal end of the duct, which you cannot get out adequately by other approaches. Most of the patients on whom we are now doing sphincteroplasties are patients who have gallstones, since I have a very large practice in pancreatitis patients. Most of the patients with acute pancreatitis have the pancreatitis, I believe, on the basis of complications of gallstone disease. I think the best approach to treating it is to cut the sphincter. Dr. Zollinger, would you do choledochoduodenostomies or nothing at all?

Dr. Zollinger: I don't know. Sphincterotomies scare me. I might do one once in a while.

Dr. White: Dr. Zollinger, what are you going to do if you have a patient who has recurrent stones and the common bile duct is 12 mm in diameter? Are you just going to take the stones out and let it go at that?

Dr. Zollinger: I expect that I would, yes. I would do a cholangiogram. I might determine the patency of the ampulla of Vater with a catheter, but I wouldn't overstretch it. Yes, I think I would stop at that.

Dr. White: Dr. Zollinger, would you dilate it up?

Dr. Zollinger: No, I would not. It might assure the patency, but I would never rip the sphincter apart.

Dr. White: Dr. Zollinger, what if no contrast went into the duodenum on x-ray?

Dr. Zollinger: Then I would do a Kocher maneuver and put my thumb and finger on the duct, and put a curette down at the bottom and twist it and get the stone out. I'll show you how to do that sometime.

Dr. White: Dr. Zollinger, after you have done that and you haven't gotten a satisfactory cholangiogram?

Dr. Zollinger: I haven't got the stone out?

Dr. White: You have the stone out but no dye goes into the duodenum. Do you accept that as being the whole answer?

Dr. Zollinger: I would push harder on the syringe. I would make dye go through. That's all. I don't think that happens very often. In my experience, it hasn't happened very often, to tell you the truth.

Dr. White: Dr. Zollinger, what if you just keep getting little pieces of cholesterol? As you keep scooping away down there, it is sort of mushy.

Dr. Zollinger: I would stop scooping; I would give it up. I have had enough. I always get it. After the method of Keever, upward and downward, and determine the patency of the ampulla of Vater with small French rubber catheters. But there is no way that I would pass through the big metal dilators, having great respect for the ampulla of Vater.

Dr. White: Dr. Zollinger, I agree with you about the big metal dilators. What are you going to do about that obstructed duct, if you can't relieve it by all this scooping?

Dr. Zollinger: The only thing I can conclude is that the stones are much harder in Washington than they are in Ohio. I think you can get them out most of the time without opening the duodenum.

Dr. White: Dr. Zollinger, let us say that they have had the stones for the third time. What are you going to do then?

Dr. Zollinger: I have never seen it or heard of it before. No, I don't think you see that very often. Maybe you do. But I don't think I see third and fourth times. Do you think that common duct stones keep coming back, lithogenic bile keeps making them?

Dr. White: Do you want to comment, Dr. Hofmann?

Dr. Hofmann: The idea is emerging that whenever a small amount of bile acids go through the liver, which happens in all of us during the night, the liver makes supersaturated bile. Then, during the day, when we have a lot of bile acids going through the liver, the liver makes good bile. This idea really came from McSherry, Glenn and Javitt in New York, but it was then confirmed in Boston by Doctors Small, Dowling and Mack. The idea is emerging that cholecystectomy is a very complicated operation in terms of biliary physiology. It probably means that we have more hours of the day when a lot of bile acids are going through the liver and, therefore, bile is better for more hours of the day. That is one factor. The other factor is that you have lost the storage area. You can't keep your crystals. And even if you nucleate, you probably wash them out. If this is true, it seems to me that there is a very obvious reason why the sphincteroplasty should help people who have recurrent common duct stones. I think that one of the justifications that we sometimes have in our more experimental departments is to rationalize certain surgical procedures. So I hope, now that we can measure serum bile acids by radioimmunoassay, that we can, in fact, get some insight into what the enterohepatic circulation is doing in patients whohave sphincteroplasties. And I think we ought to be able to show that it is a rational operation. I never thought that I would come to your defense, Dr. White, but I am doing so.

Dr. White: Dr. Alan Boyden takes a bead on me every time I talk about sphincteroplasties. He says that it is a terrible operation.

Dr. Sosin: Dr. Schwartz, do you use the sphincteroplasty?

Dr. Schwartz: Yes, we occasionally do sphincteroplasty. Actually, I think we utilize the choledochoduodenostomy more frequently. We use it for the reasons that Dr. White indicated. We will never do a choledochoduodenostomy, however, when the common duct is not significantly dilated. Confronted with the circumstances that Dr. White finally pressed forth on his chess board maneuvers, one, two, and three, that is, an insecurity at the distal duct and a duct which was not markedly distended, we would do a sphincteroplasty. We would not utilize the terms sphincterotomy and sphincteroplasty interchangeably. A sphincterotomy is an inappropriate operation which really accomplishes nothing. Dr. Eiseman showed in early studies that it just grows back and you get the same pressure phenomena that you had before. So you do have to remove a wedge.

Dr. Sosin: This question is for me, but I shall refer it to the panel, assuming that each panel member does cholecystectomies. Would you perform cholecystectomy for an asymptomatic stone discovered at the time of an anterior resection for carcinoma of colon?

Dr. White: I do if it's easy.

Dr. Schwartz: I think you presented a patient who is undergoing elective surgery of carcinoma of the colon, I take it, with a prepared bowel, so that doesn't disturb me, as far as the bacteriology. I am concerned by the postoperative incidence of cholecystitis in a patient with a stone and, therefore, would remove it. I don't know of any reason not to remove it, if it looks like a straightforward procedure.

Dr. Sosin: Anterior resection for carcinoma.

Dr. Zollinger: You would have to make a modest incision, like a filet, to get to both sides. Isn't that what he said?

Dr. Sosin: A big operation has never stopped you, in the past, Dr. Zollinger.

Dr. Zollinger: Yes, I know. Well, I walked out on Dr. Michael Debakey once when he was doing his fourth aneurysm because he was doing the gallbladder operation first. So I would walk out on Dr. Schwartz for the same reason. I don't think that any of us see that much acute cholecystitis complicating cancer surgery. If you were to look it up and did a series of cases, you would probably, Dr. Schwartz, have more difficulty, more complaints than if you left it in. I seriously feel that way about it, although it is very tempting, always, to remove the gallbladder. I would routinely do it with splenectomy. I look around for spare parts on other conditions. But not with a low anterior resection. We are way down in the pelvis and I think that would be about enough.

Dr. Sosin: Is it because the patient has a malignant disease that you resist, or is it simply because of the topography or the location?

Dr. Zollinger: I think topography. I would have to extend the incision pretty high. nless I became a gallbladder ferret and could sneak up underneath the thing to get it out, it would take a much longer incision than I would be willing to make, I think, in most patients.

Dr. Sosin: Dr. Goodale, what would you do?

Dr. Goodale: I am young, I think I would remove the gallbladder.

Dr. Sosin: Dr. White, what would you do?

Dr. White: I think that if I had to really stretch to get up to the gallbladder, I would probably not try.

Dr. Sosin: I think I would take the gallbladder out, too.

There have been several questions regarding a term used earlier today, and apparently the members of the audience do not see much of it, because they want to know what splenosis is, how common it is, and, even if splenosis occurs, is it functional.

Panelist: That is a good question. I think the term is abused. I have never seen functional splenosis. There have been two major reviews on the subject. I was suprised at Dr. Jacob's remark of this being a complication. I have never heard of it and I have not personally seen it. What splenosis means, by definition, is implantation of the spleen onto the peritoneal surface. We see it very commonly in dogs who have been run over and have multiple spleen implants. It is not an uncommon feature in dogs. But in patients, you just don't see it. And the question as to whether it is contributory to symptoms of hypersplenism has never been shown. The symptoms attributable to splenosis are different. The writeups concerning this and the experiences that we have had have been related to intestinal obstruction and adhesions, but not a functioning spleen. I would be interested to hear whether Dr. Zollinger has ever seen functional splenosis. We have looked at our records very closely and have never had a case in our hospital.

Dr. Zollinger: No, we have never seen this. Dr. Curtiss, when he was doing a lot of splenectomies for Dr. Doane, worried about it and produced it in rabbits. But this is the only time I have ever seen or heard of it.

Dr. Sosin: It is a shame that Dr. Jacobs is not here. It is not often that surgeons get to wag the tail of hematologists. I would have liked to have had him answer this question.

Dr. Schwartz, are there increased numbers of platelets after splenectomy for immunologic I.T.P.? And are they of normal or of poor quality?

Dr. Schwartz: I.T.P. is an immunologic disorder by definition. The reason that you do the operation is that the platelets will increase. So the answer to that is yes, the platelets always increase; 88%-90% of the time they will increase after splenectomy for I.T.P. Are they different? There have been studies done concerning the life span, and the answer is yes, their life span has been proven. Is their sticky quality altered? Is adhesiveness changed? The answer is no, it is the same in both circumstances. If platelet aggregation is stimulated, the answer is no, it is the same both before and after. Are we worried about the increased platelet count? Dr. Zollinger capsuled my opinion when he said that the answer generally is no, and even when it reaches levels over 1,000,000 or 1,500,000, we give the patient aspirin or, occasionally, dextran, 1 unit of 500 to 600 ml of dextran without heparin. So the answer is yes, they increase. Do they increase after other diseases? Occasionally they do, and it is not predictable. The ones in whom we see the most extraordinary increases, actually, are the myeloproliferative disorders. Some of these patients are initially thrombocytotic. They have increased platelets which may go up to very high levels. After a traumatic splenectomy, you may have a patient who runs to the 1,500,000 level, but that is somewhat unusual. We do anticipate platelets increasing after all splenectomies for immunologic disease, particularly the I.T.P.s.

Dr. Zollinger: I think myelofibrosis is where we see the very high count. Sometimes we have to worry about it and give aspirin and dipyridamole.

Dr. Sosin: Dr. Zollinger, what do you feel is an indication for the use of, or is there a need for, dipyridamole?

Dr. Zollinger: I just answered that. In myelofibrosis, there are a few unusual indications for a splenectomy and platelet levels go up rapidly.

Dr. Sosin: Is there a place for staging or splenectomy in the patients with non-Hodgkin's lymphoma?

Dr. Schwartz: The answer to that question has to be yes, with a modification of the question, why? The reasons Hodgkins staging came about via the suggestion of Dr. Kaplan, a radiation biologist, was because of the unusual circumstances of the pathologic entity. Hodgkin's disease is a disease which spreads by contiguity. Other sarcomas, such as lymphosarcoma, and reticulum cell sarcoma, do not grow by contiguity. There is an argument on both sides. Some people have seen the Reed Sternberg cell right in the blood, which would argue against contiguity. And the fact that a person can have Hodgkin's disease in the neck and in the abdomen and with no involvement of the mediastinum is against the concept of contiguity, because you can't see how it goes down that duct against the stream. There are a few people, and this is in the early experimental stage, staging lymphosarcomas and reticulum cell sarcomas. The data are not in. The number of alterations in stage is not as great as in Hodgkin's disease, where it approaches 50%. But staging is advantageous because splenectomy in lymphosarcoma patients improve prognosis. Life is extended for a long period of time and the hypersplenism is eliminated early. So the case for "staging" is beginning to rise, but all that we read about in the staging procedures pertains specifically to Hodgkin's disease.

Dr. Sosin: Are you staging for non-Hodgkin's lymphoma in Ohio, Dr. Zollinger?

Dr. Zollinger: Rather rarely, I believe. I think that Dr. Schwartz stated it accurately.

Experiences in Operative Cholangiography

Robert M. Zollinger, M.D.

Primary operations for cholelithiasis rank third among the general surgical procedures carried out in all hospitals, regardless of their size or location [1]. While patients do not seem to fear the risks of these procedures, they often express reservations about the long-term results. The surgeon must therefore not only determine unequivocal indications for operation, but also minimize the incidence and severity of post-operative complications, as well as the necessity for secondary biliary procedures. The consequences of overlooked biliary tract calculi are embarrassing to the surgeon and a source of discouragement to his patient. The implication of this complication is a second major surgical procedure whose mortality and morbidity are apt to exceed those of the original operation. This unhappy situation can best be avoided by the *routine* use of operative cystic duct cholangiography during cholecystectomy. Some experiences with operative cholangiography in more than 3,000 patients undergoing cholecystectomy for benign biliary tract disease will be presented.

The Surgical Service at The Ohio State University Hospitals became interested in operative cholangiography about two decades ago after studying 500 cholangiograms which were reported as showing normal-sized ducts. A filling defect was observed in one case of 11 [2]. Common duct exploration was carried out in 49 of these patients with recovery of calculi in 27. The incidence of unsuspected common duct stones was one case in 20. It might be said that this is a low yield; but if these stones had not been found, it would mean that five patients out of 100 would have continued to have symptoms caused by these retained common duct stones. As a result of these findings, operative cholangiography was

---

Robert M. Zollinger, M.D., Department of Surgery, The Ohio State University College of Medicine, Columbus.

performed with increasing frequency. At first the incidence was only about 5%, but this has increased every five years until between 88% and 95% of all patients undergoing cholecystectomy have an operative cholangiogram [3].

Operative cystic duct cholangiography is ordinarily not performed when there are clear-cut indications for exploration of the common duct. These include the finding of a palpable common duct stone, the presence or past history of jaundice and a dilated or thickened common duct. Patients who have suffered attacks of pancreatitis or cholangitis should invariably have a careful exploration of the common duct. In addition, the presence of a very small stone in a gallbladder which could easily pass through a somewhat enlarged cystic duct suggests a strong need for exploration of the common duct without preliminary cholangiography. Finally, if the gallbladder is free of calculi in a patient with a typical history of colic, exploration of the common duct is mandated. In the face of these indications, the percent recovery rate is as follows:

Palpable stone	88%
Jaundice (Present)	72
(History)	34
Pancreatitis	26
Small Stones/Dilated Ducts	24

If the operative cholangiogram demonstrated a definite stone, the recovery rate was 87%. When it was only "suspicious," calculi were recovered in 38% of the cases.

Many of the aggravations of operative cholangiography have been dealt with in the past 20 years, and this experience may be of benefit to other surgeons. To begin with, it has been a standard practice to elevate the patient's left thorax 15°-20° with a small sandbag or pad. This maneuver rotates the thorax so that the region of the ampulla of Vater is not over the spine and allows a clearer picture. The feet are lowered a little more than the head to take advantage of gravity during the procedure. A preliminary scout film must be made to check the positioning, and when the patient is obese, several check films may be required before the best combination of adjustments is achieved. All radiopaque instruments and pads must be removed from the peritoneal cavity, since their presence in the x-ray is distracting and can prevent the surgeon from evaluating the true status of the complete ductal system.

It has been our practice to immobilize the gallbladder, tie the cystic artery, close the liver bed and leave the gallbladder attached to the cystic duct in preparation for cystic duct cholangiography. Many feel that it saves time to clamp the lower end of the gallbladder and perform the cholangiogram early in the procedure, so that the results are back from the radiologist by the time cholecystectomy has been completed. We prefer to leave the cystic duct attached because of the risk that undue traction on the region of the ampulla of Vater may tear the cystic duct and require clamping of the common bile duct with possible injury to it as well.

A polyethylene catheter (PE-190) is introduced through the cystic duct just into the common duct and secured with a single ligature. It should not be forgotten, as Coller pointed out, that in an area the size of a 50 cent piece at the junction of the cystic and common ducts, there is more normal anatomical variation than anywhere else in the body. On one occasion, the catheter was introduced into what was thought to be the cystic duct only to find that an excellent arteriogram had been taken. The consequences could have been disastrous if the patient had been sensitive to the dye.

The dye used must not be so concentrated that it masks the presence of small stones. A 15%-20% solution of diatrizoate (Hypaque) has been preferred since experiences with several patients in which calculi were not seen during cholangiography, but showed up only on the T-tube cholangiogram done at the end of the procedure. This dilution can be obtained by adding 30 ml of normal saline to 20 ml of a 50% Hypaque solution (Fig. 1). It shouldn't be necessary to duplicate the cholangiogram before the T-tube is removed if the study has been done correctly the first time.

The polyethylene tube is connected to two 50 ml syringes. Saline is irrigated through these until the dye is injected. This will avoid introducing air bubbles into the ductal system which will show up as peculiar and ambiguous shadows. Most surgeons have had the experience of trying to talk themselves into believing that the shadows on the film were air bubbles rather than calculi.

Just before the film is taken, the surgeon must displace the duodenum laterally and the hepatic flexure of the colon downward. This is especially important if the patient has recently had barium contrast studies. Not only barium but air in the colon can obscure the cholangiogram, and it is only when the duodenum and colon are displaced that a clear view of the lower end of the common duct can be achieved.

After the cystic duct is tied and the tube in place, 5 ml of dye at room temperature is injected and an x-ray film is taken immediately. A second film is exposed after injection of an additional 15-20 ml of dye. During this time, the distal bile duct is compressed temporarily by the surgeon's fingers to ensure filling of all the hepatic radicals, the ampulla of Vater and

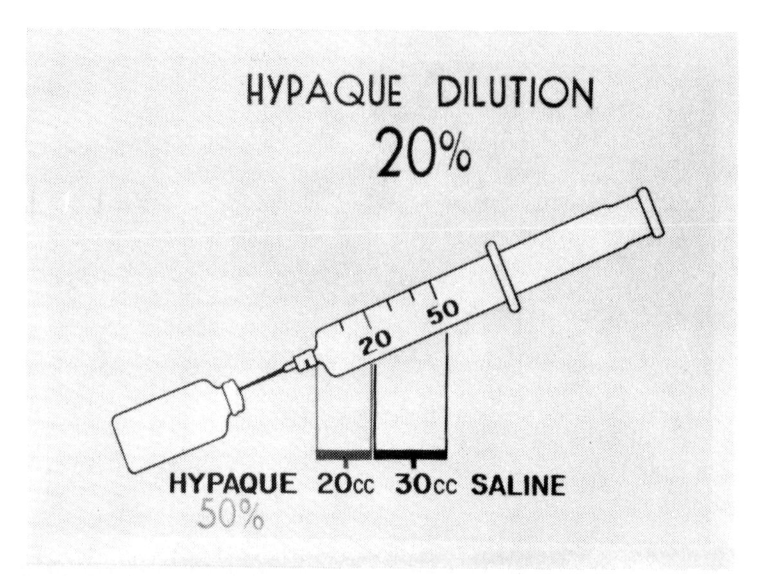

FIG. 1. The dye used in cystic duct operative cholangiography must not be so concentrated that it masks the presence of small stones.

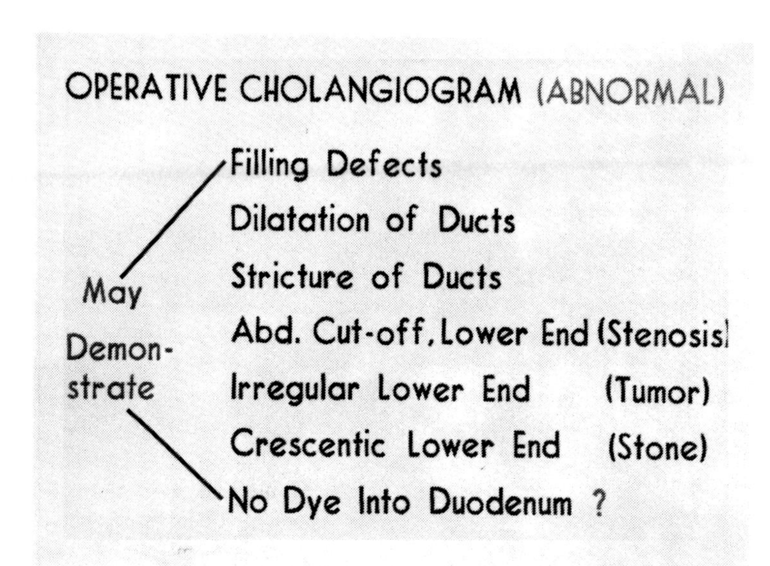

FIG. 2. In the presence of these abnormal findings on cholangiography, calculi have been recovered in as many as 87% of the patients.

the duodenum. After this, the gallbladder bed is closed and the appendix removed, if desired, as the roentgenograms are developed, read by the surgeon and his assistant and then sent to the radiologist for confirmation.

In a normal cholangiogram, there should be no filling defects, and the common duct should not be larger than 12 mm in diameter. The hepatic duct should be well filled and not distended, and dye should enter the duodenum readily. It doesn't matter if the pancreatic duct is filled, although it may well be visualized after the second injection of dye if there is a common channel present.

The abnormal cholangiogram may show filling defects, dilatation or stricture of the ducts and abnormal distention or irregularities at the distal end of the common duct, suggesting stenosis, tumor or stone (Fig. 2). If dye did not enter the duodenum, a repeat film must be made. If a calculus is suspected at the lower end of the common duct, it is well to repeat the injection with some pressure and added dye to see if the shadow can be obliterated.

The responsibility for interpreting the films should be commonly shared by the surgeon and the roentgenologist. There should be general agreement that the examination is negative, since any overlooked pathology will be the surgeon's ultimate responsibility. The challenging presence of small, rounded shadows, which tend to be labeled air bubbles, is an indication for irrigation of the ductal system followed by the addition of Hypaque injections until both the surgeon and the roentgenologist have come to terms, beyond a question of doubt, that the duct is unobstructed and free of all offending shadows.

Wiethoff and Glover [4] have recently suggested a simplification of cholangiography in which stones are milked up in the region of the cystic duct and the ampulla of Vater. After this, they use a needle and syringe to inject 50% Hypaque directly into the lower end of the gallbladder. Good pictures can indeed be obtained; however, we are hesitant to use such a high concentration of dye since the calculi might be quite small. Various types of metal gadgets with bulbous ends have been tried to facilitate introduction into the cystic duct with ligation to hold it in place; but, in general, we have reverted to the plain polyethylene tube and the simple, if exacting, steps discussed here to achieve a satisfactory operative cholangiogram.

The procedure of percutaneous cholangiography has recently been employed with specific reference to recurrent symptoms following repair of a stricture of the common duct. A polyethylene tube is left in place to provide decompression of the ductal system with immediate relief of the distressing symptoms of pruritus, which is commonly associated with

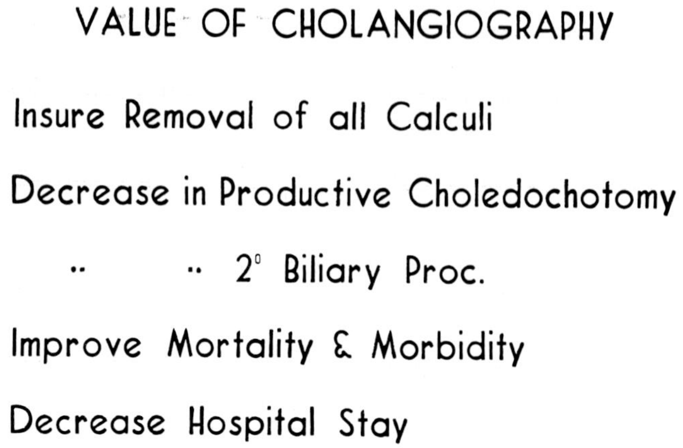

VALUE OF CHOLANGIOGRAPHY

Insure Removal of all Calculi

Decrease in Productive Choledochotomy

" " 2° Biliary Proc.

Improve Mortality & Morbidity

Decrease Hospital Stay

FIG. 3. The routine use of operative cholangiography provides the double benefit of eliminating substantial numbers of unnecessary common duct explorations and assuring that overlooked stones are detected and removed.

obstructive jaundice. This technique permits culture of the bile with sensitivity studies to determine the best type of antibiotic therapy. Furthermore, defects suggestive of multiple calculi have been noted within the dilated bile ducts. A few patients have been observed in whom the tube used in percutaneous cholangiography permitted repeated irrigations of the duct with dissolution of the pseudocalculi. On occasion, the tube has been left in place for months during which time the patient's general condition has markedly improved in preparation for re-exploration.

Summary

The routine use of operative cystic duct cholangiography at Ohio State University has aided in reducing the number of nonproductive choledochotomies from 72% in the early 1950s to 38% at present (Fig. 3). In addition, common duct calculi were discovered in 4% of the patients in whom they were completely unsuspected on clinical grounds during operation. Furthermore, cholangiography is the only way to be certain that all calculi have been removed. Hospital stays have been reduced by three to five days and certainly the long-term end results of biliary surgery have been improved. Cholecystectomy is so common that we must do everything possible to improve our results. The individual surgeon should review his own experience as well as that of the hospital in order to determine whether or not he is offering his patients the most effective and efficient biliary surgery possible.

References

1. Professional Activity Study: Commission on Professional and Hospital Activities. Ann Arbor, Michigan, 1965, vol. 3, p. 9.
2. Zollinger, R. M., Boles, E. T. and Crawford, G. P.: The diagnosis and management of biliary tract disease. New Eng. J. Med., 252:203, 1955.
3. Kakos, G. S., Tompkins, R. K., Turnipseed, W. et al: Operative cholangiography during routine cholecystectomy. A review of 3,012 cases. Arch Surg., 104:484, 1972.
4. Wiethoff, C. A., Wiethoff, R. A. and Glover, J. L.: Operative cholangiography in a rural surgical practice. Arch. Surg. (In press.)

Progress in Radiology of the Biliary Tract

H. Joachim Burhenne, M.D.

Significant advances have occurred in the field of radiology during the past decade, primarily due to the introduction of new special procedures. This is also true for the radiology of the liver and biliary tract. Angiography, transduodenal pancreatocholangiography and nonoperative extraction of biliary tract stones represent major advances in diagnostic techniques. Refinements of cholecystography and cholangiography have also occurred. We have acquired better understanding of the pharmacology of contrast media [1]. The newcomer of ultrasonography has extended into the field of liver and biliary tract roentgenology for the differentiation of cystic and solid masses.

Angiography

The rapid advance in angiography with selective studies of major vessels of the arterial tree supplying liver, bile ducts, gallbladder and duodenum made diagnostic investigation easier. Alfidi [2] and Baum [3] see the main diagnostic indications for hepatic arteriography in the diagnosis of primary and metastatic neoplasms. Cavernous hemangiomas of the liver [4], hydatid cysts [5], abscesses, hepatic trauma, hereditary hemorrhagic cholangiectasia and even necrotizing angiitis associated with drug abuse have been diagnosed [6] (Fig. 1).

Transduodenal Pancreatocholangiography

This new endoscopic technique with peroral cannulation of the papilla of Vater is practiced under fluoroscopic control by gastroenterologists or radiologists. Most experienced investigators are able to cannulate the ampulla in 75%-90% of the cases, although it is easier to obtain pancreatograms than retrograde cholangiograms [7, 8]. Primary indica-

H. Joachim Burhenne, M.D., Clinical Professor, Department of Radiology, University of California School of Medicine; Chairman, Department of Radiology, Children's Hospital and Adult Medical Center, San Francisco, Calif.

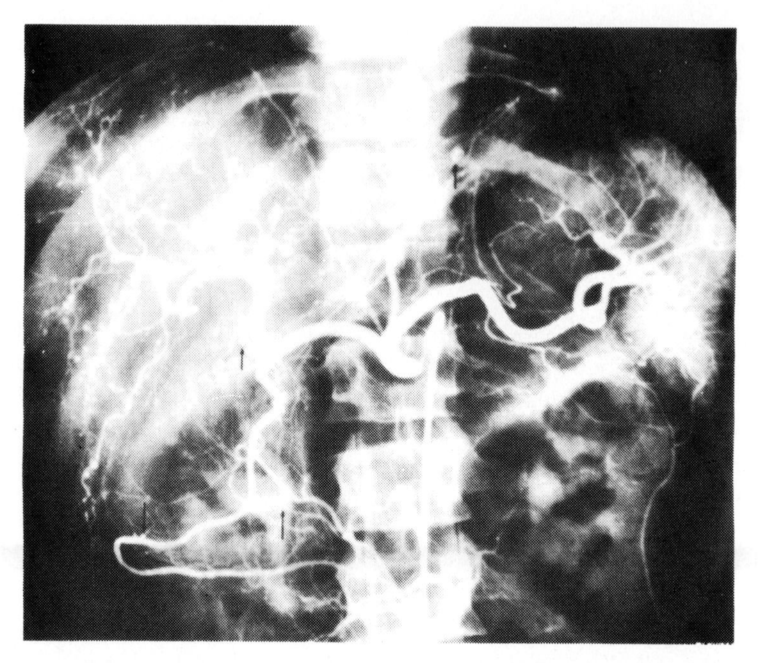

FIG. 1. Celiac arteriogram showing necrotizing angiitis of drug abuse. Many small aneurysms are present throughout the liver. (From Halpern [6].)

tions are in the jaundiced patient when cholecystography and intravenous cholangiography are impossible.

Transhepatic Cholangiography

Percutaneous transhepatic cholangiography is now more commonly practiced for the differential diagnosis of parenchymal and obstructive jaundice. Complications such as puncture of the gallbladder, bile pancreatitis, septic shock and bile blood fistula have been reported. They occur in about 5% of cases [9]. Two deaths have been reported [10].

Even though percutaneous cholangiography will probably be supplanted by transduodenal cannulization and retrograde cholangiography within the next years, the percutaneous approach will remain as the diagnostic method of choice in some common duct problems (Fig. 2), particularly if complete obstruction due to dissection of the common duct in trauma, stone or tumor prevents filling of the proximal duct system.

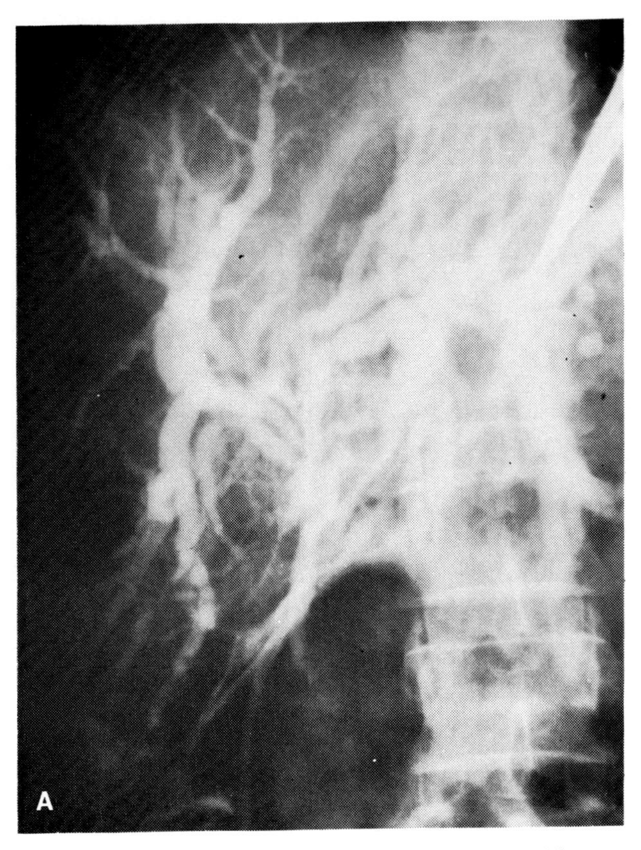

FIG. 2A. Percutaneous transhepatic cholangiography in patient with transection of the extrahepatic bile ducts. Preoperative information was needed as to the length of extrahepatic duct available above the point of dissection.

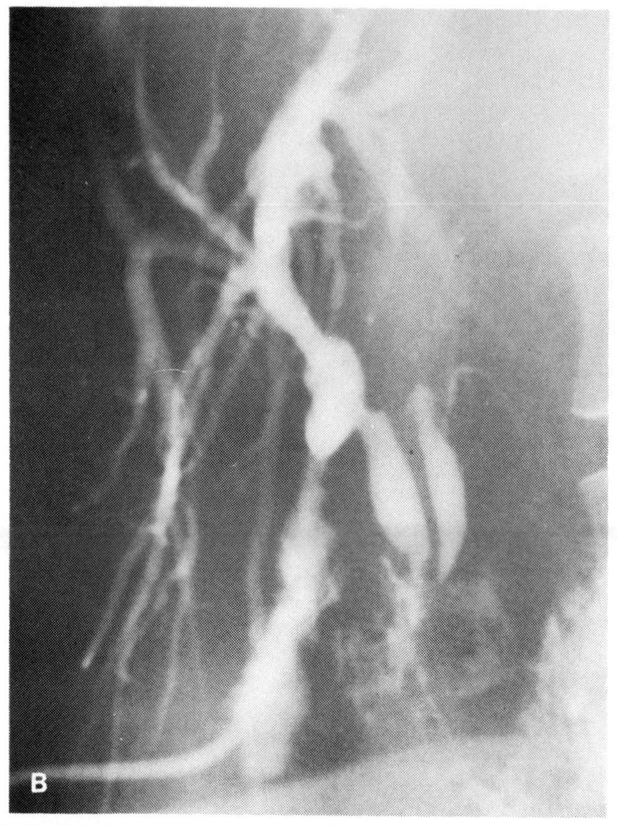

FIG. 2B. Same patient after extrahepatic bile duct anastomosis with T-tube in place.

Operative Cholangiography

The discussion of routine versus selective operative cholangiography continues in the literature, but the more convincing evidence is supplied by authors favoring routine operative cholangiography in patients undergoing cholecystectomy. In the hand of the experienced surgeon, cholangiography adds only five to ten minutes to the time of anesthesia if practiced routinely [11-16]. The number of unnecessary common duct explorations has been decreased significantly [13, 15, 17].

The same authors have stated that operative cholangiography is more accurate than any other criteria for choledochotomy and is more accurate than conventional common duct exploration. Clinically unsuspected stones may only become evident on cholangiography. False negative cholangiography has been reported to be less than 4% [13, 15, 18-20].

The percentage of retained, forgotten or missed stones in the duct system is hard to assess but does amount to at least the same 4% reported for false negative cholangiography. The combination of routine operative cholangiography, clinical judgment and possible addition of choledochoscopy should decrease the number of retained common duct stones.

Good radiographic technique is essential for successful operative cholangiography [17]. In our 115 cases of retained stones from 78 different hospitals, with operative cholangiograms available for review in 109 patients, we have noted as the most common technical mistakes:

1. Preliminary films were not obtained.
2. Poor beam collimation.
3. The distal common duct is overlapping the lumbar spine. The patient was not rotated 10° to the right.
4. Vertical grid lines. In order to permit patient rotation, laterally oriented grids should be used.
5. Inadequate communication between radiologists and surgeons at the time of interpretation. We recommend that roentgenologic readings be written on the cholangiogram before it is returned to the surgical theater (Fig. 3).
6. Reliance on preoperative intravenous cholangiography instead of precholedochotomy routine operative cholangiograms (Fig. 4).
7. Inadequate interpretation of cholangiograms (Fig. 5).

Operative cholangiography is also useful in the identification of variations in biliary duct anatomy (Figs. 6 and 7).

Oral Cholecystography

Accuracy of at least 98% in the diagnosis of gallstones has been repeatedly reported [21-23]. This figure should be applied only to patients with positive oral cholecystograms undergoing surgery. No figures are available for follow-up concerning cholelithiasis in patients with a radiographic interpretation of normal gallbladders.

Staple and McAlister have shown in vitro that 8% of gallstones were obscured by contrast material [24]. Ashmore placed gallstones in canine

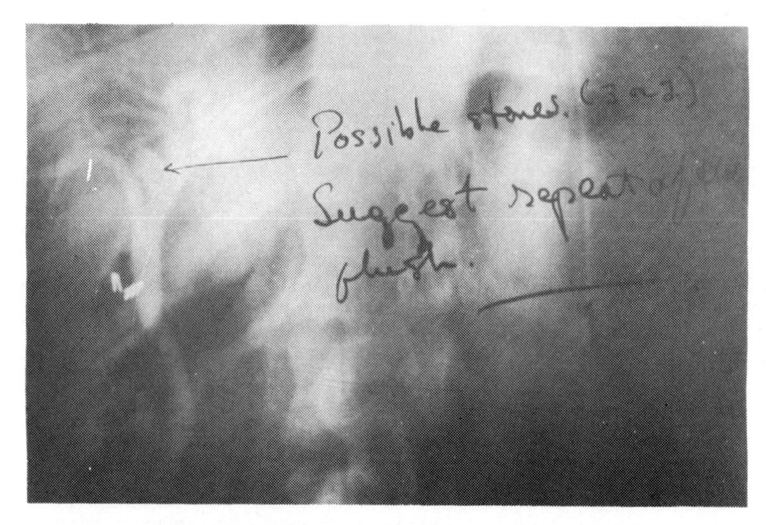

FIG. 3. The immediate reading by the radiologist should be written on the operative cholangiogram films before returned to surgery.

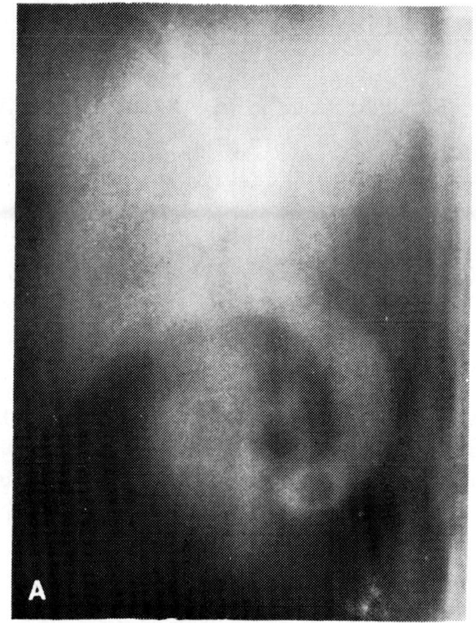

FIG. 4A. Intravenous cholangiography obtained two weeks before common duct exploration shows distal common duct stone.

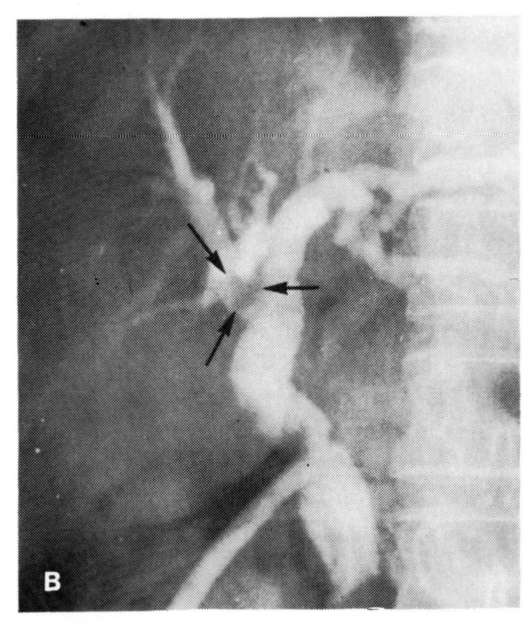

FIG. 4B. No operative cholangiogram was obtained before common duct exploration in the same patient. The stone could not be palpated and was considered to have passed. Postexploration T-tube cholangiogram demonstrates that the stone has moved proximally into the right hepatic radical since the time of intravenous cholangiography.

common ducts [25]. All 6 mm stones were seen by radiologists, but the accuracy decreased for 5 mm stones to 75%, 3 mm stones to 50% and 2 mm stones to 20%.

Furthermore, plain films of the abdomen are not routinely obtained in patients undergoing oral cholecystography. If the latter study is considered negative [26], and if clinical symptoms persist indicating gallstones, plain films should be obtained one week after oral cholecystography. They may indicate the presence of calcified gallstones previously hidden by the same density as the contrast-filled gallbladder.

On the other hand, multiple small gallstones may *disappear* from the gallbladder, passing through the cystic duct and common duct into the duodenum (Fig. 8). Disappearing gallstones have been reported in the absence of fistulas [27]. Gardner et al reported 7 cases and reviewed 15

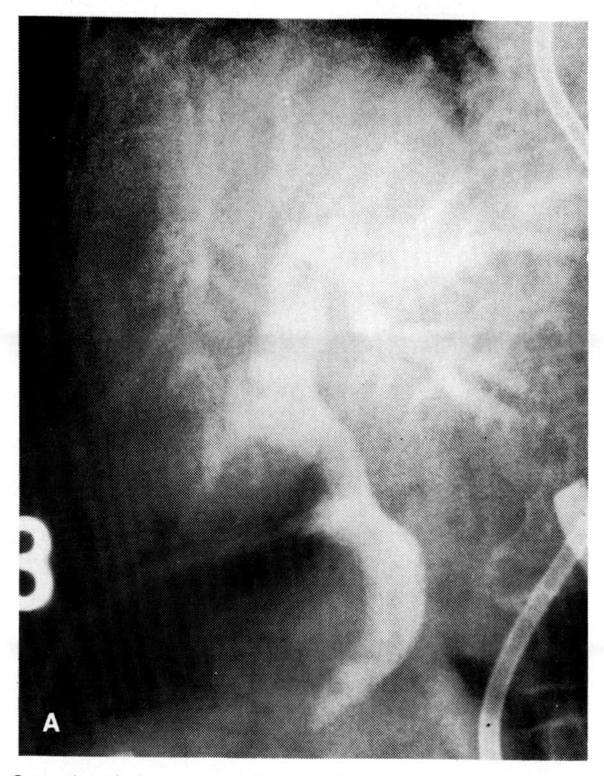

FIG. 5A. Operative cholangiogram after completion of duct exploration was wrongly interpreted as normal. (The absence of contrast passage into the duodenum is probably due to instrumentation of the ampulla. This is commonly seen and requires routine pre-exploratory cholangiograms.)

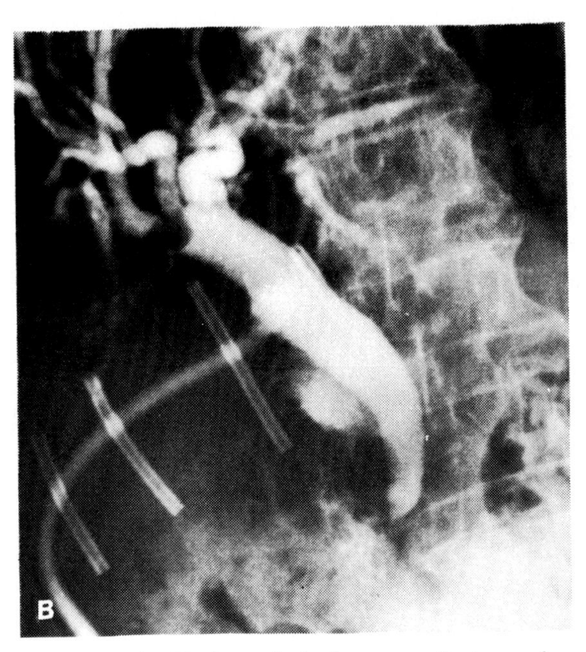

FIG. 5B. The postoperative T-tube study in the same patient now shows a retained stone in the right hepatic radical. Amputation due to stone obstruction of this bile duct was missed on the operative study.

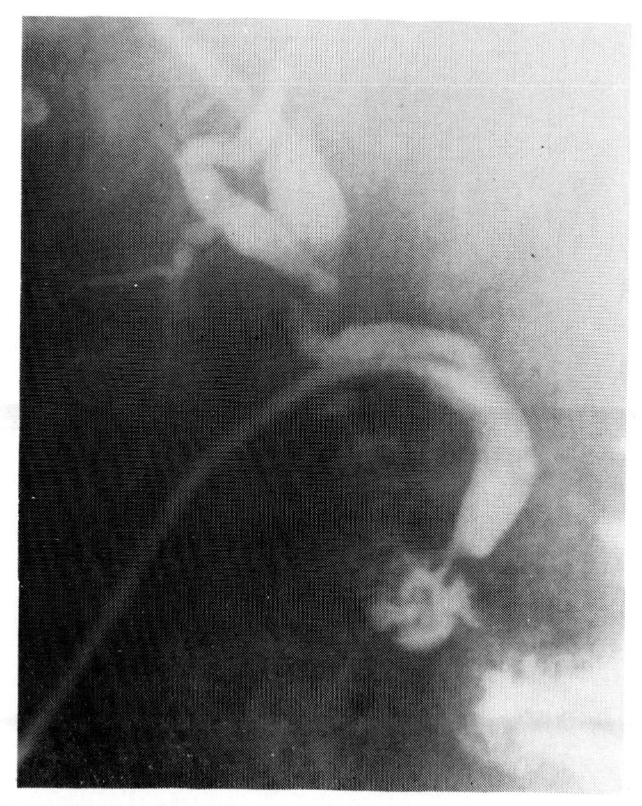

FIG. 6. Variations in bile duct anatomy with medial or low insertion of the cystic duct into the common duct occurs in about 25% of the cases.

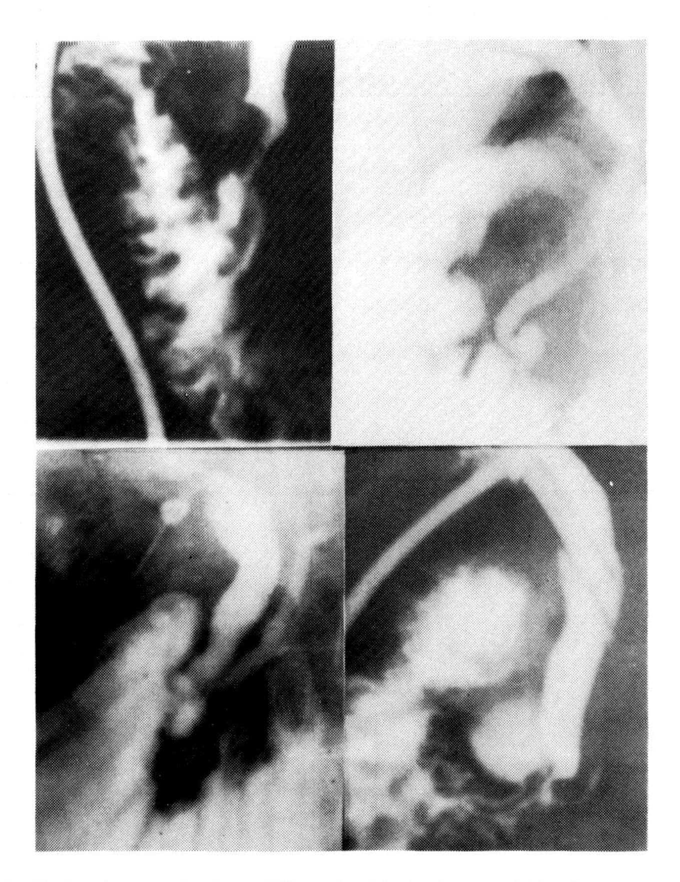

FIG. 7. Cholangiograms in four different patients show variation in anatomy with insertion of the duct into the fundus or the neck of a duodenal diverticulum. This variation of anatomy is also more common than previously thought.

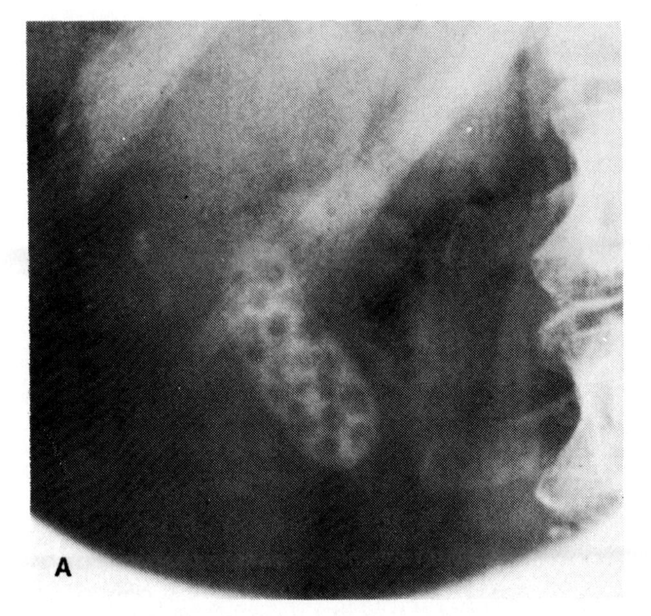

FIG. 8A. Oral cholecystogram demonstrates multiple small gallstones.

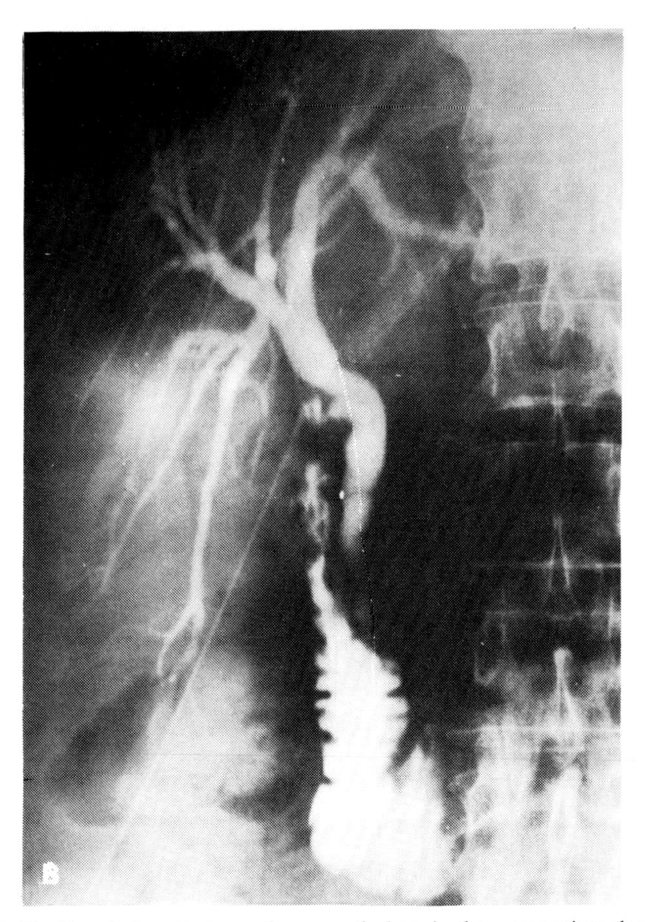

FIG. 8B. Elective cholecystectomy three months later in the same patient showed no evidence of stones in either gallbladder or bile ducts. The stones apparently all passed through the cystic duct and common duct into the duodenum. This entity of "disappearing gallstones" is not uncommon. Repeat oral cholecystogram is required before cholecystectomy.

previously reported cases. Seven of the 22 cases showed some relationship to pregnancies [28]. Calabrese reported 33 patients undergoing cholecystectomy for cholecystitis under the age of 21. All patients were girls and there was a history of previous pregnancy in 84% of the cases [29]. It has been recommended that surgery be postponed for several months when cholesterol stones are found during pregnancy or post partum [30].

Most gallstones are *asymptomatic.* The majority of gallstones discovered at autopsy are asymptomatic. Indeed, common duct stones are often asymptomatic (Fig. 9). We were surprised to find that almost all patients with retained common duct stones tolerate clamping of their T-tube during the five-week waiting period between operation and nonoperative stone extraction. The majority of these patients experience no symptoms. This might explain why surgeons opposing the routine use of T-tubes after choledochotomy do not realize that they also experience the common complication of retained stones in their patient material.

Nonvisualization of the gallbladder continues to be a problem in oral cholecystography. About 25% of patients require a second dose of contrast and re-examination of the gallbladder on the subsequent day. The majority of patients will show normal gallbladder visualization on the

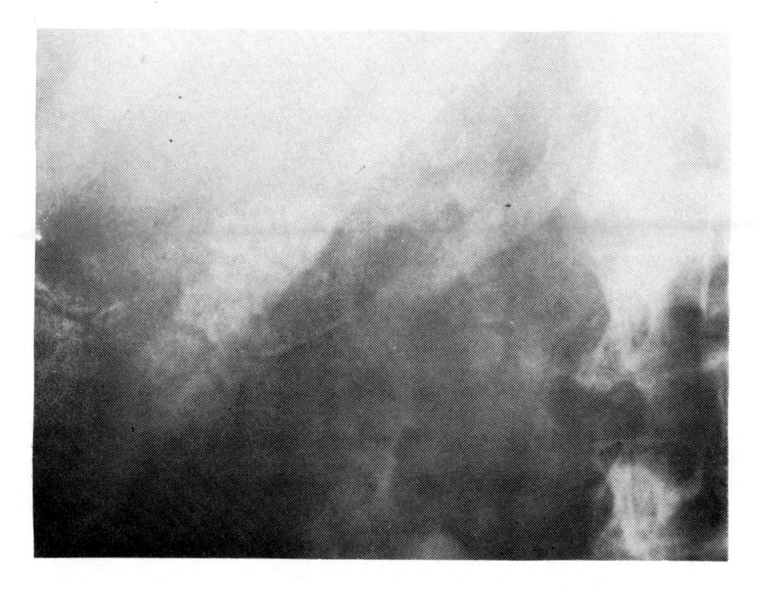

FIG. 9. Multiple stones in gallbladder and common duct were detected coincidentally in patient undergoing other abdominal radiographic examination. There were no past or present symptoms of common duct obstruction.

second day. This two-day examination is time consuming, expensive and confusing to the patient and the referring physician.

We have had excellent experience with a modification of oral cholecystography. The opaque medium is fractionated over a 48-hour period and only one patient visit and one radiographic examination is obtained on the third day. This is easily accomplished as an outpatient procedure, but is not practical for hospitalized patients. During the five-year period 1968 through 1972, 611 patients underwent this new technique of "single-visit oral cholecystography." Nonvisualization occurred only in 20 patients. Follow-up showed that nonvisualization was due to extrinsic or intrinsic causes in all of these patients, except for one patient lost to follow-up. This new approach reduces the expense for oral cholecystography significantly. It also permits a definitive roentgenologic interpretation on the first examination.

Intravenous Cholangiography

Previous uses for intravenous cholangiography included visualization of the common duct for stone evaluation and examination after cholecystectomy. The accuracy of intravenous cholangiography is limited with regard to detection of stones in the gallbladder.

More recently, intravenous cholangiography has proven quite reliable in the diagnosis of acute cholecystitis [31, 32]. The operative findings corresponded in almost all patients to the preoperative diagnosis of acute cholecystitis if the gallbladder failed to visualize four to six hours after intravenous injection of the contrast medium. This is only true in the presence of common duct visualization.

Adverse reactions, however, to intravenous cholangiography are more common than with oral cholecystography or even intravenous urography [33]. Caution is required if intravenous cholangiography is scheduled to follow two-day oral cholecystography. A two- to three-day interval should be scheduled between these two examinations.

The mortality rate reported by Ansell [33] is 1 in 5,000 intravenous cholangiograms for the United Kingdom. Acute renal failure has been described complicating intravenous cholangiography [34] and oral cholecystography [35]. More pharmacologic studies on all contrast media are required to assess possible nephrotoxic effects.

Hypotonic Duodenography

Medication without intubation [36] and with intubation [37] has been used for better radiographic visualization of the contour and mucosa in the duodenal loop. Catheterization of the duodenum using a selective catheter system is advantageous [38].

Although hypotonic duodenography has received prominent attention in recent years for evaluation and detection of small neoplasms in the duodenum and in the region of the papilla of Vater, it appears indicated only in selected cases. A second routine barium examination with aimed spot radiographs of the duodenum and with air contrast technique usually supplies the needed information.

References

1. Berk, R. N., Loeb, P. M., Goldberger, L. E. et al: Oral cholecystography with iopanoic acid. New Eng. J. Med., 290:204, 1974.
2. Alfidi, R. J., Rastogi, H., Buonocore, E. et al: Hepatic arteriography. Radiology, 90:1136, 1968.
3. Baum, S.: Hepatic arteriography. Amer. J. Gastroent., 51:151, 1969.
4. Pantoja, E.: Angiography in liver hemangioma. Amer. J. Roentgen., 104:874, 1968.
5. McLoughlin, M. J. and Hobbs, B. B.: Selective angiography in the diagnosis of hydatid disease of the liver. Canad. Med. Ass. J., 103:147, 1970.
6. Halpern, M.: Arteriography of the alimentary tract. *In* Margulis, A. R. and Burhenne, H. J. (eds.): Alimentary Tract Roentgenology, ed. 2. St. Louis:Mosby Co., 1973.
7. Kasugai, T., Kuno, N., Kobayashi, S. et al: Endoscopic pancreatocholangiography. I. The normal endoscopic pancreatocholangiogram. Gastroenterology, 63:217, 1972.
8. Vennes, J. A.: Peroral retrograde cholangiography and pancreatology. *In* Margulis, A. R. and Burhenne, H. J. (eds.): Alimentary Tract Roentgenology, ed. 2. St. Louis:Mosby Co., 1973.
9. Zinberg, S. S., Berk, J. E. and Plasencia, H.: Percutaneous transhepatic cholangiography: Its use and limitations. Amer. J. Dig. Dis., 10:154, 1965.
10. Drake, C. T. and Beal, J. M.: Percutaneous cholangiography. Arch. Surg., 91:558, 1965.
11. Ferris, D. O. and Sterling, W. A.: Surgery of the biliary tract. Surg. Clin. N. Amer., 47:861, 1967.
12. Kourias, B. and Stucke, K.: Atlas der per- und postoperativen Cholangiographie. Stuttgart:Thieme, 1967.
13. Schulenburg, C. A. R.: Operative cholangiography. London:Butterworth, 1966.
14. Ferguson, H. L. and Sampliner, J. E.: Operative needle cholangiography. Amer. Surg., 35:476, 1969.
15. Allen, K. L.: Routine operative cholangiography. Amer. J. Surg., 118:573, 1969.
16. Griffin, T. F. and Wild, A. A.: The case for peroperative cholangiography. Brit. J. Surg., 54:609, 1967.
17. Jolly, P. C., Baker, J. W., Schmidt, H. M. et al: Operative cholangiography. Ann. Surg., 168:551, 1968.

18. Hermann, R. E. and Hoerr, S. O.: The value of the routine use of operative cholangiography. Surg. Gynec. Obstet., 121:1015, 1965.
19. Edmunds, M. C., Jr., Emmett, J. M. and Clark, W. D.: Ten-year experience with operative cholangiography. Amer. Surgeon, 26:613, 1960.
20. Bardenheier, J. A., Kaminski, D. L., Willman, V. L. et al: Ten-year experience with direct cholangiography. Amer. J. Surg., 118:900, 1969.
21. Alderson, D. A.: The reliability of Telepaque cholecystography. Brit. J. Surg., 47:655, 1960.
22. Ochsner, S. F.: Reliability in diagnosing calculi approaches 98 per cent. Southern Med. J., 63:1, 1970.
23. Baker, H. L. and Hodgson, J. R.: Oral cholecystography: An evaluation of its accuracy. Gastroenterology, 34:1137, 1958.
24. Staple, T. W. and McAlister, W. H.: In vitro and in vivo visualization of biliary calculi. Amer. J. Roentgen., 94:495, 1965.
25. Ashmore, J. D., Kane, J. J., Pettit, H. S. et al: Experimental evaluation of operative cholangiography in relation to calculus size. Surgery, 40:191, 1956.
26. Kolodny, M., Colker, J. L., Callahan, E. W. et al: Falsely negative cholecystography and cholangiography. Amer. J. Dig. Dis., 13:669, 1968.
27. Dworken, H. J.: Recent experiences with spontaneously disappearing gallstones. Gastroenterology, 38:76, 1960.
28. Gardner, A. M. N., Holde, W. S. and Monks, P. J. W.: Disappearing gallstones. Brit. J. Surg., 53:114, 1966.
29. Calabrese, L. and Pearlman, D. M.: Gallbladder disease below the age of 21 years. Surgery, 70:413, 1971.
30. Ochsner, S. F.: Disappearing gallstones. Amer. J. Surg., 99:336, 1960.
31. Brewster, H. O., Beall, A. C., Jr., Noon, G. et al: Intravenous cholangiography in acute cholecystitis, use in differential diagnosis. Arch. Surg., 88:585, 1964.
32. Change, F. C.: Intravenous cholangiography in the diagnosis of acute cholecystitis. Amer. J. Surg., 120:567, 1970.
33. Ansell, G.: Adverse reactions to contrast agents. Scope of problem. Invest. Radiology, 5/6:374, 1970.
34. Craft, I. L. and Swales, J. D.: Renal failure after cholangiography. Brit. Med. J., 2:736, 1967.
35. Harrow, B. R. and Winslow, O. P.: Renal toxicity following oral cholecystography with Oragrafin (ipodate calcium). Radiology, 87:721, 1966.
36. Porcher, P.: La stase duodènale provoquèe, procèdè simple, rapide et fiele d'amèliorer la visibilitè radiologique et les dètails de l'image du bulbe ulcèreux. Arch. Mal. Appar. Dig., 33:24, 1944.
37. Liotta, D.: Pour le diagnostic des tumeurs du pancrèas: la duodènographie hypotonique. Lyon Chir., 50:445, 1955.
38. Wendth, A. J., Jr., Cross, V. F., Moriarty, D. et al: Hypotonic duodenography. Radiology, 108:274, 1973.

The Use of Drains and T Tubes in Biliary Surgery

Marvin L. Gliedman, M.D. and Clarence J. Schein, M.D.

Present day techniques in biliary surgery represent only slight modifications of those already established in the first decade of this century. They have their source in the practices of Robson, Moniyhan in England, Kehr in Germany and Halsted and Mayo in the United States. References and attitudes referable to the specific use of tubes and drains have run and rerun the triangular route from primary closure to external fistulous decompression, to internal biliary enteric anastomosis.

The attitudes presented here are those employed for the past seven years at Montefiore Hospital and Medical Center. We have chosen to consider the problems under five separate headings:

When and How Should the Common Bile Duct Be Drained?

Our experience justifies the concept that the opened common duct should always be closed over a T tube. That tube should be short limbed, guttered, of good rubber and be of the largest bore that the duct will comfortably tolerate. A size 14F is the usual.

The tube can be used as a portal for intra-operative and postoperative cholangiography. The latter procedure, performed in the Department of Diagnostic Radiology, under image intensification, employing cine filming offers the most accurate and permanent record of the postoperative status of the duct.

A further use of the tube is that it offers a portal for the extraction of retained choledochal stones that occur in even the most experienced hands. This is no small advantage.

Marvin L. Gliedman, M.D., Professor and Chairman, Department of Surgery, Albert Einstein College of Medicine (MHMC); Chief of Surgery, Montefiore Hospital and Medical Center and Clarence J. Schein, M.D., Professor of Surgery, Albert Einstein College of Medicine, Montefiore Hospital and Medical Center, Bronx, N.Y.

Intra-operatively, the tube serves as a guide to suturing the choledochostomy site. Inaccurate duct suturing with ectropion or leak can present as a late subhepatic collection that is the source of a subhepatic abscess. The short tube is utilized, the limbs just long enough to prevent extrusion. A short tube is used because there is no advantage to a long one and there is the potential that a long transampullary intubation may provoke pancreatitis.

There is no advantage to retaining the full lumen of the T limb and when the tube is "guttered" (split with a segment removed from the T limb wall) this arrangement provides an additional advantage, perhaps more theoretical than real, of allowing a small calculus that is caught above the upper limb of the T tube to come down through the gutter and to be passed spontaneously. The rubber tube is employed because it promotes a fibroblastic reaction. The silastic tube is avoided just because it does not promote this reaction.

In those instances in which the hepatic artery lies on the anterior surface of the hepatic duct, the tube is positioned away from this area or else the angulated sump T tube is positioned posteriorly. This is done to avoid the disadvantage of having a rubber tube in proximity to the artery with the possibility of damaging the latter. A posteriorly positioned T tube has the further advantage of allowing for dependent drainage of biliary silt or small calculi through a gravity favored opening.

There are instances in which primary closure can be used for the completely normal duct. Our attitude has been, why take the chance? The possible risk is not worth the advantage of the shorter hospital stay. The T tube must be used properly. Where this is not done, it is the faulty use of the instrument which is indictable rather than the disadvantage of the procedure [1]. T tube accidents and malpositions are shown in Figure 1. The tube serves as a guide to the site of cystic duct closure in certain complicated cholecystectomies (Fig. 2).

How Is the T Tube Managed?

If the T tube is to serve its maximum function, it should not be removed until the postoperative cholangiogram is determined to be normal. This examination is done on the fifth to seventh day. After that study, the tube is usually allowed to drain freely for 24 hours. Where this has not been the policy, there has been an occasional instance of postcholangiography chill. This is presumed to be a bacteremia associated with cholangiovenous reflux. When there is no such reaction, the tube is removed from the normal duct 24 hours after the x-ray examination. When the cholangiogram shows spill of contrast material out of the duct

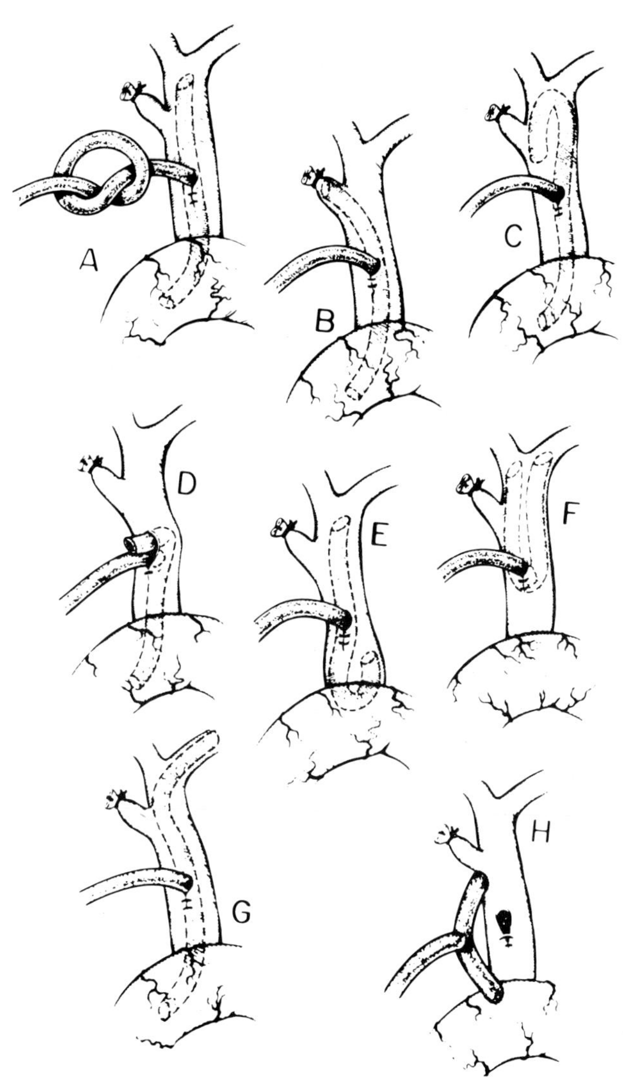

FIG. 1. This depicts some problems that have complicated the use of T tubes. (*A*) The tube has knotted: there will be no bile drainage. (*B*) The proximal limb is in the cystic duct remnant. If this tube is not multifenestrated, there will be no bile flow. (*C*) The proximal limb of the tube is too long and it has buckled. (*D*) When the arm of a T tube herniates out through the choledochostomy incision, it will initiate and maintain a biliary fistula. (*E*) Distal buckling of the T tube. (*F*) A U turn of both limbs of the tube prevents drainage. (*G*) If the proximal limb of the tube is long, it tends to enter the left hepatic duct. (*H*) This is the worst problem because if complete extrusion of the T tube is not recognized, there will be a temporary biliary fistula. If the distal duct is normal, this will close, provided a tube is maintained in the extra choledochal position. (Reproduced from Reference #1, courtesy Charles C Thomas.)

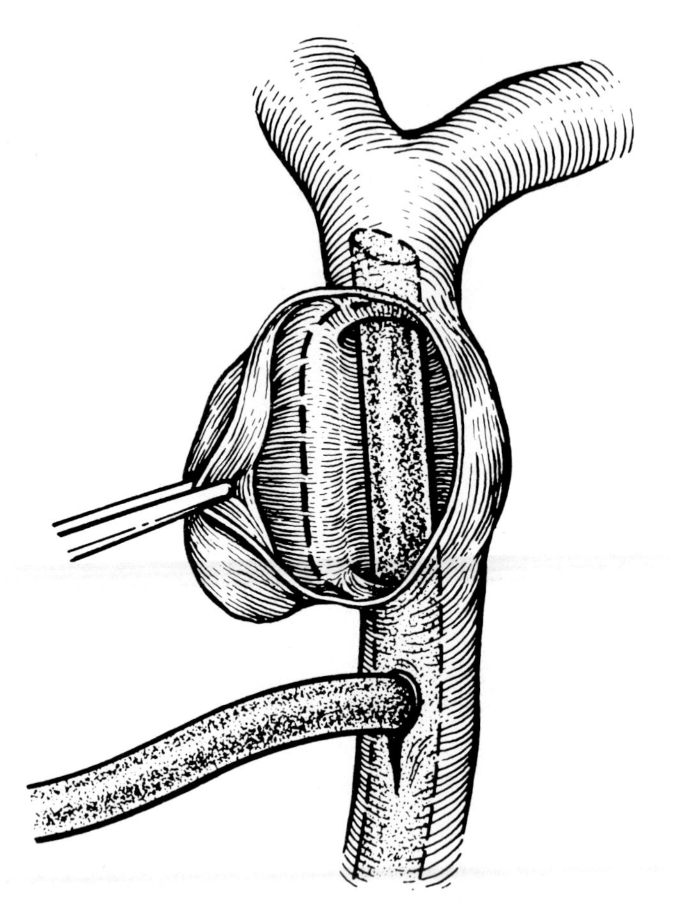

FIG. 2. The T tube offers a guide to the site of amputation of the Mirizzi type gallbladder. The cystic duct has been completely effaced and the gallbladder exists as a wide mouth diverticulum encasing the stone as the shell of an egg.

into the subhepatic space, the fistulous tract is temporarily intubated with a small red rubber catheter down to, but not into, the duct. This acts as a drain for that area.

An alternate policy is pursued if the cholangiogram is abnormal. If a small stone is present – one under 3 mm in size – in a dilated duct – greater than 1.4 mm – we accept Millbourn [2] and Lindskog's [3] data that such stones will probably pass spontaneously. This is especially to be anticipated if the choledochoduodenal passage pressure is normal. In three such instances, the tube has been removed and there were no sequelae.

The T tube can also be utilized as the portal for measuring the postoperative passage pressure. This measurement, under the stable conditions of the eighth postoperative day, gives some idea of the prognosis. An elevated transit pressure at this time is presumed to be associated with an ampullary pathology and potential for a postcholecystectomy syndrome.

Does a Choledochoduodenostomy Require a Stent?

To this primary consideration there is the collateral query of whether there is an advantage to intubating this anastomosis. Our experience is based on an increasingly liberal application of this procedure to the problem of choledocholithiasis. We are now using it as a method of decompression for almost all ducts which are wider than 1.5 cm with multiple stones, for all cases of secondary choledochal exploration and in all cases with primary duct stones. Many of the wide ducts formerly managed with T tubes are now anastomosed side-to-side to the duodenum (Fig. 3). This series now includes 108 cases. There has been one mortality due to advanced liver disease. There have been no anastomatic complications and no leaks.

The first 11 cases were splinted by a T tube exiting at the proximal duct or through the distal duodenum. The reasons for intubation appeared superfluous; there were no leaks and the infected bile could drain duodenally without causing problems. It did not have to be exteriorized (Fig. 4). The anastomosis can be evaluated by a simple barium swallow postoperatively.

When there is no liver bed area to consider (accompanying cholecystectomy), the peritoneal cavity is not drained. There is no more reason for draining this than there is for draining an enteroenterostomy. In general, the concept about the use of drains for this procedure is that when the anastomosis is well made it is not necessary and when it is necessary then such simple drainage will probably not solve the problem. The juxta anastomatic drain may actually favor a fistula. The benignity of these procedures, as far as the constitutional reaction of the patient is concerned, is related to the fact that they are performed in the supracolic compartment of the abdomen. There has been little or no ileus and there have been no subhepatic collections.

Our use of choledochoduodenostomy for stone disease has become so broad and the results so satisfactory that indications for procedures on the sphincter have been limited to delivering the incarcerated stone according to the original concept of McBurney [4].

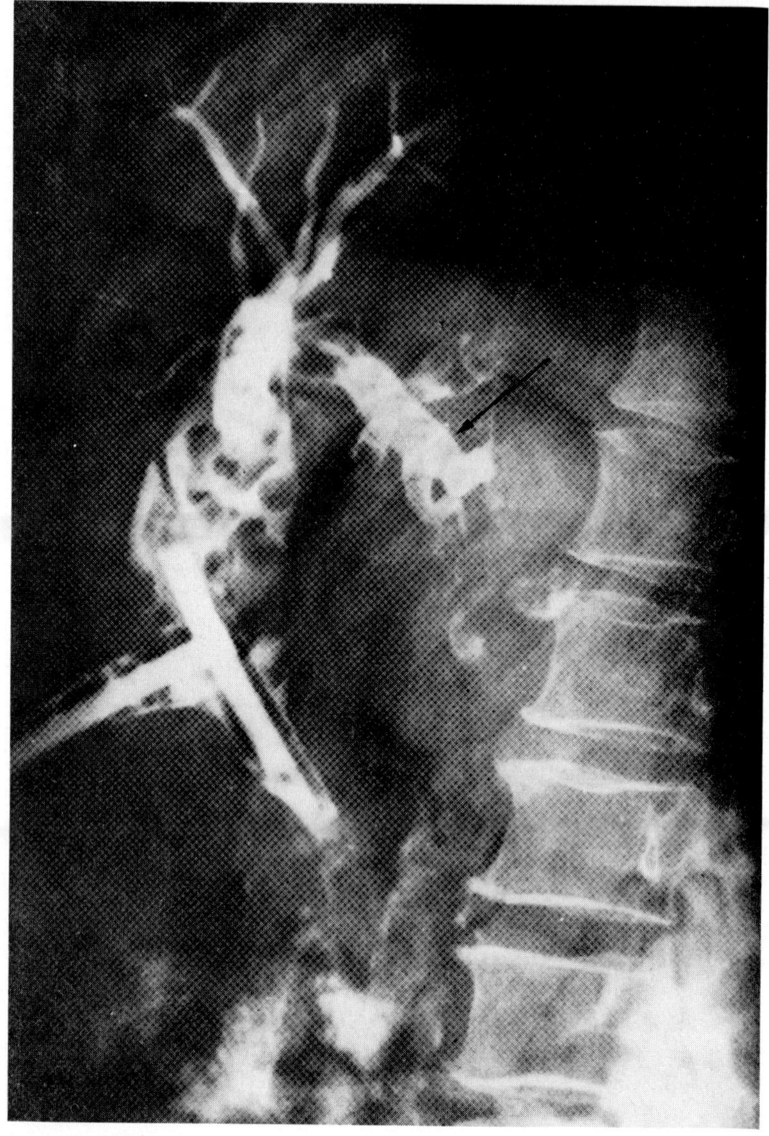

FIG. 3. It should be an abuse of principle to treat this problem by any procedure other than choledochoduodenostomy.

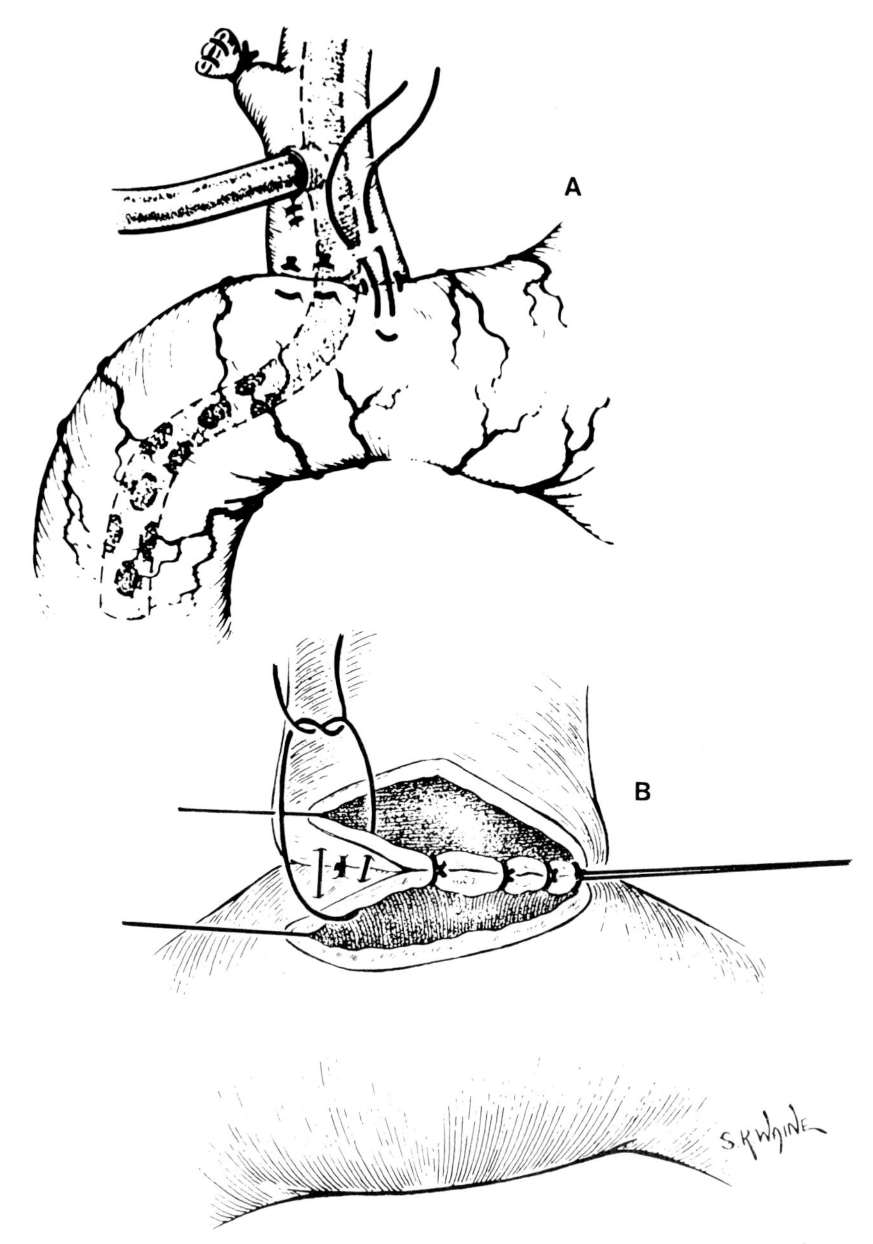

FIG. 4. (*A*) This type of stenting has been abandoned in favor of (*B*) type of anastomosis.

Is Drainage Required or Indicated After Routine Cholecystectomy?

The purpose of drainage in this instance is to provide an exit for the subhepatic collection of blood, bile and lymph that can accumulate in the subhepatic space. These fluids are the media in which a subhepatic abscess can be nurtured. The bacteria have their source in the infected bile. Technical factors, as well as the pathologic state of the organs, determine the likelihood of such a sequence of events. A postoperative febrile response is an indication of the presence of a cellulitis in the area.

Essentially all cholecystectomies are drained at our institution. The drains are generally soft rubber, Penrose type, and are exteriorized through a stab wound brought out laterally. In general, twisting the drain on the first postoperative day and then removing it within three more days when drainage is minimal (the normal circumstance) has been satisfactory.

The drain is often unnecessary. However, it is probably the safest procedure. There have been little regrets from its use. There has been a rare drain site hernia and the occasional fever associated with drain manipulation. On rare occasion, manipulation of the drain can fracture intraperitoneal synechia, with the release of small amounts of loculated bile. This produces a virulent peritoneal reaction manifested as diffuse or right sided rigidity, fever and leucocytosis that simulate a perforated viscus. The reaction usually subsides in 12 hours.

The Use of Tube Splints in the Surgery of Hepatic Duct Cancers

There are 18 cases in this category in which the tumors began north of the cystic duct junction and extended into the carina. Seventeen of these attempted palliations utilized intubation through the tumor and one had a left sided Longmire type hepaticojejunostomy. In the former cases, the tumor was bored through and intubated by a long catheter inserted proximally through the tumor through the liver and out the skin of the right upper quadrant. The distal end was introduced through the common bile duct into the duodenum via the ampulla of Vater or into a loop of adjacent bowel. Four of these patients survived over two years and required reinsertion of the tube, a procedure which could be done through the already established fistulous tract.

The Longmire procedure worked well in one patient because we could demonstrate a communication between the right and left duct systems. One cannot rely on such a communication between the ducts because in the majority of instances each lobar unit drains separately. However, in the presence of obstruction it would appear that some of the dilated radicles on the obstructed side communicate with the normal system or with the subsequently dilated radicles in the other lobe. While there has been a survival in terms of years, these patients have not been free from bouts of cholangitis and pruritis even with the tube in and functioning.

In those instances, where a resection of the carina was performed for a carcinomatous obstruction, a multifenestrated transhepatic tube was placed across the anastomatic line well down into the jejunum. The stents remained in position, but it is truly not possible to evaluate their role in maintaining clinical patency. In at least one patient the silastic stents fell out and the patient has remained with normal liver function for six months.

References

1. Schein, C. J., Stern, W. Z. and Jacobson, H. G.: The Common Bile Duct. Operative Cholangiography, Biliary Endoscopy and Choledocholithotomy. Springfield, Ill.:Charles C Thomas, 1966.
2. Millbourn, E.: Klinische Studien uber die Choledocholithiasis. Acta Chir. Scand., 86 (suppl. 45), 1948.
3. Lindskog, B.: Evaluation of Operative Cholangiography in Gall Stone Surgery with Special Reference to Residual Stones. Lund, 1970.
4. McBurney, C.: Removal of biliary calculi from the common duct by the duodenal route. Ann. Surg., 28:481, 1898.

Surgical Implications of Cholangitis

Frank G. Moody, M.D.

Bacterial cholangitis is a common problem in patients with advanced biliary tract disease. Upper abdominal pain, chills and fever, the hallmarks of the disease, present a clinical syndrome so distinct that the diagnosis can usually be made over the telephone. While such patients are first seen by their primary physician, they eventually filter into the surgeon because bacterial cholangitis is a consequence of biliary lithiasis, or benign strictures, resulting from operative injury to the bile ducts during cholecystectomy. Occasionally, patients with acute cholecystitis present with apparent cholangitis, but the mechanism of liver dysfunction in this circumstance appears to be related to lymphangitis; the bile is usually sterile in these patients. Stones in the common duct, for some reason, allow the biliary tree to become contaminated with enteric organisms which either ascend through the papilla of Vater or arrive by the portal route. These stones should be removed when identified. As has been pointed out, this can be accomplished by dissolution, ensnarement under radiologic control or by surgical means. In addition, the biliary tree must drain freely. Bile that has free egress from the bile ducts is bacteriostatic. You can inoculate such a biliary tree and it will clear itself of all bacteria within a period of several hours. Obstruction to the flow of bile, however, will lead to proliferation of bacteria and their eventual movement into the bloodstream.

I do not plan to discuss further cholangitis associated with stones in the lower bile ducts, since problems of this nature can be easily managed. I plan to focus on problems that occur at or above the bifurcation of the bile ducts. Cholangiography is a very important tool in terms of managing these patients. Figure 1 is a retrograde cholangiogram, a supercholangiogram, if you will, since it shows how much of the biliary tree we really don't see with our usual cholangiography. This is a cadaver cholangiogram [1]. I show this to emphasize that in doing cholangiography in

Frank G. Moody, M.D., Professor and Chairman, Department of Surgery, University of Utah School of Medicine, Salt Lake City.

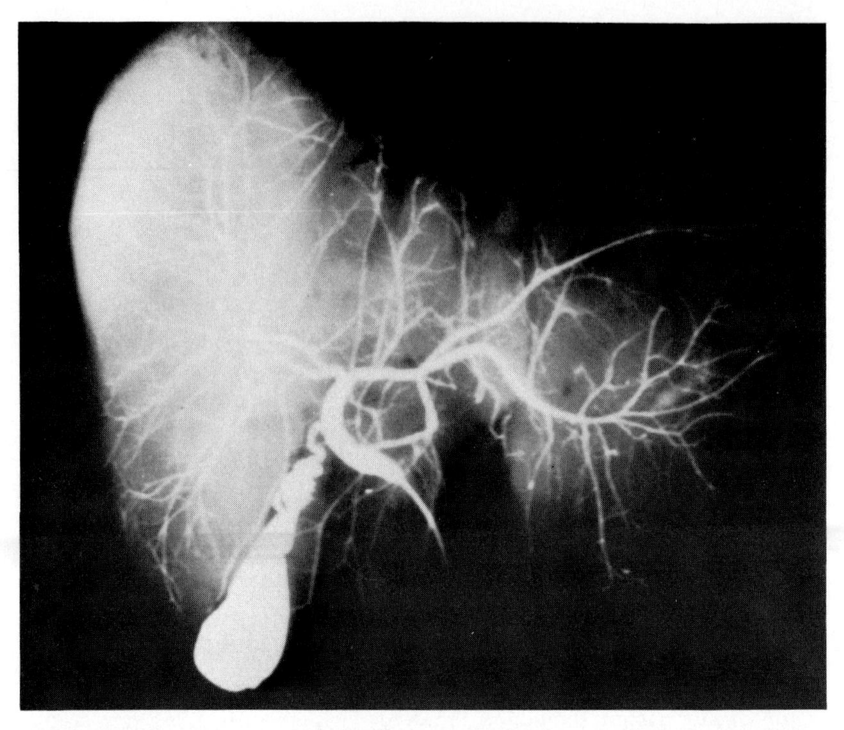

FIG. 1. This postmortem cholangiogram reveals the extensive nature of the intrahepatic biliary tree. Visualization of this extent in life may lead to cholangitis or pancreatitis. (From Moody et al [1].)

patients who have contaminated bile, one must be very careful not to introduce the material under pressure. Yet, it is essential that the proximal biliary tree be well visualized. In addition, with patients who have had recurrent episodes of cholangitis, it is most important that they be covered by broad-spectrum antibiotics prior to examination of the biliary tree.

An explanation for the episodes of cholangitis which accompany manipulation of the biliary tree may reside in the fact that bacteria in bile are very close to the bloodstream. Any increase in intralumenal pressure will allow these organisms free egress into the bloodstream. This has been demonstrated many times both clinically and in the laboratory. Figure 2 is a cholangiogram of a 53-year-old male with Caroli's disease; ectasia of the intrahepatic biliary tree. He presented with a history of several years of recurrent episodes of cholangitis. His cholangitis would occur every month, always responding to ampicillin. But with time, he began to lose weight and the frequency of the cholangitic attacks forced him to quit his

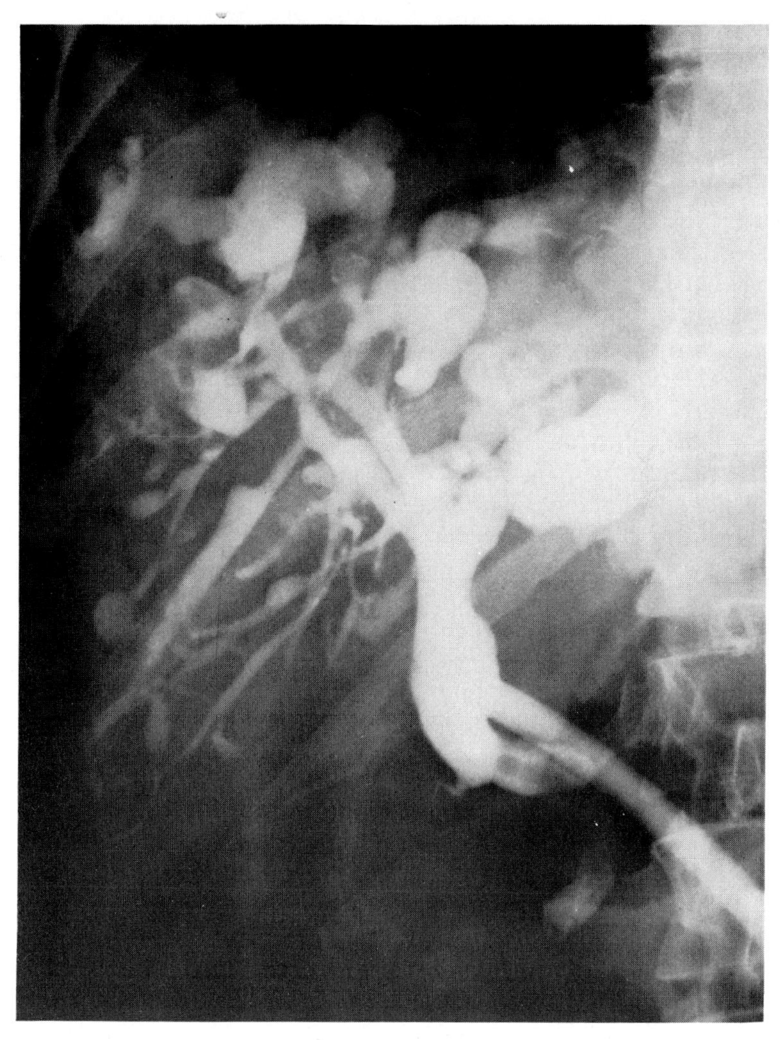

FIG. 2. Postoperative cholangiogram of a patient with Caroli's disease. Note the intrahepatic sacculation with radiolucent areas which presumably represent intrahepatic stones.

job. Numerous stones were removed from his biliary tree with only moderate relief of cholangitis. Klebsiella and pseudomonas were grown from both bile and bloodstream. As can be seen, his intrahepatic biliary tree has numerous little sacs, some of which have obvious stones in them. We have managed this patient by leaving a T-tube in place. As the stones come down into the bile duct, a radiologist removes them by a Dormier basket. We haven't come up with a better way of approaching his problem. We have tried all types of flushes including secretin and bile salts. We have also tried chenodeoxycholic acid by the oral route without success. It is curious that all of the organisms that we have been able to recover from either duodenal aspirate or from his bloodstream have been resistant to ampicillin, the drug which controlled his episodes of cholangitis for at least a year. It is very important to establish bacteriology in these patients. If one cannot do so by duodenal aspirate or retrograde aspiration of the bile duct, then one should take a needle liver biopsy. In fact, the parenchyma of the liver often will harbor organisms that are not recoverable from bile.

I still prefer to use ampicillin for the garden variety cholangitis patient, because it is a relatively safe agent and readily gains access to bile. It is excreted across the blood-bile barrier in high concentrations. Unfortunately, *E. coli,* which is the most common organism recovered from the bile, happens to be resistant to ampicillin in 50% of cases in our hospital. Patients who present with frank cholangitis and sepsis are best treated with the combination of gentamycin and clindamycin. The gentamycin covers almost all the organisms which reside in the obstructed biliary tree. Chloromycetin is also an excellent choice, since it has a broad spectrum and permeates freely into the hepatic parenchyma. We tend to use it as a drug for chronic suppression of patients who, for one reason or another, cannot be relieved of their intrahepatic source of sepsis. I, personally, like to gain bacterial control of patients with advanced biliary tract disease prior to retrograde cholangiography or operation. Sometimes it takes several days, but with the availability of numerous drugs, and the ability to establish specific antibiotic sensitivity, we are usually successful. However, there is still an occasional case that will not respond to antibiotics and early operation is required [2].

Figure 3 represents the clinical course of a patient with so-called suppurative cholangitis. This occurs when the biliary tree, or a segment of the biliary tree, is totally obstructed. Pus, then, accumulates under pressure within the biliary tree. The patient complains of severe right upper abdominal pain, chills and fever; progressive jaundice ensues. Figure 4 is a cholangiographic representation of this patient's bile ducts [3]. This type of biliary tree is one that is very difficult to keep clear of stones.

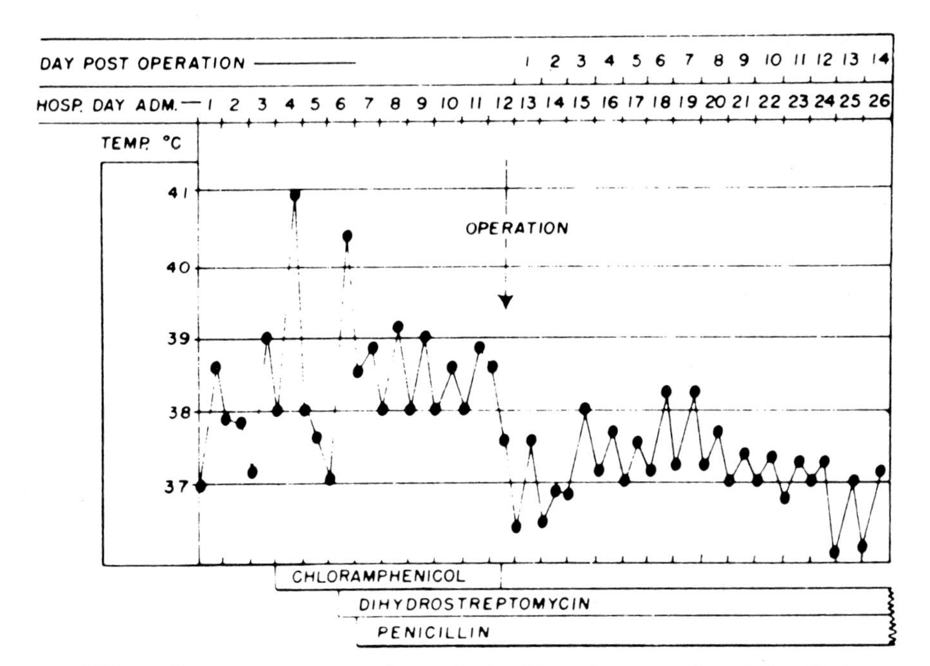

FIG. 3. Temperature course of a patient with acute suppurative cholangitis in association with common duct obstruction secondary to stone. The septic course was not interrupted by chemotherapy. Dramatic response to T-tube decompression of common duct and choledocholithotomy on 12th hospital day is shown. (From Glenn and Moody [2].)

There is controversy as to whether some type of procedure should not be done to improve drainage of this dilated, thick-walled duct where bile obviously pools. In addition, this patient happens to have an anomaly which is not too uncommon, that is, a duct that drains the right lobe of the liver into the cystic duct. If this patient, two years previously, had had a drainage procedure done, she may have been spared the episode of suppurative cholangitis depicted here. What I recommend in this type of situation is to divide the duct and to do an end-to-end choledocho-jejunostomy.

Patients with bile duct injuries and inadequate repairs are prone to develop cholangitis. This is exemplified by a patient who, at the time of cholecystectomy, had a suture placed through his common hepatic duct. The patient was reoperated upon at two weeks, the suture was removed and a T-tube was placed through the area of injury. The T-tube was removed at two weeks; it should have been left in place for at least three months, and possibly longer, to see the fate of the duct in that area.

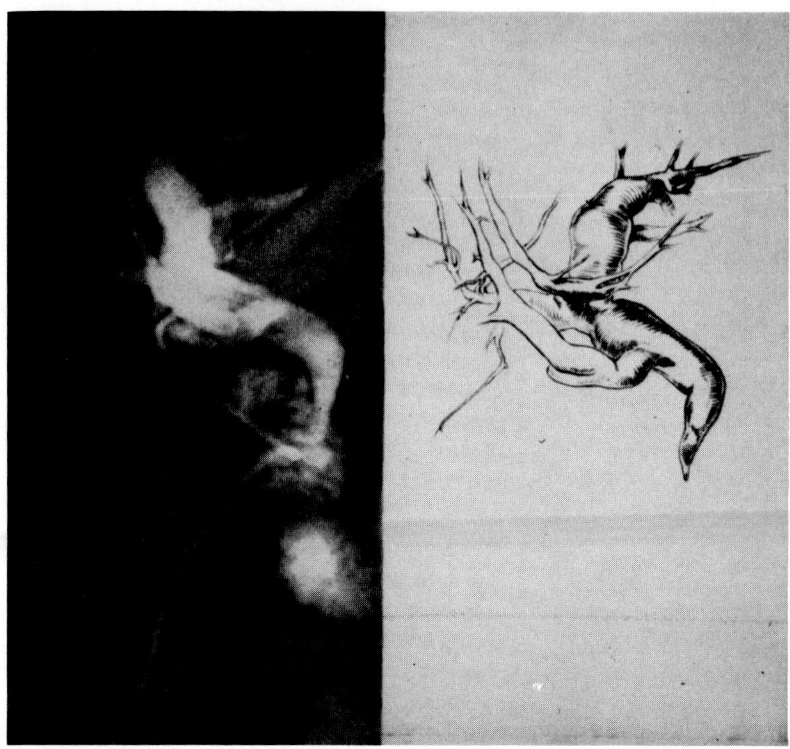

FIG. 4. A delayed postoperative cholangiogram and line drawing revealing enlargement of the left hepatic and common ducts together with an anomalous hepatic duct from the right lobe entering a cystic duct remnant. Calculi had previously been removed from the left intrahepatic common and cystic duct remnant. (From Glenn and Moody [3].)

Possibly, the patient should have had a resection of the area or a primary hepaticojejunostomy; I think that that is debatable. But certainly the tube should have been left in place for a longer period of time.

Figure 5 represents what can happen following even a minor intervention in patients who have bacteria in their biliary tree. As can be seen, the patient's temperature rose to 104°F. He became very shaky with chills and profound jaundice with his bilirubin rising to 20 mg%. The liver enzymes and bilirubin don't necessarily have to change in patients who have cholangitis. I believe that this is a function of the level of obstruction. We have observed several patients who had very little change in liver chemistries during rather severe episodes of cholangitis and sepsis. This individual, I believe, bled into his biliary tree and developed a small clot at

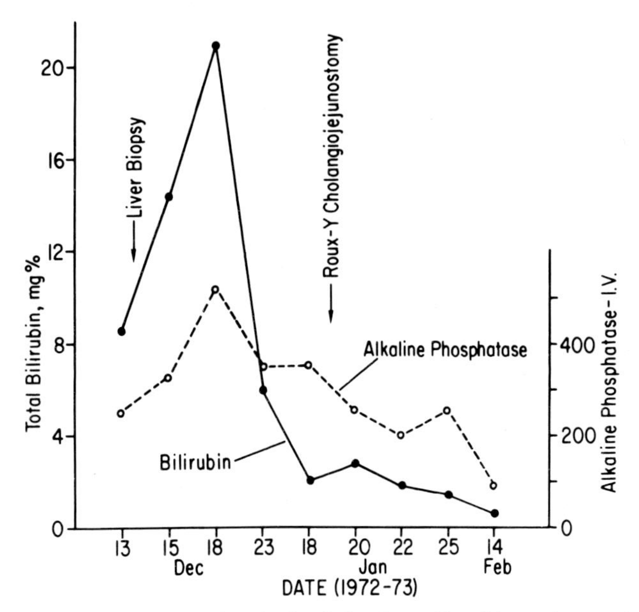

FIG. 5. Time course of liver chemistries following a liver biopsy in a patient with posttraumatic bile duct stricture and hepaticoduodenal fistula. Percutaneous cholangiogram was obtained at zenith of hyperbilirubinemia (Fig. 6).

the point where the bile ducts emptied into the duodenum, since a defect was found on a subsequent cholangiographic study (Fig. 6). He appeared otherwise to have a very adequate communication between the bifurcation of his bile ducts and the duodenum. He had prolonged, symptom-free periods, in which he was afebrile and liver chemistries were close to normal. These patients, however, will invariably go on to develop progressive episodes of sepsis and rather profound but subtle injury to the liver, culminating in biliary cirrhosis. For this reason, I believe that all of these patients deserve to have some type of surgically created biliary enteric anastomosis. A Roux-en-Y hepaticojejunostomy was performed in this case.

Sclerosing cholangitis may be associated with bacterial cholangitis. Figure 7 reveals by operative cholangiography the bile duct of a patient with such a problem. It demonstrates complete obstruction to the lower end of the common bile duct. To overcome the problem of biliary drainage internally, we did an anastomosis between the gallbladder and a Roux Y limb of jejunum. His intrahepatic biliary tree is also involved as

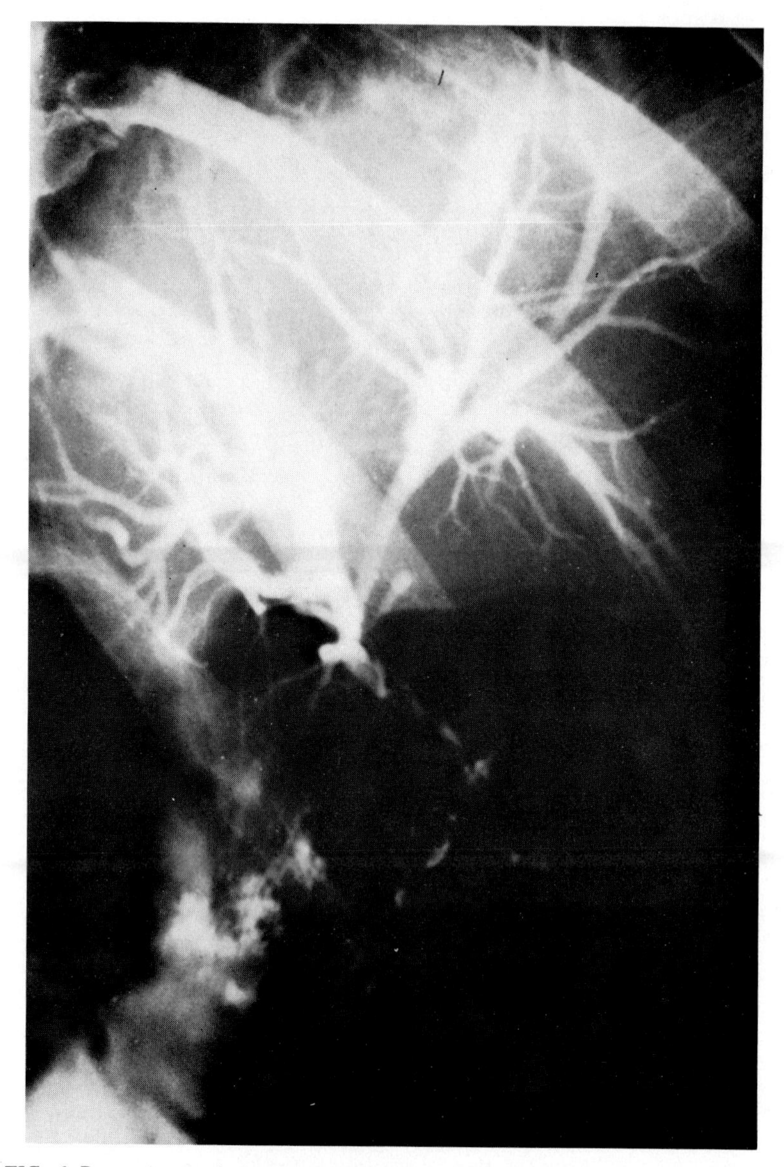

FIG. 6. Percutaneous cholangiogram demonstrating a biliary enteric fistula between the bifurcation of the primary radicals and duodenum. Radiolucency in the region of the communication may represent a blood clot.

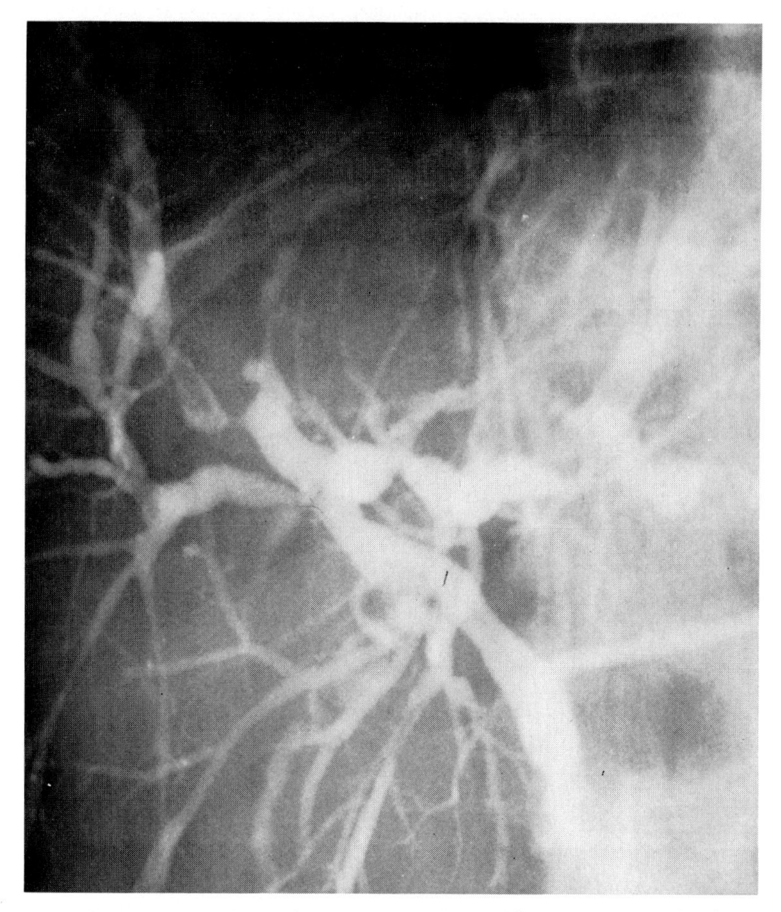

FIG. 7. Postoperative cholangiogram in a patient with suppurative and sclerosing cholangitis. Note the areas of dilatation and narrowing within the intrahepatic biliary tree.

you can see. The disease extensively involves all of the biliary radicals. His tube remained patent for a period of about two months. I find that these patients really don't like to have tubes in place and keep asking you to remove them. So, since this one wasn't working, we took it out. He went on for eight months relatively symptom-free on chloromycetin as a chronic suppressive antibiotic. He then returned with frank sepsis, not controlled by antibiotics. At reexploration we found an area of complete stricture in the lateral segment of the left lobe. This segment was removed with relief of symptoms.

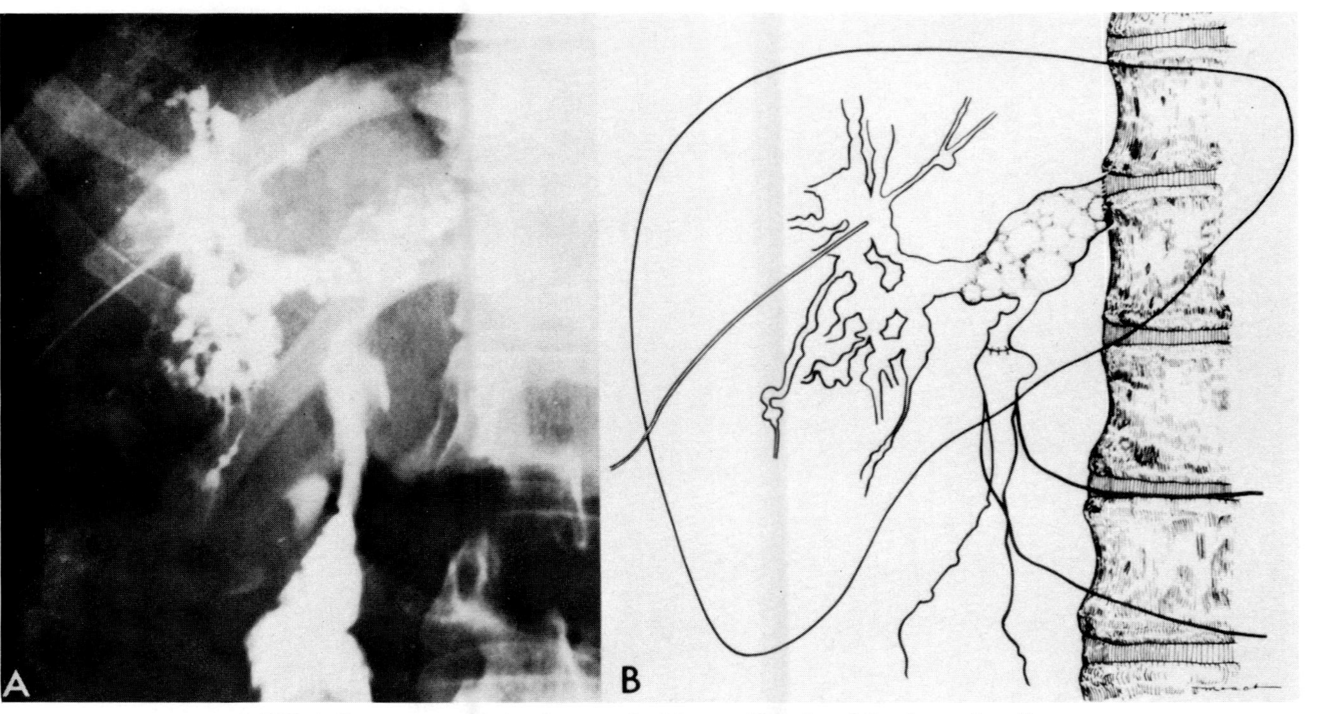

FIG. 8. Percutaneous cholangiogram of a 24-year-old patient following an hepatico-duodenostomy for atresia of the extrahepatic biliary tree. Soft concretions have filled areas of saccular dilatation in the left hepatic ductal system, contributing to cholestasis and cholangitis. (From Berensen et al, *Gastroenterology*, 66:262, 1974.)

Some people get along very well with a rather make-shift anastomosis. We recently cared for a patient with extrahepatic biliary atresia, who at age 2 months had an anastomosis between the duodenum and the apparent bifurcation of the bile ducts. The surgeon cored out a little hole in the liver, placed the duodenum up to that area and told the parents that the child had no chance of survival. Well, she did live. She is now 24 years old, a lovely lady with a family. But she still continues to have episodes of cholangitis.

Figure 8 is a cholangiographic representation of her biliary tree. As you can see, it is very similar to Caroli's disease. She has saccular dilatations. The saccular dilatations in the left lobe are filled, not with calculi, but with black sticky crankcase oil. We have operated on her twice, now, to scoop out these areas and reestablish bile flow. In addition, we have modified the anastomosis in order to provide an extra wide opening into the intestinal tract. I am not prepared to discuss the role that the duodenum in continuity may be contributing to her problem. I believe that she actually has done quite well with this arrangement. The important consideration is to ensure free flow of bile.

In summary, the management of chronic sepsis from the liver requires the establishment of free bile egress from liver to intestinal tract. Foreign bodies such as stones or rubber tubes should be removed as early as feasible. Potent, specific antibiotics such as gentamycin or chloromycetin should be employed prior to manipulation or operation upon the obstructed and infected biliary tree.

References

1. Moody, F. G., Asch, T. and Glenn, F.: Intrahepatic cholangiography. Arch. Surg., 87:475, 1963.
2. Glenn, F. and Moody, F. G.: Acute obstructive suppurative cholangitis. Surg. Gynec. Obstet., 113:265, 1961.
3. Glenn, F. and Moody, F. G.: Intrahepatic calculi. Ann. Surg., 153:711, 1961.

Primary Sclerosing Cholangitis

M. Michael Eisenberg, M.D.

Sclerosing cholangitis, of primary nature, is an extremely rare condition of unproven etiology and, using the strict criteria advocated in the literature, there appear to be fewer than 60 cases reported in the world literature up to the present time. The disease is manifested primarily by abdominal pain and progressive jaundice, in the absence of malignancy. The peak incidence tends to occur during the fourth or the fifth decades of life. Most authors writing on this subject have emphasized that it is an especially dominantly male disease [1]. It is chiefly of interest to the surgeon because of the confusion which may arise in the differentiation between primary sclerosing cholangitis and carcinoma of the extrahepatic biliary ducts, or with benign extrahepatic biliary stricture.

Etiology

A good deal of speculation has been advanced that some bacterial or metabolic alteration in bile acid metabolism may play some etiologic role. It has been suggested, for example, that lithocholic acid, which is formed in the intestine by bacterial dehydroxylation of kenodeoxycholic acid, a very highly corrosive agent, may be a fundamentally responsible factor, since it is known to produce intense desquamation in the mucosa of the common duct. Students of primary sclerosing cholangitis, and there have really only been one-half dozen good articles on the subject, have also suggested that there may be an association of the disease with other processes of an inflammatory or basically unknown etiology, such as ulcerative colitis, retroperitoneal or retromediastinal fibrosis (so-called Armand's disease) and Riedel's struma. Finally, there have been some reports of primary sclerosing cholangitis with retro-orbital fibrotic tumors.

M. Michael Eisenberg, M.D., Professor of Surgery, University of Minnesota Medical School, Minneapolis.

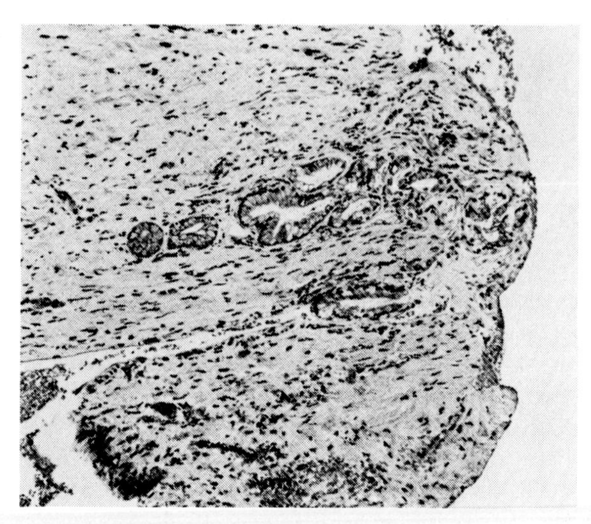

FIG. 1. Biopsy of the common bile duct showing extensive fibrosis and denuded epithelium. Ductal patterns suggest possibility of adenocarcinoma. Diagnosis: 49-year-old white male with primary sclerosing cholangitis [1].

Histopathology

Histopathologically, the disease is characterized by a very diffuse, extremely dense and extensive involvement of the bile ducts, with fibrotic thickening which may be nodular, giving the duct a thick cordlike feel (Fig. 1). The ductal diameter, however, is usually normal, with an intrinsic thickening of the wall, sharply compromising the lumen [1]. To the palpating hand of the surgeon, although the duct is clearly fibrotic, it is usually not enlarged. Histologically, there may be some lymphocytic and plasma cell infiltrate, along with hypoplasia of ductal epithelium and, sometimes, squamous metaplasia as well.

Nonspecific inflammation of a chronic type may be found in adjacent lymph nodes and in other structures including the gallbladder. Associated liver pathology is very variable and may range from mixed extrahepatic or intrahepatic cholestasis to pericholangitis and fibrosis (Fig. 2).

Clinical Characteristics

Symptomatology is vague and the diagnosis, therefore, is an extremely difficult one to make. In fact, it cannot be made outside of the operating

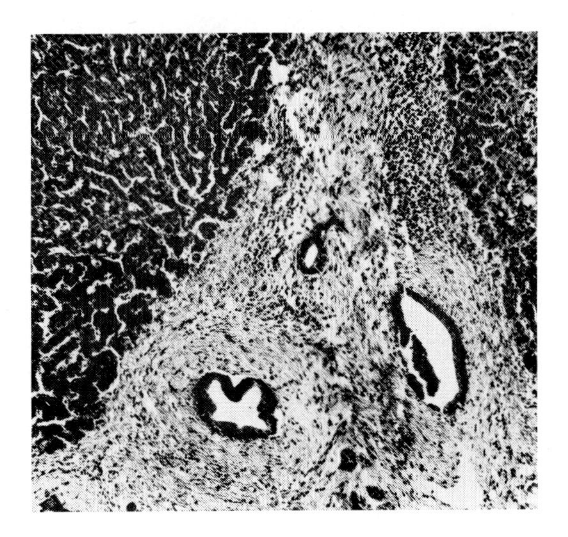

FIG. 2. Liver biopsy of portal zone showing concentric periductal fibrosis and inflammatory infiltrate. Diagnosis: Primary sclerosing cholangitis [1].

room. The patient may have some abdominal pain. There may be some associated fever, probably related to a bacterial cholangitis. There is, invariably, a progressive jaundice. The patient is frequently toxic and ill with intermittent episodes of remission. Liver function studies frequently suggest simple extrahepatic obstruction and are nonspecific for the disease. Antibody studies, as well, have proven to be unreliable, although there is continuing investigation in this area. With a patient population as small as the one available, it is self-evident that studies of this nature are difficult to execute.

While the condition may be suggested by the demonstration of a narrowed and diminutive radiographic configuration of extrahepatic biliary tree (Fig. 3), the diagnosis is essentially made on surgical grounds only, during exploration and with biopsy.

Differential Diagnosis

Of primary concern to the operating surgeon is differentiation between primary sclerosing cholangitis and carcinoma of the bile ducts. In fact, while there is little direct evidence to support the contention that primary sclerosing cholangitis may lead to carcinoma of the biliary tree, malignancy of the extrahepatic bile ducts often proves to be the correct

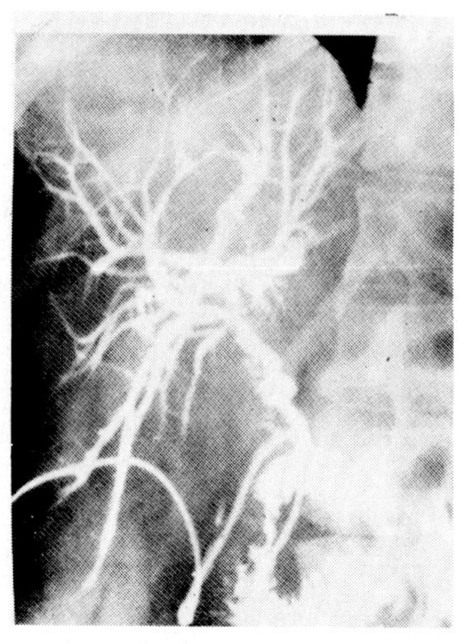

FIG. 3. T-tube cholangiogram. There is a narrowing of the main hepatic ducts with proximal dilatation. Finger branches are absent, said to be a characteristic but not a diagnostic feature of sclerosing cholangitis [2].

diagnosis. Studies reported from Cincinnati, for example, by Altmeier and his associates [3] in which 18 cases were reviewed, 11 of which were their own, it was found that 8 of the 18 cases which originally carried the diagnosis of primary sclerosing cholangitis, in fact, turned out to be carcinoma of the bile ducts. The pathologist was unable, on repeated study of histologic specimens, to make a differentiation between the two, and only following clinical experience with the patient was the final diagnosis made in retrospect.

Manesis and Sullivan [4] have suggested that in establishing the diagnosis of primary sclerosing cholangitis, the intense fibrotic reaction surrounding remnants of bile canaliculi is helpful. The pathologist, however, is very hard put to differentiate between the sclerosing process of carcinoma and the sclerosis associated with primary sclerosing cholangitis.

It is most important, if we are going to treat the subject with the respect which is its due, that we conform to very strict criteria for making the diagnosis. Manesis and Sullivan [4], as well as Schwartz [5] in their respective reports, have emphasized very nicely the high points. In establishing the diagnosis the following criteria must be adhered to: (1) it is required that there be a generalized, rather than localized narrowing of the extrahepatic biliary tree; (2) physical biopsy is required for evidence of the sclerosing process; (3) radiologic criteria should be present, but they are not, in and of themselves, diagnostic; (4) an additional criterion – and the one which eliminates most of the cases which have previously been incorrectly identified as primary sclerosing cholangitis – is that there be *no* history of previous surgery or inflammatory process in the area, including calculus disease of the gallbladder or the extrahepatic biliary tree; (5) finally, and most obviously, there should be no malignancy identifiable in the area.

Treatment

The treatment of primary sclerosing cholangitis is not a particularly rewarding subject for discussion. Therapy is fundamentally surgical since the diagnosis must be established by histologic study of the tissue involved. There is some evidence that bypass procedures to relieve biliary tract obstruction may be worthwhile, provided that one can decompress the tree proximal to the obstructive process. Obviously, if the obstructive process and the sclerotic tissue extend deeply into the intrahepatic biliary radicals, there is no proximal area which can be satisfactorily decompressed with present known procedures. The passage of a transhepatic tube to drain the biliary tree in a retrograde fashion should be attempted. On the other hand, however, should decompression be mechanically feasible there is some evidence that one may contribute significantly to the patient's welfare over a long period of time. At least one survivor, who meets all of the criteria outlined, has lived for 19 years with the disease. The vast majority, however, are dead within two to five years, a circumstance based primarily upon repeated bouts of bacterial cholangitis and jaundice, with subsequent cirrhosis and, ultimately, liver failure.

In some series, antibiotics, such as tetracycline, may offer a measure of relief, suggesting the possibility of a bacterial origin. It is my impression, from going through this small but somewhat confused literature, that the potential beneficial effects of antibiotics probably derive from control of secondary bacterial infection and cholangitis, rather than as a result of treatment of the primary disease. However, some authors are adamant that a trial of antibiotic therapy be tried, even in the absence of fever and/or evidence of bacterial contamination.

The administration of corticosteroids has been used in a number of instances with, unfortunately, variable and unpredictable results. But, here again, some authors strongly suggest that the use of steroids to suppress the inflammatory process and, in addition, to act as a choleretic agent has some benefit in these patients [1]. Schwartz [5] has reported that nine of his patients showed good to excellent results, at least on a short-term basis, while on steroid therapy. It appears reasonable, because of the nature of the prognosis in this disease, that a trial of steroid therapy be attempted in these patients.

Prognosis

In general, following establishment of the diagnosis and even after exclusion of carcinoma, the prognosis is considered to be very poor. It depends, in large measure, upon the availability of surgical options. One should always attempt to bypass these patients if possible, and the best results in the literature have, in fact, been shown to come under those circumstances in which bypass procedures, using either gallbladder, proximal common hepatic duct, or intrahepatic duct are available.

Summary

In review and summary then, primary sclerosing cholangitis is a very rare disease. Certainly fewer than 100 and probably fewer than 60 cases in the world literature meet the outlined criteria. It is dominantly a male disease. It is of completely unknown etiology, although it has been associated with other cholangitic, inflammatory and autoimmune processes. It is of special consideration and interest to surgeons because of the very common confusion made with carcinoma of the bile ducts or with benign stricture. In any event, however, the same kinds of surgical treatment are appropriate in all these instances. Unfortunately, the prognosis, with the exception of benign strictures, is also similarly discouraging.

The diagnosis must be established by biopsy, but it seems certain that only time will tell whether, in fact, the pathologist has given an accurate appraisal of the disease with which one is dealing.

The treatment is basically surgical, but antibiotics should be used and a course of steroids is clearly recommended. The temporal prognosis is in the two to five year range for most patients, although long-term survivors have been recorded.

References

1. Whelton, M. J.: Sclerosing cholangitis. *In* Clinics in Gastroenterology. Philadelphia: W. B. Saunders, 1973, pp. 163-173.
2. Thorpe, M. E. E., Scheuer, P. J. and Sherlock, S.: Primary sclerosing cholangitis, the biliary tree and ulcerative colitis. Gut, 8:435, 1967.

3. Altmeier, W. A., Gall, E. A., Culbertson, W. R. et al: Sclerosing carcinoma of the intrahepatic (hilar) bile ducts. Surgery, 60:191, 1966.
4. Manesis, J. G. and Sullivan, J. F.: Primary sclerosing cholangitis. Arch. Intern. Med., 115:137, 1965.
5. Schwartz, S. I.: Primary sclerosing cholangitis: A disease revisited. Surg. Clin. N. Amer., 53:1161, 1973.

Chronic Acalculous Cholecystitis

John P. Delaney, M.D., Ph.D.

Chronic acalculous cholecystitis and acute acalculous cholecystitis are probably quite unrelated. About acute acalculous cholecystitis there are no real controversies, although the pathogenesis remains uncertain. On the other hand, chronic biliary tract disease in the absence of stones has been the source of wide differences of opinion among thoughtful clinicians.

Some very well known surgeons [1-8] have addressed themselves to the topic of acalculous gallbladder disease (Table 1). The last general survey of the subject was by Glenn [8], almost 20 years ago. The argument regarding the existence of chronic acalculous cholecystitis as a significant entity has subsided in recent years, not because it has been resolved but because it is almost impossible to resolve with the types of supporting data that are acceptable in present day surgical discourse.

The results of an informal questionnaire survey of surgeons from the St. Paul-Minneapolis area are shown on Table 2. Most believed that biliary tract symptoms can occur without stones. Two thirds of the responding surgeons have done elective cholecystectomies in these circumstances during the past two years.

Eight members of the University of Minnesota Surgery Department responded to the questionnaire. Three thought that biliary tract pain does not occur in the absence of stones. Five gave the opposite response. Only three could recall ever having done an elective cholecystectomy for relief of pain without demonstrated stones and only three such operations were done in the preceding two years among these eight surgeons. Thus, the University group appears to be more conservative in this regard than the practicing surgeons in the Twin Cities. While the question is not one to be solved by the democratic process, current opinions and policies of these surgeons are of interest.

From a practical point of view, the clinician is confronted with a patient complaining of upper abdominal pain and a normal cholecystogram. Thorough x-ray studies have largely ruled out other intra-abdominal

---

John P. Delaney, M.D., Ph.D., Associate Professor of Surgery, University of Minnesota Health Sciences Center, Minneapolis.

Table 1.

Lord Moynihan	1909
Allen Whipple	1926
John Deaver	1927
E. Starr Judd	1927
Frank Lahey	1927
James Priestley	1932
Warren Cole	1938
Frank Glenn	1956

sources of the symptoms. The pain pattern is consistent with biliary tract origin. The issue separates itself into two questions: (1) With what degree of certainty does the normal cholecystogram rule out gallstones? (2) Does pain originate from the biliary tract even though no stones are present? Two further questions evolve from the second. Does the gallbladder wall harbor pathologic changes which can give rise to pain even though stones are absent? Can motor abnormalities cause pain from a stoneless, histologically normal gallbladder? The question of occult pathology is not the main problem for the surgeon for it can be answered only after the fact, that is, the gallbladder must be removed before the pathologist can assess microscopic changes.

Let me first turn to the question of the accuracy of cholecystography. There are in the literature extensive studies which conclude that gallstones are present with a perfectly normal cholecystogram in approximately 2% of cases [9-11]. Other reports admit to as much as a 6% incidence of stones missed by x-ray [12]. This seems a relatively insignificant rate of error. However, considering the numbers of cholecystograms done each year, it actually represents a sizable number of patients.

Table 2.

	Yes	*No*
Do you believe that chronic recurrent abdominal pain can originate from the biliary tract in the absence of gallstones?	46(89%)	6
Have you done elective cholecystectomies for relief from pain of biliary tract origin in the presence of a normal cholecystogram?	35(66%)	18
If Yes, approximately how many such operations have you done in the past two years?	Range (0-6) Average 3	

A paper from the University of Kentucky, entitled "An Evaluation of the Reinforced Oral Cholecystogram," reviewed 3,000 x-ray studies done over a five year period [13]. In 141 cases, the gallbladder was not seen on the first cholecystogram, but repeat study the next day showed a normal or faintly visualized gallbladder. Ten of these patients were operated upon because of persistent pain typical of biliary colic and all ten had stones. It should be emphasized that these patients were selected for operation from a subgroup in which the gallbladder did not visualize on the first examination.

There are other anecdotal reports of three or four patients who proved to have gallstones at operation after normal cholecystograms. The most extensive series has been reported by White [14]. At his hospital, 38 patients were operated upon because of persisting biliary pain in the face of normal x-rays. Particularly noteworthy in White's series is the fact that every patient had at least three normal cholecystograms. Thirty-four of the 38 had stones in the gallbladder. Almost all of the stones were under 5 mm in diameter. Only four of the 38 patients had normal gallbladders.

Figures of 2% for falsely negative cholecystograms are necessarily underestimated because the great majority are never assessed by operation and, therefore, the absence of stones is not definitively established. The dilemma is to attempt to pick out from a rather large group of individuals with upper abdominal pain and normal x-ray studies those few patients who do, in fact, have gallstones. White [14], among others, has suggested the value of duodenal drainage. This consists in aspiration of duodenal contents after stimulation of bile flow by either topical magnesium sulfate, systemic secretin or cholecystokinin. The recovery of cholesterol crystals from the duodenum is nearly pathognomonic of the presence of stones in the biliary tree. This diagnostic modality was popular in an earlier era and probably still has a useful place.

Now let us set aside the question of stones missed on x-ray examination and turn to the situation in which stones are truly absent, but pain does seem to originate from the biliary tract. One must look to the literature of 30 and 40 years ago to find sizable series dealing with the results of cholecystectomy done in the absence of stones. In recent years, wholesale removal of acalculous gallbladders is either not being done or is not being talked about. Warren Cole [7] in 1938 estimated that approximately one third to one half of all gallbladders removed in the United States contained no stones. Excluding acute acalculous cholecystitis, a present day figure would probably be well under 5%.

One of the best papers on the subject was written by W. Arthur Mackey [15] who, visiting the Department of Evarts Graham at Washington University in the years 1932-1933, reviewed the ten previous years at that institution and found 264 cholecystectomies done in the absence of stones. He carried out a follow-up regarding relief of the symptoms for which the operation was done. He was able to obtain valid information from about two thirds of these patients. The results were almost evenly divided: 31% were free of symptoms after operation, 31% claimed to be improved and 38% had no relief of the symptoms for which the procedure was done. Mackey attempted to correlate the results with a variety of clinical, operative and pathologic findings. Only two features proved to be helpful in predicting the probability of successful symptomatic relief. Among the patients with typical, episodic biliary colic as the presenting complaint, approximately three fourths were either completely or partially relieved. If the symptoms were atypical, more than 40% were not helped by the operation. The other predictive factor was the finding of extensive adhesions around the gallbladder at the time of the operation. In those patients in whom the surgeon reported marked adhesions, three fourths were substantially relieved of symptoms. In those individuals without adhesions, about half were not relieved. A provocative finding in this study was that histologic findings showed no correlation with the probability that symptoms would be relieved.

Glenn [8] surveyed a 22-year experience in which just over 3,000 cholecystectomies were done at Cornell. In 135 patients, no stones were present. One hundred twenty-one of these had sufficient follow-up to allow assessment of results. Two thirds were relieved of symptoms while the remainder were classed as either poor or fair results. One hundred of the gallbladders were said by the pathologist to show cholecystitis. The remainder were interpreted as normal. Comparing the patients relieved of pain with those who had persistent symptoms, there were no differences in the character of the pathologic changes – thus confirming Mackey's observations of 20 years earlier.

In 1933, Noble [16] examined gallbladder changes in routine autopsies. His criterion for diagnosing cholecystitis was that the wall of the gallbladder be infiltrated with lymphocytes and in some instances with granulocytes. Forty percent of the gallbladders without stones were interpreted as showing histologic cholecystitis. The incidence of pathologic changes was just as high in the group of patients under 30 as it was in the older age group. There are other studies suggesting much the same point, namely, that histologic changes in the gallbladder wall probably have little significance.

The conclusions that I draw from these observations are *first*, in the absence of stones the frequency of the pathologic changes interpreted as cholecystitis will depend somewhat upon the enthusiasm and the prejudices of the pathologist and *second*, the histologic changes bear little, if any, relationship to the probability that symptoms arose from the biliary tract.

How can patients be selected who really do have pain originating from the biliary tree and who might be relieved by cholecystectomy, even though no stones are present? As surgeons, we are all familiar with the symptoms of gallbladder disease: food dyscrasias, heartburn, epigastric distress, flatulence and fatty food intolerance. W. H. Price [17] from Edinburgh examined the relationship between "dyspepsia" and gallbladder disease. To do so, he surveyed all women between the ages of 50 and 70 in a general practice population of 3,000. One hundred forty-two women were interviewed and then underwent cholecystograms. Neither the patient nor the doctor knew whether gallstones were present at the time the history was taken. Twenty-four of the 142 had gallstones. The histories of these 24 were compared with those of the 118 women who had normal cholecystograms. There were no differences regarding complaints of food intolerance, heartburn or flatulence. Surprisingly, the complaint of fatty food dyscrasia was more frequently elicited from controls than from the women with cholelithiasis. Price concluded: "In practice, therefore, a history of chronic dyspepsia in women of this age group should not be taken to indicate gallbladder disease. It would clearly be unjustifiable to regard chronic dyspepsia as an indication for cholecystectomy."

How then can patients be identified who have no stones but might be relieved of biliary colic by cholecystectomy? Since 1961 cholecystokinin has been available in a form sufficiently pure to administer to humans. A number of reports [18-21] have emphasized its diagnostic usefulness. The technique starts with a conventional oral cholecystogram. After the initial films are developed, an intravenous dose of cholecystokinin is given. A major feature in a positive result is that the typical pain pattern is reproduced by the administration of this agent. Most of the studies have claimed delayed or incomplete emptying of the gallbladder in those patients whose symptoms were reproduced. From this has evolved the concept of the cystic duct syndrome or partial noncalculous obstruction of the cystic duct leading to pain when the gallbladder contracts. Each of these authors states that the cystic duct was found to be narrow or partially obstructed. The evidence cited was as follows: (1) The gallbladder did not empty readily when squeezed at operation. (2) Adhesions or kinking of the cystic duct were found. (3) The pathologist reported fibrosis or abnormal valves in the cystic duct. If one can judge from the difficulty involved in passing a catheter into the common duct via the cystic duct, most patients have narrow cystic ducts. If the surgeon starts with the premise that pain is due to a narrow cystic duct, he almost certainly will be able to confirm his belief at the operating table.

The most impressive feature in the reports on cholecystokinin is the total relief of symptoms in almost all of the patients following cholecystectomy. In a report by Camishion [18] from Jefferson Medical College, 13 of 13 patients with the cystic duct syndrome were completely relieved of pain by operation. Nora [19] from Northwestern reported that 12 of 14 experienced complete relief. Valberg [20] from Kingston, Ontario, reported 12 of 12 obtaining complete relief. McFarland [22] from Denver reported ten of ten to be completely relieved by cholecystectomy.

Dunn [23] ,and colleagues carried out a systematic study of cholecystokinin x-ray exams, which included normal control subjects. Three radiologists interpreted the films independently with no clinical information available to them. The investigators did not tell the referring surgeon the results of the cholecystokinin test and made no recommendations regarding cholecystectomy. There were 44 patients with what was thought to be typical biliary colic, 25 with so-called dyspepsia and 44 normal controls. Twenty-nine symptomatic patients eventually underwent cholecystectomy. The authors concluded that their "results showed that cholecystokinin cholecystography was of little value in the diagnosis and management of patients with possible acalculous biliary tract disease." They gave four reasons for this assertion: "*First*, the incidence of 'abnormal' gallbladder contractions in normal subjects is high (14% to 36%). *Second*, cholecystokinin cholecystography does not help predict which patients with symptoms suggestive of gallbladder disease will be cured by cholecystectomy; our results show that patients with both normal and abnormal cholecystokinin cholecystograms usually claim to be cured or improved by cholecystectomy. *Third*, cholecystokinin cholecystography does not help predict histologic findings in the gallbladder; patients with normal and abnormal cholecystokinin cholecystography had similar histologic findings in their gallbladders. *Fourth*, there is a high degree of observer disagreement (approximately 28%) in the roentgenographic interpretation of the result of the test."

They noted further that 80% of the symptomatic patients who underwent cholecystectomy claimed to be cured or improved and cited two possible reasons for the excellent results. "*First*, the gallbladder may have been the cause of pain, and its removal brought about a cure. *Second*, the response to surgery may have been mainly a placebo effect. A controlled group with a placebo surgical procedure would be required to decide this issue, but it seems unlikely that such a study will ever be conducted."

Finally, these investigators noted that approximately 60% of their patients with possible acalculous gallbladder disease considered themselves cured or definitely improved 6-24 months later, even though cholecystectomy had not been done. Many such patients improved in time even without operation.

Conclusions

1. Most importantly, the normal cholecystogram does not insure the absence of stones. In the face of the typical symptoms of biliary colic, the cholecystogram should be repeated at intervals. Aspiration of duodenal contents for cholesterol crystals may have a place in identifying patients who have stones but normal x-ray studies.

2. Chronic vague upper abdominal distress, dyspepsia, flatulence and food intolerance should not be indications for cholecystectomy. Discrete recurrent attacks of acute, severe epigastric or right upper quadrant pain radiating to the back preferably accompanied by tenderness or vomiting *may* suggest that pain really is arising from the biliary tree.

3. Pathologic changes in the gallbladder wall do not correlate with symptoms and are not a justification, even in retrospect, for cholecystectomy.

4. Induction of pain by administration of cholecystokinin may help identify patients with acalculous biliary tract pain, although this issue is in doubt.

References

1. Moynihan, B. G. A.: A disease of the gallbladder requiring cholecystectomy. Amer. Surg., 50:1265, 1909.
2. Whipple, A. C.: Surgical criteria for cholecystectomy. Amer. J. Surg., 129:39-40, 1926.
3. Deaver, J. B. and Bortz, E. L.: Gallbladder disease, a review of 903 cases. JAMA, 88:619, 1927.
4. Judd, E. S.: Cholecystitis. Coll. Papers Mayo Clin., 19:324, 1927.
5. Lahey, F. H.: Cholecystitis, the cholesterol gall bladder and silent gall stones. Boston Med. Surg. J., 196:677, 1927.
6. Judd, E. S. and Priestley, J. T.: Ultimate results from operations on the biliary tract. JAMA, 99:887, 1932.

7. Cole, W. H.: Noncalculous cholecystitis. Surgery, 3:824, 1938.
8. Glenn, F. and Mannix, H., Jr.: The acalculous gallbladder. Ann. Surg., 144:670, 1956.
9. Baker, H. L. and Hodgson, J. R.: Further studies on the accuracy of oral cholecystography. Radiology, 74:239, 1960.
10. Shehadi, W. H.: Radiologic examination of the biliary tract. Plain film of the abdomen. Oral cholecystography. Radiol. Clin. N. Amer., 4:463, 1966.
11. Kolodny, M., Colker, J. L., Callahan, E. W. et al: Falsely negative cholecystography and cholangiography. Amer. J. Dig. Dis., 13:669, 1968.
12. Twiss, J. R. and Oppenheimer, E.: Liver, biliary tract, and pancreas. Philadelphia:Lea and Febiger, 1955.
13. Eadie, E., Jr., Nighberg, E. H. and Griffen, W. O., Jr.: An evaluation of the reinforced oral cholecystogram. Amer. Surg., 38:546, 1972.
14. White, T. T.: Gallbladder stones in patients with negative gallbladder x rays. Amer. Surg., 37:518, 1971.
15. Mackey, W. A.: Cholecystitis without stone. Brit. J. Surg., 22:274, 1934-1935.
16. Noble, J.: Cholecystitis in routine postmortems. Amer. J. Path., 9:473, 1933.
17. Price, W. H.: Gall-bladder dyspepsia. Brit. Med. J., 2:138, 1963.
18. Camishion, R. C. and Goldstein, R.: Partial, noncalculous cystic duct obstruction (cystic duct syndrome). Surg. Clin. N. Amer., 47:1107, 1967.
19. Nora, P. F., McCarthy, W. and Sanex, N.: Cholecystokinin cholecystography in acalculous gallbladder disease. Arch. Surg., 108:507, 1974.
20. Valberg, L. S., Jabbari, M., Kerr, J. W. et al: Biliary pain in young woman in the absence of gallstones. Gastroenterology, 60:1020, 1971.
21. Nathan, M. H., Newman, A., Murray, D. J. et al: Cholecystokinin cholecystography. Amer. J. Roentgen., 110:240, 1970.
22. McFarland, J. O. and Currin, J.: Cholecystectomy and the cystic duct syndrome. Amer. J. Gastroent., 52:515, 1969.
23. Dunn, F. H., Christensen, E. C., Reynolds, J. et al: Cholecystokinin cholecystography. JAMA, 228:997, 1974.

Acute Acalculous Cholecystitis

Richard J. Howard, M.D. and John P. Delaney, M.D., Ph.D.

Cholelithiasis is found in 90% to 95% of patients with acute cholecystitis and is believed to be a major etiologic factor. Little attention, however, has been directed to those cases where acute cholecystitis occurs in the absence of stones. We review here all cases of acute acalculous cholecystitis occurring at the University of Minnesota and allied hospitals during a 16-year period 1954 through 1969.

Chart Review

In the years 1954 through 1969 780 patients underwent cholecystectomy for acute cholecystitis at the University of Minnesota Hospitals and affiliated teaching hospitals. In each instance the diagnosis was confirmed by pathologic examination. No calculi were found in 34 (4.4%) specimens. The patients' ages ranged from 18 to 87 years (average 57).

Medical History

Only four patients had symptoms suggestive of gallbladder disease, fatty food intolerance. Eight patients developed acute acalculous cholecystitis while recovering from operative procedures, only two of which were intra-abdominal. Four others had suffered extensive trauma in automobile accidents, and two of these had operations related to the injuries.

Four other patients were alcoholics, and one of these developed cholecystitis while being treated for bleeding esophageal varices. Nine patients had been treated for cancer including lung, stomach, prostate, thyroid, cervix, breast and testis. Other associated medical problems included ulcerative colitis, heart disease, arteriosclerotic peripheral vascular disease and gastric ulcer.

Richard J. Howard, M.D. and John P. Delaney, M.D., Ph.D., Department of Surgery, University of Minnesota Hospitals, Minneapolis.

Symptoms and Signs

Right upper quadrant pain was the most common complaint, noted in 26 of the 34 case records. In two the pain was diffuse throughout the abdomen and in one it was periumbilical. Three patients had no pain and one patient was comatose.

Right upper quadrant tenderness was detected in 28 patients. Two had diffuse abdominal tenderness and three had none. Twenty-two patients vomited. Six of the 34 had a palpable right upper quadrant mass. Abdominal distention was present in 12, bowel sounds were decreased or absent in 14 and clinical jaundice was detected in seven instances. Twenty-seven patients had fever.

Laboratory Studies

The white blood cell count ranged from 4750 to 29,000 cell per cu mm, exceeding 10,000 in 23 instances. The serum bilirubin was measured in 25 patients and was elevated in 12, exceeding 3 mg/100 ml in seven. The serum glutamic oxalic transaminase was elevated in six of ten measurements, and the alkaline phosphatase was increased in eight of 18 patients.

Roentgenographic Studies

Biliary x-ray studies were done in 12 patients. The gallbladder did not visualize in 11 examinations. Air was seen in the gallbladder lumen in one.

Preoperative Diagnosis and Operation Performed

There was a delay of 1 to 67 days from the onset of symptoms to operation. Acute cholecystitis was not suspected in 12 instances. Incorrect diagnoses included subhepatic abscess, hepatic abscess, acute appendicitis, "inflammatory mass," ruptured spleen and mesenteric vein thrombosis.

Cholecystectomy was performed in all cases, although cholecystostomy was done initially in three instances because inflammatory reaction obscured the anatomy. Elective cholecystectomy was performed one to two months later. Common bile duct exploration was carried out in four patients because of jaundice. Common duct exploration was not performed in three jaundiced patients, one of whom had a normal operative cholangiogram.

Pathology and Bacteriology

Acute cholecystitis was confirmed histologically in all cases of acalculous cholecystitis. The gallbladder wall showed areas of gangrene in 14 specimens. There were three instances of empyema and three of localized perforation.

The bile was cultured from 17 patients and the surrounding peritoneal fluid from eight. Eight of the 25 specimens were sterile. *Escherichia coli,* the most common organism, was cultured eight times. Other organisms included alpha hemolytic streptococcus, coagulase negative staphylococcus, klebsiella, aerobacter, pseudomonas, clostridium, and bacteroides. In three instances the organism found in the bile had previously been cultured from the blood. One patient had a urinary tract infection caused by the same organism found in the bile.

Morbidity and Mortality

There were seven deaths. Two occurred in patients who had been involved in automobile accidents and had extensive injuries. Cholecystitis developed 5 and 35 days after injury. A 20-year-old man was brought to the University of Minnesota Hospitals five days after treatment in another hospital for injuries sustained in an automobile accident. He was comatose and was operated upon because blood was found in the peritoneal aspirate. He died in the early postoperative period with pneumothorax and adrenal hemorrhage. A 66-year-old woman died of congestive heart failure one month following cholecystectomy, vagotomy and gastrectomy.

Three deaths occurred in patients who developed acute cholecystitis while recovering from other surgical procedures. A 63-year-old man who had the onset of symptoms 20 days after insertion of an aortic valve prosthesis died of cardiac arrest shortly after cholecystectomy. A 79-year-old woman developed pneumonia after radium insertion for carcinoma of the cervix. She developed cholecystitis 27 days later and died of continuing pneumonia and septicemia one month following cholecystectomy. The third patient was a 73-year-old man who had gram negative sepsis and cholecystitis following thyroidectomy and radiation for lymphoblastoma of the thyroid. A bleeding dyscrasia developed after cholecystectomy, and death resulted from gram negative sepsis.

Two other patients, both alcoholic, also succumbed. One had cholecystectomy for acute cholecystitis discovered during emergency portacaval shunt. He died 15 days postoperatively of recurrent upper gastrointestinal hemorrhage and hepatic coma. An 85-year-old male developed congestive heart failure following cholecystectomy and died.

Three nonfatal complications related to cholecystectomy. Two patients had prolonged bile drainage which ceased spontaneously. A 78-year-old man developed hepatitis six months following cholecystectomy, was treated medically and recovered.

Incidence

In large series of acute cholecystitis 90%-95% of the patients have gallbladder stones and two thirds are women [2, 6, 8]. Conversely, three fourths of the patients with acalculous cholecystitis are male. In the present series also, when six male patients from the Veterans Administration Hospital are excluded, 71% of the patients were male. The incidence of the acalculous variant is significantly higher when cholecystitis occurs in the postoperative period [10, 12], after trauma [11] or in children [3, 7].

Pathogenesis

Experimental work indicates that bile stasis, impairment of blood supply and cystic duct obstruction are the most important factors in the development of acute cholecystitis [13].

Infection has also been proposed as a cause of cholecystitis. Lindberg et al [11] found infected bile in nine of 12 wounded soldiers with acute acalculous cholecystitis. Six of the nine had wounds infected by the same organism subsequently found in the bile. Cole et al [4] have proposed that infection is a late event imposed upon an already inflammed gallbladder. A lower incidence of positive cultures of bile and gallbladder wall is found if the specimen is obtained in the early, rather than late, phase of acute cholecystitis [1, 8].

Reflux of pancreatic secretions into the gallbladder has also been implicated in the etiology of cholecystitis. Colp et al [5] found amylase and trypsin in the bile of inflammed gallbladders and Wolfer [14] produced cholecystitis by injecting pancreatic juice into the gallbladder of dogs.

Clearly, no single explanation can account for all cases of acute acalculous cholecystitis. Most of our patients were being treated for other illnesses at the time of onset of acute cholecystitis. Eight developed cholecystitis while recovering from operations and four following extensive injuries. Several previous reports have implicated surgery and trauma as predisposing to acute acalculous cholecystitis [10-12].

Many of our patients had arteriosclerosis. Their gallbladder blood flow may have been decreased to a level where further minor insults could lead to cholecystitis. No cystic duct obstruction was evident in these patients.

Summary

Thirty-three patients developed acute cholecystitis without gallbladder stones. There were 25 males and eight females. Three fourths were older than 50 years. Only four patients had prior symptoms referable to the biliary tract. Eight developed acute cholecystitis while recovering from surgery, and four had suffered extensive trauma.

Their symptoms did not differ appreciably from patients with acute acalculous cholecystitis. Right upper pain and tenderness, vomiting, abdominal distention, decreased bowel sounds, jaundice and fever were frequent.

Fourteen specimens showed gangrene. There were three instances of empyema and three of localized perforation. Seventeen of 25 specimens were infected; *E. coli* was the most common organism.

We believe that decreased gallbladder perfusion caused by arteriosclerosis possibly combined with a low cardiac output contributed to the development of cholecystitis. It is not clear if cystic duct occlusion was a factor.

References

1. Andrews, E. and Henry, L. D.: Bacteriology of normal and diseased gallbladders. Arch. Intern. Med., 56:1171, 1935.
2. Becker, W. F., Powell, J. L. and Turner, R. J.: A clinical study of 1060 patients with acute cholecystitis. Surg. Gynec. Obstet., 104:491, 1957.
3. Brenner, R. W. and Stewart, C. F.: Cholecystitis in children. Rev. Surg., 21:327, 1964.
4. Cole, W. H., Novak, M. W. and Highes, E. O.: Experimental production of chronic cholecystitis by obstructive lesions of the cystic duct. Ann. Surg., 114:682, 1941.
5. Colp, R., Gerber, I. E. and Doubilet, H.: Acute cholecystitis associated with pancreatic reflux. Ann. Surg., 103:67, 1936.
6. Glenn, F.: A 26 year experience in the surgical treatment of 5,037 patients with nonmalignant biliary tract disease. Surg. Gynec. Obstet., 109:591, 1959.
7. Glenn, F. and Hill, Jr., M. R.: Primary gallbladder disease in children. Ann. Surg., 139:302, 1954.
8. Goldman, L., Morgan, J. H. and Kay, J.: Acute cholecystitis: Correlation of bacteriology and mortality. Gastroenterology, 11:318, 1948.
9. Judd, E. S. and Phillips, J. R.: Acute cholecystic disease. Ann. Surg., 98:771, 1933.

10. Levin, J. F.: Death due to gangrenous cholecystitis and peritonitis following unrelated surgery. JAMA, 160:1040, 1956.
11. Lindberg, E. F., Grinnen, G. L. B. and Smith, L.: Acalculous cholecystitis in Viet Nam casualties. Ann. Surg., 171:152, 1970.
12. Schwegman, C. W. and DeMuth, Jr., W. E.: Acute cholecystitis following operation for unrelated disease. Surg. Gynec. Obstet., 97:167, 1953.
13. Thomas, Jr., C. G. and Womack, N. A.: Acute cholecystitis, its pathogenesis and repair. Arch. Surg., 64:590, 1952.
14. Wolfer, J. A.: The role of pancreatic juice in the production of gallbladder disease. Surg. Gynec. Obstet., 53:433, 1931.

Reprinted from *Minnesota Medicine* (55:549-551, 1972).

Strictures of the Bile Duct

Rodney Smith, M.S.

Various strictures in the biliary apparatus may be recognized. I do not propose to deal today with malignant strictures at the lower end of the common bile duct, the radical surgical cure of which involves a pancreatic resection. Nor do I propose to discuss nonmalignant stenosing lesions in the same area and I certainly do not intend to become involved in an argument around the old topic of sphincteroplasty versus choledocho-duodenostomy.

Carcinoma of the common hepatic duct is not a particularly uncommon lesion. Patients are usually in the 50-70 age group and present with a deepening obstructive jaundice without other major symptoms and, in particular, without pain. A carcinoma of the head of the pancreas or periampullary region is often suspected but the gallbladder cannot be felt on examination. Together with the deepening jaundice, certain general symptoms may be observed, such as pruritus, anorexia and weight loss and, should the biliary obstruction be accompanied by cholangitis in the obstructed bile duct, intermittent febrile episodes, sometimes with rigors. Clinical examination will often reveal no abnormality apart from deep jaundice and an enlarged and sometimes tender liver.

Laboratory investigation having supported a diagnosis of obstructive jaundice, the most useful radiologic investigation is percutaneous trans-hepatic cholangiography, performed immediately before surgical exploration in order to minimize the chances of bile leakage (Fig. 1).

As regards treatment, resection is seldom possible but can sometimes be carried out. In the majority of cases, the surgeon has to be satisfied with some form of palliative surgery. If, having opened the empty common bile duct below the tumor the malignant stricture can be dilated from below, the simplest technique is to insert a long Cattel T tube, the upper limb of which lies through the carcinoma in the dilated bile duct within the liver, the lower limb within the common bile duct. Patients may often live a year or more after their jaundice has been palliated in this way (Fig. 2, A and B).

Rodney Smith, M.S., F.R.C.S., Senior Surgeon, St. George's Hospital, London, England.

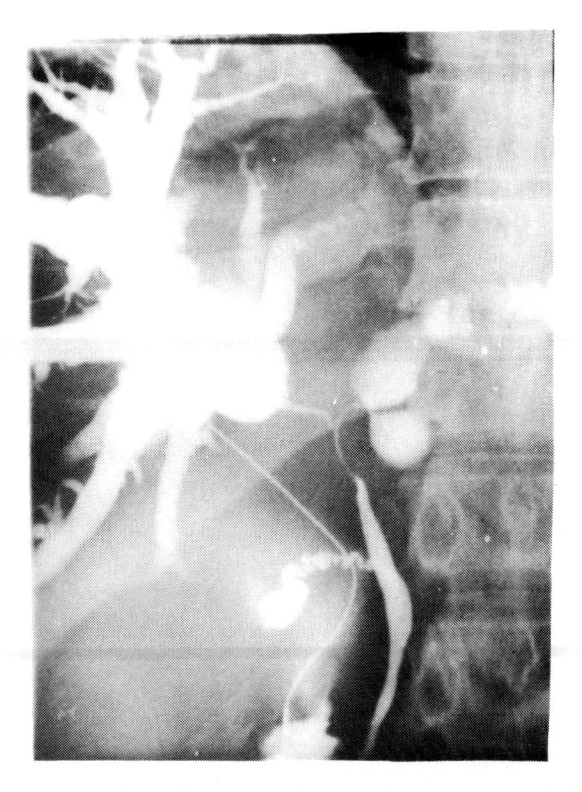

FIG. 1. Transhepatic cholangiogram showing a typical carcinoma of the common hepatic duct.

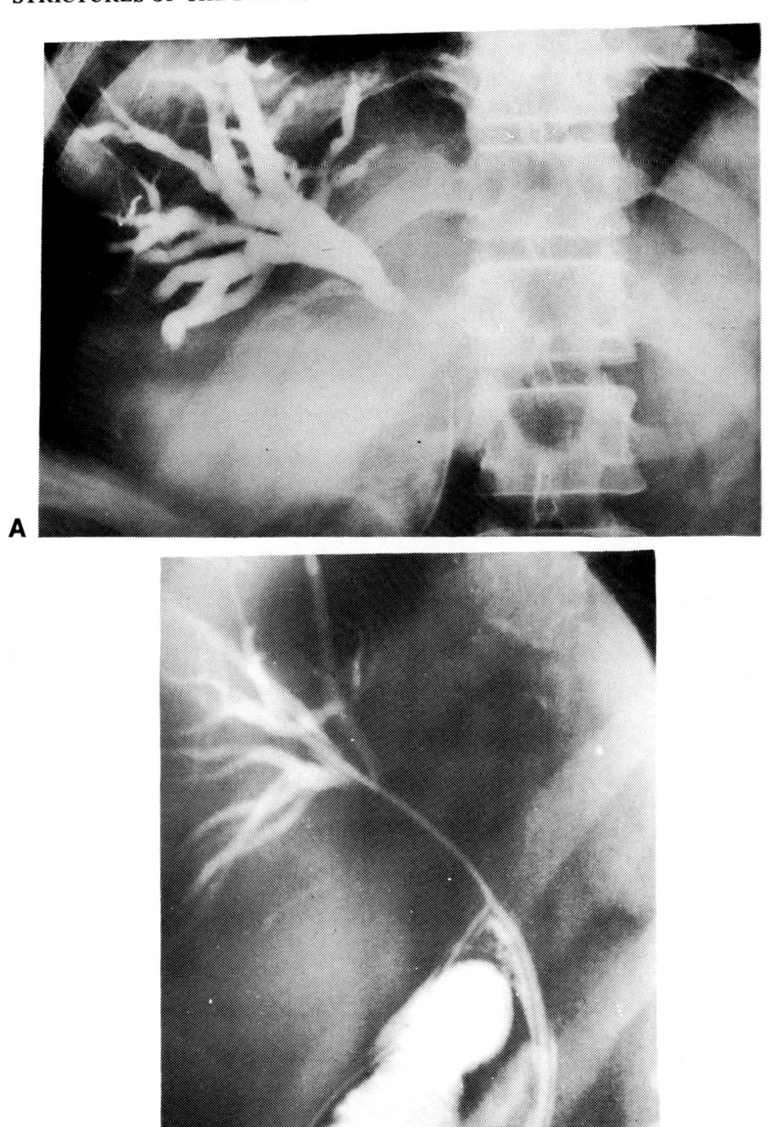

FIG. 2. (*A*) Carcinoma of the common hepatic duct dilated and tube inserted for cholangiography. (*B*) Same case four months after intubation with a long T-tube.

Palliation may also be effected by some form of biliary short-circuit, the dilated bile ducts within the liver being anastomosed to a loop of jejunum (Fig. 3) or, if the gallbladder is present and is normal, to the gallbladder itself (Fig. 4).

Diffuse sclerosing cholangitis is an inflammatory condition producing multiple strictures throughout the biliary apparatus, outside and inside the liver, and if adequate cholangiograms are available, should not cause any confusion in diagnosis, for the picture is characteristic (Fig. 5). The treatment is medical. Therapy with steroids is quite often effective for a period of time and more recently treatment with Azothioprine has been used.

Traumatic stricture following cholecystectomy. Regrettably, the most common traumatic stricture of a major bile duct is that following an operation, in particular cholecystectomy.

Diagnosis

Damage to a major bile duct may be recognized during an operation, diagnosed in the immediate postoperative period or identified at a later date, after the patient has left the hospital.

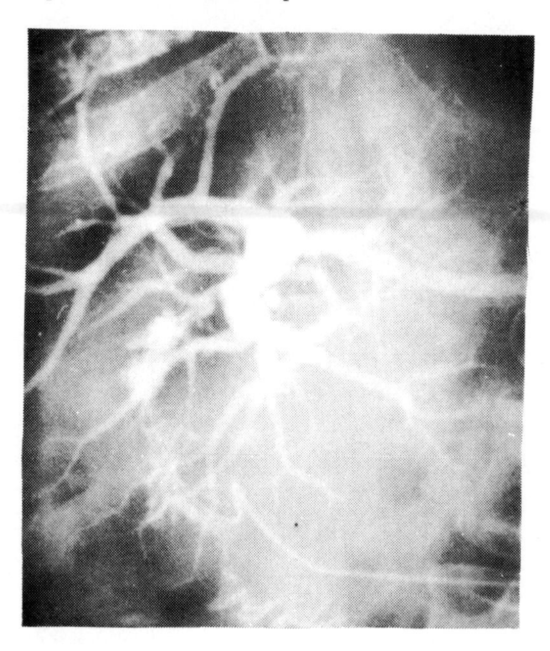

FIG. 3. Intrahepatic cholangiojejunostomy for nonresectable carcinoma of the common hepatic duct.

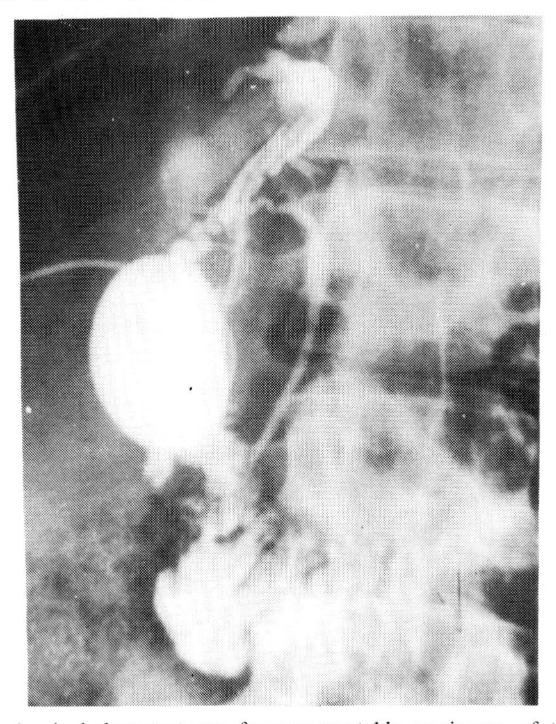

FIG. 4. Cholangiocholecystostomy for nonresectable carcinoma of the common hepatic duct.

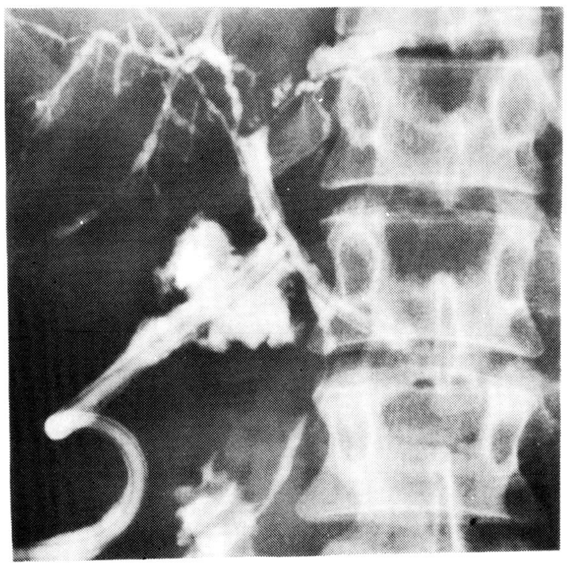

FIG. 5. Cholangiogram showing typical diffuse sclerosing cholangitis.

If the operation has been completed without evidence that anything untoward has occurred, the early onset of a deepening obstructive jaundice will naturally arouse suspicions that the common bile duct or common hepatic duct has been accidentally ligated. More commonly a main extrahepatic bile duct may have been incised, torn, crushed or even divided. In this circumstance, from the day of the operation a profuse discharge of bile will indicate a serious duct injury. In a high proportion of cases of this kind, the discharge of bile eventually stops, but optimism on this score is shown to be an illusion as the patient slowly becomes icteric. Sometimes the fistula will reopen with relief of the jaundice and then close again with return of the jaundice. This sequence of events is a not uncommon way for a bile duct injury to present. The picture may be further complicated by subphrenic or subhepatic sepsis as the result of infection in bile pooling under the liver or above.

A relatively minor ductal injury may result in a temporary fistula which eventually dries up completely leaving a patient who is apparently perfectly well. Later a stricture develops at the site of the injury; the existence of biliary stasis is signalled by the onset first of attacks of cholangitis and later by the slow development of obstructive jaundice. Occasionally, this may occur after the main common hepatic duct has been totally divided and the patient develops a spontaneous internal fistula into the duodenum. Such a fistula does not result in a spontaneous cure, for being small and not lined with epithelium, the stoma is inadequate from the start and tends to contract with the passage of time. Biliary stasis is further complicated by the development of stones and biliary sludge within the intrahepatic bile ducts; clinically, the patient develops intermittent jaundice and recurrent cholangitis with bouts of high fever, perhaps with rigors.

One further way in which a duct injury may manifest itself should be mentioned. Leakage of bile into the peritoneal cavity does not always produce a severe peritonitis. The evil reputation of biliary peritonitis is probably due to the fact that leakage of bile has so often been infected bile, leading to a rapidly spreading bacterial peritonitis, rather than merely chemical irritation. Occasionally, a cholecystectomy has been followed by a slow progressive distention of the abdomen in a patient who remains remarkably well. It is possible for 4-5 liters of bile to collect in a greatly distended abdomen in this way, the patient complaining merely of the increase in abdominal size and pressure and the difficulty of breathing caused by this, a mild icterus developing from the absorption of bile pigment.

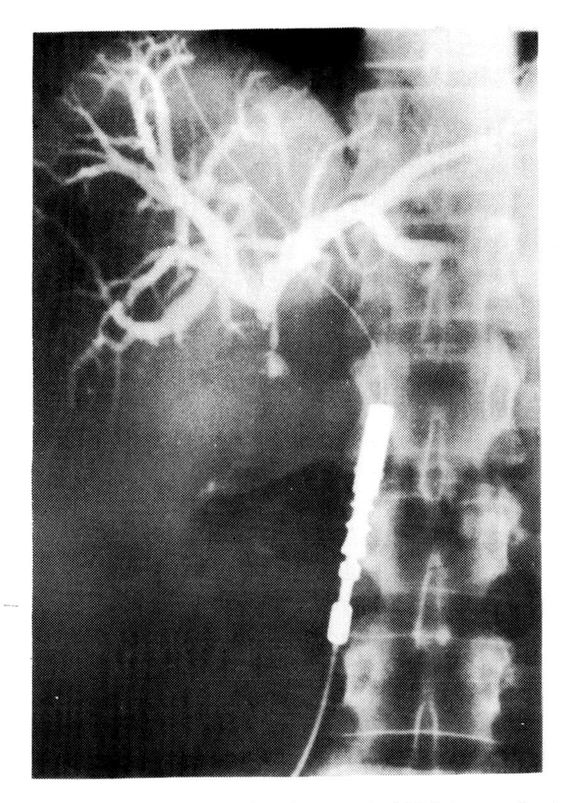

FIG. 6. Transhepatic cholangiogram showing a typical high traumatic stricture of the common hepatic duct.

Investigations and Preoperative Management

The presence of major injury to a bile duct is usually evident and the necessity for a further operation clear. Preoperative investigations should include a full blood picture, liver function tests, electrolyte estimation and an estimate of renal function. Correction of any deficit brought to light must include administration of vitamin K by intramuscular injection. The patient will often be pyrexial with a high leukocyte count and it is important to decide whether the infection lies within the bile ducts, in other words, whether the patient has cholangitis, or whether it is due to a subphrenic abscess which should be drained, leaving the repair of the bile duct injury to a later date. Immediately before operation percutaneous transhepatic cholangiography is useful to outline the dilated bile ducts within the liver and to demonstrate the site of the stricture (Fig. 6).

It should be borne in mind that the two major hazards of surgery to repair a bile duct stricture are renal failure and septicemia. The use of mannitol in the deeply jaundiced patient may reduce the risk of renal failure. The hazard of septicemia requires cover with antibiotics. Bile will be taken for culture during operation, but if preoperatively the patient has a severe cholangitis with rigors it is probable that blood culture will reveal the responsible organisms and their sensitivities.

The Surgical Technique of Repair

Immediate end-to-end anastomosis of a divided bile duct can be carried out if during the course of an operation it is recognized that the accident has occurred. More commonly, the stricture develops later and the surgeon may be faced with a difficult technical operation, often to repair a stricture which has already recurred on a number of occasions in a patient who has had multiple operations. To have any chance of success, the surgeon should routinely mobilize thoroughly both lobes of the liver and the whole of the right colon so that the latter can be removed completely from the right upper quadrant of the abdomen and packed away downwards and to the left in order to secure a wide exposure in the area where the stricture lies. Few surgeons today believe that excision of the stricture and end-to-end anastomosis of the duct is the best technique for the late repair of a lesion of this kind. Most believe that a better long-term result is likely to be obtained by anastomosis of the common hepatic duct to the jejunum. There are a number of different techniques for performing such an anastomosis. The center of the problem is how to prevent further stenosis after an operation of this kind, for while it is true that complete success may follow the restoration of a free flow of bile through a hepaticojejunal anastomosis, the restenosis rate is high and if restenosis does occur a further operation is imperative, for without a free unimpeded passage of bile the patient will eventually develop chronic biliary sepsis and before long irreversible biliary cirrhosis. The problem is how to perform an anastomosis of this kind with the maximum chance of success and the minimum likelihood of recurrent stenosis. It is easy to state the principles most to be desired: a large anastomosis, accurate apposition of epithelium to epithelium at all points and no tension. But the injury to the duct is in many instances so high and the duct itself so encased in dense scar tissue, particularly if there have already been multiple operations, that these principles are impossible to achieve by direct suture.

High Ductal Stricture

Trauma to the bile duct during cholecystectomy often does occur at a very high level. Moreover, if the injury leaves, say, 0.5 cm of common hepatic duct below the liver, this 0.5 cm of usable common hepatic duct may disappear as a result of repeated unsuccessful attempts at repair. It is thus far from uncommon for a surgeon to explore a stricture of the bile duct and to find that the normal criteria for success cannot possibly be achieved, and that in particular it does not appear possible to appose accurately the lining of the common hepatic duct above the stricture either to the lining of the distal duct below or to the epithelium of a loop of jejunum brought into the porta hepatis. It is little use in these cases to core out of the thickened capsule of the liver a cylinder of scar tissue and to call this a duct, because anastomosis of a cylinder of scar tissue without an epithelial lining to the jejunum, while it will serve for a while, is bound to restenose at a later date. If this cylinder of scar tissue is partly lined by epithelium, then sometimes a permanent satisfactory result can be achieved by splinting the anastomosis with an indwelling tube, either a T-tube passed from below or, probably better, by one or two transhepatic tubes, one through the right hepatic duct and the other through the left hepatic duct.

Principles of the "mucosal graft" operation. If access to the epithelial lining of the bile duct is so inadequate through the mass of scar tissue in the porta hepatis that accurate suture to the epithelial lining of the jejunum appears to be impracticable, a successful repair can still be achieved if in some way the epithelial lining of the jejunum can be placed through the zone of fibrosis and in contact with the duct lining. This is the principle of the "mucosal graft" operation. It is effected by cutting away a disc of the seromuscular coat of the jejunum in order to expose the mucosa and make a diverticulum which can be used as a mucosal graft to line the area where the epithelium is missing. A variety of methods have been employed in order to place this graft in situ. At the present time it is believed that the most effective technique is to attach the mucosal graft to a transhepatic tube (Fig. 7), using this to draw up the sleeve of mucosa through the scar tissue and well into the intrahepatic duct system. It is believed that the combination of the mucoscal graft with a transhepatic tube is a useful one for the following reasons:

1. However high the ductal injury, the mucosa of the jejunum can be placed in contact with the lining of the duct epithelium.

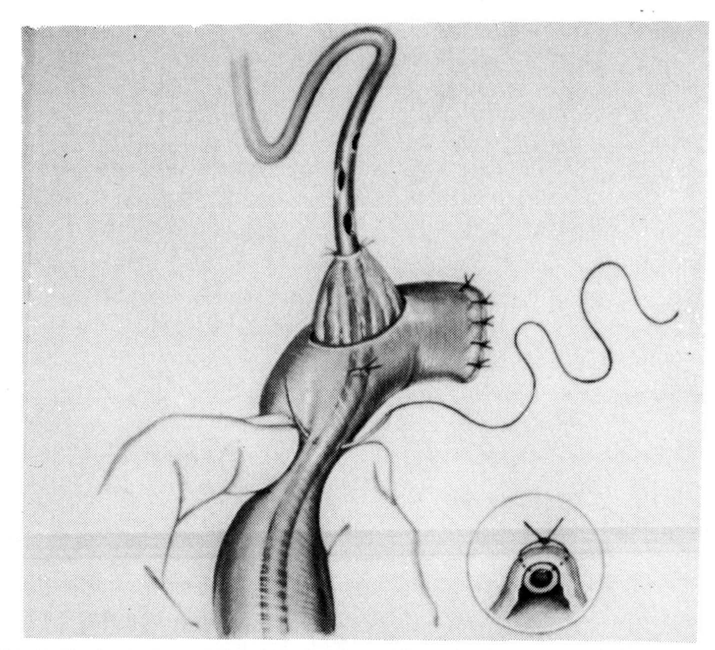

FIG. 7. Method of attaching "mucosal graft" to the lower end of the transhepatic tube. Note holes cut in that part of the tube about to be drawn back into the intrahepatic duct system.

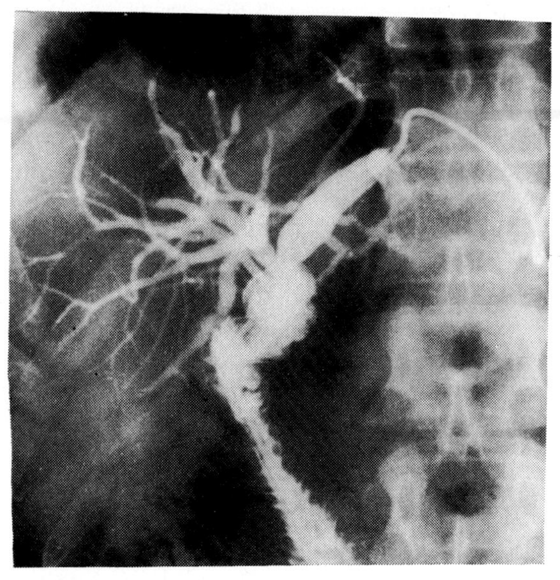

FIG. 8. Postoperative cholangiogram via transhepatic tube. Striation of the jejunal mucosal graft well shown.

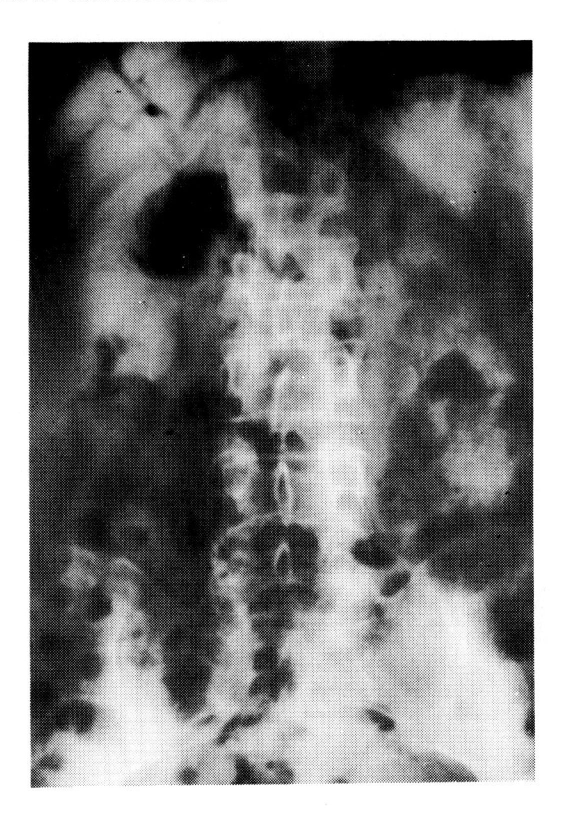

FIG. 9. "Pepsicolagram" one year postoperatively in an asymptomatic patient. Junction of bile ducts, which are not dilated, to the jejunum well shown.

2. Splinting the junction of duct to jejunum with an indwelling tube is probably useful and the transhepatic tube can be left in as long as is desired.

3. The only stitches employed are those anchoring the Roux loop to the capsule of the liver and the junction of bile duct epithelium to jejunal epithelium is sutureless.

4. Diversion of bile from the healing junction is achieved in the postoperative period by connecting the transhepatic tube to a low tension electric pump.

5. The transhepatic tube allows the duct system to be washed out postoperatively as well as at operation. It further allows radiologic studies and bile to be taken for culture at any moment that is desired (Fig. 8).

Prognosis in Traumatic Structure of the Bile Duct

The late Dr. Richard Cattell of Boston in discussing the problem of the damaged common bile duct often used to say that there was only one good treatment for this and that was not to have it, meaning of course that surgeons never should risk damaging a common bile duct because of the serious effects. It has already been stated that the major problem in repair is the prevention of restenosis and the "mucosal graft" procedure described represents an attempt to counter this very common problem of restenosis which, it is believed, is related to the absence of an epithelial lining if repair is carried out using a normal suture technique. Many years must pass before an accurate appraisal can be made of the method but in the hands of the author the incidence of early restenosis, that is during the first year after operation, has been considerably lower than that following any other type of surgical repair that has been employed (Fig. 9).

Bibliography

Cattell, R. B.: Benign strictures of the biliary ducts. J. Amer. Med. Ass., 134:235, 1947.

Smith, R.: Strictures of the bile ducts. Proc. Roy Soc. Med., 62:131, 1969.

Smith, R. and Sherlock, S.: Surgery of the Gallbladder and Bile Ducts. London: Butterworth, 1964.

Nonoperative Instrumentation of the Postoperative Biliary Tract

H. Joachim Burhenne, M.D.

Patients with indwelling tubes after surgery on the biliary tract experience a variety of complications. Instrumentation under roentgenologic control is now available to correct these conditions with the use of catheters, guidewires, wirebaskets and other equipment. The indwelling tube or its sinus tract is used for access to the biliary tract (Fig. 1). A steerable catheter is used for negotiation of the sinus tract and selective instrumentation of the intra- and extrahepatic bile ducts* (Fig. 2) [1, 2]. In order to facilitate postoperative instrumentation of the biliary tract, no T-tubes or straight-tubes with a caliber less than #14 French should be placed after choledochotomy (Fig. 3).

We have used postoperative instrumentation of the biliary tract with excellent results in a variety of conditions:

Obstruction of Indwelling Tubes

Long-term indwelling tubes in the extrahepatic ducts may become obstructed due to bile encrustation. A guidewire is then introduced through the tube in order to re-establish drainage [3]. This procedure is done during contrast cholangiography under fluoroscopic control. It is difficult in some cases to negotiate the angulation at the junction of the short and long arm of the T-tube. The tip of the guidewire tends to protrude through the wedge-shaped cut at the T-junction. Steerable guidewires or pre-shaped tips facilitate manipulation into the short arms of

---

*Medi-Tech, Inc., Watertown, Mass.

H. Joachim Burhenne, M.D., Clinical Professor, Department of Radiology, University of California School of Medicine; Chairman, Department of Radiology, Children's Hospital and Adult Medical Center, San Francisco, Calif.

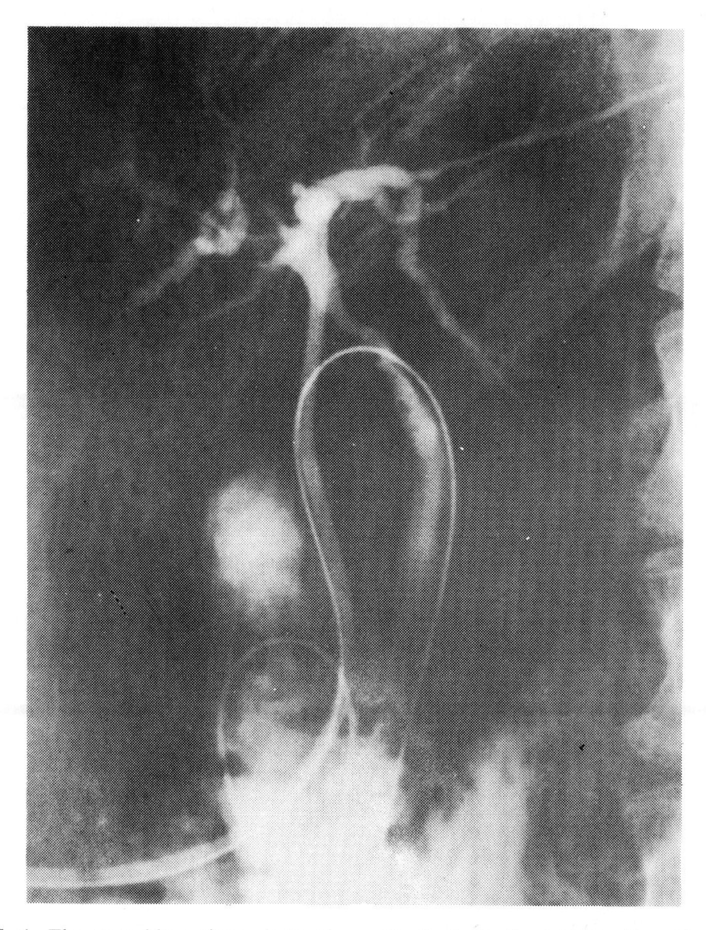

FIG. 1. The steerable catheter is in place with its tip in the left hepatic radical. A stone in the right hepatic radical was successfully extracted. A second stone just above the ampulla of Vater was also extracted. A guidewire was placed alongside the stone into the duodenum. Note the separation of catheter and guidewire at the entrance into the duct system, the point of previous T-tube placement. The folding short arms of the T-tube usually widen the opening in the duct during extraction.

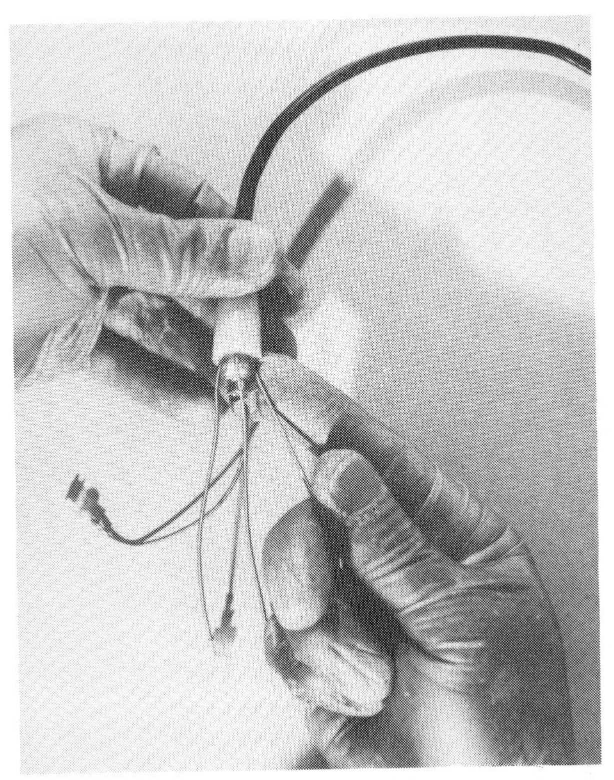

FIG. 2A. Wires embedded into the wall of the steerable catheters permit manipulation through turns in the sinus tract and bile ducts.

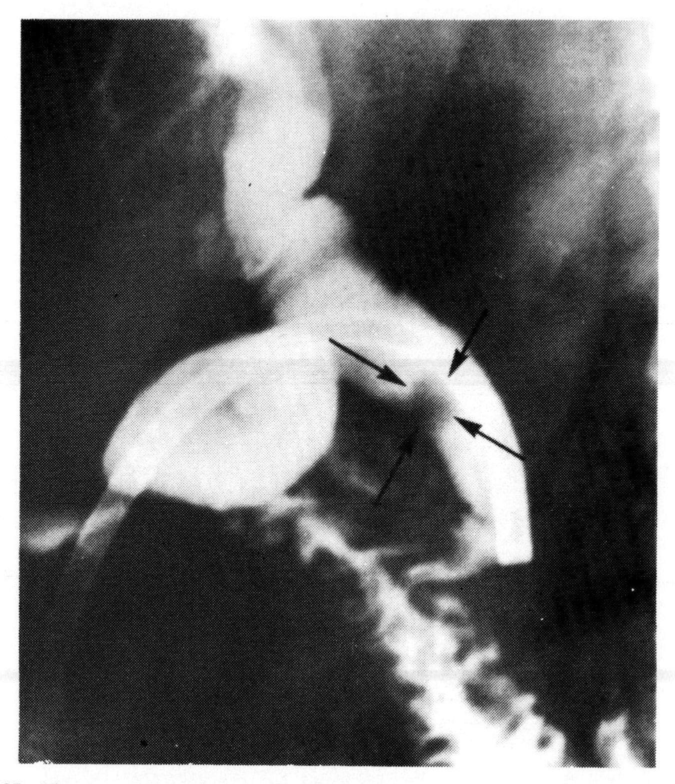

FIG. 2B. The steerable catheter has been placed beyond the retained common duct stump.

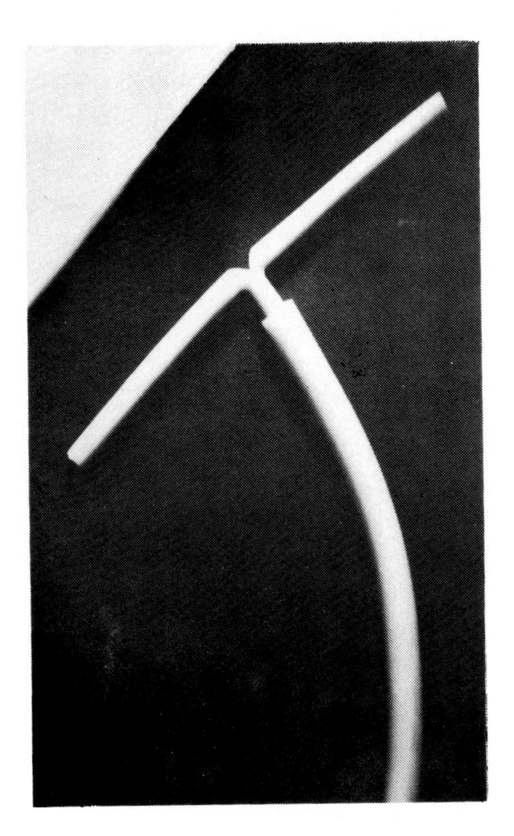

FIG. 3. Large sinus tracts for postoperative instrumentation are created by slipping a larger catheter over the long arm of the T-tube.

the T-tube. Slight traction on the T-tube is another maneuver to facilitate guidewire insertion, stretching the tube junction into a more obtuse angle (Fig. 4).

Inadvertent Tube Extraction

If the tube is inadvertently extracted, the patient is brought to the radiologic special procedure room, and a straight tube is reinserted into the extrahepatic bile duct. This can be accomplished readily within the first day or two after inadvertent extraction. The sinus tract is first negotiated with the steerable catheter. After the tip of the catheter has been placed into either the common hepatic duct or the common duct, a guidewire is inserted and the steerable catheter is extracted. A straight, preferably opaque tube is then inserted over the guidewire into the duct system. The guidewire is extracted. The straight tube may be anchored to the skin with a stitch or with a loop of adhesive tape and adhesive spray (Fig. 5).

Retained Stones

If the postoperative T-tube cholangiogram demonstrates retained intrahepatic or extrahepatic stones in the bile ducts, the T-tube is left in place for five weeks in order to accomplish a fibrous-lined tract [4]. At that time, the T-tube is extracted and the sinus tract is used for access with the steerable catheter into the bile ducts. A ureteral stone basket is then manipulated through the steerable catheter and opened distally to the retained stone (Fig. 6). The Dormia* wire basket was first used for biliary stone extraction in 1969 [5]. Stones up to 8 mm size may be extracted through a sinus tract of a #14 French T-tube. Larger stones are fragmented within the duct system using a double-sling of guidewires (Fig. 7). The fragments are extracted separately (Fig. 8). Small stones or fragments up to 4 mm in size may be expelled with a small catheter through the ampulla of Vater into the duodenum (Fig. 9). Most stones are relatively soft and fragmentation by the wire basket also occurs at the entrance to the sinus tract with the use of moderate traction (Fig. 10). Retained stones in cystic duct remnants are moved distally by erect positioning of the patient on the fluoroscopic table. They are then extracted from the distal common duct (Fig. 11). If the T-tube was placed through the cystic duct stump, manipulation is more difficult during extraction (Fig. 12). It is not recommended to place the T-tube through cystic duct remnants, although Mazzariello has had considerable success in stone extraction through the cystic duct [6].

*V. Mueller, Chicago, Ill.

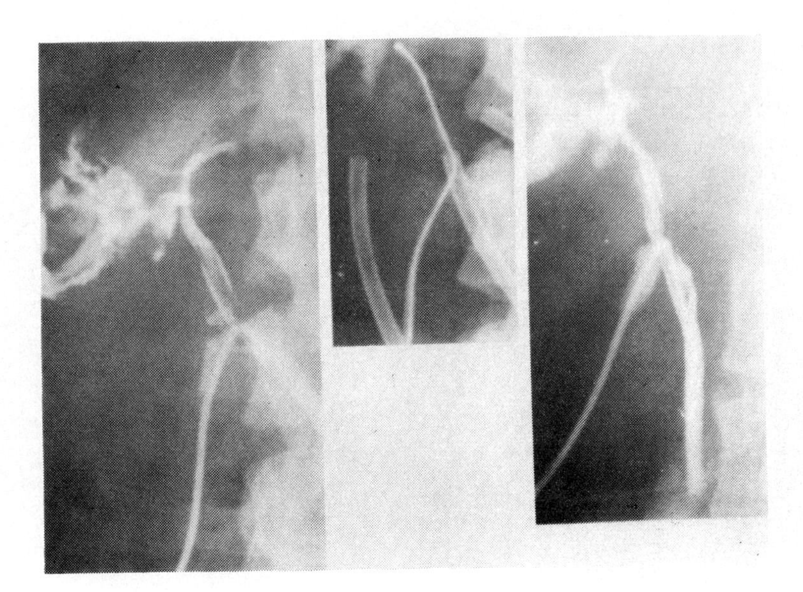

FIG. 4. A long-term indwelling T-tube for drainage of an intrahepatic abscess shows obstruction of the proximal arm. A guidewire was placed through the plugged branch of the T-tube. The final radiograph on the right shows drainage re-established. (From Margulis et al [3].)

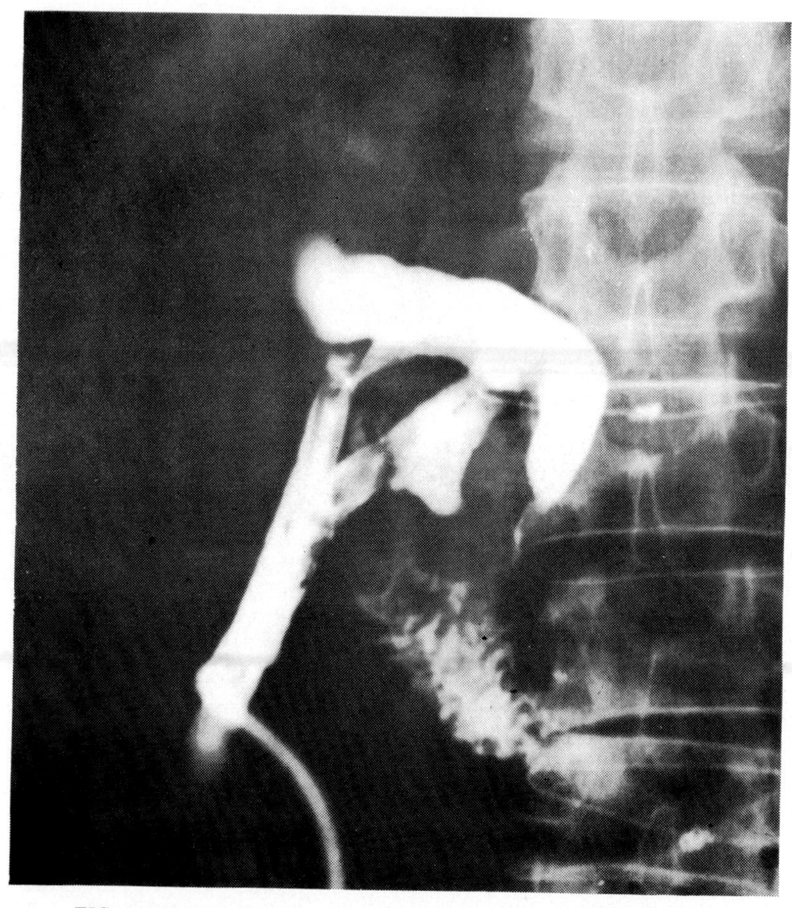

FIG. 5A. Both arms of the T-tube have slipped from the common duct.

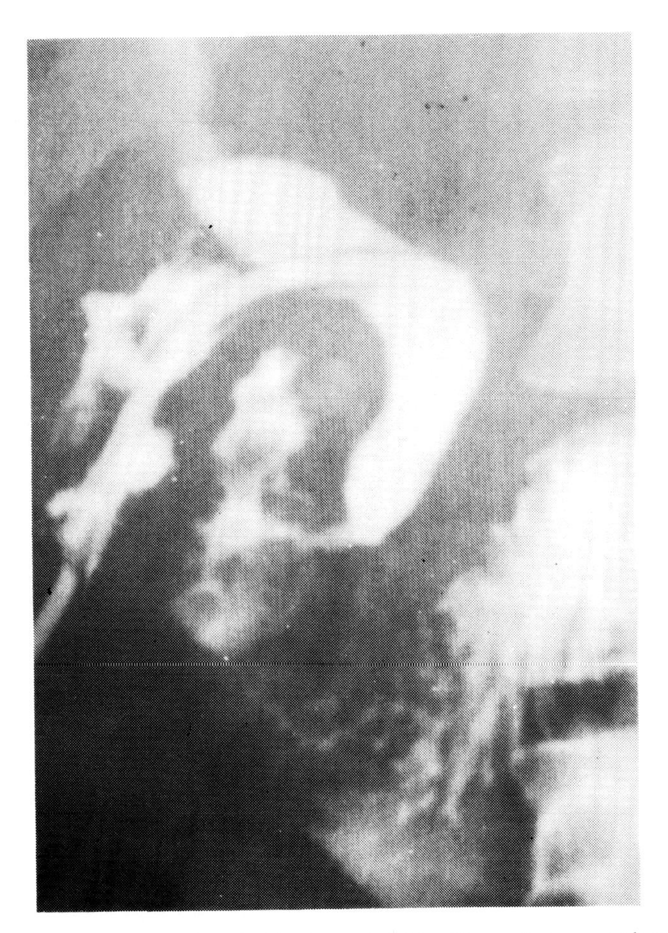

FIG. 5B. After withdrawal of the T-tube, a straight rubber catheter was placed into the common duct with the use of a steerable catheter and guidewire.

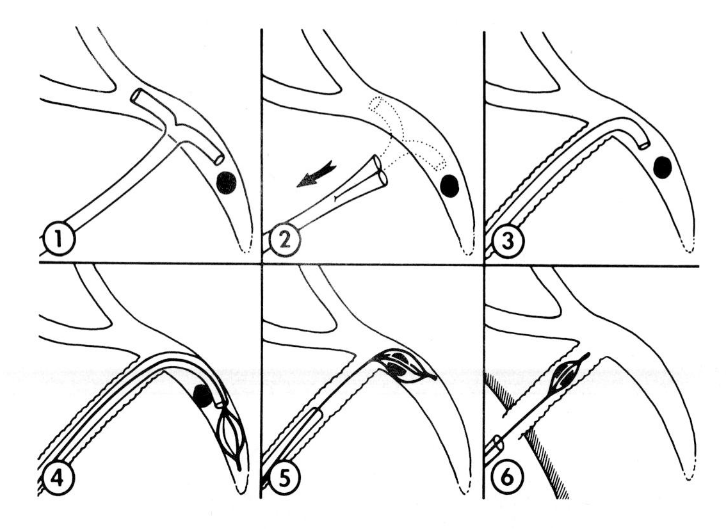

FIG. 6. Technical steps for the Burhenne stone extraction technique: 1. Repeat T-tube cholangiogram is obtained on the day of stone extraction four to five weeks after choledochotomy. 2. After the location of the retained stone has been ascertained, the T-tube is withdrawn. 3. Using the sinus tract of the T-tube, the steerable catheter is guided into the bile duct and its movable tip is advanced beyond the retained stone. 4. The basket is inserted through the steerable catheter, the catheter is withdrawn and the basket is opened. 5. The open basket is withdrawn in order to engage the stone. The basket is only retracted, never advanced, outside the enclosure of the steerable catheter. 6. The stone is extracted through the drain tract. (Reproduced with permission from *American Journal of Roentgenology, Radium Therapy and Nuclear Medicine* [117:388, 1973].)

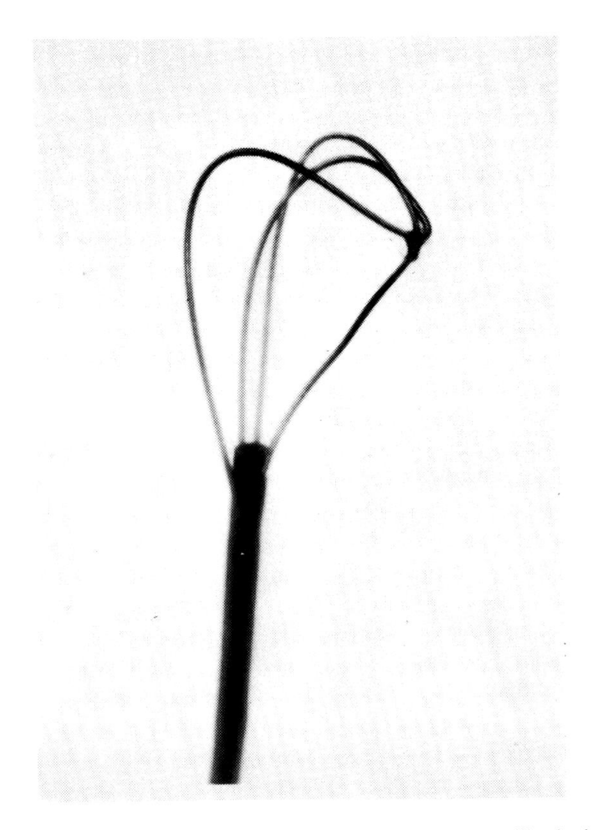

FIG. 7. A double sling formed from two guidewires with a silk tie is used for fragmentation of large stones. (From Burhenne [2].)

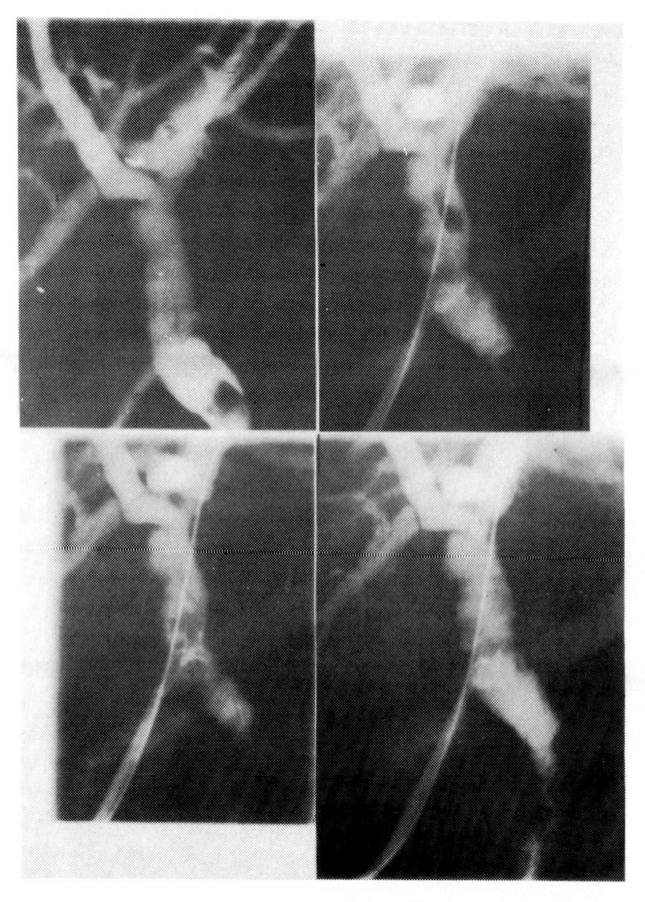

FIG. 8. A large retained common duct stone was fragmented within the duct with the use of a guidewire sling. Final radiograph shows the common duct clear after extraction of both fragments.

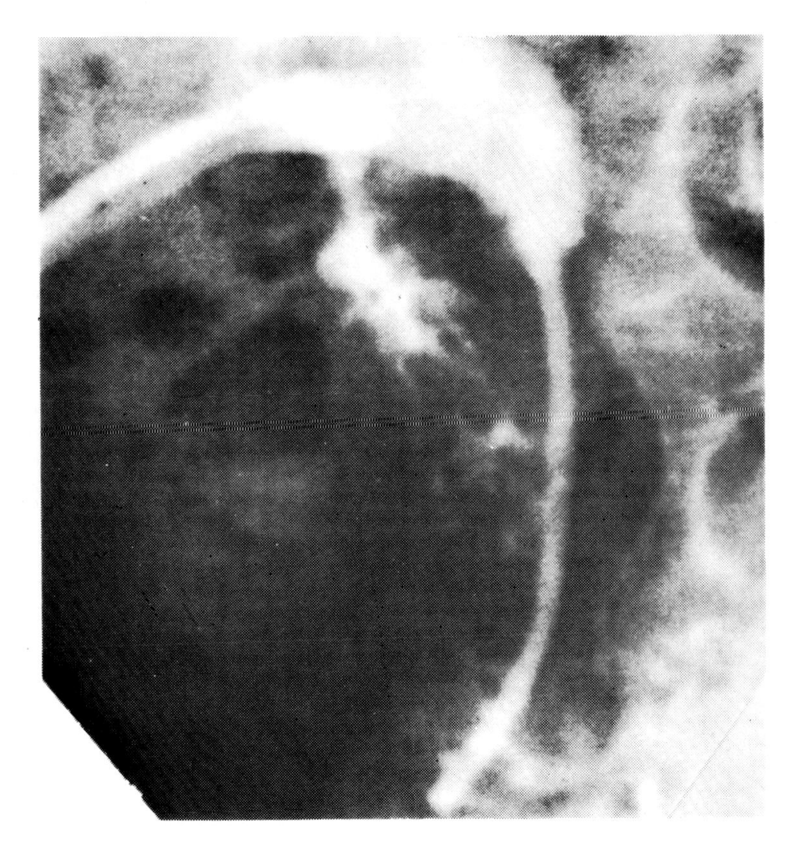

FIG. 9. A small caliber catheter may be used to expel small stones or fragments through the ampulla of Vater into the duodenum.

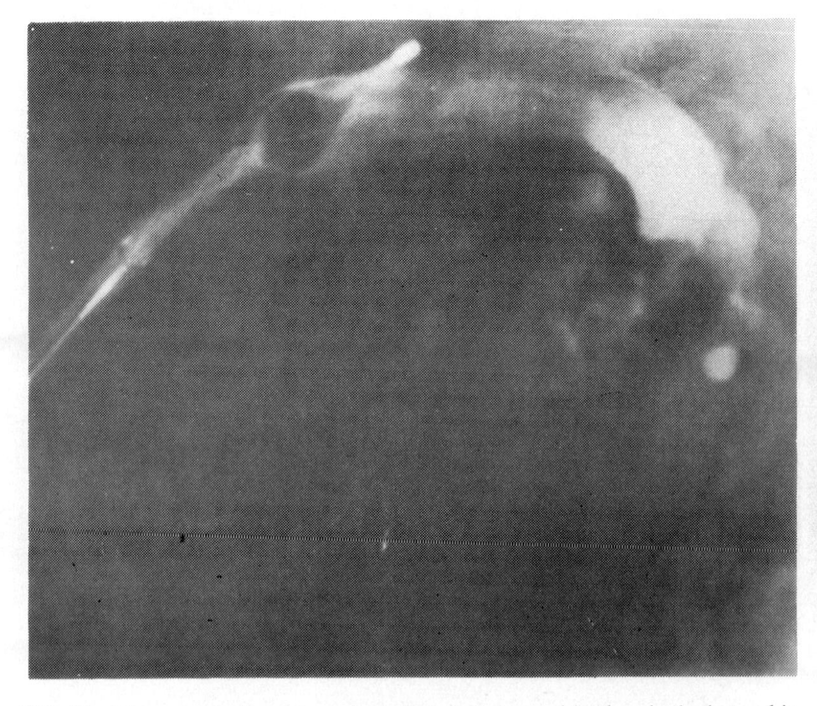

FIG. 10. A large retained common duct stone is entrapped in the wire basket and is located at the entrance to the sinus tract. Traction on the wire basket resulted in fragmentation. All fragments were successfully extracted.

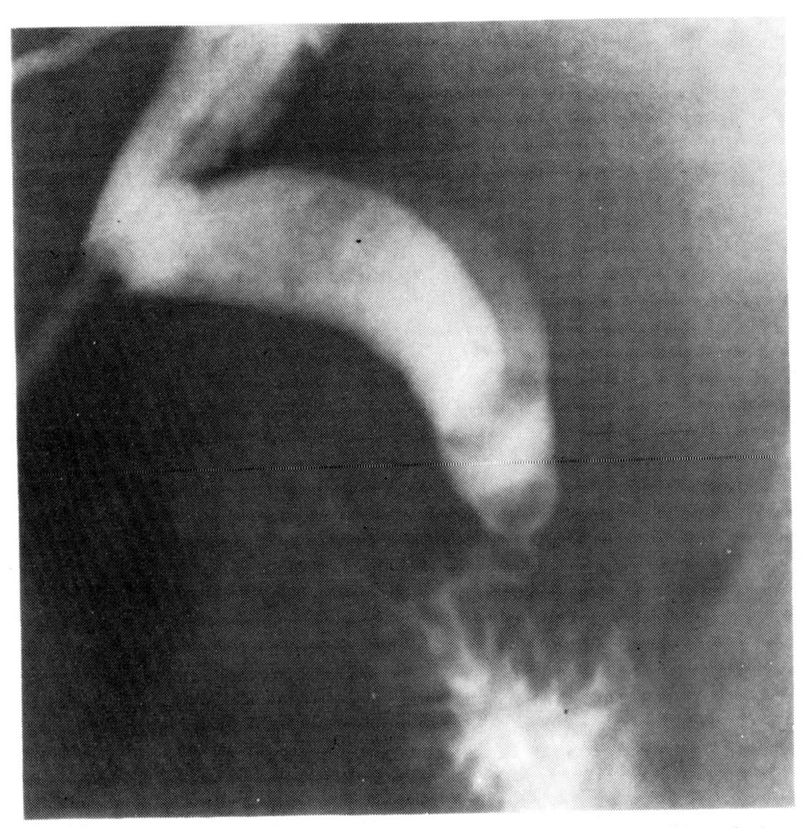

FIG. 11A. Two retained common duct stones. One of the stones moved into the large cystic duct remnant during the procedure. It was moved again into the common duct by upright positioning of the patient.

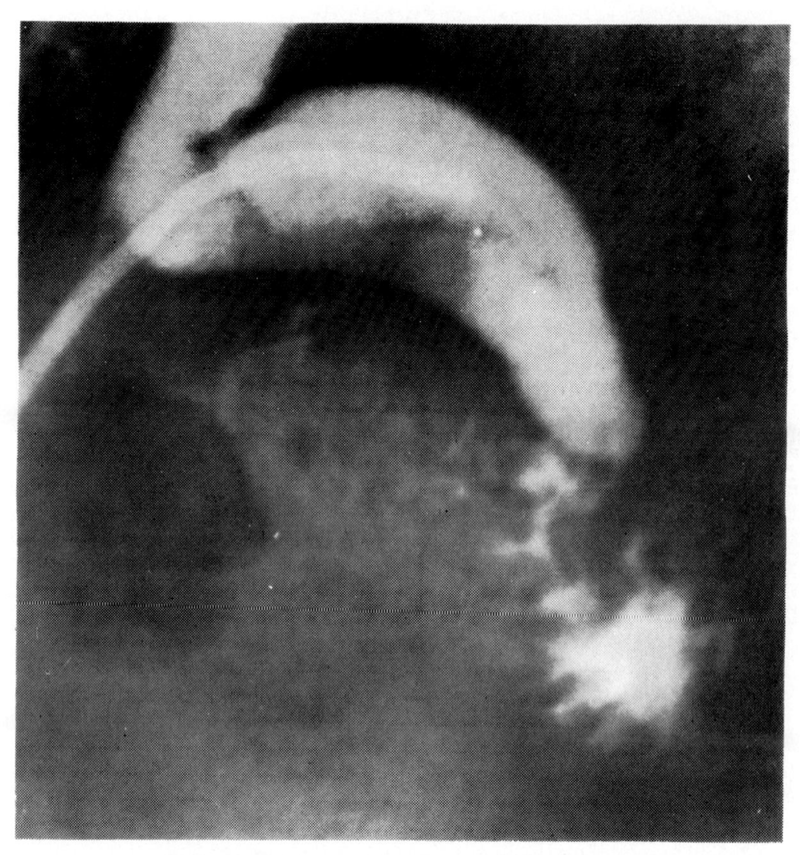

FIG. 11B. Both stones were successfully extracted.

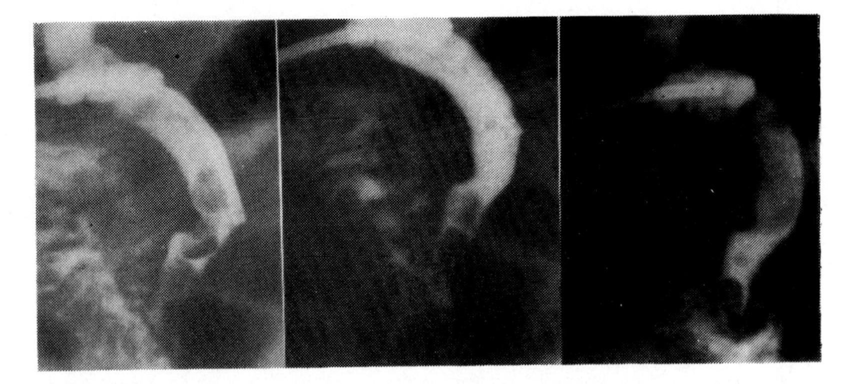

FIG. 12. Three stones were extracted from the common duct but manipulation was difficult due to T-tube placement through cystic duct remnant. Note the edema at the papilla of Vater on the final film.

Encrustation on the outside of the short arms of the T-tube within the bile ducts occurs. This material may stay behind as the catheter is extracted and is dealt with in the same way as retained stones (Fig. 13). Stones in hepatic radicals are extracted with the same technique (Fig. 14).

If the completion cholangiogram after extraction is not conclusive due to air or blood clots, a straight catheter is placed and the patient is returned one week later for a final study. This also gives small retained pieces after stone fragmentation a chance to clear spontaneously into the duodenum.

Partially impacted stones in the distal common duct are a somewhat more difficult problem. The basket is passed alongside into the duodenum before it is opened. Suction and Fogarty balloons are also helpful in these instances (Figs. 15 and 16).

We have now extracted one or more stones in all but five out of 115 patients. These five patients underwent reoperation for stone extraction. Reasons for failure were the operative use of T-tubes smaller than #12 French caliber and the placement of T-tubes through midline incisions (Fig. 17).

Complications consisted of three cases with extravasation from the sinus tract after repeated stone manipulation and extraction (Fig. 18). Two patients developed septicemia after prolonged manipulation, primarily with multiple intrahepatic stones. These patients were the only ones to receive antibiotics. No further symptoms developed. In none of the other patients was either premedication or anesthesia used. All procedures were done ambulatory.

Gallbladder Stones

Nonoperative instrumentation after surgery on the gallbladder may be of help if a cholecystostomy tube is present. Stones from the gallbladder can be removed, particularly if the patient is a poor surgical risk. We have introduced the steerable catheter through the cholecystostomy tract into the gallbladder for removal of a partially impacted gallstone in the neck of the gallbladder causing obstruction and acute cholecystitis. This was accomplished two weeks after surgery. We could not engage the stone with the wire basket. Suction through the steerable catheter was applied for successful stone removal (Fig. 19).

Biopsy

The Dormia wire basket may be used for biopsy of mucosal lesions. Postoperative instrumentation through the T-tube tract is accomplished,

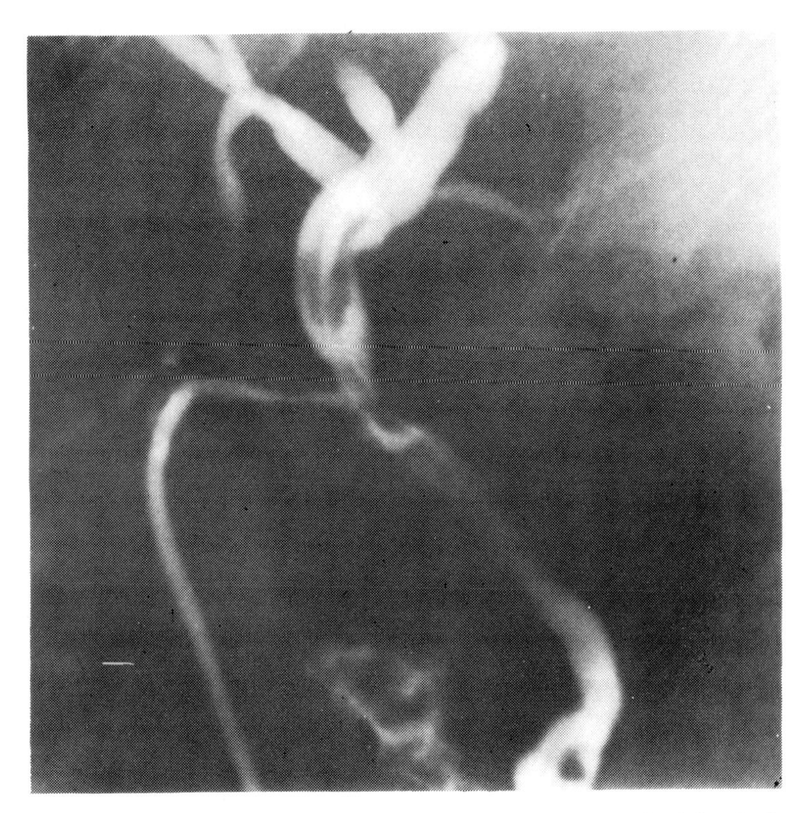

FIG. 13. Single small retained stone in the distal common duct. The defect in the common hepatic duct represents encrusted bile material on the short arm of the T-tube which remained behind after T-tube extraction.

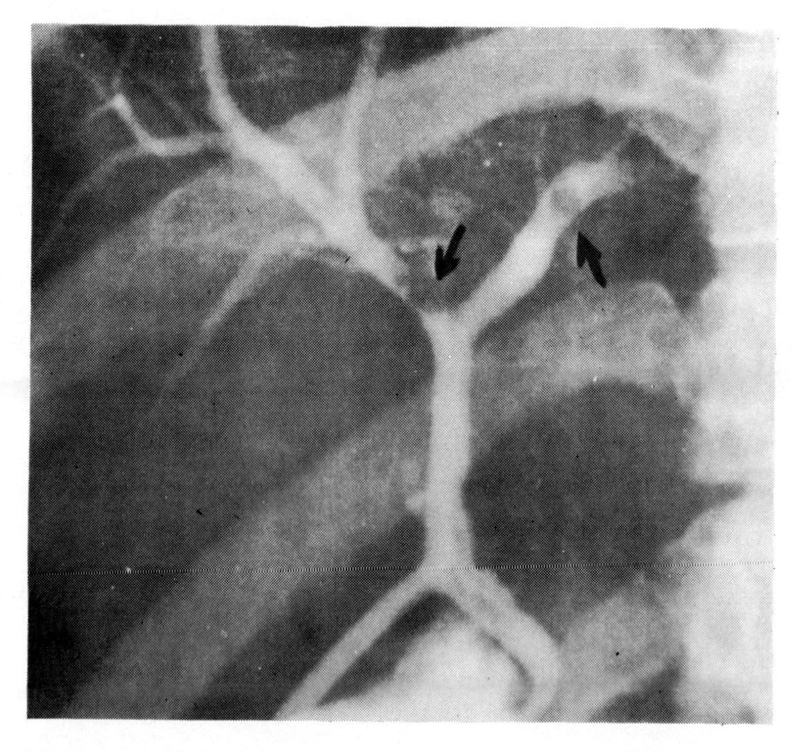

FIG. 14. Two small stones in the major hepatic radicals were successfully removed.

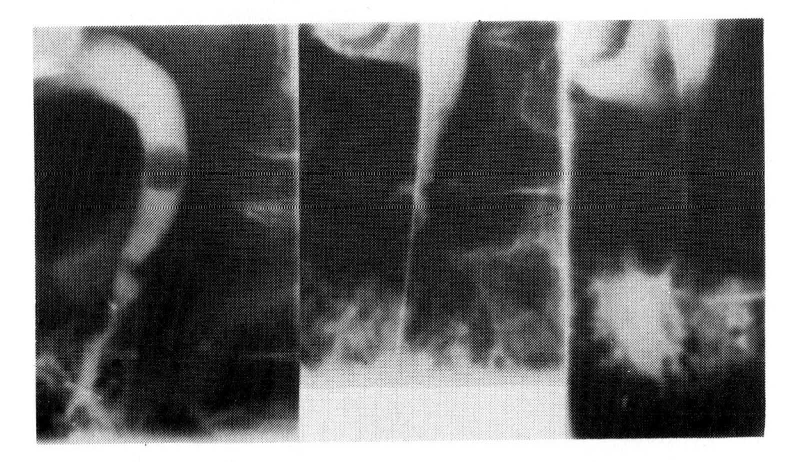

FIG. 15. Distal common duct stone impacted during the procedure was entrapped after the basket was opened within the duodenum and was successfully extracted.

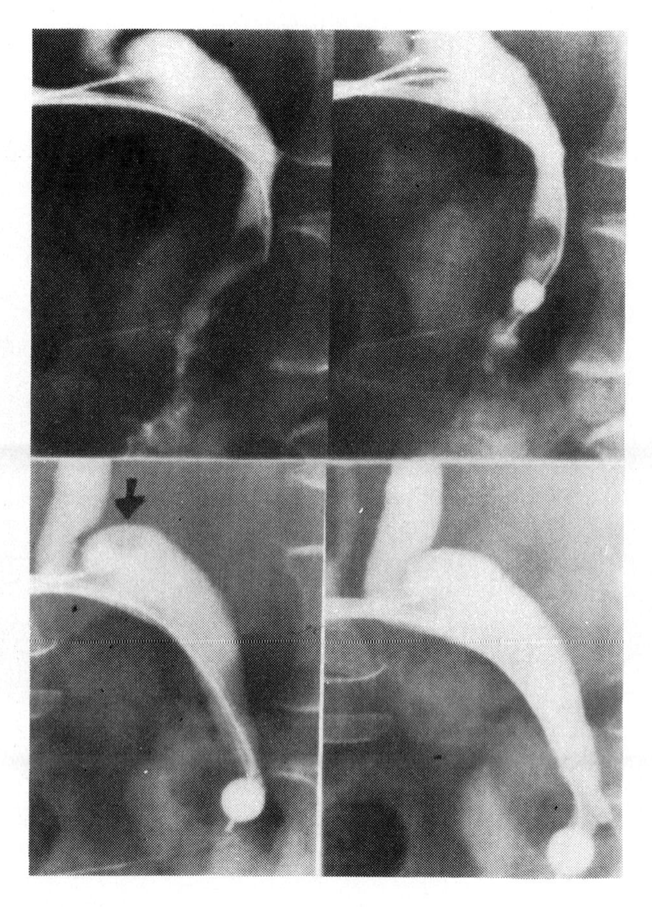

FIG. 16. A small Fogarty balloon in the distal common duct prevented stone impaction. The stone had to be moved out of the cystic duct remnant with upright patient positioning.

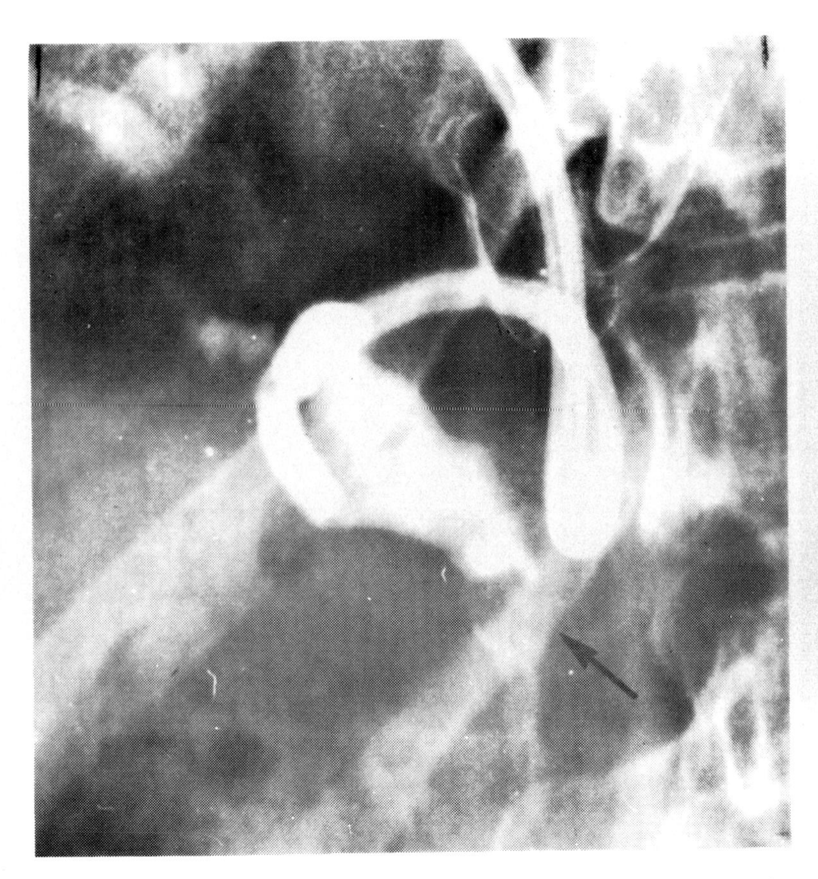

FIG. 17. Failure to extract common duct stone due to tortuous sinus tract after operative positioning of the T-tube through a midline incision.

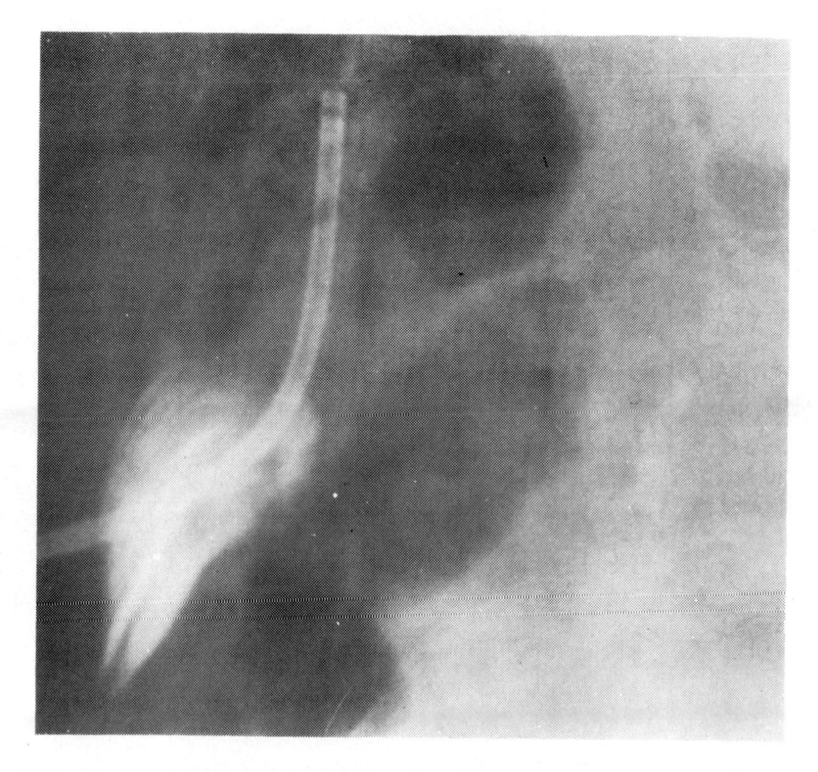

FIG. 18. Extraction of a large stone through a small sinus tract resulted in extravasation from the sinus tract, but no further complication occurred.

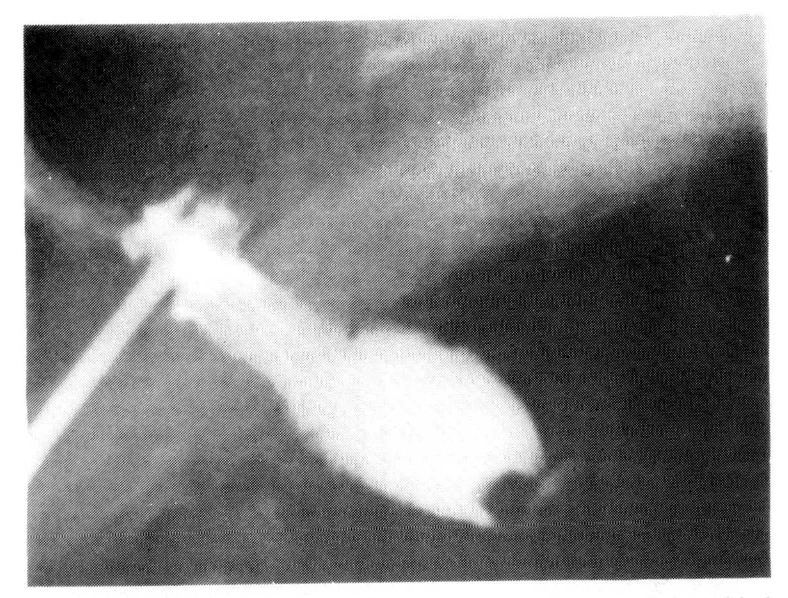

FIG. 19A. Cholecystostomy tube in place after drainage for acute cholecystitis due to impacted stone in the neck of the gallbladder.

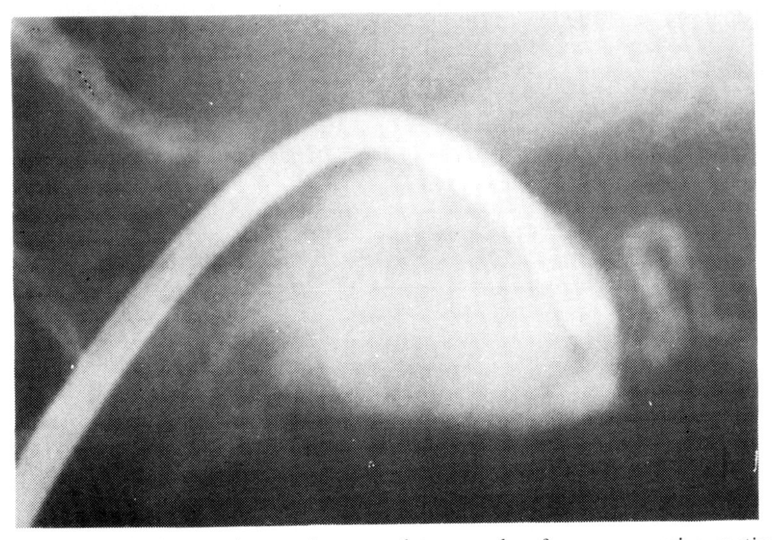

FIG. 19B. The impacted stone is removed two weeks after surgery using suction through the steerable catheter. Second surgical intervention was avoided in this patient with a poor operative risk.

and the wire basket is positioned over the lesion and then closed. The specimen is extracted (Fig. 20). We have successfully used this technique in a case with a mucosal flap in the distal common duct, which was apparently raised during operative bougienage and instrumentation of the distal common duct. This procedure clarified the differential diagnosis between retained stone and mucosal injury. A second surgical intervention was avoided.

Strictures

Nonoperative instrumentation with small dilatation balloon catheters through the steerable catheter lends itself to the treatment of bile duct strictures. We have used this technique in eight patients. Two patients had iatrogenic strictures of the extrahepatic bile ducts, three had strictures of the intrahepatic left main radical and three patients had strictures at hepatojejunostomy sites.

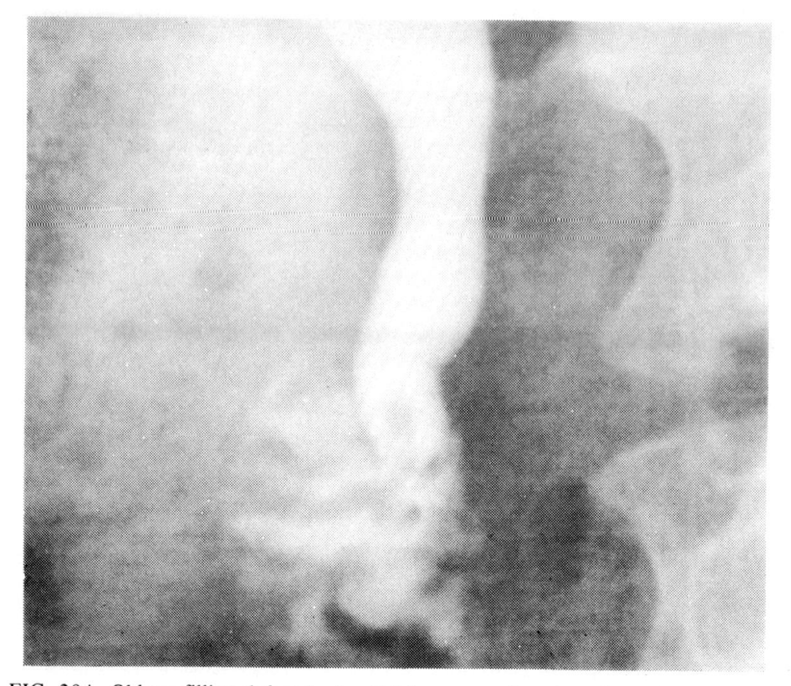

FIG. 20A. Oblong filling defect in the distal common duct just above the ampulla of Vater.

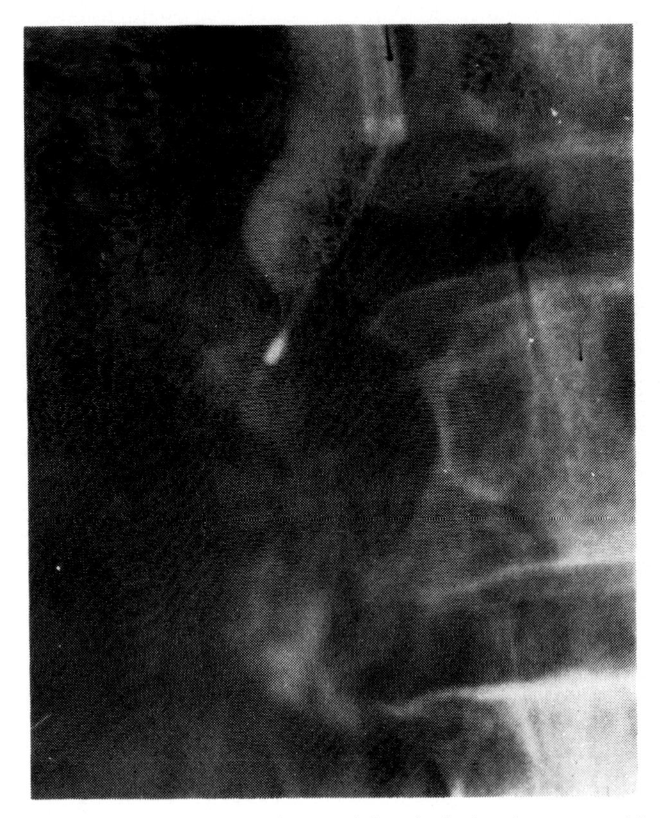

FIG. 20B. Biopsy of the lesion by closure of the wire basket demonstrated it to be a raised mucosal flap after operative instrumentation.

The steerable catheter is first manipulated through the sinus tract to the stricture. The balloon catheter is then advanced through the first catheter and is inflated within the stricture. The use of contrast within the dilatation balloon* permits controlled expansion visible on the fluoroscopic screen. Some strictures need two or three sessions in order to dilate to a normal caliber of 6 or 8 mm. Balloon retention catheters are then left in place for long periods of time in order for the scarring at the stricture or anastomosis to mature (Fig. 21). Two of our patients with previous strictures at hepatojejunostomy sites have had the indwelling catheter in

*Edwards Laboratories, Santa Ana, Calif.

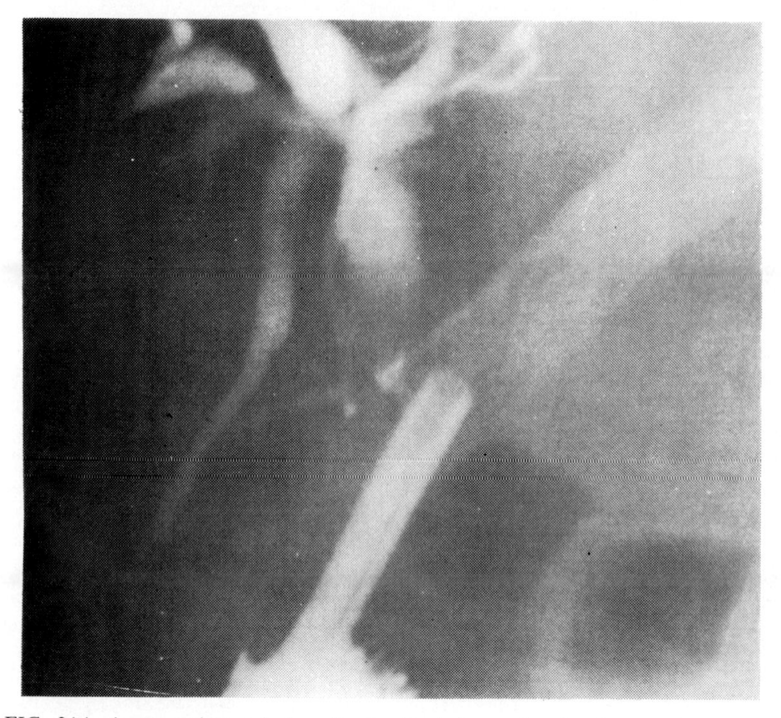

FIG. 21A. 1 mm stricture in jaundiced patient six weeks after hepatojejunostomy. The straight catheter splint had moved into the jejunum.

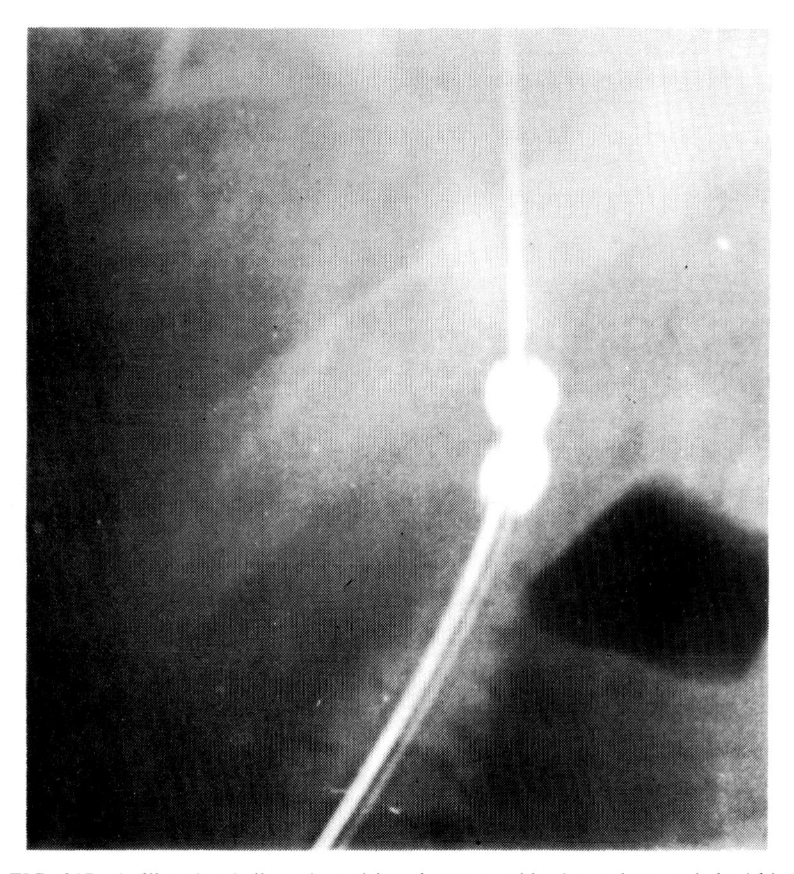

FIG. 21B. A dilatation balloon is positioned over a guidewire and expanded within the stricture. In two separate sessions, the stricture was dilated to a caliber of 8 mm.

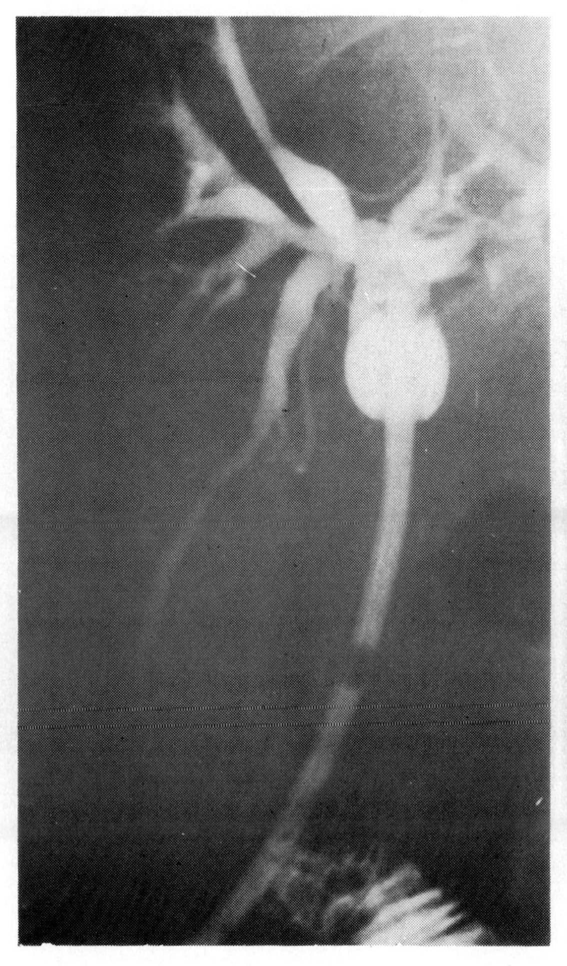

FIG. 21C. Plastic-coated retention catheter in place 12 months after stricture dilatation with the contrast-filled retention balloon above the hepatojejunostomy. Bile drainage into the jejunum is established through a side-hole in the catheter.

place for slightly over one year. Plastic coated catheters* are used for this purpose with side-holes for internal drainage. The catheter is changed every three months. It extrudes from the jejunostomy site and is closed with a plastic plug permitting irrigation.

Further experience is needed to see if the caliber of the dilated previous strictures can be maintained. We contemplate withdrawing the retention catheters into the jejunum after about 18 months to see if a stricture should recur. Repeat of the nonoperative instrumentation would be feasible in this way if indicated.

References

1. Burhenne, H. J.: Extraktion von Residualsteinen der Gallenwege ohne Reoperation. Fortschr. Roentgenstr., 117:425, 1972.
2. Burhenne, H. J.: Nonoperative retained biliary tract stone extraction: A new roentgenologic technique. Amer. J. Roentgen., 117:388, 1973.
3. Margulis, A. R., Newton, T. H. and Najarian, J. S.: Removal of plug from T-tube by fluoroscopically controlled catheter. Amer. J. Roentgen., 93:975, 1965.
4. Mazzariello, R.: Removal of residual biliary tract calculi without reoperation. Surgery, 67:566, 1970.
5. Lagrave, G. et al: Lithiase biliaire résiduelle. Extraction à la sonde de Dormia par le drain de Kehr. Mem. Acad. Chir., 95:430, 1969.
6. Mazzariello, R.: Transcholecystic extraction of residual calculi in common bile duct. Surgery, 75:338, 1974.

*Dow Corning Corp. Med. Prod., Midland, Mich.

Panel Discussion

Moderator: **J. P. Delaney, M.D.**

Panelists: **R. M. Zollinger, M.D.** **M. L. Gliedman, M.D.**
F. G. Moody, M.D. **M. M. Eisenberg, M.D.**
R. Smith, M.D. **H. J. Burhenne, M.D.**

Dr. Delaney: Let us poll the panelists on the clinical significance of adenomyomas in the gallbladder.

Mr. Smith: I think that there is a variety of adenomyosis which can certainly assume formidable proportions. I operated on a girl in her 20s with a gallbladder wall literally 2 cm thick. Now, that is gross pathology, even without gallstones. Nobody could really argue about performing cholecystectomy. If, however, I operate on a patient because I think on clinical grounds that the x-rays may be wrong, that there might be stones, and if having removed the gallbladder, a cooperative pathologist describes some mild inflammatory changes in its wall, I feel very unhappy about the results. In general the results of removing a gallbladder in this group without stones are bad.

Dr. Delaney: Dr. Zollinger, if you see a patient with supposed biliary tract pain and an adenomyoma on the x-ray, is that cause to make you operate?

Dr. Zollinger: I think I would probably fudge on that for a little while. I certainly would look over the rest of the GI tract. I would get somebody to hold my hand, such as a gastroenterologist, I suppose, and then I would put it off for a while. I don't think that I would be in a hurry to operate on such a patient.

Dr. Moody: I think that one of the things that we overlook is the fact that many patients evacuate their gallbladders continuously. Studies from South America reported (*New Eng. J. Med.,* 290:484-487, 1974) a few months ago support this possibility. I guess that an acalculus gallbladder may have discharged its stones.

Dr. Delaney: Dr. Eisenberg, there are several questions about how one should go about biopsying the common bile duct. It is already narrow in the circumstance of sclerosing cholangitis.

Dr. Eisenberg: I am glad that somebody asked that question. There is frequently a sclerotic reaction surrounding the bile duct that can be biopsied but, in any event, you are operating on a patient for jaundice and the bile duct has to be opened and explored; cholangiography has to be done. There really should be no problem in getting a full thickness biopsy of the wall during the course of exploration of the common bile duct. In addition, there are frequently lymph nodes to be found surrounding the sclerotic process and they, too, can be sent for biopsy. I hope that I emphasized in my presentation that even biopsy is a nonspecific way of making the diagnosis. The diagnosis is a retrospective one, in most instances. It is only after a number of years, when the patient has been shown not to have carcinoma, that one can safely say that one is dealing with primary sclerotic cholangitis.

Dr. Gliedman: I took care of one patient, who fulfilled all of Dr. Eisenberg's criteria. This patient is a young man who had asymptomatic ulcerative colitis and then went on to develop jaundice. He had, first, a cholecystojejunostomy, with the diagnosis of primary sclerosing cholangitis. This closed off, and he went on to have a t-tube passed into the liver through the sclerotic extrahepatic biliary tree; that eventually became encased. He then had an anastomosis up higher between his jejunum and one of the ducts to one lobe; that closed off. An attempted Longmire procedure was unsuccessful, because the entire liver was a mass of scar. He then had 17 bleeds from varices, which we controlled through a variety of mechanisms. He represents one of the patients whom I shall present with an "H" shunt as a prelude to a liver transplant. The point that I want to make is that he was treated with steroids to the extent that he couldn't get out of bed because he was so osteoporotic. At that time, we reviewed what the objective effects were of steroids in this group of patients and felt convinced that they did nothing. In this patient, it did nothing except to keep him totally bedridden during the brief time he had.

Dr. Delaney: Another question for you, Dr. Gliedman: Has the minilaparotomy, as a diagnostic tool, been replaced by the retrograde cholangiogram?

Dr. Gliedman: I am not sure that it has because on occasion, you can't do things with the retrograde cholangiogram that you do with the minilap. In our area, the minilap is a relatively popular procedure. Either in x-ray or in the operating room, you make a small incision under local anesthesia, do a transhepatic cholangiogram or liver biopsy. You can extend the procedure as much as your vigor allows and then, on this basis, you proceed either immediately or subsequently to a bigger operation. The rationale for the procedure, particularly by Dr. Del Gercio at the Albert Einstein College of Medicine, was that there just wasn't enough time to formally explore all the patients who had undiagnosed jaundice. So this became a popular approach. However, I do think that the retrograde approach reduces the number needing the approach. The typical case is the patient we saw within the last two weeks with icterus up to 25 mg%, almost all of it direct. The patient had a markedly elevated alkaline phosphatase. He had longstanding lymphosarcoma and was on a number of drugs. The argument as to diagnosis went on and on. Before exploration we asked for a retrograde study. The retrograde study showed a perfectly normal extrahepatic ductal system. He then had a needle liver biopsy. It showed noncaseating granulomas. He then had a bone marrow biopsy. It showed the same thing. The diagnosis did not require a laparotomy or minilap.

Dr. Eisenberg: Just recently, we returned from San Francisco, where I heard a report on 42 retrograde cholangiographic studies. It brought home to me the fact that we here, in Minnesota, are so completely at home with the retrograde study that we have come to take it for granted. I don't know Dr. Vennes' exact figures. But I would believe that we have seen many retrograde cholangiograms. Many are done every week. I no longer operate on any jaundiced patient, without asking for a retrograde study. I see no reason, with the availability of that technic, to "fly blind" in the abdomen.

Dr. Delaney: Here is a question which has been asked many times, so I am going to poll the panel, as to whether a cystic duct cholangiogram should be done, if definite indications for common bile duct exploration are present. If so, does a normal study then eliminate the need for doing the common bile duct exploration?

Dr. Zollinger: I think that if there is an indication for exploration of the common duct (and there are at least eight or ten), I wouldn't do a cholangiogram first. In the presence of little stones, I would go ahead and explore the common duct. If the stones are good sized, then I might do a cholangiogram, feeling that maybe the ductal system had deviated a little bit in the presence of a nonfunctioning gallbladder.

Dr. Gliedman: We do more and more cystic duct cholangiograms. It has several advantages. One is that it sometimes will tell you what you are going to look for. The other thing that it does, which hasn't been mentioned to this point, is demonstrate patency into the duodenum. On some cholangiograms that you get after instrumentation, you can't document that there is emptying into the duodenum. At that point, the surgeon may be prompted to do a choledochotomy. With the cystic duct cholangiogram showing free passage before there is a lot of playing around with the distal end of the common duct, you've got some benefit in not proceeding further with big surgical maneuvers.

Mr. Smith: I would do a cystic duct cholangiogram, first, in most cases. The reason would be similar to the one just given. If one knows that there is a stone or several stones in the common bile duct, and you open that duct and you get the stones out, and then, just to be thorough, you pass a probe down the duct and it won't go into the duodenum through the sphincter, you may have to do a sphincterotomy. The one thing about which you can be quite sure is that after there has been any interference with the biliary apparatus, the duodenal wall will go into spasm at the lower end, and you will have lost all chance of seeing clearly that important segment of the lower end. If you do a preliminary cholangiogram, before you have interfered with the biliary tree at all, this gives you your best chance of having an accurate radiological guide of what the distal duct looks like. Even if I know that there are several stones present, I would like to have a cholangiogram at the start of the operation.

Dr. Moody: I agree with Mr. Smith's reasoning, except that there is a new wrinkle, now, with the retrograde cholangiogram – the catheter goes through the lower end. We have usually accepted the fact that, in these cases, it is spasm. Do you agree, Mr. Smith?

Mr. Smith: You don't always get a good cholangiogram from below, with this retrograde technique. Quite often, the catheter goes into the pancreatic duct, and you get a beautiful pancreatogram. Try as you will, you cannot always engage the end in the duct that you really want to see.

Dr. Delaney: Dr. Burhenne, since you don't operate, at least, in the fashion that we do . . .

Dr. Burhenne: Dr. Delaney, perhaps I should answer this question because I don't operate. What the question really refers to is: What does routine operative cholangiography mean? What it means, in surgical terms, is to do operative cholangiography in every single case of cholecystectomy, before you make a decision as to whether to explore the common duct or not. In the surgical literature, you will find that the accuracy of operative cholangiography is higher than that of clinical signs. So if you had to rely on only one test, you would rather rely on the x-ray. Why not get the full yield and combine the two? No radiologist and no surgeon, for that matter, should be asked to interpret an x-ray after exploration of the common duct system. Spasm at the distal end is particularly bothersome.

Retrograde studies, even if they are done on the day before surgery, fall into the same category as intravenous cholangiograms done 24 hours before surgery. Stones may move in the duct system from one hour to the next. I can show you a good number of cases where the surgeon relied on the position of the stone in the distal common duct from the intravenous cholangiogram, explored the duct and couldn't find the stone. It had moved in one of the hepatic radicals. It was even missed on the postexploration, or so-called postcholedochotomy cholangiogram. It was only on the t-tube study that it became apparent. I think that surgeons interested in this topic will tell you that routine operative cholangiography means doing it in every single patient from whom you remove the gallbladder.

Dr. Delaney: To pursue that a little further, how confident can you be when the radiologist assures you that it is a normal operative cholangiogram?

Dr. Burhenne: The false negative and the false positive, about 4% each, should not disturb you. You are still talking about a 90%-92% accuracy of x-ray, alone. Why don't you combine the x-ray with the clinical indications and get all the information you can get? Besides, all you need is one good case to remember, where the radiologist on the precholedochotomy cholangiogram showed you the right radical entering the cystic duct, and you were ready to cut that duct close to the common duct. You will never forget that case as an indication for routine operative cholangiography.

Dr. Eisenberg: At the risk of disagreeing with Dr. Zollinger . . .

Dr. Delaney: That is risky!

Dr. Eisenberg: I really can't add much, except to emphasize what was just said. The point that I wanted to make is that I am uncomfortable operating on the biliary tree, beyond simple cholecystectomy, without knowing what kind of anatomy I am dealing with. I like, therefore, to have a completely satisfactory retrograde cholangiogram, which I do think has value. In the very ill, very jaundiced and the very toxic patient, it can save a lot of valuable operating and anesthesia time. I am willing to risk the movement of stone and take that (retrograde cholangiography) as a satisfactory preliminary study. But I virtually never open the common duct without knowing first what anatomy I am dealing with.

Dr. Moody: What I hear coming out of this is that cholangiography should be used on almost every cholecystectomy. If that is so, shouldn't we have modern equipment, with all of the nice things they have in the x-ray department?

Dr. Burhenne: Yes, I am glad to have the opportunity to answer that. We use the image intensifier, of course, for removal of these retained stones. The stone, however, that is 3 mm or 4 mm is not seen on the television screen. But if you take one spot film, it hits you in the eye! Detail can be seen in the ratio of 10:1, spot films compared to television. The television helps you in gauging your contrast injection to get more optimal films. But I don't think that you will pick up more stones by having a television in surgery. The spot film device will still be your critical attachment on that machine, if you have the money to buy it.

The best book on operative cholangiography was written by Dr. Schulenburg, a surgeon from South Africa. He used a 15-MA portable machine, outdated equipment, but he has a routine that works: He has a tunnel under the patient. He takes a preliminary film, as was mentioned by Dr. Zollinger, which is so important. It is done before anesthesia is started, so you don't prolong anesthesia and the technician has a chance to adjust his films. The operative cholangiogram consists of two films, exchanged through the tunnel, the patient is not moved, the anesthetist can rotate the patient 15° to the right. Of those 115 patients, where we have extracted stones, we insisted upon getting the operative cholangiograms. We were successful in slightly over 100 patients. I was surprised to learn that that many were taken. But the main reason, we found, that stones were missed was poor operative cholangiography technique. They were underexposed, they were poorly collimated, no lateral grids were used, the vertical grid lines obscure detail as you rotate the patient. The contrast was not properly diluted. It is not the fancy equipment that is so important. The important thing is to develop a routine that both the surgeon and the radiologist can live with and use it every day, not only just occasionally.

Mr. Smith: Dr. Delaney, may I comment? You know, I am, myself, an enthusiastic operative cholangiographist. But we mustn't get too technology minded. However good the pictures, however good the apparatus, it is only one element in diagnosis. I am sure that all radiologists would agree with that. The radiologist can only tell you what he thinks he sees. It must be put against the previous history of the patient and what the surgeon sees at operation. He can say what he sees, but he cannot tell the surgeon whether he ought or ought not to open the common bile duct. It is very important to say this because, in some centers, not in Minneapolis of course, a radiologist may tend to confuse having the last word with being the last word.

Dr. Burhenne: I shall accept this challenge for the last word. I think what we were talking about is not whether the radiologist says that the cholangiogram gives you all the information. The question was, will you do a cholangiogram in every case where you explore the common duct? And that answer is affirmative because why should you deprive yourself of extra information?

Dr. Delaney: I am sure that the pathologists would challenge you two as having the true last word. Mr. Smith, is there such a thing as fibrosis or stenosis of the sphincter of Oddi which causes symptoms, causes pain, but nothing else?

Mr. Smith: I am sure that fibrosis of the sphincter of Oddi exists but usually when it exists, it is because somebody else has been much too enthusiastic with metal dilators on a previous occasion. This lesion is common. Spontaneous fibrosis of the sphincter of Oddi, or localized inflammatory reaction, Odditis, perhaps has some place. But I think that it is extremely rare. I was impressed with a paper about two or three years ago in a British journal, where a group had gone to the trouble of examining a series of removed duodenums with the attached lower end of the bile duct at a large number of autopsies. Sections through the sphincter of Oddi and papilla had shown various things, papillitis, fibrosis, and so forth. Then they correlated these findings against the past histories of the patients and found that there was no relation whatsoever between what the pathologist said that he had seen and the symptoms. I don't believe that primary fibrosis or papillitis is a common condition at all. If, however, a surgeon when he has opened the common duct passes metal dilators down, and if the dilator doesn't drop through, forcibly dilates the sphincter of Oddi, I think in a proportion of these cases a false passage is made between the common duct and the duodenum. Submucosal extravasation can then lead to quite a dense stricture. You can, if you wish, call this fibrosis of the sphincter of Oddi. In other words, patients at the beginning of the operation may not have fibrosis of the sphincter, but many of them may have it as the result of surgery.

Dr. Delaney: Dr. Zollinger, would you like to comment?

Dr. Zollinger: Dr. Charles Branch, of Peoria, Illinois, and I studied this in animals "right after the Civil War," and we found that, indeed, every time we passed a big probe through the papilla, we had hemorrhage and a much higher perfusion pressure, and ended up with marked scarring. Since that time, we have had great respect for the sphincter and never do anything more than determine its patency. We make no effort to dilate it forcibly, and we certainly never push through a large dilator. We use a very firm French woven catheter, maybe a No. 8 or a No. 10, but certainly no bigger than a No. 12, and we do it very gently. I agree with Mr. Smith; I think that a lot of damage is done by overdilatation of the ampulla. Certainly this room would be pretty empty if we said we were going to pass a No. 50 sound up the urethra of those in attendance. I think the same thing should apply to the papilla of Vater as well.

Dr. Eisenberg: I cannot argue with anyone who says that mechanical dilatation of the sphincter or dilatation of the sphincter or stone passing through the sphincter can cause fibrosis. But, on the other hand, Dr. Richard Egdahl did report 12 or 13 cases of primary papillitis or Odditis. While I was initially skeptical about the description of the patients in the pathologic studies that he presented, I have since seen such a patient that I think meets his criteria. I agree with Mr. Smith that it is rare. But I think that, probably, it does occur and it should not be simply discarded as a nonentity.

Dr. Moody: I don't think that you should overlook Dr. Nardi's data that came out about ten years ago (*Ann. Surg.,* 164:611-617, 1966). They did find, in patients who had gallstones, and presumably the stones had passed on through the sphincter of Oddi, that there was scarring, histologically. They did do an autopsy series in patients who did not have demonstrable biliary tract disease and they found no scarring in the papilla. So there is that little piece of evidence to suggest that people with stones may develop a papillitis.

Dr. Gliedman: I am curious to know whether the next step from this is: Is there such an entity as ampullary stenosis? The characterization in our institution is the patient who has had a previous cholecystectomy, has not had a common duct exploration, returns later with an elevated bilirubin, an elevated alkaline phosphatase, a dilated common duct, and, on intravenous cholangiography, shows progressive opacification of the common bile duct lasting for hours. That is, the duct gets progressively more dense with time rather than tapering off within an hour. Does the panel think that there is an entity of ampullary stenosis, as I have described it?

Dr. Moody: I would like to comment on that, if I may. I think that there is such an entity in patients who have had stones residing at the lower end of the common bile duct for a long period of time. They are unusual, but I believe that they do exist. Dr. White would probably jump up and say, "Yes, they are the ones on whom I do a sphincteroplasty." I have certainly seen such cases.

Mr. Smith: I think that the evidence, as presented, would undoubtedly make one decide that there must be an obstruction at the lower end. If you have icterus and you have a duct that is wider than normal, you have a high alkaline phosphatase, and you have a delay in emptying, then I would say, yes, certainly, I would accept that. I would be suspicious that at the last operation, when the gallbladder was removed, that there had been instrumentation. But if one is quite certain that that is not so, then, all right, we have one of those rare lesions. The only thing that I would say is that they are rare.

Dr. Delaney: Dr. Gliedman, this question is for you: The statement is that the Penrose drain is a two-way street. It lets serum and blood out and it lets bacteria in. What is your comment on that?

Dr. Gliedman: I think that the statement is correct. The best data, I think, would be that at 48 hours, it seems like you are clearing from inside out, but by somewhere around four or five days, the odds are better that you are moving from outside in. Certainly, the rapid removal of drains is appropriate. I won't take issue with the statement. It really is correct. If you don't really feel that there is a need to drain, you probably should not do so. The general idea of draining the peritoneal cavity is, in my opinion, a useless concept. We really use drains under limited circumstances, just because of the very statement that you have made.

Mr. Smith: I was glad to hear someone in the audience say "Hemovac." There is a great deal of difference between a Penrose drain and a very small vacuum drain left in for 24 hours and then taken out again if there is nothing significant coming out of it. I, personally, do not use a Penrose drain. I nearly always use a suction-type drain.

Dr. Zollinger: How can you afford to use it, Mr. Smith?

Dr. Gliedman: Aside from affording it, I don't think that hard catheters are innocuous. They can erode into bowel or vessels. I think that there are areas where it should be used, but not as a routine. I, personally, had a disaster as a result of my early enthusiasm for suction catheters. I have therefore become much less enthusiastic. This is not a problem with the soft drain.

Dr. Delaney: I have a number of questions about the significance of cholesterol crystals in duodenal aspirate. Would the panel care to comment on that?

Dr. Zollinger: I don't know anything about it.

Mr. Smith: I have had no experience, at all, with this.

Dr. Gliedman: Not in the surgical department, but our gastroenterology department does a large number, dropping through a Rehfuss' tube, and collecting the effluent from the duodenum. They are quite good. Once the resident can identify a cholesterol crystal, which is a very specific thing, a rectangle with a little corner broken off, it is an excellent test. I commend its use to everyone. It is just that it is better if someone else has to do it. But if you do get the data, it is useful.

Dr. Zollinger: But you have never seen one, Dr. Gliedman?

Dr. Gliedman: No, on the contrary, I have seen them countless times.

Dr. Zollinger: Dr. Gliedman, do you go and look at these things?

Dr. Gliedman: Yes, I do, on occasion. However, I trust the group that does the studies.

Dr. Zollinger: I thought only the fellow in medicine did that?

Dr. Gliedman: He does the study – I look at them because we have a not uncommon controversy about whether a cholangiogram is normal or not normal in the presence of crystals. So a discussion evolves as to whether or not there are cholesterol crystals. We will operate on the basis of cholesterol crystals. If the surgeon is going to operate on a patient, because of the test, he ought to see the crystals at least often enough to trust the people who say they are present.

Dr. Zollinger: Dr. Gliedman, what kind of a case are you talking about? Are you talking about the old-time duodenal drainage?

Dr. Gliedman: Yes, that is correct.

Dr. Zollinger: Dr. Gliedman, what type of case would you do this on? When Hadacol fails? Or Lydia Pinkham's fails? Why do you need that to make a diagnosis?

Dr. Gliedman: For one reason or another, we have symptomatic patients who, on repeated oral cholangiograms, show opacification of the gallbladder without showing stones. As well, some people are allergic to the contrast material and can't have roentgen studies. The follow-up on those patients may use a Rehfuss' tube passage into the duodenum to collect the aspirate. Then, if the aspirate shows cholesterol crystals, we are confident that that patient does, in fact, have an abnormal gallbladder.

Dr. Delaney: This question is directed to Dr. Burhenne: A stricture is so hard to cut with a knife, why is it easy to dilate with a balloon filled with fluid?

Dr. Burhenne: I can see where any surgeon would have question marks on anything that the radiologist does. All you have to do is to measure the balloon pressure between your fingers. Actually, the Edwards Company will tell you how much pressure you can apply before the balloon will burst. We have to push quite hard with a small syringe to distend this balloon. In the first session, as I mentioned, we usually cannot bring it further than from 1 mm to 3 mm, which is about 10 or 12, French. There is a lot of pressure to overcome.

Dr. Moody: Dr. Burhenne, you don't anticipate a long-term result from this, do you?

Dr. Burhenne: The patient that I showed you is now 14 months after his stricture dilation. In the preceding 14 months, he had three operations for recurrent stricture. We will let these patients go for 16 to 18 months, then withdraw the catheter from the stricture into the jejunum and see if they restricture. At that time, we could redilate them. We contemplate that they may live with this potential catheter in place for 1½ years. After that we hope to put a button into the jejunostomy so that we can keep the jejunostomy open, in case we have to redilate that stricture. We now have three patients over nine months.

Mr. Smith: May I comment, Dr. Delaney? I think, surely, it would be better if the patient had had a successful operation and no button in his jejunum. I am naturally interested in this method and obviously, it is possible to dilate a stenosis of this kind. If the patient is a particularly bad risk patient, on whom you really hesitate to perform any major operation, then perhaps it can be right to dilate his stricture every 12 months or 14 months or 16 months. On the other hand, it would be overoptimistic to think that there is any reasonable chance that you are going to cure anybody this way. Restenosis, I am sure, occurs because fibrous tissue contracts progressively, if there is no epithelial lining. To say that, perhaps, if you stretch it enough, a new epithelial lining will grow all the way around again, is to deny something that our surgical forefathers knew very well years ago. If you have a urethral stricture, where there is a total circumferential destruction of the lining epithelium, it really doesn't matter how long you leave a catheter in. When you take the catheter out, you soon have the stricture back again. In surgery, you know, the rules of the game apply to the body as a whole. What applies to the urethra and to the ureter and to the bronchial tree and every other hollow system applies to the biliary apparatus. If you haven't got any epithelium, you'll have another stricture. This technique may be a way of temporizing. It may even be a way of treating a patient intermittently, if the risk of another operation is prohibitive. But I would have thought, in most cases, that if the patient's general condition is reasonable, the aim should be to cure him.

III

Pancreas

The Pathogenesis of Pancreatitis

Thomas Taylor White, M.D.

Just exactly what causes pancreatitis is still unknown. There appear to be, however, two main types: Acute pancreatitis follows intraductal activation of pancreatic juice proteases in the pancreatic duct [1], and chronic pancreatitis follows obstruction to the outflow of pancreatic juice by strictures, protein plugs or tumors [2, 3]. There is considerable confusion relative to the definition of the two main clinical types. Acute pancreatitis is a disease which occurs acutely without prodrome and resolves completely with no sequelae. This can occur several times, each episode followed by complete resolution of the process. This disease is usually related to gallstones and is completely arrested by removal of a gallbladder containing stones and/or common bile duct stones. Only occasionally does chronic pain and fibrosis follow, then usually in conjunction with a stricture of the sphincter of Oddi secondary to passage of common bile duct stones and/or instrumentation. Chronic pancreatitis is a disease in which the patient has chronic pain with occasional exacerbations in which the pain becomes much more acute. Figure 1 is a diagram of various possible courses. The average age of patients with acute pancreatitis is 53, with most of the patients being women, while the average age of patients with chronic pancreatitis is 38, with the bulk of the patients being men.

The mechanism of interaction between the pancreas and its secretory products to produce activation of trypsinogen, chymotrypsinogen, and other zymogens to their active forms is unclear. Experimental studies using the injection of bile, India ink and other foreign substances into the pancreatic duct will produce acute pancreatitis, but in most instances the intraductal pressure must exceed 37 cm of water before the ductal and acinar membranes are ruptured [4]. Because the pressure required to cause pathology is above the physiologic range, this type of experiment has been

---

Thomas Taylor White, M.D., Clinical Professor of Surgery, University of Washington School of Medicine; Active Staff, Swedish and University Hospitals, Seattle, Wash.

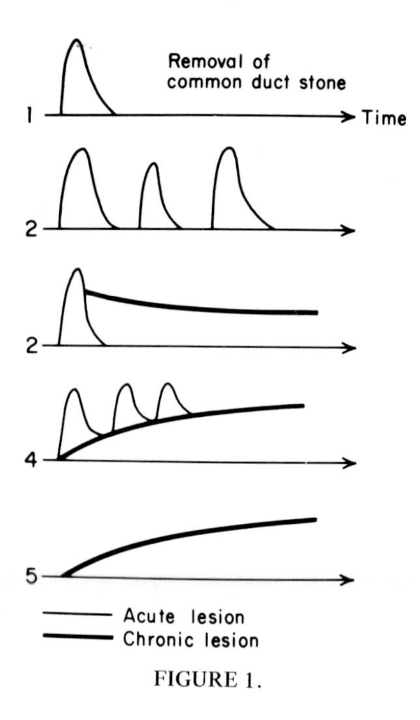

FIGURE 1.

somewhat discounted as phenomenology. While it was once thought that the common biliary pancreatic passageway at the ampulla of Vater might cause reflux of bile into the pancreatic duct, which in turn might activate the zymogens, perfusion of bile, with or without duodenal contents through the goat or dog pancreas, does not produce pancreatitis. Since the dog pancreatic secretory pressure is normally higher than bile secretory pressure, it is unlikely the bile would normally enter the dog pancreas. While it is admitted that the majority of patients having acute pancreatitis have gallstones, the theory that bile reflux into the pancreatic duct is responsible for this catastrophe is no longer generally accepted. There is also a question as to whether or not studies carried out on dogs, cats, goats, guinea pigs, hamsters, and other animals who eat a diet quite different from that which humans eat would be applicable to man [4-6].

The zymogens, trypsinogen and chymotrypsinogen, must be activated by enterokinase from the duodenum, or by trypsin, in order to be transformed into their active trypsin and chymotrypsin form, by the splitting off of an activation peptide (Fig. 2). It is thought that premature activation of these pancreatic proteases occurs in most types of pancreatitis and in cancers of the head of the pancreas. Detection of pancreatic

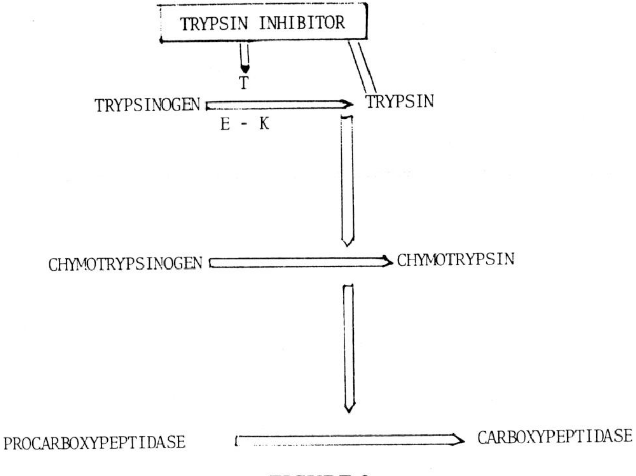

FIGURE 2.

enzymes and their inactive zymogen precursors, first carried out on specimens obtained at autopsy, segments of pancreas removed at operation, and stimulated duodenal secretions did not tell us much about mechanism. Later studies on human ductal secretions have been more revealing. When Troll and Doubilet studied a patient's pancreatic juice following an attack of acute pancreatitis, a large proportion of the proteases in the secretions collected were active [7]. Later studies have been on patients with fistulas following biopsy of a pancreatic carcinoma, fistula fluid from surgically drained pseudocysts, direct puncture of the pancreatic duct during operation for chronic pancreatitis, secretions obtained from a T-tube placed in the pancreatic duct to decompress the distended duct behind a cancer of the head of the pancreas [8] and from tubes left in the pancreatic duct following sphincteroplasty or anastomoses between pancreas and intestine (Figs. 3 and 4) [3, 9-14].

These studies show that there are variations in human pancreatic trypsin inhibitor levels, with the trypsin inhibitor levels being lowest in patients with pancreatitis. We were able to show that there was a significantly lower trypsin inhibitor activity in the pancreatic juice on the first postoperative day, which returned toward normal by the fourth postoperative day (Fig. 5) [4, 5]. Further, we were able to show that Trasylol infused intravenously during the postoperative period resulted in a significant rise in the trypsin inhibitory levels in pancreatic juice. In one patient this rise was accompanied by marked clinical improvement and clearing of the previously bloodstained juice from the pancreatic duct following a sphincteroplasty for acute pancreatitis. This suggested to us, as

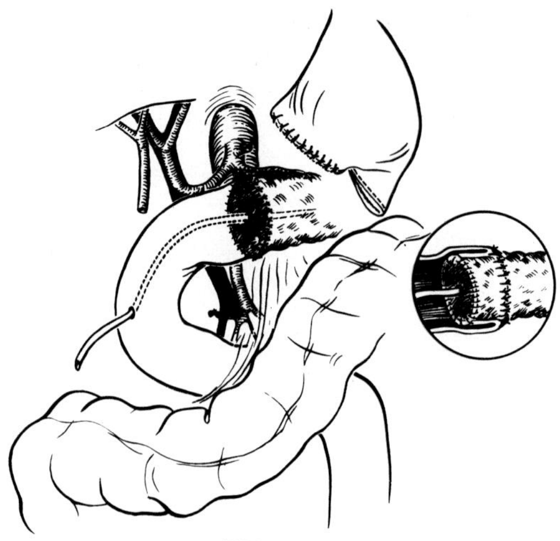

FIGURE 3.

it had to German investigators before, that Trasylol could significantly reduce the incidence of morbidity and mortality in patients with attacks of acute pancreatitis. It was felt that this substance might prevent further conversion of trypsinogen to trypsin by binding trypsin. Still, extensive studies by Trapnell [15] and Nardi [16] have shown no significant benefit from the administration of these drugs, perhaps because they were given too late after the onset of the acute, inflammatory process, and to the fact that there was a mixture of perhaps as many as 23 proteins in the commercial substance. This substance was completely withdrawn from investigation in the United States in October 1969, but, because of further purification, has been recently reintroduced for investigative purposes.

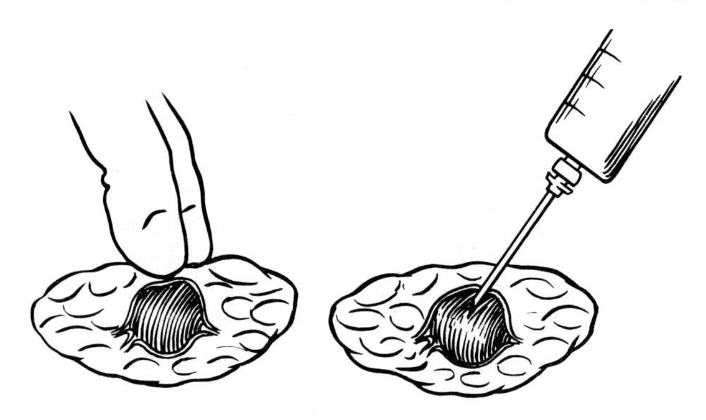

FIGURE 4.

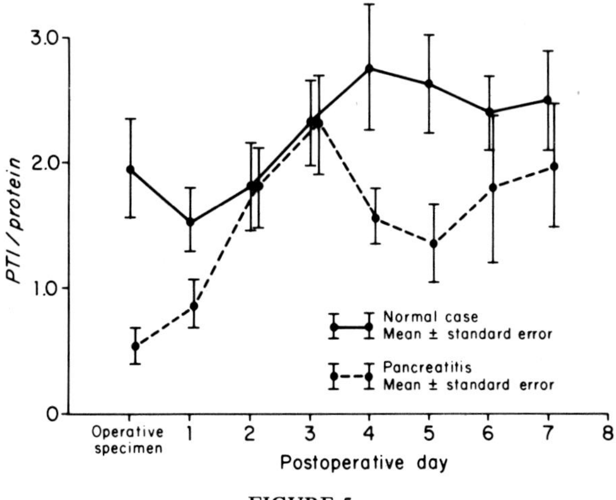

FIGURE 5.

Specimens of pancreatic juice obtained from patients during the postoperative period and by duodenoscopy by a number of investigators have shown that there are approximately 23 enzymes in the pancreatic juice and two trypsin inhibitors [9, 12, 14]. The most interesting feature of these studies is that the human enzymes are quite different from those of the cow and the pig, and that active trypsin is formed much more slowly from human trypsinogen than it is in the cow and the dog, perhaps due to higher levels of trypsin inhibitor present in human pancreatic juice than in other species (Fig. 6).

While there are a number of different explanations as to why acute pancreatitis appears most commonly in conjunction with gallstone disease, the passage of gallstones into the duodenum through the sphincter of Oddi seems to be the most likely explanation. The suggestion that reflux of duodenal contents into the pancreatic duct is responsible for the activation has been made by many authors, most energetically by Pfeffer and Byrnes. The relative infrequence of common bile duct stones in patients operated two to three weeks following an attack of acute pancreatitis has made this theory open to question. The recent observation of Acosta [17] that 34 out of 36 patients with acute pancreatitis and known gallstones passed stones in the stool during the ten days following an attack, has revised this thought. It seems reasonable that during the passage the duct could be propped open by the stone, allowing activated pancreatic secretion and duodenal contents to pass upward into the pancreatic duct, at the same

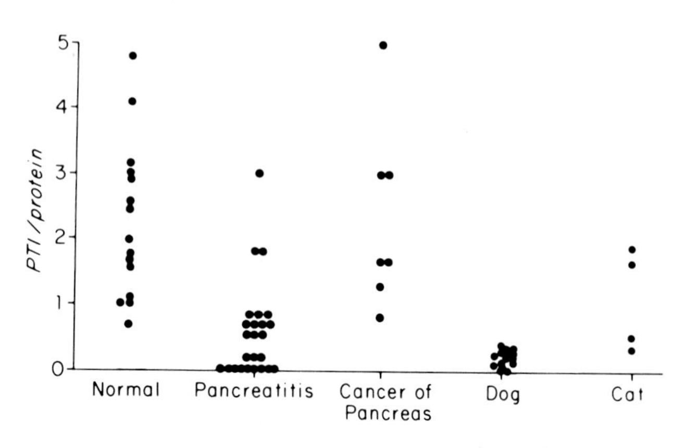

FIGURE 6.

time as the bile and pancreatic ducts are partially obstructed. The partial obstruction would induce further passage of these substances upwards into the bile and pancreatic ducts, perhaps producing the acute lesion by the mixture of enterokinase with the pancreatic juices and subsequent intraductal activation of the enzymes.

While reflux of enterokinase into the pancreatic duct is probably the main cause of intraductal activation of pancreatic enzymes in patients with nonmalignant disease, this does not explain the acute pancreatitis found in patients with carcinoma of the head of the pancreas. In a recent study, pancreatic secretions were collected from a patient with carcinoma of the head of the pancreas who had a T-tube left in the pancreatic duct to relieve pain from ductal distention behind a tumor [1]. Because the tumor totally blocked the duct to the left of the duodenum there was no possibility of activation of juice by enterokinase. The secretions were collected one week postoperatively, no traces of chymotryptic activity were found in the juice and no active phospholipase A or elastase was present. Later, the patient had an attack of acute abdominal pain. The secretions became bloody and decreased in volume and output. Active chymotrypsin was present in all the bloody specimens, but at lower specific activities than those initially seen. When the pain subsided, secretions appeared normal again as to flow rate and protein output. Again, no free chymotrypsin could be found. When these materials were analyzed biochemically, it was found that the pancreatic juice trypsin inhibitor had started to fall just before the onset of pain, dropped to insignificant levels while the juice was bloody and then started to rise as the juice cleared, rising again to normal levels. This again suggests to us that injected human or bovine trypsin inhibitor may reverse the process of acute pancreatitis.

Human pancreatic trypsin inhibitor has been recently shown by Dr. Lewis Greene at Brookhaven Laboratory to contain 55 or 56 amino acid residues [18]. It is conceivable that this substance, when synthesized, will be more effective in suppressing the activation of zymogens within the pancreatic ducts than Trasylol. We hope that this substance will be available soon.

This leaves us with the speculation as to whether the pancreatitis seen in our cancer patient and the acute pancreatitis seen in patients with gallstone disease develop by the same mechanism. Relative to the activation which took place in our cancer patient, Reich and his colleagues [19] have found that some tumor cells produce a proteolytic enzyme which will break down plasminogen. A substance of this type might have activated the zymogens. Nardi and Lees' [16] observation of elevated serum trypsin in patients with pancreatic cancer is compatible with this idea. The possibility exists then that unusual trypsin-like enzymes are present in the secretions from cancer patients which may cause the activation of the proteases. A second possibility is that cancer cells may secrete the trypsin-like enzymes into the circulation [20] which, in turn, may leak from the capillaries into the duct and initiate premature activation of trypsinogen. It is possible, of course, that trace levels of pancreatic trypsin may be present in the juice, which would be responsible for this activation, because the inhibitor does not completely inhibit human trypsin.

As to the lesion of chronic pancreatitis, a protein precipitate is frequently found in pancreatic juice obtained during and after a surgical operation for this disease, which has the same histochemical features as the intraductal protein plugs found throughout the pancreatic system by Nakamura, Sarles, and Payan [2]. The alcoholic rat and humans have an increased enzyme concentration in the juice with decreased total fluid output [2, 3]. This suggests that protein plugs might form from this material in the small ducts of patients with chronic pancreatitis which later may be calcified. The alcoholism itself may cause the conversion of some of the zymogens into active forms by direct action on the acinar cells [21], but not to the same degree as in patients with acute pancreatitis. This may cause the persistent chronic pain with protein precipitation and plugging of the ducts.

Patients with acute pancreatitis unrelated to cancer and alcoholism may have a spontaneous drop in trypsin inhibitor levels for some as yet unknown metabolic reason such as occurs in the immediate postoperative period following a surgical operation for duodenal ulcer or gallstones, without accompanying pancreatitis. They also may have circulating trypsin-like substances which will initiate the activation. Still, the same mechanisms responsible for pancreatitis associated with gallstone disease or cancer may play a part in the causation of the chronic disease. There also may be alterations in the cells caused by alcoholism which are responsible for the intermittent leakage of active substances from damaged cells into the duct.

Conclusions

Acute pancreatitis is caused by activation of the pancreatic zymogens, probably usually due to reflux of duodenal secretions into the pancreatic duct during the passage of gallstones.

Acute pancreatitis may also be caused by the release of trypsin-like substances secreted by cancer cells or due to the breakdown of the acinar cellular membrane by alcoholism.

Depression in pancreatic secretory inhibitor secondary to various metabolic diseases may also result in activation of the zymogens.

Obstruction to the pancreatic duct may produce another type of chronic pancreatitis, either by stricture of the sphincter, a cancer or scarring of the ducts.

References

1. Allan, B. J., Tournut, R. and White, T. T.: Intraductal activation of enzymes behind a carcinoma of the pancreas. Gastroenterology, 65:412, 1973.
2. Nakamura, K., Sarles, H. and Payan, H.: Three-dimensional reconstruction of the pancreatic ducts in chronic pancreatitis. Gastroenterology, 62:942, 1972.
3. Tournut, R. and White, T. T.: Water, electrolyte, and protein secretions of the human exocrine pancreas in the early postoperative period. Surg. Gynec. Obstet., 135:17, 1972.
4. White, T. T.: Pancreatitis. Baltimore:Williams & Wilkins, 1966.
5. Morgan, A., Robinson, L. A. and White, T. T.: Postoperative changes in the trypsin inhibitor activities of human pancreatic juice and the influence of infusion of Trasylol on the inhibitor activity. Amer. J. Surg., 115:131, 1968.
6. White, T. T., Morgan, A. and Hopton, D.: Postoperative pancreatitis: A study of seventy cases. Amer. J. Surg., 120:132, 1970.
7. Troll, W. and Doubilet, H.: The determination of proteolytic enzymes and proenzymes in human pancreatic juice. Gastroenterology, 19:326, 1951.

8. Cattell, R. B.: Anastomosis of the duct of Wirsung: Its use in palliative operations for cancer of the head of the pancreas. Surg. Clin. N. Amer., 27:636, 1947.
9. Figarella, C.: Revue Generale: Les proteines du suc pancreatique humain. Arch. Mal. Appar. Dig., 62:337, 1973.
10. Geokas, M., Rinderknect, H., Wilding, P. et al.: Proteolytic enzymes in human pancreatic juice in acute pancreatitis. Presented at the Western Section of American Federation of Clinical Research, February 2, 1968, Carmel, California.
11. Haverback, B. J., Dyce, B., Bundy, H. et al: Trypsin, trypsinogen and trypsin inhibitor in human pancreatic juice. Amer. J. Med., 29:424, 1960.
12. Keller, P. J. and Allan, B. J.: The protein composition of human pancreatic juice. J. Biol. Chem., 242:281, 1967.
13. Robinson, L. A., Churchill, C. L. and White, T. T.: Electrophoretic analysis of twenty-four specimens of human pancreatic juice. Biochim. Biophys. Acta, 222:390, 1970.
14. Robinson, L. A., Kim, W. J., White, T. T. et al: Trypsins in human pancreatic juice: Their distribution as found in 34 specimens. Two human pancreatic trypsinogens. Scand. J. Gastroent., 7:43, 1971.
15. Trapnell, J. E., Talbot, C. H. and Capper, W. M.: Trasylol in acute pancreatitis. Amer. J. Dig. Dis., 12:409, 1967.
16. Nardi, G. L. and Lees, C. W.: Serum trypsin: A new diagnostic test for pancreatic disease. New Eng. J. Med., 258:797, 1958.
17. Acosta, J. M. and Ledesma, C. L.: Gallstone migration as a cause of acute pancreatitis. New Eng. J. Med., 290:484, 1974.
18. Greene, L. J., Roark, D. E. and Bartelt, D. C.: Human pancreatic secretory trypsin inhibitor. Proceedings of the Second Symposium on Proteinase Inhibitors. New York:Springer Verlag, 1974.
19. Ossowski, L., Quigley, J. P., Kellerman, G. M. et al: Fibrinolysis associated with onogenic transformation. Requirement of plasminogen for correlated changes in cellular morphology, colony formation in agar, and cell migration. J. Exp. Med., 138:1056, 1973.
20. Nardi, G. L.: Pancreatitis, current therapy. New Eng. J. Med., 268:1065, 1963.
21. Sarles, H., Lebreuil, G., Tasso, F. et al.: A comparison of alcoholic pancreatitis in rats and men. Gut, 12:377, 1971.

Partially supported by NIH Grant CA-AM 14380 and American Cancer Society CI 82.

Serum Amylase Removal Mechanisms

Michael D. Levitt, M.D. and William C. Duane, M.D.

The serum amylase level represents the net result of the rate that amylase enters the serum and the rate that the enzyme is removed from the serum. Most studies have been concerned with various factors that result in amylase deposition in the serum. In contrast, this paper will review available data concerning amylase removal mechanisms.

Most measurements of amylase turnover in animals are of questionable relevance to the human situation, since many of these investigations have utilized common laboratory animals which have very high serum amylase levels and have very little amylase in the urine. In addition, heterologous amylase was used in many of these studies. To obviate these criticisms, we [1] studied amylase kinetics in the baboon, an animal that has a serum amylase level and renal clearance of amylase similar to that of man. Amylase isolated from the salivary glands or the pancreas of the baboon was employed in these studies.

Figure 1 shows typical results of serial measurements of serum amylase and renal clearance of amylase (C_{Am}) after the serum amylase of the baboon was markedly elevated by intravenous injection of a bolus of amylase. Of particular interest is the very rapid fall-off in serum amylase activity which had a half time of about 80 minutes. This rapid disappearance of amylase can be contrasted with albumin, a protein of roughly similar molecular weight, which has a serum half time of about 20 days. This rapid removal of amylase from the serum no doubt accounts for the rapid fluctuation in serum amylase levels that may occur in pancreatitis.

It can also be observed from Figure 1 that the renal clearance of amylase remained relatively constant throughout a wide range of serum amylase levels. Since C_{Am} = Urinary Amylase/[Amylase]$_{serum}$, it is apparent that the urinary amylase always varies in a fixed relation to the

Michael D. Levitt, M.D. and William C. Duane, M.D., University of Minnesota Hospitals, Minneapolis.

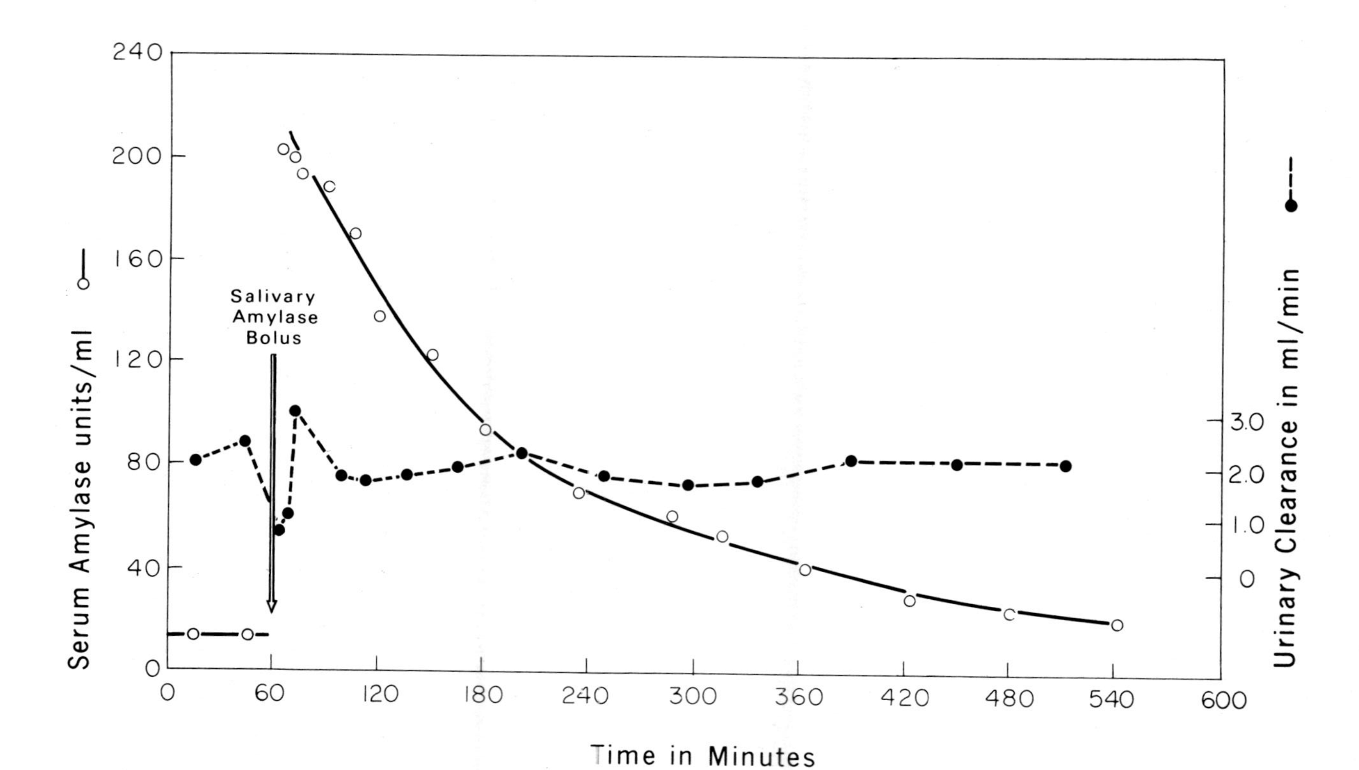

FIG. 1. Study of the fall-off of serum amylase activity and renal clearance of amylase after intravenous injection of a bolus of salivary amylase.

serum level. This type of relation is typical for an excretory mechanism in which there is glomerular filtration without tubular reabsorption. Additional evidence for this mechanism of renal excretion of amylase were observations on the influence of mannitol diuresis on the renal clearance of amylase. Mannitol reduces tubular reabsorption by hastening the passage of fluid through the tubules and by reducing the concentration of amylase in the tubule. Amylase clearance was not influenced by a mannitol diuresis, thus supporting the concept that there is no tubular reabsorption or destruction of amylase.

The relatively minor role played by the kidney in serum amylase removal is illustrated in Figure 2. Following intravenous injection of a bolus of salivary amylase, only about 20% of the total amylase which disappeared from the serum appeared in the urine. The remaining 80% was cleared by some extraurinary mechanism. The clinical application of this information is that renal insufficiency should not cause a marked elevation in serum amylase activity. A uremic patient with a high serum amylase level probably has pancreatitis. Studies with iodinated amylase [2] suggested that the liver and spleen removed amylase from the serum.

The urinary amylase measurement has been used for many years because it is thought that the urinary amylase is a more sensitive indicator of pancreatitis than is the serum level. If the urinary amylase is elevated out of proportion to the serum level in pancreatitis, then there should be an elevation of the ratio of urinary amylase/serum amylase in pancreatitis. Since this ratio represents the renal clearance of amylase, what we are actually postulating is that the kidney clears amylase more rapidly in the patient with pancreatitis than in the normal subject.

That such an increase in C_{Am} occurs in pancreatitis is shown in Figure 3, which depicts the C_{Am}/C_{Cr} of various groups of subjects [3]. In order to normalize for differences in renal function, C_{Am} is expressed as a percentage of C_{Cr} in this figure. This ratio, C_{Am}/C_{Cr}, is of value in distinguishing causes of hyperamylasemia and is easily calculated in the clinical situation since:

$$\frac{C_{Am}}{C_{Cr}} = \frac{\dfrac{[Am]_{urine} \times V/T}{[AM]_{serum}}}{\dfrac{[Cr]_{urine} \times V/T}{[Cr]_{serum}}}$$

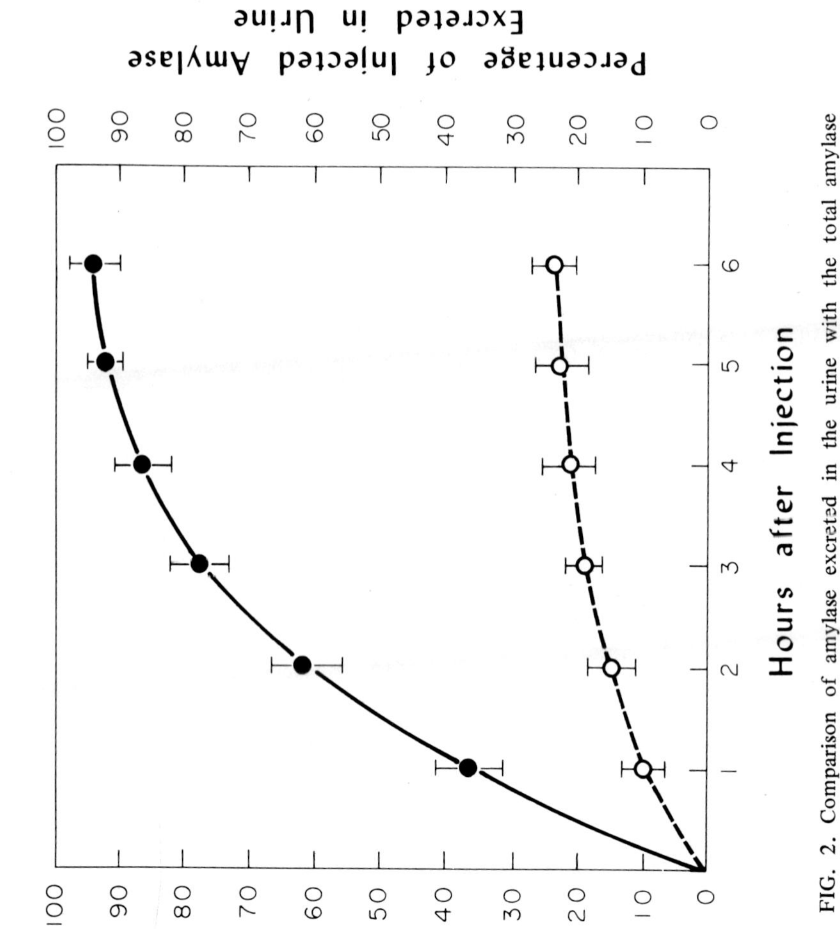

FIG. 2. Comparison of amylase excreted in the urine with the total amylase calculated to have disappeared from serum after a bolus injection of salivary amylase.

Note that the urine volume (V) and time of urine collection (T) cancel out and this ratio reduces to:

$$\frac{C_{Am}}{C_{Cr}} = \frac{\dfrac{Am_{urine}}{Am_{serum}}}{\dfrac{Cr_{urine}}{Cr_{serum}}}$$

Thus, a timed urine sample is not needed and this ratio is calculated from measurements of amylase and creatinine concentration in a simultaneously collected serum and "grab" urine specimen.

Normal subjects clear amylase about 2.5% as rapidly as they clear creatinine. Since it is likely that amylase is excreted by the mechanism of glomerular filtration without tubular reabsorption, amylase must be filtered about 2.5% as fast as is creatinine. This rate is consistent with the molecular size of amylase (molecular weight = 55,000) which makes it possible for amylase to slowly squeeze through the glomerular pores. As shown in Figure 3, the C_{Am}/C_{Cr} of hospitalized subjects and patients with renal insufficiency is comparable to normal. On the other hand, early in the course of acute pancreatitis, there is a dramatic increase in C_{Am}/C_{Cr} to about three times the normal level. What this indicates is that for any given level of serum amylase and renal function, the patient, early in the course of acute pancreatitis, will excrete urinary amylase three times faster than will the normal subject. For this reason, the urinary amylase is a more sensitive indicator of pancreatitis than is the serum level.

As shown in Figure 3, patients with the condition termed macroamylasemia [4] have a very low C_{Am}/C_{Cr}, usually less than 1%. In this condition, normal amylase is bound by another serum protein to form a macromolecular complex. This complex is too large to pass through the glomerular pore and hence the low C_{Am}/C_{Cr}. In addition, this complex is slowly removed by extrarenal mechanisms and thus is often associated with persistently elevated serum amylase levels. While asymptomatic and not injurious to health, macroamylasemia may be confused with pancreatitis because of the elevated serum amylase values. As shown in Figure 3, measurement of C_{Am}/C_{Cr} provides a simple means of clearly differentiating between these two conditions.

The elevated C_{Am}/C_{Cr} observed in pancreatitis is not dependent upon the existence of an elevated serum amylase level but is commonly seen when the serum amylase value is within normal limits. How is it possible

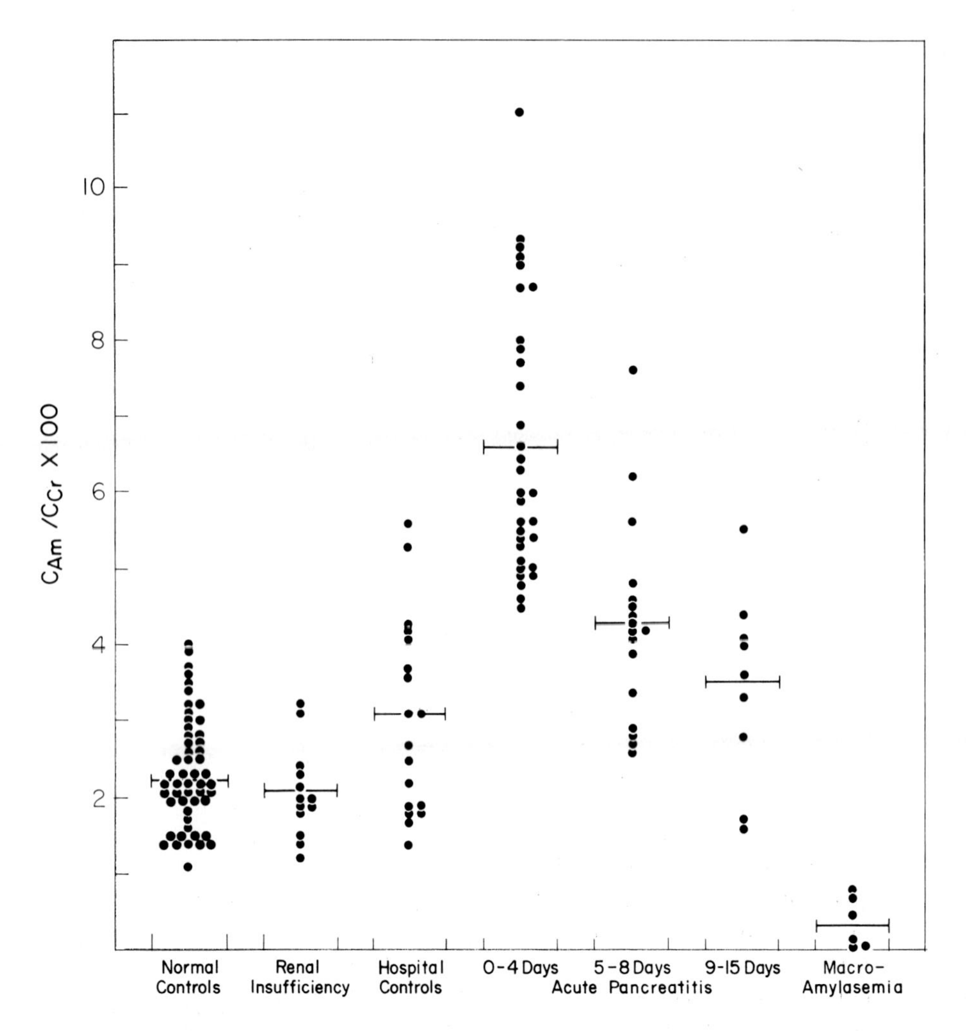

FIG. 3. Measurements of C_{Am}/C_{Cr} in various groups of subjects. Measurements in patients with acute pancreatitis have been arbitrarily divided into studies performed 0-4, 5-8 and 9-15 days after onset of attack.

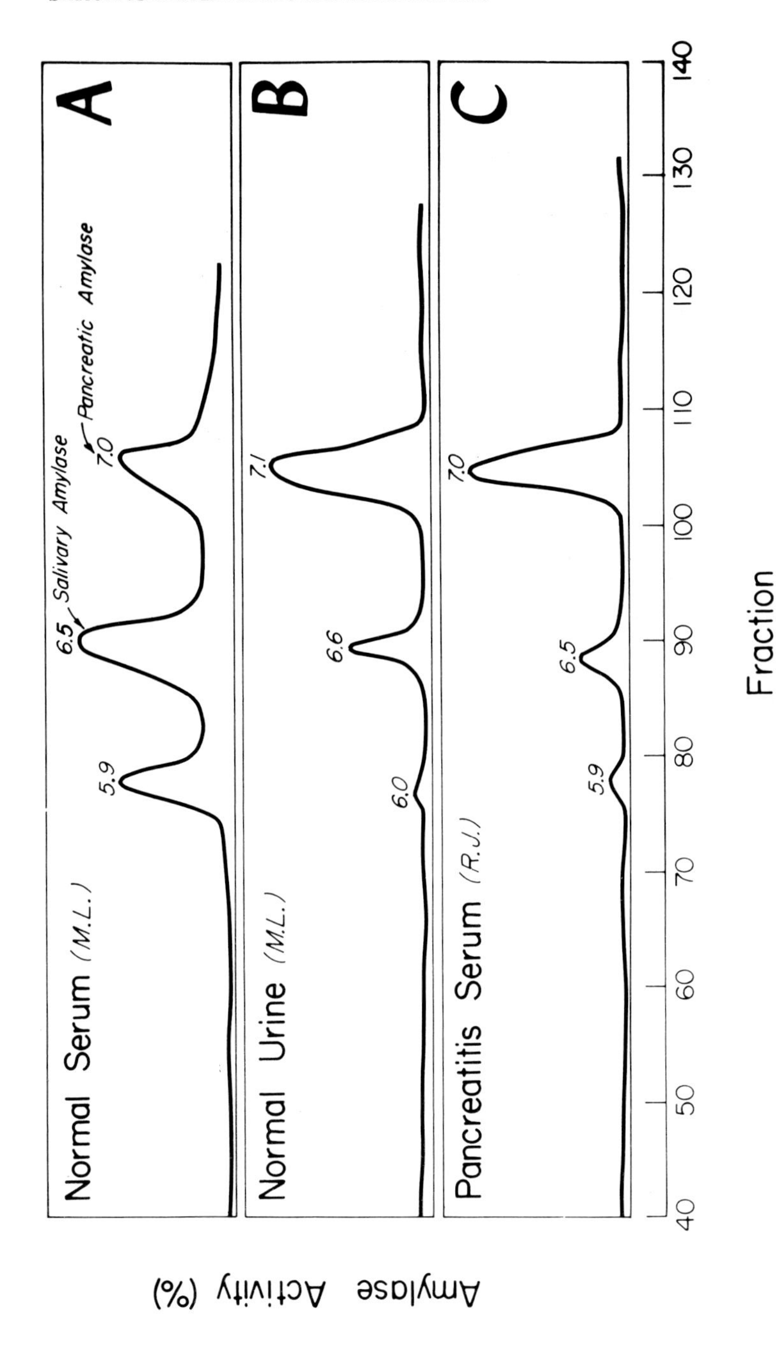

FIG. 4. Isoelectric focusing of serum isoamylases. (*A*) The isoelectric point of the three major peaks are shown as are location of pancreatic and salivary amylase. (*B*) Isoamylases of a normal urine obtained simultaneously with the serum sample shown in (*A*). (*C*) Isoamylases of a serum sample obtained from a patient who had a normal serum amylase and an elevated urinary amylase.

that the kidney in pancreatitis receives amylase at a normal rate (judged by the serum amylase level) yet excretes amylase at a supranormal rate? A possible answer to this question was provided by a study in which amylase clearance was measured when the baboon's serum amylase was markedly elevated by a constant infusion of either salivary or pancreatic amylase. Salivary amylase was consistently cleared less rapidly than was the baboon's endogenous amylase while pancreatic amylase was consistently cleared more rapidly than endogenous amylase. Thus, a supranormal amylase clearance might be expected in pancreatitis, since most of the circulating amylase would be of pancreatic origin.

To determine if pancreatic amylase is more rapidly cleared by the human kidney than is amylase of other origins, isoelectric focusing of human serum and urine samples was performed to separate the various isozymes of amylase. Figure 4 shows the results of these preliminary studies. Normal serum (Fig. 4A) has three major peaks with isoelectric points of about 7.0, 6.6 and 5.9. Amylase in pancreatic drainage migrates as a single peak at pH 7.0. This peak at 7.0 appears to be entirely of pancreatic origin as evidenced by its complete disappearance after total pancreatectomy. The peak at pH 6.6 is primarily salivary amylase and the source of the other peaks remains to be identified.

Whereas pancreatic amylase represents about one third of the amylase of the normal serum, it makes up about 70%-80% of the total urinary amylase (Fig. 4B). Thus, pancreatic amylase is excreted three to four times more rapidly than is the remainder of the serum amylase. This rapid renal clearance explains why the urinary amylase is elevated out of proportion to the serum amylase when the serum amylase activity is markedly elevated by pancreatic amylase in pancreatitis.

Figure 4C shows the serum isoamylase pattern of a patient who was recovering from acute pancreatitis. This patient had a normal total serum amylase level but an elevated urinary amylase (ie, an elevated C_{Am}). It is apparent that despite the normal serum amylase level, the bulk of this patient's serum amylase was still of pancreatic origin thus explaining the rapid renal clearance. It also follows that the absolute quantity of the nonpancreatic amylases in the serum must be reduced in this patient, since most of the amylase was of pancreatic origin. Apparently, the presence of pancreatitis either inhibited the entrance of the nonpancreatic amylases into the serum, or, alternatively, the extrarenal clearance of amylase from the blood might have been enhanced in pancreatitis.

It is apparent from Figure 4A and B that salivary amylase is cleared much more slowly by the kidney than is pancreatic amylase. This finding is supported by the observation that parotitis is usually associated with an elevated serum amylase level and a normal urinary amylase excretion (ie, a low C_{Am}). This clearance difference between salivary and pancreatic amylase is not attributable to a demonstrable difference in molecular weight and may represent a difference in configuration or charge.

Measurement of C_{Am}/C_{Cr} appears to provide a "poor man's" means of obtaining a serum isoamylase determination. A high C_{Am}/C_{Cr} indicates that a large proportion of serum amylase is of pancreatic origin while a low C_{Am}/C_{Cr} indicates that a high proportion of the serum amylase is salivary amylase or macroamylase.

References

1. Duane W. C., Frerichs, R. and Levitt, M. D.: Distribution, turnover and mechanism of renal excretion of amylase in the baboon. J. Clin. Invest., 50:151, 1971.
2. Duane, W. C., Frerichs, R. and Levitt, M. D.: Simultaneous study of the metabolic turnover and renal excretion of ^{125}I-salivary amylase and ^{131}I-pancreatic amylase in the baboon. J. Clin. Invest., 51:1504, 1972.
3. Levitt, M. D., Rapoport, M. and Cooperband, S. R.: Renal excretion of amylase in renal disease, pancreatitis and macroamylasemia. Ann. Int. Med., 71:919, 1967.
4. Berk, J. E., Kizu, H., Wilding, P. et al: Macroamylasemia: Newly recognized cause for elevated serum amylase activity. New Eng. J. Med., 277:941-946, 1967.

Supported by U. S. Public Health Service Grant AM13309.

Retrograde Pancreatic Ductogram

Stephen E. Silvis, M.D. and Jack A. Vennes, M.D.

Endoscopic retrograde pancreatocholangiography is performed with side-viewing duodenoscope that is 125 cm in length and 1 cm in diameter. The 1 cm diameter of the scope can be used to identify the size of the pathology seen on the x-rays when the scope is also shown in the field and allows correction for magnification on the film. The technique requires patience, persistence and practice [1]. The endoscope is passed through the esophagus, stomach and duodenum and into the second portion of the duodenum. The papilla of Vater is identified and a cannula is passed into the papilla with injection of 30%-60% renografin as a contrast agent. The injection must be carefully monitored on fluoroscopy to prevent over-filling of ducts. It is believed to be hazardous to overinject the pancreatic duct for fear of producing pancreatitis. The patients will experience pain if the pancreatic or biliary ducts are overfilled. Success in the procedure depends upon adequate premedication of the patient, identification of the papilla and ductal orifices or orifice, position of the cannula, injection of the desired duct, careful x-ray monitoring with film recording of the adequately filled ductal system and interpretation of results.

Our current premedication routine consists of rather heavy sedation with intravenous Valium as necessary. If large amounts of Valium (ie, over 30 mg) are necessary, a synthetic narcotic such as Nisentil may be added very slowly intravenously. The patient should be relaxed and cooperative. The duodenal atony is obtained with intramuscular Bentyl of 60 mg, atropine 0.4 mg and intravenous glucagon 0.5 mg as necessary [1, 2]. Relaxation of the duodenum is required to find the papilla and to relax papillary smooth muscle so it will admit a cannula. The anatomic location of the papilla varies widely; it is usually 6-8 cm from the duodenal bulb and is frequently on a vertical fold. It may be at the lower end of this fold, in the middle, or at the upper end and is usually seen in profile from

Stephen E. Silvis, M.D., Chief, Gastroenterology Section, Minneapolis VA Hospital and Associate Professor of Medicine, University of Minnesota, Minneapolis, and Jack A. Vennes, M.D., Chief, Endoscopist, Minneapolis VA Hospital and Associate Professor of Medicine, University of Minnesota, Minneapolis.

above. The papilla frequently appears slightly more reddened than the duodenal mucosa. When the papilla has been located, it must be viewed very closely to identify the duct orifice. There is usually a very fine reticular pattern in the orifice of the duct, and occasionally the papilla will have two ductal orifices: one leading to the common bile duct and one to the pancreatic duct.

Table 1 shows the analysis of our first 300 cases which were studied before August 1973. There were 139 patients studied for suspected pancreatic disease and 161 were studied for biliary disease. The success rate increases with experience from 67% in the first 150 to 93% in the second 150. Categorizing pancreatic disease is somewhat difficult. We have rather arbitrarily divided these patients into four disease states, shown in Table 2: (1) acute recurrent pancreatitis; (2) chronic pancreatitis; (3) pancreatic neoplasm: (4) pancreatic pseudocyst. Only 82 of these patients fit into the four preceding categories.

Acute Recurrent Pancreatitis

Definition: Previously Elevated Serum or Urine Amylase Accompanied by Abdominal Pain

Figure 1 shows an entirely normal pancreatic duct. The pancreatic duct courses superiorly, then passes laterally to cross the spine. The duct tapers gradually and smoothly toward the tail and gives off fine lateral branches. There is marked variation in position and shape of the major pancreatic duct; we doubt if diagnostic interpretations can be made of the position of the main duct. This is the most characteristic finding of

Table 1. Endoscopic Cholangiograms and/or Pancreatograms

A. Indication for Study:		
Suspected pancreatic disease	139	
Suspected biliary disease	161	
Total studies attempted		300
B. Successful Studies:		
Cholangiogram and pancreatogram	155	
Pancreatogram only	48	
Cholangiogram only	62	
		265 (88%)
C. Desired Duct Obtained:		
Of first 150 cases	100 (67%)	
Of second 150 cases	139 (93%)	

Table 2. Diagnostic Requirements

A. Acute Recurrent Pancreatitis
1. Elevated serum or urine amylase and presence of abdominal pain
B. Chronic Pancreatitis
1. Depressed pancreatic exocrine function with either history of previous pancreatitis or presence of pancreatic calcification
2. Tissue diagnosis of chronic pancreatitis
C. Pancreatic Neoplasm
Tissue Diagnosis of Neoplasm
D. Pancreatic Pseudocyst
Surgical Proof of Pseudocyst

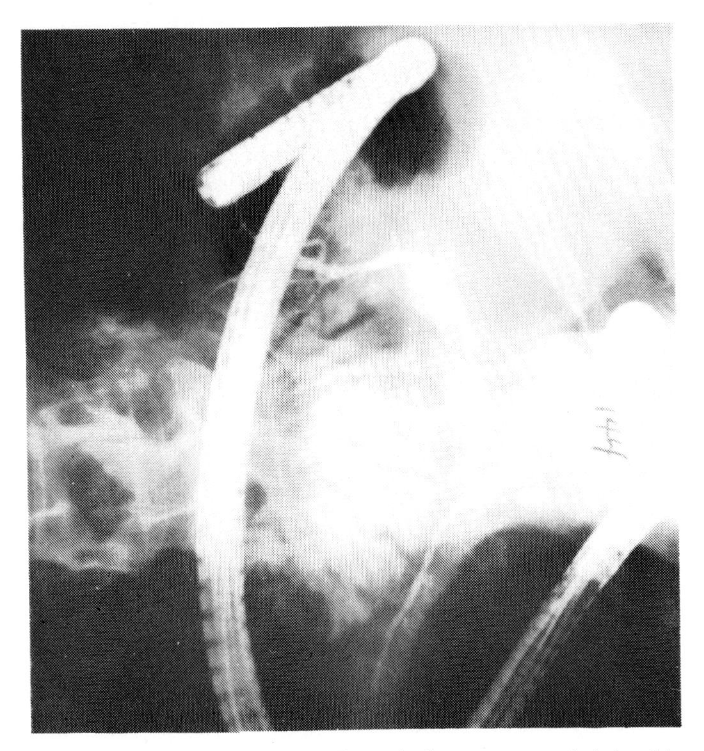

FIG. 1. This is a normal pancreatogram. The main duct courses cephalad and turns to pass over the spine. It tapers gradually and gives off fine branches.

patients with acute recurrent pancreatitis. Figure 2 shows a dilated common bile duct with entrapment of the distal portion of a duct in pancreatic inflammation in a patient with acute recurrent pancreatitis.

Table 3 shows the findings in 21 patients with acute recurrent pancreatitis. There were 19 successful studies with 14 normal pancreatograms. Four patients (such as the one shown in Figure 2) had abnormal cholangiograms. This is probably the most important finding in this patient group. Various changes of ductal irregularity, stenosis, obstruction or nonfilling of the duct were seen in four patients. We will discuss these findings further under chronic pancreatitis and carcinoma.

Chronic Pancreatitis

Definition: (1) Depressed Pancreatic Exocrine Function With Either History of Previous Pancreatitis or Presence of Pancreatic Calcification, or (2) Tissue Diagnosis of Chronic Pancreatitis at Surgery

Figure 3 shows a pancreatogram in a patient with chronic pancreatitis. Massive dilatation of the main pancreatic duct, lateral branches and branches to the head are seen. These changes appear to be characteristic of severe chronic pancreatitis. Localized abnormalities have been seen in patients with chronic pancreatitis. These changes have consisted of irregularity in the duct with cystic lateral spaces in one area of the pancreas with the rest of the duct appearing normal. Table 4 shows the findings in patients with chronic pancreatitis. Only a single patient out of 15 had a normal pancreatogram. The most characteristic changes are in the caliber and irregularity of the main duct and branches in ten of 15 cases. Five of the 15 patients had calculi and/or obstruction. Abnormal cholangiograms were seen in three of the 15 patients. Because of the surgically correctable nature of this abnormality, visualization of the common bile duct is very important in these patients.

Pancreatic Neoplasm

Definition: Diagnosis of the Neoplasm on Tissue Biopsy

Figure 4 shows obstruction of the pancreatic duct with a long tapering stricture shown at the small arrows. The cholangiogram is abnormal with an irregular mass shown at the long arrows. This represented tumor in the hilum of the liver. Figure 5 shows obstruction of the common duct by a long narrowed stricture. There is stricturing of the pancreatic duct shown at the arrows. Typical changes of chronic pancreatitis are seen above the strictured pancreatic duct. At surgery the patient had tumor in the area of

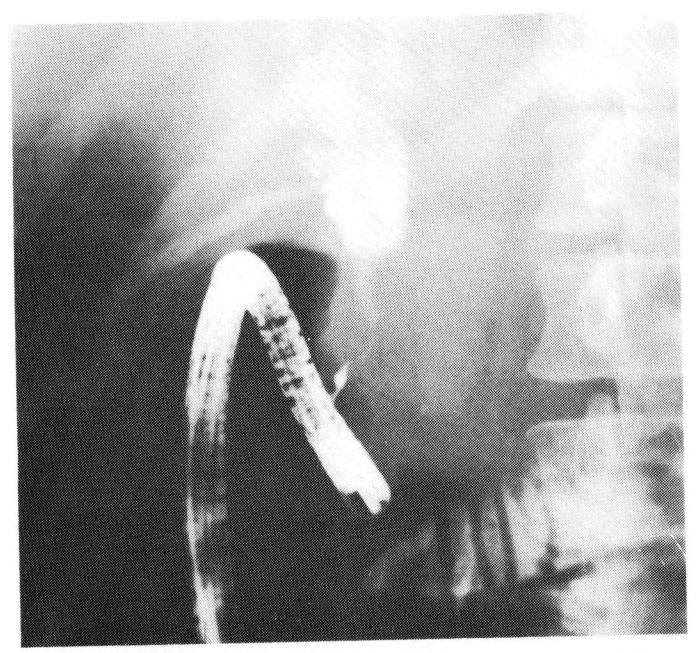

FIG. 2. This patient with acute recurrent pancreatitis has obstruction of the common bile duct by entrapment of the distal duct in pancreatic fibrosis. Surgery demonstrated only the fibrosis with obstruction. Choledochoduodenostomy has relieved her symptoms.

Table 3. Pancreatic Findings in Patients With Proven Acute Recurrent Pancreatitis

Number of patients	21
Satisfactory studies	19
Normal pancreatograms	14
Extraductal cavity filled	0
Mass effect	0
Abnormal endoscopic cholangiogram	4
Main Pancreatic Duct	
Caliber irregularity	3
Increased caliber	2
Stenosis	1
Obstruction or nonfilling	4
Ductal calculi	0
Ductal Branches	
Nonfilling or obstruction	3
Caliber irregularity	6

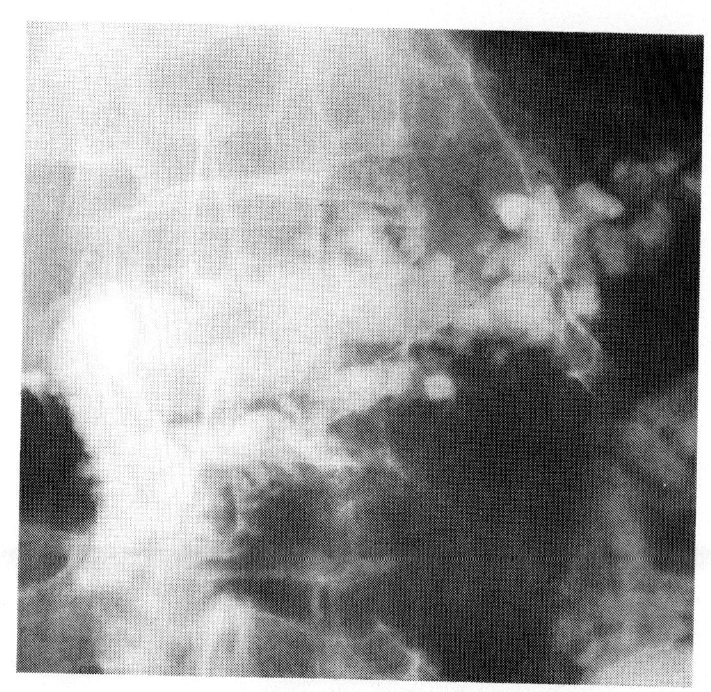

FIG. 3. This is the pancreatogram in a patient with alcoholic pancreatitis and calcification of the pancreas. There is massive dilatation of the main duct and lateral branches with cystic dilatation of the terminal portion of the lateral branches.

Table 4. Pancreatographic Findings in Patients With Proven Chronic Pancreatitis

Number of patients	15
Satisfactory studies	15
Normal pancreatograms	1
Extraductal cavity filled	2
Mass effect	0
Abnormal endoscopic cholangiogram	3
Main Pancreatic Duct	
Caliber irregularity	5
Increased caliber	6
Stenosis	0
Obstruction or nonfilling	5
Ductal calculi	5
Ductal Branches	
Nonfilling or obstruction	1
Caliber irregularity	10

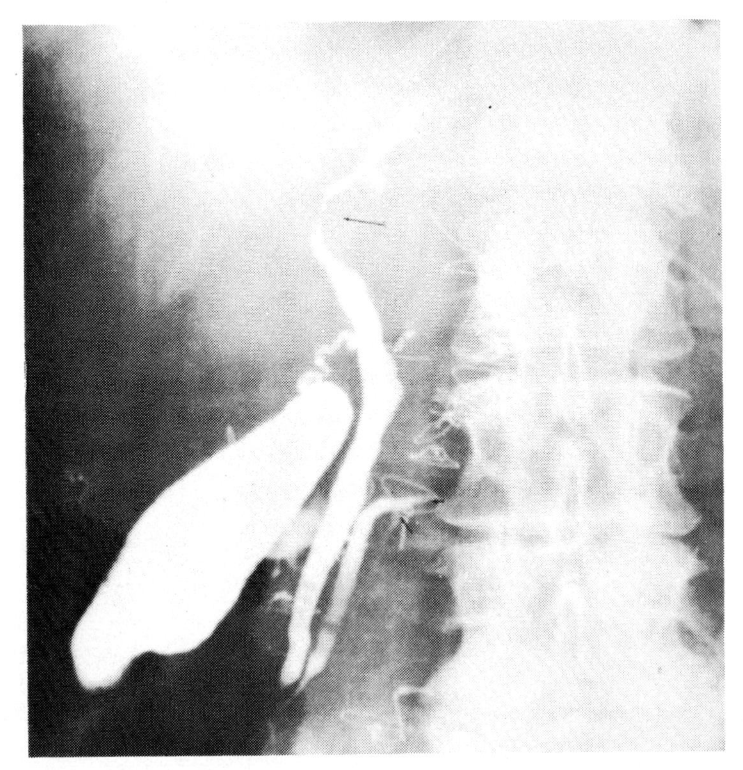

FIG. 4. This patient had biopsy proven adenocarcinoma of the pancreas. The main pancreatic duct has a long tapering stenosis ending in the obstruction shown at the short arrows. There is an impression on the bile duct shown at the long arrow which was tumor in the hilum of the liver. In our experience this long stenotic lesion is most characteristic of carcinoma.

stricture and chronic pancreatitis in the remainder of the gland. We do not know whether these changes developed after the carcinoma or the carcinoma developed in a patient with chronic pancreatitis.

Table 5 shows the findings in 23 cases with carcinoma of the pancreas. There were satisfactory studies in 22 patients. It should be emphasized that six of these patients had normal pancreatograms; therefore, a normal pancreatogram does not rule out carcinoma. The six patients with normal pancreatograms all had abnormal cholangiograms. The most characteristic finding in carcinoma of the pancreas was a long stenosis. There are caliber changes and irregularity was seen in four and five patients, respectively. Obstruction of the pancreatic duct is noted in eight patients. Changes in the lateral branches seen in carcinoma of the pancreas are probably related

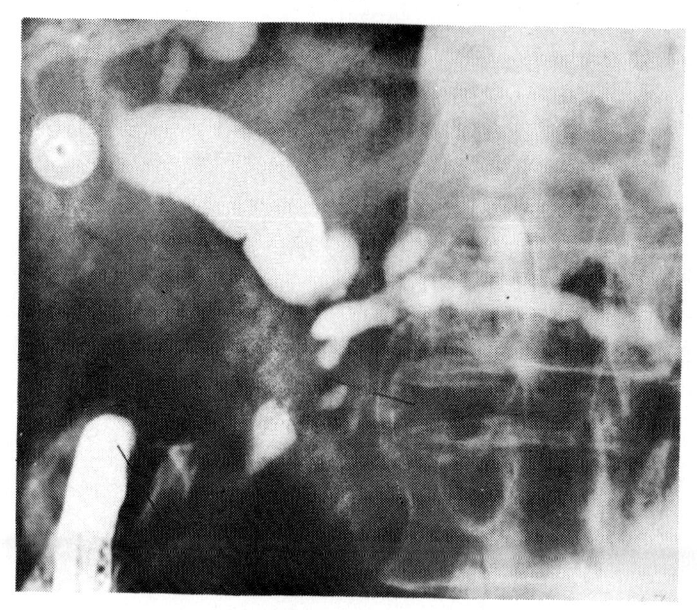

FIG. 5. This pancreatocholangiogram shows obstruction of the common bile duct with a long stenotic area. A very long stenotic area is seen in the pancreatic duct between the arrows. The changes in the body of the pancreas are similar to those seen in chronic pancreatitis. At surgery, adenocarcinoma of the pancreas was found in the area of the stenotic duct and chronic pancreatitis in the remainder of the gland.

Table 5. Pancreatographic Findings in Patients With Proven Neoplasm Involving Pancreas

Number of patients	23
Satisfactory studies	22
Normal pancreatograms	6
Extraductal cavity filled	4
Mass effect	0
Abnormal endoscopic cholangiogram	11
Main Pancreatic Duct	
Caliber irregularity	4
Increased caliber	5
Stenosis	10
Obstruction or nonfilling	8
Ductal calculi	1
Ductal Branches	
Nonfilling or obstruction	2
Caliber irregularity	4

to coexisting pancreatitis. Obstruction or nonfilling of the pancreatic duct must be interpreted with great caution because it is observed in all disease groups and has been seen as a low pressure filling artifact.

Pancreatic Pseudocysts

Definition: Surgical Proof of Pseudocyst by Drainage

Figure 6 shows faint filling of the pseudocyst with obstruction of the duct. There is a second nonfilling pseudocyst indenting the antrum of the stomach. Knowledge of this complex anatomy preoperatively was important to the surgical drainage of these lesions. Large nonfilling pancreatic pseudocysts have been seen stretching the common duct and displacing the duodenum. Lack of involvement of the duct suggests benign nature of these masses. Table 6 shows the findings in 16 patients with proven pancreatic pseudocyst. Eleven of the cysts filled with contrast. Three had a mass effect and three had an abnormal cholangiogram. The diagnosis could be suspected in 15 of the 16 patients from filling of the cyst in 11 cases and a prominent mass effect in 4 additional patients. Changes in caliber, irregularity and obstruction of the main duct and the ductal branches are probably related to coexisting chronic pancreatitis.

Miscellaneous Cases

We have seen two patients with apparent spontaneous healing of pancreatic pseudocysts. These patients were not treated by surgical drainage because they were relatively asymptomatic at the time of the initial study and the contrast drained promptly from the cyst. On repeat studies, the cystic space no longer filled with contrast and the impression on the upper GI series had disappeared. These cases were not included in the group of pseudocyst because of lack of surgical proof.

Figure 7 shows the pancreatogram on a patient that we have referred to as "pancreatic pseudo-pseudocyst" [3]. This was a 56-year-old alcoholic man who developed pancreatitis and became jaundiced during the pancreatitis. Approximately six weeks later, the jaundice had cleared but a palpable mass remained. At the time of the first study, shown on the right, there is attenuation of the common duct with displacement of the duodenum. The pancreatic duct is poorly filled and displaced from the common duct. In the second study, shown on the left, the common bile duct now courses along the duodenum without dilatation and the pancreatic duct back along the common duct, and the duodenal displacement is no longer present. The upper GI series at the time of the

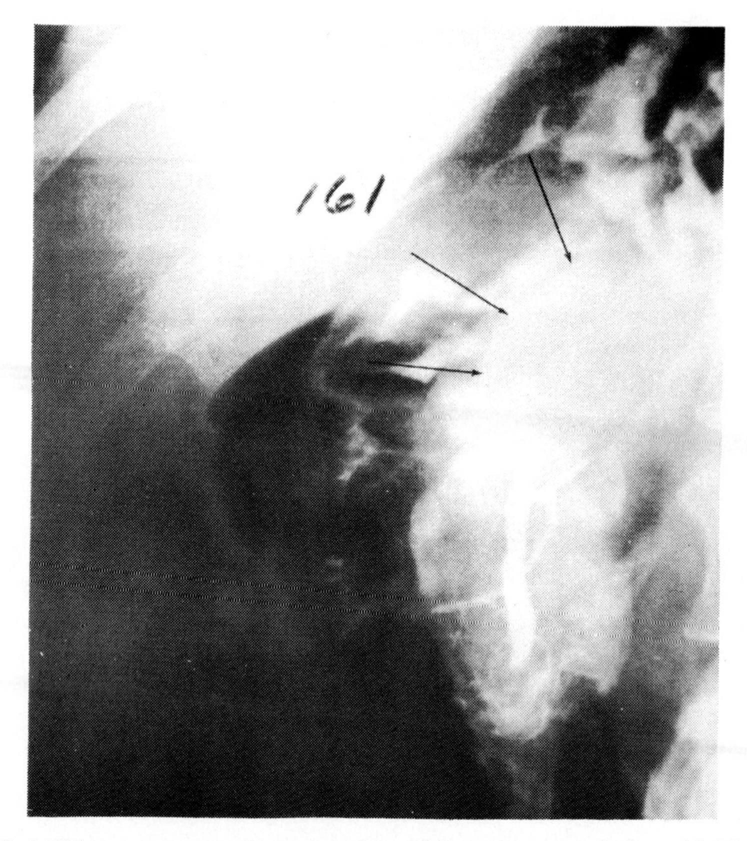

FIG. 6. This pancreatogram shows obstruction of the main pancreatic duct with faint filling of a cystic space. An impression on the antrum by a mass is shown at the arrows. These areas were shown to be pancreatic pseudocysts at surgery.

Table 6. Pancreatographic Findings in Patients With Proven Pancreatic Pseudocyst

Number of patients	16
Satisfactory studies	16
Normal pancreatograms	0
Extraductal cavity filled	11
Mass effect	3
Abnormal endoscopic cholangiogram	3
Main Pancreatic Duct	
Caliber irregularity	2
Increased caliber	4
Stenosis	0
Obstruction or nonfilling	12
Ductal calculi	1
Ductal Branches	
Nonfilling	2
Caliber irregularity	8

initial study showed a mass impressing on the antrum. This was no longer present at the time of the second study and the palpable mass had disappeared. We felt that this most likely represented pancreatic edema.

Figure 8 illustrates some attenuation of the pancreatic duct near the papilla with displacement of the major and accessory pancreatic duct, shown at the arrows. This was interpreted to represent a mass in the area between the main and accessory pancreatic duct. At surgery a true cyst of the pancreas was drained from this area. We have studied two true cysts; as anticipated, neither filled with contrast agent.

Table 7 shows the complications of the procedure in these 300 patients. The nine patients with cholangitis all had a delay in surgical relief of the obstruction. We have not observed cholangitis in patients without an obstructed common bile duct. Our current policy is to have them operated on within 24 hours, if they have had no previous cholangitis. If they have had symptoms suggestive of cholangitis, we feel that the procedure should be done immediately before operation. There were ten patients with clinical pancreatitis, which we have defined as pain for more than four hours following the procedure with an elevated serum or urine amylase. None of these patients developed severe pancreatitis. We injected dye into the duodenal wall on one occasion without difficulty. One patient had a respiratory arrest from the premedication and one had sepsis following the injection of a pancreatic abscess. Asymptomatic hyperamylasuria occurs in 40%-60% of the patients studied [4].

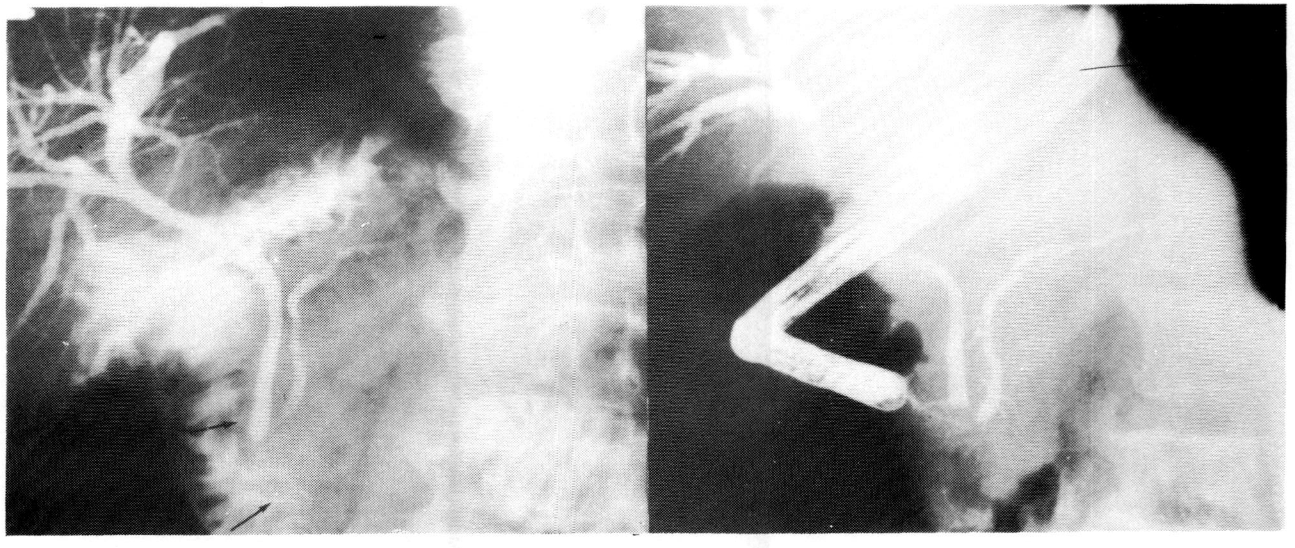

FIG. 7. On the right: This pancreatico-cholangiogram shows displacement of the common bile duct and pancreatic duct from each other and the duodenum. The bile duct above the pancreas was slightly dilated. (This finding is not well shown in the picture.) A mass impressing the duodenum seen at the arrows. On the left: When studied 6 weeks later, the displacement of the ducts and evidence of mass impressing the duodenum at the arrows is no longer present. Dilatation of the common bile duct is no longer seen. The mass felt on physical examination had disappeared and the deformity on the upper gastrointestinal series was no longer present. We believe this sequence of events is best explained by resolving pancreatic edema.

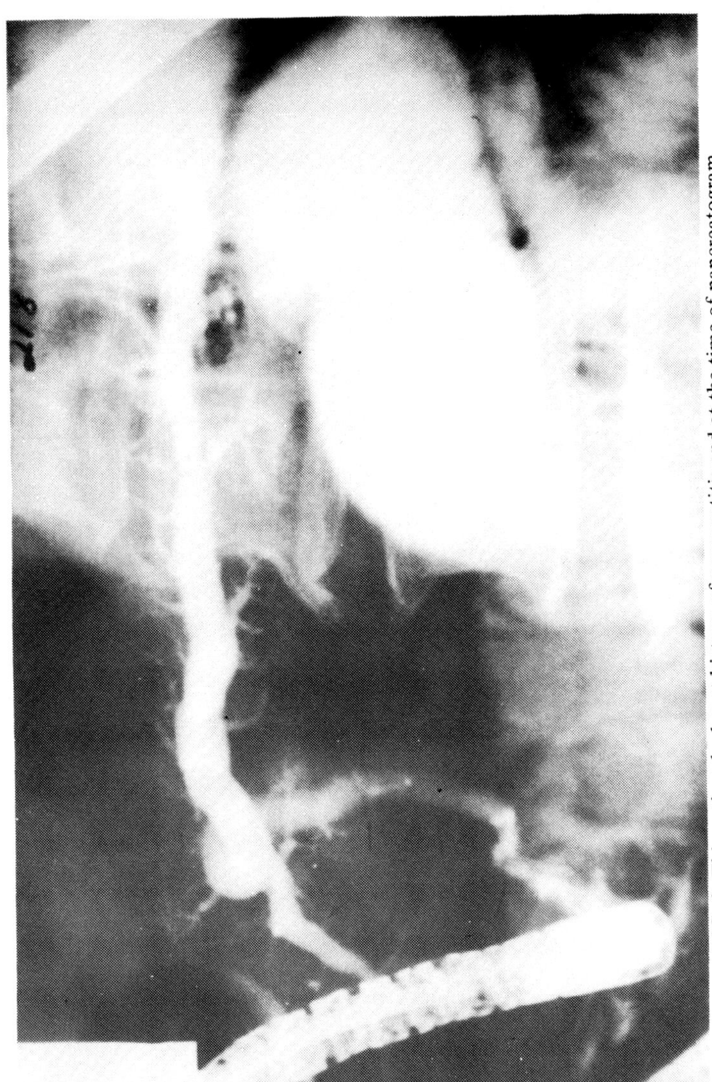

FIG. 8. This patient had past history of pancreatitis and at the time of pancreatogram had chronic abdominal pain. There is stretching and attenuation of the main and accessory pancreatic duct shown by the arrows. At surgery this mass was shown to be a true cyst of the pancreas which was drained into the duodenum. The remainder of the pancreatic duct shows dilatation with some clubbing of the lateral branches, either related to chronic pancreatic or partial obstruction by the true cyst. After surgery the patient had marked decrease but not complete disappearance of the abdominal pain.

Table 7. Complications of Ductal Cannulation Procedures (300 patients)

Cholangitis	9
Pancreatitis	10
Dye injected into duodenal wall	1
Respiratory depression	1
Sepsis following injection of pancreatic abscess	1
Total	22
(Hyperamylasuria 40%)	

The data on pancreatography are inconclusive. Many more cases need to be carefully analyzed. In our experience, a cholangiogram, along with the pancreatogram, is very important. The problem of chronic pancreatitis versus carcinoma of the pancreas remains difficult, as it is to the surgeon at the operating table. We are hopeful that the analysis of a number of cases in careful detail will help to resolve this problem. Results in pancreatic pseudocyst look quite promising.

We would urge caution in the interpretation of pancreatograms. One must be certain that a good study was obtained before action is taken and if necessary repeat the study if findings are equivocal. There needs to be some reevaluation of the question: Can we tailor surgery in the treatment of chronic pancreatic pain on the basis of the findings on the pancreatogram? Notwithstanding these limitations, we feel that pancreatography will advance our knowledge of pancreatic disease.

References

1. Vennes, J. A. and Silvis, S. E.: Endoscopic visualization of bile and pancreatic ducts. Gastroint. Endosc., 18:149-152, 1972.
2. Silvis, S. E. and Vennes, J. A.: The role of glucagon in endoscopic pancreatography, abstracted. Gastroint. Endosc., 20:185, 1974.
3. Shafer, R. and Silvis, S. E.: Pancreatic pseudo-pseudocyst. Amer. J. Surg., 127:320, 1974.
4. Blackwood, W. D., Vennes, J. A. and Silvis, S. E.: Elevations of urine amylase following upper gastrointestinal endoscopy. Gastroint. Endosc., 20:56-58, 1973.

Bibliography

Classen, M.: Fibreendoscopy of the intestines. Gut, 12:330, 1971.

Cotton, P. B.: Cannulation of the papilla of Vater by endoscopy and retrograde cholangiopancreatography (ERCP). Gut, 13:1014, 1972.

Cotton, P. B., Salmon, P. R., Blumgart, L. D. et al: Cannulation of papilla of Vater via fiber-duodenoscope; Assessment of retrograde cholangiopancreatography in 60 patients, Lancet, 1:53, 1972.

Doubilet, J., Poppel, M. and Mulholland, J. H.: Pancreatography: Techniques, principles and observation. Radiology, 64:325, 1955.

Doubilet, H., Poppel, M. H. and Mulholland, J. H.: Pancreatography. Ann. N. Y. Acad. Sci., 78:829, 1959.

Ogoshi, K., Niwa, M., Hara, Y. et al: Endoscopic pancreatocholangiography in the evaluation of pancreatic and biliary disease. Gastroenterology, 64:210, 1973.

Oi, I.: Fiberduodenoscopy and endoscopic pancreatocholangiography. Gastroint. Endosc., 17:59, 1970.

Okuda, K., Someya, N., Goto, A. et al: Endoscopic pancreatocholangiography: A preliminary report on technique and diagnostic significance. Amer. J. Roentgen., 117:435, 1973.

Rohrmann, C., Vennes, J. A. and Silvis, S. E.: Evaluation of the endoscopic pancreatogram. Radiology. (In press.)

Silvis, S. E., Rohrmann, C. and Vennes, J. A.: Diagnostic criteria for the evaluation of endoscopic pancreatograms. Gastroint. Endosc., 20:51-55, 1973.

Silvis, S. E., Vennes, J. A. and Rohrmann, C.: Endoscopic pancreatography in the evaluation of the patients with suspected pancreatic pseudocyst. Amer. J. Gastroent. (In press.)

Takagi, K., Ikeda, S., Nakagawa, Y. et al: Retrograde pancreatography and cholangiography by fiber duodenoscope. Gastroenterology, 59:445, 1970.

Vennes, J. A.: Peroral retrograde pancreatography and cholangiography. *In* Margulis, A. R. (ed.): Alimentary Tract Radiology, ed. 2. St. Louis, Mo.:C. V. Mosby Company, 1973.

Vennes, J. A., Jacobson, J. R. and Silvis, S. E.: Endoscopic cholangiography in the evaluation of the biliary system. Ann. Int. Med., 80:61-64, 1974.

Figures 5 and 6 are reproduced with permission from *Gastrointestinal Endoscopy* (20:51, 1973).

Acute Pancreatitis: The Toxic Effects

Marvin L. Gliedman, M.D.

This is a compilation of data from over 2,000 patients seen during a 13-year period [1], handled by the same staff giving therapy under a fairly set regimen. These patients give insights rarely appreciated by the individual physician caring for the "occasional" pancreatitis patient.

I shall start with the conclusion, that is, the cause of death from pancreatitis really falls into two categories (Fig. 1). In the first, the patient develops necrosis and gangrene of the pancreas. He develops a large lesser sac collection. It is either properly drained or the patient goes on to die from sepsis. The second group of patients has signs and symptoms that tend to be progressive from the time of admission for severe pancreatitis, with shock, electrolyte imbalances, abnormal electrocardiograms, neurasthenias, toxic encephalopathies (DTs), renal shutdown, hyperkalemia and, finally, respiratory failure and death. These may be characterized as toxic phenomena and are probably due to denatured protein products, active enzymes and other breakdown products that should not be intraperitoneal, retroperitoneal or systemic.

The incidence of pancreatitis in this experience was almost 200 cases per year. Even late in the course of this series, 22 patients in a single year were identified only at autopsy. Today, the great surgical mimic is acute pancreatitis. Within the last few months, a patient was in our hospital for two months. Finally, when he came to surgery, for another reason, he was found to have a still acute pancreatitis.

These patients follow fairly set patterns. There are the "chronic" acute pancreatitis; they tend to be admitted, get their analgesia and leave after a brief stay. The treated group we have divided into either "benign" or so-called malignant type. The overall mortality runs about 9% and has

---

Marvin L. Gliedman, M.D., Professor and Chairman, Department of Surgery, Albert Einstein College of Medicine (MHMC); Chief of Surgery, Montefiore Hospital and Medical Center, Bronx, N. Y.

DEATH FROM PANCREATITIS

TOXIC	SEPTIC
Shock (Hypovolemia) Hypocalcemia Abnormal ECG Neurasthenia Sensorium (D.T.'s Hallucinations) Renal shutdown (Azotemia, Oligueria, Hyperkalemia) Resp. failure	Pancreatic abscess Lesser Sac collection

FIGURE 1.

remained relatively unchanged over the years. If you decide, within 12 to 24 hours of admission that the patient is in the "malignant" category, one third of this group will die. A considerably smaller percentage of those who appear benign on admission will succumb (Fig. 2). You must successfully treat the "malignant cases" to significantly change the mortality from acute pancreatitis. The benign case is what you would expect it to be. The patient has mild pain, needs little electrolyte or colloid solution, has a mild temperature and leukocyte elevation, has mild amylase elevation and has a relatively mild ileus that rapidly abates.

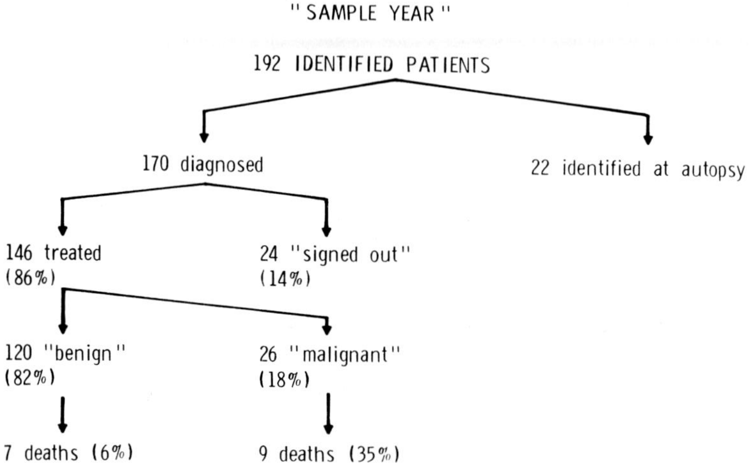

"SAMPLE YEAR"

192 IDENTIFIED PATIENTS

170 diagnosed

22 identified at autopsy

146 treated
(86%)

24 "signed out"
(14%)

120 "benign"
(82%)

26 "malignant"
(18%)

7 deaths (6%)

9 deaths (35%)

FIGURE 2.

Contrariwise, the malignant form is accompanied by severe abdominal findings, and the need for large amounts of colloid and electrolyte. There is higher fever and a higher leukocytosis and, very importantly, tachypnea and dyspnea. Patients commonly have left pleural effusions and free peritoneal fluid; sometimes, they have profound ileus. Operation is common in this group of patients.

This distinction may be made more objective by looking at some of the features for each group. There is an age difference that relates to the higher incidence of older patients with biliary tract disease in the malignant groups. There are more females in the malignant group. We ordinarily think of pancreatitis as being a "seven day" disease. If the patient is not well and on his way home by that period of time, we begin to worry about the complications or the progressions of these toxic signs and findings. It is interesting to note that in a sample group of "benign" patients, only one was operated upon – a 72-year-old man with his second admission for gallbladder disease and pancreatitis. He appeared "benign," but the disease progressed. He was operated upon and died, one week later, following cholecystectomy and choledochotomy, with azotemia and acute respiratory failure, which is a very typical end for these patients. In the sample year group (Fig. 2), 15 patients characterized as malignant required surgery.

In looking at statistics for causes of pancreatitis, you can switch the percentage back and forth between biliary disease and alcoholism, depending upon your institution. In a city hospital population they are primarily alcoholic. At the present time at Montefiore Hospital, we see more biliary tract-caused pancreatitis. This does not refer to people who enter with acute gallbladder disease with an elevated amylase. The group discussed enters with acute pancreatitis without obvious acute biliary pathology. Patients present with the syndrome of acute pancreatitis. They are often found to have biliary tract pathology later or retrospectively.

There were some 370 deaths in our series. A high proportion of the biliary tract induced pancreatitis patients fell into this group. Many think that pancreatitis caused by biliary tract disease is a milder disease. This series showed quite the contrary. This group of patients has a soft, succulent enzyme-rich gland. As well, in our opinion, these patients are more liable to die, being older than the alcoholic patient who has the tougher fibrotic gland which has probably had many mild insults previously from alcoholic debauches and is perhaps more enzyme depleted.

Laparotomy resulted in this series (1) when biliary tract disease did not get better, with nonoperative care, (2) when we thought that the patient had, or when we could document a lesser sac abscess or collection and (3) when the diagnosis was in question and surgery was indicated clinically. Finally, a very common indication for operation for acute pancreatitis in our group was "desperation" surgery based on the hope something could be accomplished.

The results of operating in our group showed that if you operated for a specific reason, you lost about one half of the patients; if you operated in desperation and did nothing, the patient's downhill course was hastened, with essentially universal mortality.

Biliary tract surgery is most difficult in this group of patients. In 12 patients, we attempted to remove stones from a common bile duct, knowing they were there. In only four instances could we retrieve the stones. There is considerable distortion of the anatomy by edema and inflammation, making successful operation most difficult.

One might think that the diagnosis of choledocholithiasis would be obvious in the group of patients with gallstones. Jaundice, however, was more commonly associated with alcoholic pancreatitis. Only 20% of the patients who had stones in the common bile duct had objective signs which could lead to the diagnosis of a common duct stone. Practically, one has to go on the premise that the patient has acute cholecystitis or he has a stone in the common duct if his disease is not due to alcoholism. People with simple chronic cholelithiasis, in this series, rarely had severe acute pancreatitis.

What about toxic factors? Ordinarily, we think that shock in pancreatitis is simply due to hypovolemia with peritoneal and retroperitoneal fluid; perhaps other pharmacologically active materials are involved. Certainly, however, if the patient goes into shock, he is in the malignant category. It is an ominous prognostic indicator. If you take a series of patients with shock that have been reported, the mortality is high [2]. Whether this blood pressure depression is due to one of the 'kinins remains unanswered. In treating large numbers of patients for shock with colloid, suspicion arises that there is something other than simple colloid depletion that is at fault. Similarly renal failure, in this group, appears to be not simply a feature of shock. The presence of renal failure is also an ominous sign although it is well handled in the majority of patients; people who have renal failure with acute pancreatitis have a high mortality [3]. Thal identified patients with anuria, who did not have preceding shock [4]. It is unfortunate that biopsy data on the kidneys are relatively meager because it is clear that the group with shock will have acute tubular necrosis. There is a small group of patients, however, who had their renal pathology reviewed during their acute pancreatitis episode. That group of patients, interestingly enough, also had glomerulitis, an entity that we ordinarily relate more to toxic phenomena than to hypotension [5].

There was a subgroup of pancreatitis patients that clearly had considerable respiratory problems. Recognizing that this group of over 2,000 patients was relatively young and considering that the biliary group was relatively small, we had a disproportionate number of patients who had such trouble. You can separate from the respiratory pathology group a subgroup that had a rather identifiable syndrome. Usually there was a 24-hour period with the patient having a rising pulse, a rising blood pressure, a rising temperature, tachycardia, acute dyspnea and, finally, cardiorespiratory arrest.

Ranson has measured blood gases serially on a group of acute pancreatitis patients, from the time of admission. He has demonstrated that early blood gas changes parallel the severity of the attack [6]. We think that this particular respiratory syndrome is similar to, if not exactly the same, as the acute respiratory overwork syndrome that Burke [7] described for patients with peritonitis. Burke described high output failure as a vicious circle, with an increased need for oxygen, the patient increasing his respiratory rate, ending with shallow breathing and a low alveolar opening pressure, resulting in atelectasis and shunting. To maintain a high oxygen uptake the patient increases his cardiac and respiratory work. There is an added facet, of course, in the patient with acute pancreatitis; he has active ferments, including lecithinase, that can act on surfactant. Surfactant is needed for alveolar integrity and is rich in lecithin. The lecithinase can destroy surfactant and so aggravate the alveolar factor in the respiratory failure syndrome.

Another common "toxic" finding is an abnormal electrocardiogram from myocarditis and sometimes neurasthenia. We also see toxic encephalitis (DTs), renal shutdown and respiratory failure. How should this kind of patient be treated? We have used the usual regimen, giving lots of fluid, lots of colloid, at one point Traysolol, and antibiotics. However, nothing really seems to reach this group of people, and they progress to respiratory failure and death.

Peritoneal Lavage

It is interesting to note that the experimental data for the treatment of acute pancreatitis with peritoneal lavage are rather clear [8, 9]. All of the studies using peritoneal dialysis or peritoneal lavage with experimental pancreatitis show either that the animals have an improved survival rate or that the progression of the disease stops. In 1966 we thought lavage promising experimentally and tried it. At that time Dr. Wall had published information on a group of three patients with toxic signs [10]. Gjessing [11], as well, published on patients who survived with peritoneal lavage.

Hemodialysis in this group of patients does not seem to offer much [12]. Simply treating azotemia does not, apparently, have a lasting effect. It would appear that the lavage with the removal of the ferments from the peritoneal cavity is the useful feature. We have utilized a high volume (30 liters/24 hours) of 4¼% dialysate containing 5 mg heparin sulfate, 4 mEq potassium and 40 mg of Keflin per liter.

These case summaries illustrate a fairly common sequential pattern in the malignant group. They show the progression illustrated in Figure 1.

Illustrative Case Summaries

Case #1 – 43-Year-Old Male

Admission –	Severe abdominal pain, temp. 103°F, pulse 120, WBC 12,000, serum amylase 550 Somogyi units
10th day –	Stuporous Dialysis: in 24 hours awake Postdialysis out of bed (2nd day)
25th day –	Discharged

Case #2 – 37-Year-Old Female

Admission –	To psychiatry – dx. acute DTs Treated for *10 days,* hallucinating, abdominal pain, B.P. 80/60, pulse 120, CVP 0, serum amylase 280 Somogyi units
18th day –	Temp. 104°F, 46 ml paraldehyde for agitation, incoherent; postdialysis: coherent and awake, pulse down, urine output up
27th day –	Discharged

Case #3 – 22-Year-Old Female

Admission –	Alcoholic, temp. 102°F, resp. rate 28/min, pulse 100, Hct. 37%, serum amylase 277 Somogyi units
2nd day –	Temp. 105°F, pulse 140
4th day –	*Stuporous, temp. 105°F, pulse 100,* HCT 42%, WBC 11,000, *CVP 0,* with dialysis: no more colloid required, abdominal pain disappeared
11th day –	Discharged

Case #4 54-Year-Old Male

Admission –	Alcoholic, 10 day Hx., temp. 102°F, pulse 110, serum amylase 1,648 Somogyi units
4th day –	*Stuporous,* resp. rate 28/min, severe *abdominal pain*
5th day –	Dialysis: Sensorium improved. Pain decreased
6th day –	Temp. normal, wide awake
7th day –	Out of bed, oral feedings
10th day –	Normal upper GI and IV cholangiogram Discharged

Case #5 – 35-Year-Old Female

Admission –	Temp. 101°F, pulse 140, CVP 8, serum amylase 208 Somogyi units
5th day –	DTs, temp. 104°F, pulse 140 beats/min, WBC 12,000, CVP 15 cm H_2O Tachycardia
7th day –	Stuporous, temp. 104°F, resp. difficulties, B.P. down, pneumonia or atelectasis, azotemia
9th day –	Isoproterenol, mannitol for oliguria, K 6.9, Engstrom resp. B.P. 50%, CVP 25, dialysis: 16 hours, *DIED*

Somewhere in the course, stupor or a significant change in sensorium occurs. At this point the use of peritoneal lavage appears a useful adjunct, though the data are anecdotal and not statistically significant.

Patient #5 demonstrated the sequence to death. Admission findings demonstrated the malignant criteria: a progression by the fifth day to a change in sensorium, a strikingly elevated fever and, by the seventh day, stupor and the beginning of respiratory difficulties. The patient succumbed receiving isoproterenol, mannitol, respiratory therapy and a final futile attempt at dialysis. Clearly, this patient should have been lavaged on the fifth day.

In conclusion, a large group of pancreatitis patients can be divided, almost on admission, into a malignant and benign group. Those patients who have the progression of what we have called "toxic symptomatology" should have peritoneal lavage carried out at the time that there is a change in sensorium.

References

1. Gliedman, M. L., Bolooki, H. and Rosen, R. G.: Acute pancreatitis. Curr. Probl. Surg., Aug. 1970.
2. Foster, P. D.: Severe acute pancreatitis. Arch. Surg., 85:92, 1962.

3. Frey, C. F.: Pathogenesis of nitrogen retention in pancreatitis. Amer. J. Surg., 109:747, 1965.
4. Thal, A. P., Perry, J. F., Jr. and Egner, W.: A clinical and morphologic study of 42 cases of fatal acute pancreatitis. Surg. Gynec. Obstet., 105:191, 1957.
5. Sussman, H. M., Reyes, E., Caneghem, A. V. et al: Renal and hepatic pathology in hemorrhagic pancreatitis. Amer. J. Gastroent., 50:351, 1968.
6. Ranson, J. H. C., Roses, D. F. and Fink, S. D.: Early respiratory insufficiency in acute pancreatitis. Ann. Surg., 178:75, 1973.
7. Burke, J. F., Pontoppidan, H. and Welch, C. E.: High output respiratory failure: Important cause of death ascribed to peritonitis or ileus. Ann. Surg., 158:595, 1963.
8. Rogers, R. E. and Carey, L. C.: Peritoneal lavage in experimental pancreatitis in dogs. Amer. J. Surg., 111:792, 1966.
9. Rasmussen, B. L.: Hypothermic peritoneal dialysis in the treatment of acute experimental hemorrhagic pancreatitis. Amer. J. Surg., 114:716, 1967.
10. Wall, A. J.: Peritoneal dialysis in treatment of severe acute pancreatitis. Med. J. Austr., 2:281, 1965.
11. Gjessing, J.: Peritoneal dialysis in severe acute hemorrhagic pancreatitis. Acta Chir. Scand., 133:645, 1967.
12. Balslov, J. T., Jorgensen, H. and Nielsen, R.: Acute renal failure complicating severe acute pancreatitis. Acta Chir. Scand., 124:348, 1962.

Resection for Acute Hemorrhagic Pancreatitis

B. Eiseman, M.D.

This presentation summarizes the technique and role for all-but-total pancreatectomy in acute hemorrhagic pancreatitis.

Neither patient, internist, nor surgeon has enthusiasm for operative intervention in the vast majority of patients with acute pancreatitis. Most get well without the benefit of operation – even though the morbidity is significant, complications frequent and prognosis dismal. There is an occasional patient, however, who presents in the so-called malignant phase of the disease and is resistant to therapy. He is moribund.

Mortality sharply increases as acute edematous pancreatitis progresses to the hemorrhagic stage. Less than 15% of patients die from the uncomplicated disease [1]. In contrast, Foster and Ziffren [2] reported a mortality of 82% among 28 patients with acute hemorrhagic pancreatitis. Nine of 12 patients (67%) died of acute hemorrhagic pancreatitis in the series of Kaplan, Cotlar and Stagg [3]. There were no survivors in 30 patients treated nonoperatively according to Jordan and Spjut [4] whereas mortality was 57% among 21 patients treated operatively (Table 1).

A significant improvement in survival after sump drainage of the pancreas itself was reported by Waterman et al [5]. Only one of ten patients so treated died. Lawson et al [6] added tube decompression of the biliary and gastrointestinal systems to sump drainage to obtain survival in six of eight patients with acute hemorrhagic pancreatitis. Such success with drainage techniques has not been achieved either in our experience or in that of others who have reported mortalities of 50% or more.

Faced with the enormous mortality of the "maligant" form of acute hemorrhagic pancreatitis ("M"AP), sporadic attempts have been made to resect the inflamed organ. Watts in 1963 [7] made the first such suggestion.

B. Eiseman, M.D., Department of Surgery, Denver General Hospital and University of Colorado Medical Center.

Table 1. Mortality

Simple Edematous Pancreatitis ± 15%	
AHP	
Foster & Ziffrin (28)	82%
Kaplin (15 pts)	67%
Jorden (30 pts) non-op	100%
(21 pts operation)	57%

Rives, Stoppa and Lardennois [8] subsequently resected portions of the pancreas along with the spleen in three patients with acute hemorrhagic pancreatitis and all patients survived. Devic, Garde and Gelain [9] reported the use of pancreatectomy in eight patients, but only one, a survivor, had hemorrhagic disease.

The largest experience with resection for acute hemorrhagic pancreatitis is that of Hollender et al [10-13]. To date, he [14] had removed various amounts of pancreas in 23 patients with a mortality of 35%. Three patients had resection of the pancreas to the left of the portal vein and all survived. Ten had resection at the portal vein and six survived. A technique of near total pancreatectomy similar to ours was performed in six patients, two of whom died, a mortality of 33%. The head of the pancreas and the duodenum were excised in three patients, only one of whom survived. One patient survived total pancreaticoduodenectomy.

Our experience at the Denver General Hospital with the "malignant" form of acute pancreatitis was as dismal as others [15]. Operative drainage had little influence and those that did not die had a long hospitalization filled with distressing and expensive complications. We therefore instituted the policy of all-but-total pancreatectomy (Child's procedure) in established cases of "M"AP.

Our experience to date can thus be summarized:

Case 1. A 42-year-old Spanish-American woman was hospitalized 12 hours after the onset of severe epigastric pain which followed heavy ingestion of alcohol. History was significant only for chronic alcoholism. Initial examination of the abdomen revealed epigastric guarding and tenderness and absent bowel sounds. Temperature and vital signs were within normal limits. Chemistries demonstrated an amylase level of 316 Somogyi units (normal, 60 to 150 units). After 36 hours, despite nasogastric suction and fluid replacement, temperature was 39°C and amylase was 444 Somogyi units. The patient's abdomen was rigid with rebound tenderness. Urine output was less than 20 ml per hour. On exploration, hemorrhagic pancreatitis involving the entire gland was found. Two liters of serosanguineous fluid were aspirated from the peritoneal cavity. The lesser sac contained a large inflammatory mass extending from the hilum of the spleen to the second portion of the duodenum. Splenectomy, 80% pancreatectomy and cholecystostomy were performed within 1½ hours. The excised pancreas, weighing 60 gm, showed focal necrosis with hemorrhage in peripancreatic fat. The first two postoperative days were complicated by a respiratory distress syndrome which cleared gradually with ventilation and diuretic therapy. Recovery was rapid thereafter and the patient was discharged from the hospital 16 days after surgery.

Case 2. A 38-year-old black man with chronic alcoholism was admitted 12 hours after the onset of diffuse abdominal pain which followed a drinking episode. Temperature was 39°C and blood pressure was within normal limits. The abdomen was distended with guarding and rebound tenderness in the lower quadrants and absent bowel sounds. Amylase was 71 Somogyi units and white blood cell count 16,000 per mm^3. Serum calcium was within normal limits. During treatment with nasogastric suction, the patient became increasingly ill, with abdominal rigidity, fever of 40°C, tachycardia and hypotension, which was unresponsive to rapid intravenous infusion of fluids. At laparotomy 24 hours after admission, the body and tail of the pancreas were necrotic and hemorrhagic in appearance. An inflammatory mass involved the mid distal pancreas, spleen and left kidney. Only a small amount of cloudy fluid was present in the peritoneal cavity. Splenectomy, 65% pancreatectomy and cholecystostomy were performed in an operation lasting 90 minutes. The excised pancreas measured 12 cm in length and showed extensive parenchymal necrosis and hemorrhage on histologic examination. Postoperative recovery was complicated by delirium tremens occurring from the third to the seventh day. The patient was discharged 11 days postoperatively after removal of the drains and cholecystostomy tube.

Case 3. A 24-year-old albino black man was awakened by epigastric pain six hours before admission to the hospital. He denied having previous abdominal pain but admitted to having chronic alcoholism. The abdomen was rigid with rebound tenderness and no bowel sounds. Temperature, vital signs and blood cell count were within normal limits. Serum amylase was 438 Somogyi units. Despite 24 hours of treatment with nasogastric suction and fluid replacement, the patient's abdomen remained rigid and tender. Temperature was 39°C and white blood cell count was 16,000 per mm^3. Serum calcium level was normal. Tachycardia, hypotension and diminishing urine output prompted surgical exploration of the abdomen. An inflammatory mass with hemorrhage and saponification of fat surrounded the pancreas. Several liters of serosanguineous fluid were present within the abdomen. Splenectomy and 85% pancreatectomy were performed over a two hour period. The excised pancreas measured 15 cm in length and weighed 150 gm. Microscopic examination revealed acute inflammation of the parenchyma with focal necrosis and interstitial hemorrhage. A severe respiratory distress syndrome occurred on the second postoperative day and persisted for one week. There were no abdominal complications referable to pancreatectomy. Drains were removed on the eighth day and the patient was discharged from the hospital 20 days after surgery.

Case 4. A 47-year-old white woman underwent cholecystectomy, choledocholithotomy and sphincterotomy in another state. Several hours after operation she became hypotensive, requiring blood transfusion. During the next five days, bleeding occurred intermittently via peritoneal drains and a nasogastric tube. On the sixth postoperative day the patient was transferred to a Denver hospital because of bleeding (hematocrit, 15%) and anuria (blood urea nitrogen, 200 mg/100 ml). Gastric hemorrhage increased during renal dialysis. The patient became comatose with unobtainable blood pressure. Another surgeon explored the abdomen 24 hours after transfer, finding free blood and a large hematoma which filled the left gutter. The transverse mesocolon appeared to have been digested and its vessels were bleeding in several areas. The presence of hemorrhagic pancreatitis with saponification in surrounding fat was confirmed after evacuation of the hematoma. The surgeon performed splenectomy, 85% pancreatectomy, vagotomy and gastroenterostomy in an operation lasting 2½ hours. The pancreatic specimen showed focal necrosis and hemorrhage in the parenchyma.

Postoperatively, persistent anuria required repeated renal dialysis, although the patient had awakened and had normal vital signs. Gastric bleeding recurred one week after pancreatectomy. Emergency laparotomy revealed disruption of the gastroenterostomy. The lesser sac, however, contained no pus or necrotic debris. Antrectomy and gastrojejunostomy were performed. Four days later, despite improving renal function, the patient became semicomatose with evidence of sepsis. Death occurred three weeks after pancreatectomy and was attributed to sepsis caused by unsuspected leakage from a duodenotomy performed during the initial operation for choledocholithiasis. At autopsy the bed of the resected pancreas contained no pus and the cut surface of the pancreatic remnant appeared normal.

Case 5. Following a week long alcoholic debauch during a leave period, a 20-year-old airman was admitted to Fitzsimmons Army Hospital desperately ill with acute hemorrhagic pancreatitis. He had bilateral pleural effusion with amylase concentration over 1,200 units. For 24 hours the issue was in doubt but he gradually began to improve. But on the tenth postadmission day, he developed high fever, ecchymoses, scrotal fluid and severe toxicity. He looked like he would die.

Laparotomy on March 28, 1974, disclosed massive pancreatic necrosis. An all but total pancreatectomy was performed, leaving only 1 cm along the duodenum. Because the veins over the superior mesenteric vein were open, a small rim (7 mm) of pancreatic tissue was left covering the vein and bleeders cauterized.

His postoperative course was benign. He had no respiratory insufficiency and was up and eating by the fourth postoperative day. He is maintained on 25 units insulin.

Operative Technique

The technique of near total pancreatectomy, similar in all the patients described, began with mobilization of the spleen to allow left to right dissection of the pancreas. The splenic artery was ligated after division of the spleen's attachments. By retraction of the spleen anteriorly, the tail of the pancreas was identified despite surrounding inflammation. A plane of dissection posterior to the pancreas was established with surprising ease. Blunt or sharp dissection through inflammatory tissue promptly exposed the pancreas. The gland could be peeled from the surrounding edematous, hemorrhagic tissue.

Dissection proceeded rapidly to the confluence of the splenic and superior mesenteric veins. The splenic vein was divided at this point. Venous tributaries from the pancreas, very troublesome during pancreatectomy for cancer or trauma, were usually thrombosed and could often be divided without tying. Silver clips were sufficient for those small vessels which remained patent.

In the three patients with disease of the entire gland, the uncinate process of the pancreas was partially excised as dissection progressed toward the duodenum. The percentage of pancreatectomy was determined by the amount of gland left along the duodenal loop, as in Child's procedure for chronic pancreatitis [16]. A rim of pancreas measuring between 1.5 and 2.0 cm was representative of an 85% pancreatectomy. Division of the gland just to the right of the portal vein was judged to be a 65% pancreatectomy.

No attempt was made to close the distal pancreatic remnant except in Case 2 in which 35% of the pancreas remained. A sump drain and multiple

Penrose type rubber drains were placed in the pancreatic bed and lesser sac and were removed five to ten days after surgery. After cholecystostomy was judged to be of little benefit in diverting bile flow in the first two patients, it was not used in subsequent operations.

Time spent in actual dissection of the pancreas in all patients averaged 30 minutes. A clear demarcation of diseased and normal pancreas was evident in Case 2. Others had division of the pancreas through obviously diseased tissue.

Discussion

When faced with the grave condition of malignant acute pancreatitis, we advise an all-but-total pancreatectomy according to the Child's technique [16].

During the past year we had occasion to care for a 26-year-old lady who in the postpartum period developed an acute abdomen and at laparotomy had severe hemorrhagic pancreatitis. Although our experience as here recorded dictated resecting the gland, we were loath to do so in such a young nonalcoholic patient. We drained and got out. Her postoperative course has been horrible with most of the life- and happiness-threatening complications of the disease spread over three months. She subsequently has required as her fourth operation, pancreatic resection. We wish we had donc it at the original exploration.

Conclusion

Five patients with the "malignant" form of acute hemorrhagic pancreatitis have been treated by Child's procedure of all-but-total pancreatectomy. All have survived the immediate postoperative period. One died 25 days following operation of an unrelated complication.

Pancreatectomy of this type is advised for unremitting life-threatening pancreatitis in the occasional patient. Technically, it is surprisingly easy and the postoperative course is characteristically benign except for self-limiting transient respiratory distress.

References

1. Gliedman, M. L,, Boloorki, H. and Rosen, R. G.: Acute pancreatitis. Curr. Probl. Surg., August, 1970.
2. Foster, P. D. and Ziffren, S. E.: Severe acute pancreatitis. Arch. Surg., 85:252, 1962.

3. Kaplan, M. H., Cotlar, A. M. and Stagg, S. J.: Acute pancreatitis. Amer. J. Surg., 108:24, 1964.
4. Jordan, G. L. and Spjut, H. J.: Hemorrhagic pancreatitis. Arch. Surg., 104:489, 1972.
5. Waterman, N. G., Walski, R., Kasdan, M. L. et al: The treatment of acute hemorrhagic pancreatitis by sump drainage. Surg. Gynec. Obstet., 126:963, 1968.
6. Lawson, D. W., Daggett, W. M., Civetta, J. M. et al: Surgical treatment of acute necrotizing pancreatitis. Ann. Surg., 172:605, 1970.
7. Watts, G. T.: Total pancreatectomy for fulminant pancreatitis. Lancet, 384:24, 1963.
8. Rives, J., Stoppa, R. and Lardennois, B.: Traitement des pancréatites nécrotiques et hémorragiques par la pancréatectomie gauche. Acad. Chir., 95:346, 1969.
9. Devic, G., Garde, J. and Gelain, J.: Traitement des pancréatites aiguës par pancréatectomie. Lyon Chir., 66:438, 1970.
10. Hollender, L. F., Gillet, M. and Sava, G.: La pancréatectomie d'urgence dans le pancréatites aiguës. Ann. Chir., 24:647, 1970.
11. Hollender, L. F., Gillet, M. and Kohler, J. J.: Die dringliche Pankreatektomie bei der akuten Pankreatitis. Langenbeck Arch. Klin. Chir., 328:314, 1971.
12. Hollender, L. F., Kohler, J. J., Kelin, A. et al: A propos due traitement de la pancréatite aiguë nécrotico-hémorragique. Ann. Chir., 26:649, 1972.
13. Hollender, L. F. Kohler, J. J. and Klein, A.: Zur chirurgischen Behandlung der akuten, nekrotischen Pankretitis. Chirurg., 43:256, 1972.
14. Hollender, L. F.: Personal communication, 1973.
15. Trapnell, J. E.: Management of the complications of acute pancreatitis. Ann. Roy. Coll. Surg. Eng., 49:361, 1971.
16. Child, C. G., Fry, C. F. and Fry, W. J.: A reappraisal of removal of ninety-five per cent of the distal portion of the pancreas. Surg. Gynec. Obstet., 129:49, 1969.

Supported by NIH Grant No. GM20309 and No. AM 17022.

Total Pancreatectomy for Ductal Carcinoma of the Head of the Pancreas

Clayton H. Shatney, M.D., Javier Castellanos, M.D., Guillermo Manifacio, M.D. and Richard C. Lillehei, M.D., Ph.D.

Billroth in 1894 or Franke in 1900 is often credited with performing total pancreatectomy [1], but the first documented total pancreatic resection was reported by Rockey [2] in 1943. The patient survived only 15 days following surgery. The first successful total pancreatectomy was performed by Priestley in 1944 for a benign insulinoma [3]. The uneventful postoperative course of this patient suggested that total removal of the pancreas was both technically and physiologically feasible and stimulated interest in the use of this procedure for pancreatic carcinoma during the next several years (Table 1). In 1954 Ross [4] reported four cases of total pancreatectomy for carcinoma and stated that this procedure was the operation of choice for cancer of the pancreas. Nevertheless, because of the high morbidity and mortality rates and poor long-term survival, total pancreatic resection soon fell into disfavor. In the last decade, however, surgeons have renewed interest in total pancreatectomy in the treatment of ductal carcinoma of the head of the pancreas. At the University of Minnesota three patients have undergone total pancreatic resection for this disease. The results in these patients, along with a review of the literature, form the substance of this report.

Case Reports

Case 1

L. F. (UMH #115-10-83), a 66-year-old white male, was admitted to the University of Minnesota Hospitals on November 16, 1971, because of

---

Clayton H. Shatney, M.D., Javier Castellanos, M.D.,* Guillermo Manifacio, M.D.* and Richard C. Lillehei, M.D., Ph.D., Department of Surgery, University of Minnesota Health Sciences Center, Minneapolis.

*Current Address: Hospital 20 Noviembre, I. S. S. T. E. Mexico, D. F., Mexico.

Table 1. Total Pancreatectomy for Ductal Carcinoma 1943-64

Author	*Number Patients*	*Operative Mortality*	*Survival (yrs) 0-1*	*1-2*	*2-3*
Rockey [2]	1	1			
Brunschwig [5]	2	2			
McClure [6]	1	0	?	?	?
Brunschwig [7]	2	2			
Dixon [8]	1	0		1	
Gaston [9]	1	1			
Ross [4]	4	2		1	1
Chandler [10]	1	0	1		
McCullagh [11]	6	0	6		
Foster [12]	4	1	3		
Warren [13]	6	1	5		
Totals	29	10	15	2	1

epigastric pain and jaundice during the preceding month. Three years prior to admission he had undergone cholecystectomy. Evaluation revealed obstructive jaundice with extrinsic compression on the second portion of the duodenum seen on radiologic examination of the upper gastrointestinal tract.

On November 19, 1971, an exploratory laparotomy was performed. A carcinoma was found involving the head, uncinate process and body of the pancreas; total pancreatectomy and vagotomy were carried out. On pathological examination of the specimen, adenocarcinoma was present in the head and body of the gland, and tumor was seen in the peripancreatic tissue. The regional lymph nodes were free of tumor.

The patient had an uneventful postoperative course and has been maintained on 16-25 units of lente insulin and 16 Viokase® tablets daily. In March, 1973, he underwent a "second look" exploratory laparotomy. No gross recurrent tumor or other intra-abdominal pathology was found. However, microscopic examination of a small cluster of lymph nodes at the celiac axis revealed metastatic adenocarcinoma. The patient is currently alive and well without evidence of further metastatic disease 2½ years after total pancreatectomy. A "third look" is being considered.

Case 2

W. M. (UMH #116-44-13), a 63-year-old white male, entered the University of Minnesota Hospitals on April 16, 1972, with a complaint of painless jaundice of three months' duration. Shortly after the onset of these symptoms, he had undergone cholecystectomy and common bile duct exploration at an outside hospital. Jaundice had recurred whenever the T-tube was clamped, and the patient was referred to University Hospitals for evaluation. T-tube cholangiography revealed complete obstruction of the distal common bile duct.

On April 21, 1972, the patient underwent exploratory laparotomy. A hard mass was palpated in the head of the pancreas, and transduodenal needle biopsy revealed adenocarcinoma. There was no evidence of metastasis to either the liver or the regional lymph nodes, but the entire pancreas was firm. A total pancreatectomy was performed. Pathological examination of the specimen revealed adenocarcinoma of the head and body of the gland with spread to the peripancreatic lymph nodes. The tail of the pancreas was free of tumor, as was the line of resection across the common bile duct.

The patient had an uncomplicated postoperative course and was discharged on May 12, 1972. Diabetes was readily controlled with 20 units of lente and 7 units of regular insulin daily. Symptoms of pancreatic insufficiency were controlled with 12-16 Viokase® tablets per day. The patient died of probable metastatic disease in February 1973, ten months after total pancreatectomy. Permission for autopsy was denied.

Case 3

N. H. (UMH #119-94-74), a 61-year-old white male, was admitted to the University of Minnesota Hospitals on October 28, 1973, with a complaint of jaundice, right upper quadrant pain and fatty food intolerance of six weeks' duration. Just prior to admission to University Hospitals he had undergone exploratory laparotomy at an outside hospital. An open biopsy of a mass in the head of the pancreas had revealed adenocarcinoma.

On November 5, 1973, the patient underwent total pancreatectomy, including resection of a short segment of the superior mesenteric vein with end-to-end anastomosis. Pathological examination revealed adenocarcinoma of the head and neck of the pancreas with posterior extension to the peripancreatic tissue. The body and tail of the gland were free of tumor, as were the regional lymph nodes.

Postoperatively the patient experienced hemorrhagic shock due to intra-abdominal bleeding. At reexploration a leak was found and repaired in the superior mesenteric vein anastomosis. The patient subsequently developed acute renal failure. On the 15th postoperative day, he had a cardiac arrest and could not be resuscitated.

Discussion

One of the major reasons for the renewed interest in total pancreatectomy for ductal carcinoma has been the general dissatisfaction with the results of pancreaticoduodenectomy. Although there have been isolated reports of low mortality following Whipple procedures by experienced surgeons [13-15], in the hands of most surgeons this operation has been fraught with high rates of complication and mortality.

Aston and Longmire [14] reported a 14% mortality rate and listed 46 complications among 65 patients undergoing pancreaticoduodenectomy. Included in this series were the 31 patients of Longmire without an operative death. Only one of 35 patients with carcinoma of the head of the pancreas lived five years. Gilsdorf and Spanos [16] cited a 25% incidence of minor complications and a 40% rate of major complications among 88 patients undergoing Whipple procedures. Twenty-three percent of these patients died in the operative and postoperative periods. Smith [17] experienced a 20.5% operative mortality among 44 patients undergoing pancreaticoduodenectomy for carcinoma of the head of the pancreas. Only two of his patients lived five years following surgery. Monge [18] reported a 21% mortality rate among 119 patients treated by pancreaticoduodenectomy for all types of pancreatic cancer. Of 239 patients undergoing the Whipple procedure for various conditions, 156 (65%) experienced postoperative complications. Only eight of the 119 patients with cancer lived five years. Warren [19] found a 12.4% operative mortality among 89 patients undergoing pancreaticoduodenectomy for carcinoma at the Lahey Clinic. Only two patients survived five years following surgery, and neither had adenocarcinoma of the pancreas.

In addition to the immediate postoperative morbidity and mortality, pancreaticoduodenectomy is associated with a significant incidence of late complications. Warren [19] reported a 12.4% rate of diabetes and a 21.4% incidence of pancreatic insufficiency among 89 patients undergoing the Whipple operation. Miyata et al [20] recently reported the finding of glucose intolerance and an impaired insulin response to oral glucose in ten pancreaticoduodenectomized patients with normal fasting blood sugar concentrations. Four and a half percent of the patients in Warren's series developed jejunal ulceration, a problem that was subsequently eliminated by performing a routine vagotomy at the time of pancreaticoduodenectomy.

Another source of disenchantment with the Whipple procedure in the treatment of pancreatic carcinoma has been the high reported incidence of tumor beyond the line of resection in the pancreas. Monge [21] found carcinoma distal to the point of division in five (18%) of 28 patients undergoing pancreaticoduodenectomy. Hicks and Brooks [22] reported that ten of 22 patients treated for ductal carcinoma by either total pancreatectomy or pancreaticoduodenectomy had tumor in the distal gland. All three of our patients had carcinoma in either the distal pancreas or the peripancreatic tissue, which would have been left behind by a Whipple procedure. The presumed routes of spread of carcinoma of the head of the pancreas are by direct extension of the primary tumor and migration of tumor cells along the pancreatic ducts or lymphatics. In addition, carcinoma of the pancreas is often multicentric in origin [22].

Recently, several small series of patients have been reported following total pancreatectomy for ductal carcinoma (Table 2). The largest study in the literature is that of ReMine et al [23] who presented the results of treatment in 23 patients with various types of pancreatic malignancy. The operative mortality was 22%, and the complication rate was 39%. Of 14 patients surviving surgery and available for long-term follow-up, seven (50%) survived at least two years, and two lived for more than five years following operation. Hicks and Brooks [22] reported on 11 patients undergoing total pancreatectomy for ductal carcinoma during the past ten years. Their operative mortality was 9% and the complication rate was 18%. Of the ten patients surviving surgery, four have lived at least 18 months, and one has lived four years. In 1966-1967, Warren [13] performed total pancreatectomy in five patients without an operative death. No follow-up information is available on these patients. Of the three patients reported in this review, one patient died of complications 15 days postoperatively, and the other two had uneventful postoperative courses. One patient survived ten months, and the other has lived 2½ years following surgery. Thus, of 30 patients in the recent literature with sufficient follow-up information, 20 (65%) have lived at least one year and

Table 2. Total Pancreatectomy for Ductal Carcinoma 1964-74

Author	*Number Patients*	*Operative Mortality*	*Complications*	*Survival (yrs)* 0-1	1-2	2-3	3-5	5
Warren [13]	5	0	?	?	?	?	?	?
ReMine [23]	23	5	7	4*		7	5	2
Hicks [22]	11	1	2	5†	4†		1*	
U. of Minn.	3	1	0	1		1*		
Totals	42	7	9	10	4	8	6	2

*Currently alive and well.

†Two patients alive and well.

16 (53%) at least two years after total pancreatectomy. Ten of these patients are still alive and eligible for five-year survival.

Although the long-term survival following total pancreatectomy is encouraging, it is apparent from the results in our own patients and those in the literature that survival can be even further improved by the proper selection of patients for this procedure. In both of our patients who died, there was evidence at the operating table of spread of the tumor beyond the pancreas: to the lymph nodes in Case 2 and to the superior mesenteric vein in Case 3. The poor results in these two patients and the dismal results in Fortner's [24] four patients after radical total pancreatectomy would suggest that once the tumor has spread beyond the substance of the pancreas the patient's interests are best served by biliary and possibly duodenal bypass.

One of the early concerns about total pancreatectomy was the potential difficulty in physiologically and symptomatically controlling the pancreatic endocrine and exocrine insufficiency [3, 25]. However, these fears have not been borne out by practical experience. The insulin requirements can be quite variable in the early postoperative period, but usually after the patient has resumed eating the diabetes is readily manageable [22, 23]. Most patients require between 15-50 units of insulin daily. Although there have been isolated reports of diabetic vascular lesions in patients followed for more than ten years, this complication of total pancreatectomy appears to be an infrequent occurrence [26, 27]. Pancreatic exocrine insufficiency can be satisfactorily controlled by a combination of a low-fat diet and pancreatic extracts [22, 23].

Conclusions

Total pancreatectomy appears to be preferable to pancreatico-duodenectomy in the treatment of ductal carcinoma of the head of the pancreas for several reasons. First, the demonstration of distal glandular involvement in approximately 50% of patients with resectable pancreatic cancer indicates that total pancreatectomy offers the only means of cure in at least half. Second, total pancreatectomy has a lower morbidity than and, at most, the same mortality as pancreaticoduodenectomy. Third, the management of the pancreatic endocrine and exocrine insufficiency following total pancreatectomy has not been a difficult problem. Finally, although to date only a limited number of patients have undergone total pancreatic resection for carcinoma, the long-term results in recent series have been encouraging.

Current evidence indicates the need for a cooperative controlled clinical study to resolve the issue of the merits of total pancreatectomy versus pancreaticoduodenectomy in the treatment of resectable adenocarcinoma of the head of the pancreas.

References

1. Sauve, L.: Des Pancréatectomies et specialement de la pancréatectomie céphalique. Rev. Chir., 37:113, 1908.
2. Rockey, E. W.: Total pancreatectomy for carcinoma: Case report. Ann. Surg., 118:603, 1943.
3. Priestley, J. T., Comfort, M. W. and Radcliffe, J.: Total pancreatectomy for hyperinsulinism due to an islet-cell adenoma. Ann. Surg., 119:211, 1944.
4. Ross, D. E.: Cancer of the pancreas. A plea for total pancreatectomy. Amer. J. Surg., 87:20, 1954.
5. Brunschwig, A.: Surgical treatment of carcinoma of body of pancreas. Ann. Surg., 120:406, 1944.
6. McClure, quoted by Brunschwig, A.: Surgical treatment of carcinoma of body of pancreas. Ann. Surg., 120:406, 1944.
7. Ricketts, H. T., Brunschwig, A. and Knowlton, K.: Diabetes in totally depancreatized man. Proc. Soc. Exp. Biol. Med., 58:254, 1945.
8. Waugh, J. M., Dixon, C. F., Clagett, O. T. et al: Total pancreatectomy: A symposium presenting four successful cases and a report on metabolic observations. Proc. Mayo Clin., 21:25, 1946.
9. Gaston, E. A.: Total pancreatectomy. New Eng. J. Med., 238:345, 1948.
10. Chandler, G. N. and Oldfield, M.: Total pancreatectomy. Brit. J. Surg., 45:263, 1957.
11. McCullagh, E. P., Cook, J. R. and Shirey, E. K.: Diabetes following total pancreatectomy. Clinical observations of ten cases. Diabetes, 7:298, 1958.
12. Foster, J. H. et al: A ten-year experience with carcinoma of the pancreas. A cooperative study. Arch. Surg., 94:322, 1967.
13. Warren, K. W., Braasch, J. W. and Thum, C. W.: Carcinoma of the pancreas. Surg. Clin. N. Amer., 48:601, 1968.
14. Aston, S. J. and Longmire, W. P., Jr.: Pancreaticoduodenal resection: Twenty years' experience. Arch. Surg., 106:813, 1973.
15. Howard, J. M.: Pancreatico-duodenectomy: Forty-one consecutive Whipple resections without an operative mortality. Ann. Surg., 118:629, 1968.
16. Gilsdorf, R. B. and Spanos, P.: Factors influencing morbidity and mortality in pancreaticoduodenectomy. Ann. Surg., 177:332, 1973.
17. Smith, R.: Progress in the surgical treatment of pancreatic disease. Amer. J. Surg., 125:143, 1973.
18. Monge, J. J., Judd, E. S. and Gage, R. P.: Radical pancreaticoduodenectomy: A 22-year experience with complications, mortality rate, and survival rate. Ann. Surg., 160:711, 1964.
19. Warren, K. W., Cattell, R. B., Blackburn, J. P. et al: A long-term appraisal of pancreaticoduodenal resection for peri-ampullary carcinoma. Ann. Surg., 155:653, 1962.

20. Miyata, M., Takao, T., Uozumi, T. et al: Insulin secretion after pancreatico-duodenectomy. Ann. Surg., 179:494, 1974.
21. Monge, J. J., Dockerty, M. B., Wollaeger, E. E. et al: Clinicopathologic observations on radical pancreaticoduodenal resections for peri-ampullary carcinoma. Surg. Gynec. Obstet., 118:275, 1964.
22. Hicks, R. E. and Brooks, J. R.: Total pancreatectomy for ductal carcinoma. Surg. Gynec. Obstet., 133:16, 1971.
23. ReMine, W. H., Priestley, J. T., Judd, E. S. et al: Total pancreatectomy. Ann. Surg., 172:595, 1970.
24. Fortner, J. G.: Regional resection of cancer of the pancreas: A new surgical approach. Surgery, 73:307, 1973.
25. Goldner, M. G. and Clark, D. E.: The insulin requirement of man after total pancreatectomy. J. Clin. Endocr., 4:194, 1944.
26. Burton, Y., Kearns, T. P. and Rynearson, E. H.: Diabetic retinopathy following total pancreatectomy. Proc. Mayo Clin., 32:735, 1957.
27. Doyle, A. P., Balcerzak, S. P. and Jeffrey, W. L.: Fatal diabetic glomerulo-sclerosis after total pancreatectomy. New Eng. J. Med., 270:623, 1964.

Blunt and Penetrating Pancreatic Trauma

B. Eiseman, M.D. and L. Norton, M.D.

This summarizes our clinical approach at the Denver General Hospital to pancreatic injuries based on an experience with 50 patients requiring operation during the years 1968 and 1973. Emphasis is on the controversial aspects of the operative management of such lesions.

Clinical Experience

During the five years between 1968 and December 1973, 50 patients with pancreatic injury required laparotomy at the Denver General Hospital. Of these, ten were blunt (usually automobile accident) injuries and 40 penetrating. Thirty-five of the latter were caused by gunshot wounds. During this period, there was a laparotomy for trauma essentially every other day (180-212 per year or a total of approximately 1,000 laparotomies). Pancreatic injuries are not uncommon.

Forty percent (16 patients) of the perforating injuries involved the pancreatic head. Three of these 16 patients had only minor contusion of the gland without parenchymal disruption. The other 13 had penetration or laceration of the pancreatic head (Table 1).

Seven patients had penetrating trauma to the body and 13 penetrating trauma of the pancreatic tail. We do not include splenic injuries of which we have about one every six to seven days at the Denver General Hospital.

In the penetrating trauma group, 59% had other major organ involvement, emphasizing the need to look for pancreatic injury in the presence of other organ injury.

Recognition of Injury

Penetrating. Since penetrating abdominal injuries ordinarily dictate exploratory laparotomy, the only difficulty regarding diagnosing pancre-

B. Eiseman, M.D. and L. Norton, M.D., Department of Surgery, Denver General Hospital and University of Colorado Medical Center.

Table 1. Open Pancreatic Injury Site

Head	40%
Body	18%
Tail	33%
Combined	9%

atic injury is missing the injury at the time of the systematic intraperitoneal visceral operative inventory. In the presence of massive bleeding or a large retroperitoneal hematoma, the timid or careless surgeon can overlook a significant pancreatic laceration. Discovery of an unsuspected retroperitoneal pancreatic injury is one of several reasons that retroperitoneal hematomata should be explored.

Blunt. Leak of pancreatic fluid anteriorly into the peritoneal cavity declares itself by the expected florid peritonitis. It is not easily overlooked either on preoperative physical examination or on peritoneal lavage. When associated with duodenal or jejunal blow-out in a seat-belt injury, there is little excuse for much delay in diagnosis.

Retroperitoneal pancreatic injury without peritoneal disruption can be insidious. In April 1974 we cared for a patient with total transection of the pancreas over the vertebra without intraperitoneal leak. The abdomen was soft and signs of intraperitoneal injury were minimal for several hours after admission. Paracentesis was not diagnostic. After six hours the patient (who had concomitant severe extremity injuries) became sick. Serum amylase rose from an admission baseline of 200 units to 600 units. An alert surgical resident insisted on exploratory laparotomy and found the completely transected retroperitoneal pancreas, which was resected.

Duodenal blow-out, though rare in blunt trauma, can accompany pancreatic injury. We have treated three patients with nonpenetrating duodenal injuries each of whom at the least had contusion to the head of the pancreas. The extent of duodenal injury dictates the operative technique employed. The outcome depends to a large extent upon early recognition of the combined pancreatic and duodenal injury. Delayed surgical repair when both the mashed duodenum and pancreas are bathed in a pool of leaking bile, pancreatic juice, duodenal contents and blood is a predictable disaster.

Operative Management of Injury to the Body and Tail

Of the open injuries of the pancreas 18% of our five year D.G.H. experience involved the body and another 33% the tail. In 10% there were multiple sites of injury.

As our experience matures, our acceptable operative options narrow. In dealing with pancreatic injuries of the body and tail [1-3], the decision resolves itself whether to (1) resect everything to the left of the injury or (2) drain via the flank.

Such an all or none simplistic philosophy has resulted from inordinate numbers of complications where reconstructive procedures were employed at the time of trauma on sinistral pancreas. Transduodenal operative pancreatograms are theoretically appealing as a means of delineating the extent of duct injury in the body and tail of the gland, but in practice this is not realistic. Surrounded by structures such as the vena cava, aorta, portal vein, spleen and colon, pancreatic injuries seldom exist in pristine anatomic isolation. One or two other major abdominal neighbors have usually been transected. By the time the surgeon has tidied up other injuries, he seldom is willing to tempt the patient's fate with diagnostic maneuvers such as pancreatography which is more suited to the serenity of elective operative procedures than to the turmoil of repairing retroperitoneal havoc following trauma.

Enlarging experiences with all but total pancreatectomy for trauma, acute hemorrhagic pancreatitis and tumor proves that there is but little endocrinologic morbidity associated with removing large segments of normal gland. The trade-off in avoiding postoperative complication in trying to salvage a seriously damaged pancreatic body is cost-effective. We consider everything to the left of the superior mesenteric vein as pure pancreatic reserve in a normal patient. If any question of viability exists, the sinistral pancreas should go.

There are no hard and fast criteria for determining whether the left side of the injured pancreas should be resected. If either the entire gland or the duct is transected, the decision is easy – resect. If there is only a surrounding hematoma and some contusion – drain. If the parenchyma has but minimal laceration by a low velocity missile, resection is probably not necessary. It is at best a judgment call.

Blunt Injury over the Vertebra

Seat-belt injuries occasionally crush the midline pancreas where it abuts the vertebra. Characteristically, this injury is to the left of the confluence of the splenic and superior mesenteric veins where they form the portal trunk. We advise resecting all pancreas to the left of the injury rather than trying to anastomose the uninjured tail of the gland into a loop of gut or hooking the two ends of the debrided gland back together. We find it easy to avoid this temptation as we accumulate experience with the morbidity in preserving the endocrinologically unneeded pancreatic tail.

We are willing to let others [4-6] accumulate experience in anastomosing the right and left halves of the pancreas to each other or to the bowel following trauma.

Injuries of the Pancreatic Head

Injuries of the pancreatic head require both technical skill and surgical judgment for proper management [7, 8]. Both the factors dictating choice of operative repair and the techniques available are numerous. Decision is doubly difficult because the options have a wide spread in mortality and morbidity [9, 10].

Factors to be considered in the decisions are:

1) Damage to other organs.
2) Duodenal perforation or blow-out.
3) Common bile duct or pancreatic duct severance within the injured pancreas.
4) Degree of pancreatic contusion around a missile tract through the pancreatic head.
5) Degree of injury to the body and tail of the pancreas.

Operative options are:

1) Debridement and simple drainage.
2) All but total pancreatectomy saving a thin pancreatic crescent containing the vasculature along the duodenal lesser curvature according to the technique described by Child [11].
3) Resection of the duodenum and pancreatic head while preserving the body and tail either,
    a) with drainage of the pancreas into a limb of gut or
    b) without internal drainage.
4) Total pancreatectomy and duodenectomy.

Other Organ Injury

Its head nestled in the arms of the duodenum and resting lightly on the soft vena caval vascular pillow, this portion of the pancreas can hardly be jostled or skewered without stirring up serious trouble. Occasionally, a low velocity .22-calliber missile or an ice pick miraculously bores through this area without major damage to the cava, aorta or duodenum, but this is the exception. More commonly, when faced with such an injury, the surgeon spends a few lively minutes achieving hemostasis before the pancreatic damage can be assessed.

Even blunt trauma to the pancreatic head may be associated with duodenal or jejunal blow-out plus an ugly retroperitoneal and peritoneal hematoma. The right upper quadrant is a bad place to be shot, stabbed or kicked!

Degree of Associated Pancreatic Contusion

Because pancreatic head resection carries with it a high morbidity and mortality, we are willing to risk simple debridement and drainage of a low velocity bullet or stab wound of the pancreatic head if there is not extensive contusion to the surrounding gland or the duodenum. Two cases with simple drillhole gunshot wounds of the pancreatic head have thus been conservatively managed within the past six months and both have had uncomplicated postoperative recovery. In both, the missile went through the vena cava and in one the missile also transected the common duct. These concomitant injuries made operative repair more interesting but also measurably reduced enthusiasm for adding extensive pancreatic resection to an already busy laparotomy.

When, however, the missile or crushing blow makes pulp of the pancreatic head, there obviously is no recourse but to resect the head and perform a Whipple operation. Saving the duodenal vascular rim along its lesser curve – as described by Child [11] which has, in our opinion, an important occasional place in the operative management of acute hemorrhagic pancreatitis [12] – seldom can be used following trauma. The vessels are either blown away or turned to pulp, in which case resection is required, or are so unmolested that resection is unnecessary.

Internal Drainage of the Body and Tail

With isolated damage to the pancreatic head there is every theoretic reason to save and utilize the endocrine and exocrine function of the unsullied sinistral pancreatic body and tail.

Blunt trauma sufficiently severe to crush the pancreatic head beyond salvage usually also provides serious involvement of the body and tail. We have had no case of blunt injury to the head requiring resection where we were able to drain the body into the gut.

Penetrating trauma is somewhat different. Of the 16 missile wounds of the pancreatic head we resected the head in three. In each the body and tail of the pancreas were preserved and inserted into a Roux-Y limb of jejunum. One of these patients died; the others recovered without endocrine or exocrine disability. Our results are summarized in Table 2.

Table 2. Open Pancreatic Injuries

	Drained	*Resected*
Mortality	15%	10%
Morbidity	65%	60%
Sepsis	30%	30%
Pseudocyst	10%	0
Fistula	45%	10%

Conclusion

A five year summary of 50 patients with pancreatic injury requiring laparotomy has been reviewed. Ten of the injuries were for blunt and 40 for penetrating injury. Emphasized in this discussion were the following points:

a) Diagnosis following blunt injury may be difficult if there is not intraperitoneal pancreatic duodenal or biliary leak. A rising serum amylase and clinical deterioration may be the only early signal that the pancreas is injured and leaking into the retroperitoneal space.

b) Injury to the pancreatic body and tail is relatively easily managed. The sinistral pancreas must be excised. Repair of the injured pancreatic duct is not advocated.

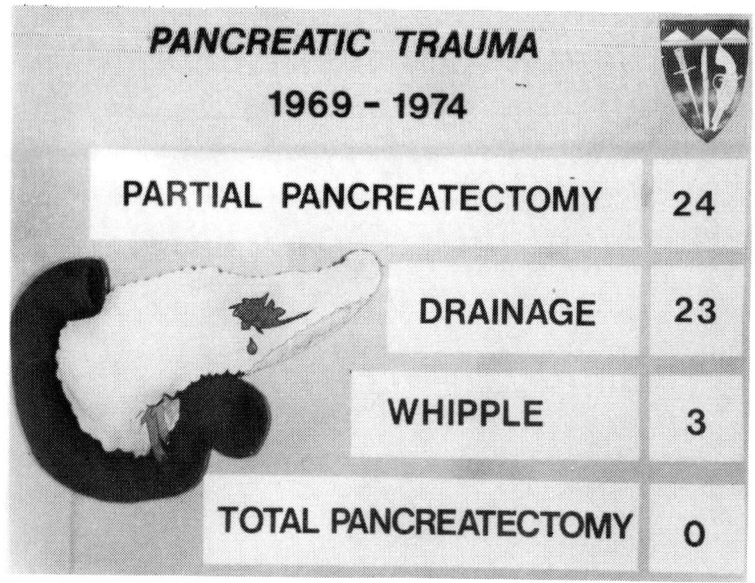

FIGURE 1.

c) Injuries to the pancreatic head are complex. In our experience they usually are associated with injuries of the duodenum, cava, aorta or bile duct. Of the various available operative techniques, we lean toward the conservative, ie, simple drainage and duodenal reconstruction if that is at all feasible. Only occasionally is it indicated to utilize complex surgical techniques for draining the intact pancreatic body and tail following resection of the duodenum and pancreatic head for trauma (Fig. 1).

References

1. Jones, R. C. and Shires, G. T.: The management of pancreatic injuries. Surgery, 96:712, 1968.
2. Thompson, R. J., Jr. and Hinshaw, D. B.: Pancreatic trauma: Review of 87 cases. Ann. Surg., 163:153, 1966.
3. Yellin, A. E., Vecchione, T. R. and Donovan, A. J.: Distal pancreatectomy for pancreatic trauma. Amer. J. Surg., 124:137, 1972.
4. Martin, L. W., Henderson, B. M. and Welsh, N.: Disruption of the head of the pancreas caused by blunt trauma in children: A report of two cases treated with primary repair of the pancreatic duct. Surgery, 63:697, 1968.
5. Pellegrine, J. N. and Stein, J. J.: Complete severance of pancreas and its treatment with repair of main pancreatic duct of Wirsung. Amer. J. Surg., 101:707, 1961.
6. Letton, A. H. and Wilson, J. P.: Traumatic severance of pancreas treated by Roux-Y anastomosis. Surg. Gynec. Obstet., 109:473, 1959.
7. Freeark, R. J., Kane, J. M., Folk, F. A. et al: Traumatic disruption of the head of the pancreas. Arch. Surg., 91:5, 1965.
8. Smith, A. D., Jr., Woolverton, W. C., Weichert, R. F. III et al: Operative management of pancreatic and duodenal injuries. J. Trauma, 11:570, 1971.
9. Berne, C. J., Donovan, A. J. and Hagen, W. E.: Combined duodenal pancreatic trauma. The role of end-to-side gastrojejunostomy. Arch. Surg., 96:712, 1968.
10. Nance, F. C. and DeLoach, D. H.: Pancreaticoduodenectomy following abdominal trauma. J. Trauma, 11:577, 1971.
11. Child, C. G. III, Fry, C. F. and Fry, W. J.: A reappraisal of removal of ninety-five percent of the distal portion of the pancreas. Surg. Gynec. Obstet., 129:49, 1969.
12. Norton, L. and Eiseman, B.: Near total pancreatectomy for hemorrhagic pancreatitis. Amer. J. Surg., 127:191, 1974.

Supported by NIH Grant No. GM 20309.

Panel Discussion

Moderator: **R. L. Simmons, M.D.**

Panelists: **T. T. White, M.D.**, **S. Silvis, M.D.**, **B. Eiseman, M.D.**, **M. Levitt, M.D.**, **M. L. Gliedman, M.D.**, **J. M. Howard, M.D.**

Dr. Simmons: Dr. Levitt, do you think that the amylase or the other pancreatic enzymes have any usefulness in the diagnosis of carcinoma? Would you like to comment on the use of amylase in other conditions discussed today?

Dr. Levitt: In general, I think that the amylase determination does not have much value in the diagnosis of carcinoma of the pancreas. Occasionally, the amylase will be elevated but, in general, the serum amylase and the urinary amylase are both normal in carcinoma of the pancreas.

Dr. Simmons: Do you feel that urinary amylase is of any use in pancreatic trauma, Dr. Eiseman?

Dr. Eiseman: I think that it is of little value in penetrating injury, since we explore anyway. Rarely in blunt injury, I think it is of value.

Dr. Simmons: What about the peritoneal lavage amylase in pancreatic trauma?

Dr. Eiseman: Occasionally it is of value in blunt trauma.

Dr. Simmons: Is it an indication for exploration in a patient who otherwise does not have an indication?

Dr. Eiseman: Occasionally it is of adjunctive help in deciding to explore.

Dr. Howard: Dr. Simmons, he didn't mention either arteriography or preoperative duodenography in diagnosing pancreatic injuries. We have no great experience, but it seems to me that this ought to be a promising area if the patient is stable at the time.

Dr. Eiseman: Dr. Howard, we do a considerable amount of arteriography for other lesions but as we reviewed our experience with injury, we seldom rely on arteriography to decide that laparotomy is required.

Dr. White: One other comment about the amylase: Just because the pancreas is transected doesn't automatically mean that the patient is going to become acutely ill. There are patients, also, who get pancreatic ascites without having an acute belly. So you might be deceived if you just went on amylase, alone.

Dr. Eiseman: In trauma, at least, my plea is: Don't get too fancy in trying to avoid laparotomy! In the long run patients are best served by an occasional negative laparotomy rather than not exploring someone with a serious intra-abdominal injury.

Dr. Gliedman: One should not assume from this discussion that all penetrating wounds should be explored. A number of large series, ie, the one by Gerald W. Shafton et al, strongly suggests that the patient is not harmed by waiting until he develops peritoneal or intra-abdominal signs that would lead us to do a laparotomy for any other surgical condition. The patient's abdominal findings would decide laparotomy, along with signs of unexplained shock, positive abdominal tap, et cetera.

Dr. Simmons: Dr. Eiseman, would you like to comment?

Dr. Eiseman: This is an area of argument. It depends upon the environment. If you can count on having only one stab wound patient that evening, you might be justified in watchful waiting. If, however, you expect to be inundated with more trauma patients, then you must liberalize indications for early exploration. I think there should be no argument about gunshot wounds, however.

Dr. Simmons: Dr. Silvis, how do you set up the operative schedule and what do you do about complications of the procedure?

Dr. Silvis: The operative schedule has to be arranged before the studies are done. This is one of the most frequent reasons for us to refuse to do a procedure on a patient, that is, they don't have operating time already designated for the patient.

Dr. Simmons: Do you do the procedure only when you think there is a surgically treatable disease, Dr. Silvis?

Dr. Silvis: Yes, certainly in the common duct, and in the jaundiced patient, the procedure should not be done in a patient whom you would not operate on, if you find the common duct obstruction. If you have a patient with very severe liver disease, that patient should not be studied.

Dr. Simmons: What kinds of symptoms and signs do you go on when deciding whether an emergency operation is indicated, when you have found no surgically treatable disease? Or don't you have the complications unless there is an obstruction?

Dr. Silvis: We have not seen problems unless we find an obstructed duct. We feel that all such patients should be operated on, promptly. The majority of the pseudocysts have had surgery. In the two that I showed that we followed, the cysts drained promptly, and the ducts drained promptly, and they had no trouble. I would think a pseudocyst that is sizable should be operated on. And, certainly, if it drains slowly, it should be operated on.

Dr. Eiseman: May I comment on pseudocysts? In our experience, a much better way of diagnosing a pseudocyst and differentiating it from phlegmon is ultrasound. Ultrasound allows one to localize the mass and to differentiate the cystic from the solid inflammatory mass. We have used both ultrasound and angiography. We like ultrasound.

Dr. White: I'll buy ultrasound, too. We use it. I have three patients in the hospital right now, all of whom were beautifully outlined by ultrasound. You cannot see very small cysts, however, if they get down much under 5 or 6 cm; they are very difficult to see in ultrasound. I would think that, as far as the discussion on retrograde examination, it is these smaller lesions, smaller cysts, which are better diagnosed by the endoscopy. I might add, also, that one of the problems that we are having with endoscopy is they find lesions, ie, a great big pancreatic duct, and at operation the pancreas is perfectly normal. So there are some side effects to retrograde cannulation, which we didn't think about, at first.

Dr. Howard: Dr. Silvis, does retrograde cannulation infect the obstructed duct converting it into an emergency? Is that the problem?

Dr. Silvis: The problem with an obstructed duct is cholangitis, yes.

Dr. White: It would be the same thing for the pancreas, too?

Dr. Silvis: Yes, I think that is probably true. We have seen essentially no trouble in the pancreas, except for one that clearly was infected before the study.

Dr. White: Do you mean that you can't infect them by stuffing that little tube up there?

Dr. Silvis: I really doubt if we are infecting, if we are carrying organisms into the common duct. The dye is bacteriocidal, diluted 1:1,000, the concentration that we are using and infection does not occur in an unobstructed duct. Though I think that we are probably stirring up organisms that are there, I don't think that anybody knows why the obstructed patient gets cholangitis.

I don't know of a good comparison series between ultrasound and ductagrams, as far as pseudocyst goes. I know people who have varying degrees of confidence in ultrasound. We are currently getting some experience with it. But really we have nothing objective to talk about, locally.

Dr. Eiseman: Dr. Silvis, what do you do if pancreatitis develops after retrograde pancreatography?

Dr. Silvis: Of the patients whom we have had, there have only been two who had what I would call moderately severe pancreatitis – both recovered without operation.

Dr. Simmons: Dr. Silvis, I have a question about whether intraductal cytology is of any use in the diagnosis of carcinoma.

Dr. Silvis: We have very little experience in this. A few groups are now collecting secretions from the duct and doing cytology on it. And there are some positive studies reported. This may be important for the future.

Dr. Gliedman: Years ago Aka, Rosen and Garret needled the dilated pancreatic duct at laparotomy in carcinomatous obstructed patients and fairly routinely could retrieve cancer cells from those ducts. They would do immediate cytology. They were quite accurate. It is laborious, however, and time consuming. It comes back to whether or not this group of patients who had Whipple procedures were, in fact, having the operative area bathed by these tumor cells.

We argue about whether or not a total pancreatectomy or a partial pancreatectomy should be done and, here we are, able to retrieve the cancer cells right out of the dilated pancreatic duct, right through the area that we are going to transect.

Dr. Simmons: The panel members have expressed unanimity primarily on the idea that you shouldn't biopsy the pancreas when the duct is obstructed. Perhaps we should get into the problem of biopsy of pancreas, anyway.

Dr. Howard: You shouldn't biopsy behind the obstruction. I think that it is all right to biopsy the tumor, itself.

Dr. Simmons: Dr. Howard, do you do a Whipple procedure, if you don't have a cancer on a biopsy?

Dr. Howard: Are you asking me, have I done it? Yes, I have done it.

Dr. Simmons: Do you do it routinely? Do you advise others to do it?

Dr. Howard: We make the diagnosis at the operating table by feeling the tumor. If we can biopsy it on the surface, we do it. But if it comes back negative, and it still feels like tumor, we call it tumor and do whatever is required.

Dr. Simmons: Dr. Gliedman, would you like to comment?

Dr. Gliedman: I think it would be unfair, in Minneapolis, not to mention the so-called Watson test that originated here and that we have used for many years, which is a qualitative fecal urobilinogen determination. I don't know if anybody else uses it, but it is extremely accurate. In our institution, 95% of the patients who have cancerous obstruction have less than 5 mg daily of fecal urobilinogen per day using the mean of a three day collection. As a matter of fact, you get down to infinitesimal amounts, which are usually under 1 mg per day. It is a very reliable determination. With a positive test, we do not biopsy the pancreas before resection.

Dr. Eiseman: I think that it is totally unjustified for those of us who don't have the track record and exceedingly low mortality as does John Howard in doing a total pancreatectomy, without tissue diagnosis. We are going to kill more people than we are ever going to save! I therefore insist on a tissue diagnosis of cancer on my service.

Dr. Howard: Dr. Simmons, this is the heart of the matter: You ought not to be operating upon them in the first place, unless you are prepared to do the definitive operation.

Dr. Simmons: Dr. Gliedman, would you like to comment?

Dr. Gliedman: I would recommend that all of you read an article by Weingartner, Hague and Elliot in *The American Journal of Surgery* in 1966 on biopsying the pancreas. A positive biopsy was obtained only 85% of the time – after multiple biopsies! Even for an experienced surgeon, I am not sure that it is as simple as Dr. Eiseman would suggest to get that positive biopsy. If you don't want to do a Whipple operation or a total pancreatectomy, for good or poor reasons, then you simply shouldn't do it. However, the biopsy should not be the excuse that you use.

Dr. White: I still find it very difficult to get a positive biopsy result, using the technique which you described earlier, by aspirating the pancreatic duct. We have done that quite a number of times and we ended up doing pancreaticojejunostomies on some six or seven patients where we were convinced that this individual had chronic pancreatitis, and not cancer. So we could neither make the diagnosis on the basis of the aspirate of the pancreatic duct, nor could we make it on the basis of taking out a long ridge or a long furrow of tissue in the front of the pancreas. So sometimes it is very, very difficult to come up with a diagnosis, and very frustrating, as Dr. Gliedman has just said. What I do think that you can do, however, and this will prevent you from operating on a lot of patients, is to biopsy the lymph nodes around the distal end of the bile duct. The pathologists much prefer this to taking pancreas, itself. While you are waiting, you then proceed on down to the superior mesenteric vessels, just below the mesocolon, and biopsy more nodes. And, then, while you are waiting, further, I might add, you have opened the gastrocolic ligament in the process of looking at the pancreas, and you take some lymph nodes from around the celiac axis. By the time you have taken the third set of nodes out, sometimes you have the answer. I do not, as a policy, do a pancreatic resection on anybody who has any one of these three sets of nodes positive. This will render unresectable 75% of the patients with carcinoma of the head of the pancreas.

The big question then arises: How are you going to find out what portion of the pancreas to biopsy? John Howard says, "I won't biopsy behind an obstruction."

Dr. Howard: And leave the obstruction!

Dr. White: And leave the obstruction, that is correct. Okay, well, a large proportion of our patients have a tumor in the head of the pancreas, which obstructs the pancreatic duct. And the entire tail is hard, also. So you really don't know exactly where to biopsy; this is where the problem lies. Do you mean, Dr. Howard, that you would biopsy a patient who had, say, a lesion in the superior edge of the pancreas obstructing the bile duct only and not obstructing the rest of the pancreas? You would be willing to do a pancreas biopsy on that?

Dr. Howard: No, I think that you can usually tell by palpation which is carcinoma and which isn't carcinoma. I think that the patient with carcinoma of the head of the pancreas has a firmness of the tail, but that tail doesn't feel like carcinoma. I think that if the carcinoma is in the head, you want to biopsy the head. The one point that I would like to make is that I believe that pancreatography, preoperative pancreatography, is going to get us in earlier on these patients than ever before. We have been saying for years that we don't have a means for diagnosing carcinoma of the pancreas. I believe that pancreatography is going to make a significant advance. I shall be disappointed if we do not find that we are delaying one year on these patients.

Dr. White: Or two years!

Dr. Howard: These patients can be diagnosed a year or two years earlier, before they get obstructive jaundice. When the symptomatology is still relatively vague, pancreatography may well get us in earlier.

Dr. Simmons: Dr. Silvis, would you do a pancreatogram on the basis of vague symptoms, with cholangiogram normal, upper GI normal?

Dr. Silvis: We have not done a large number of these patients. In the ones that we have studied, the yield has been low. I think that this is one area where possibly, as Dr. Levitt commented, the amylase may be of value; certainly, if you did have an abnormal amylase in such a patient, we would do the study and do it considerably earlier.

Dr. Simmons: Dr. Levitt, you might see a lot of these patients with mild upper abdominal distress, a little weight loss, a vague feeling of discomfort, and your work-up is negative. In such a case do you ever consider, or would you consider, ordering retrograde pancreatography?

Dr. Levitt: We do see a number of these patients and the one exception that I take is to the weight loss. If there is very much weight loss, we would be more likely to go to pancreatography. The average patient whom we see has vague discomfort and is in otherwise good general health. I don't think that we would send these patients over to Dr. Silvis.

Dr. Simmons: Dr. White, wuld you like to comment?

Dr. White: Basically, I think that the problem is one of screening the patients, of deciding on which patient you want to do pancreatography. There are a number of different approaches, none of which are too marvelous, yet. The one which Dr. Zamchek and some others would like to see used is the carcinoembryonic antigen (CEA). Do you use that type of approach, Dr. Simmons?

Dr. Simmons: We do CEAs on a vast number of patients here and I must say that we have not found it to be very helpful. It is certainly high when patients have extensive disease.

Dr. White: Patients who have cirrhosis of the liver have a high CEA.

Dr. Simmons: Dr. Gliedman, I have a lot of questions for you here, most of which relate to the technic of peritoneal lavage. Where do you put the catheters? Is this the same as putting it in the retrogastric space? How much fluid do you use? How rapidly do you infuse? When do you stop? What do you do when the patient gains 6 kg the first day and you get back that much less fluid?

Dr. Gliedman: We use one or two regular peritoneal dialysis catheters in the unoperated patient. We place one catheter high and one toward the pelvis. We are not talking about placement of catheters at the time of laparotomy, where we generally place two large bone catheters. We lavage with high volumes (30 liters in 24 hours) in and out with 2 liter aliquots. It represents a fair amount of work on the part of the nursing staff and the people committed to the care of the patient. I specifically mentioned that we usually used a hypertonic solution. We tend to get out *more* than we put in, in spite of which, the patients have a very good urinary output. By the time we get to do peritoneal lavage or dialysis, our patients are waterlogged. We have all been raised with the concept that the severe acute pancreatitis patient is hypovolemic, electrolyte-depleted, and correctly we tend to give large amounts of fluid. The group that I am describing is just sequestering that fluid. We continue to lavage until the patient wakes up, begins to improve, or dies. I can describe a case that I treated by telephone, in another institution, where the patient had already had a respiratory arrest, had a catheter placed, was lavaged for one day, with the amylase falling in the peritoneal fluid from astounding levels down to low levels. The lavage was stopped when the patient awoke. One day later, the patient was again in trouble. The peritoneal fluid was again high in amylase. The lavage was again started and continued for one more day and it was again stopped, when the peritoneal amylase, which was used as a marker, again had come down to the serum level. Then, on a third occasion, the patient was again lavaged, with final recovery. So I think that leaving the catheter in place and monitoring the fluid that is coming out of the peritoneal cavity is a good technic. If the peritoneal amylase, the marker, is rising astoundingly, there is the suggestion that those ferments or "humors" that you are really trying to prevent from becoming systemic are now increasing in quantity. You should remove them.

Dr. Simmons: Dr. Eiseman, you implied in your presentation that you might try this peritoneal lavage before you go to more radical treatment. Is that true?

Dr. Eiseman: No, we have not done it. We discussed this 1½ years ago, at the Society of University Surgeons. At that time, the consensus seemed to be that the mortality even with lavage was around 40%, so I decided to stick with resection. Prior lavage might make subtotal pancreatectomy a bit more gamy, though. What does the belly look like, Dr. Gliedman, if you have to explore after you have lavaged?

Dr. Gliedman: We have lavaged only two patients and then gone on to operate upon them. One of them was because the internist felt that the lavage should be stopped and the patient should be explored, even though we felt that there was improvement. At surgery, the pancreas looked very normal and we simply placed drains in and closed. Another patient who had been lavaged recovered and then went on to develop a lesser sac collection. At operation to drain the lesser sac collection, an area of necrotic pancreas was marsupialized.

Dr. White: We have used this procedure some. Most of our patients in which this has been done have had kidney failure, as well. This is one indication for using peritoneal lavage, quite aside from all of the others which have been mentioned. There was one complication, however: One of our nephrologists put a tube in and I said, "How do you know it is not going to go into the intestine?" And he said, "It never does!" As it turned out, we had to operate on that patient later. He had stuck the tube right into the small intestine. So this can happen, too, especially in patients who have been operated upon. Has it ever happened in Minneapolis?

Dr. Simmons: We are not very big peritoneal dialyzers. Dr. Eiseman, would you like to comment?

Dr. Eiseman: I wonder if Rodney Smith could give us his evaluation of glucagon in acute pancreatitis.

Dr. White: Speaking of glucagon, one of the interesting things is that patients who had total pancreatectomy, our patients, have no glucagon in the blood, at all. This makes plain why they don't get such high blood sugars.

Mr. Smith: The question about glucagon is such a long one that I cannot even begin to summarize this. As part of the treatment of some patients with chronic pancreatitis, we had the opportunity of having a T-tube in the pancreatic duct for varying periods of time, with pancreatic juice dripping out into a bottle. This seemed to be a very good opportunity to do some physiological studies. Right in among this was the confirmation of the observation which had been made previously, that glucagon will largely switch off pancreatic external secretion. This agent seemed a possible weapon to be used in the treatment of acute pancreatitis. The Research Council in Great Britain has now started a proper controlled trial in a number of centers in Great Britain, to see if we can prove whether this is true or whether it is an illusion. Even if it does prove to be true, my own feeling is that the benefits may, in the end, be marginal, that what we shall find is that if you are lucky enough to arrive at a position where the patient has an edematous pancreas which has not yet undergone massive necrosis and hemorrhage, possibly, some of those processes can be arrested in a phase before they cross over this important dividing line. But I would not expect the use of glucagon to have any great effect on the patient who has already suffered gross hemorrhage and necrosis.

Dr. Simmons: Thank you, Mr. Smith. Dr. Eiseman, there is a question here. How do you define pancreatitis because the pancreas we saw being removed looked normal?

Dr. Eiseman: Beauty is in the eye of the beholder. It wasn't a normal pancreas!

Dr. Simmons: Do you use the same criteria for pancreatectomy that Dr. Gliedman would use for dialysis?

Dr. Eiseman: Yes.

Dr. White: Do you mean that you operate on them, when they are almost dead?

Dr. Eiseman: That is about right.

Dr. Simmons: It would seem from what I have heard here that cerebral symptoms or signs are the most important or the most crucial, when the patient begins to get less coherent. Am I correct?

Dr. Gliedman: I think that that is about the point of changing your approach. We will stick with the routine, aggressive, nonoperative approach, except if the patient develops an acute abdomen, such that we are concerned about need for surgery. When the sensorium changes, in our clinical opinion, and that ordinarily is beyond the third day, we then would say that that is the point to interrupt the disease. The patient, in our opinion, is clearly retrievable, at that point. It gets less clear beyond the change in sensorium. I don't have the courage to do very much before then, although I think that you can predict that some will go on to that point.

Dr. Eiseman: I would answer pretty much the same way. I would say that a change in sensorium is a very grave sign. I have often wondered whether fluid overload doesn't contribute. I also wonder whether some of the respiratory distress syndromes might not also be due to water overload despite all our efforts – including Lasix – to dry the patient out.

Dr. Howard: This may be a very important point. On the other hand, it strikes me that our major objective within that first 24 hours, when the patient comes in with severe, acute pancreatitis, is to prevent acute renal failure. I would ask if any member of the panel has salvaged a patient who has acute necrosis of the pancreas, after an overt stage of acute renal failure. Has anyone pulled the patient out of acute renal failure?

Dr. White: We have had seven such patients. Of these, six died and one we managed to pull through.

Dr. Levitt: We had one recent survival, a patient with acute tubular necrosis.

Dr. Gliedman: Few survive total anuria but may survive oliguric renal failure.

Dr. Simmons: I think that Dr. Eiseman's point is well taken. By the time that the surgeon usually recognizes acute renal failure, progressive renal failure has been going on for several days, and there is a tremendous water overload.

I have several questions here about whether we shouldn't perform peritoneal lavage before the stage of "malignancy." Will it prevent the progression of the disease?

Dr. Gliedman: I visited Dr. Campbell, in Arkansas; they were undertaking an approach like that. We have not used that approach because even in the "malignant" category, only one third were going to go on to die. On that basis, I couldn't say that you should do it to all patients, because the malignant group is really a relatively small group. However, recall that we are discussing a group of "malignant" patients that represents about 18% of the whole group of acute pancreatitis patients. The non-lavage therapy group had nine of 28 patients dying. It is those nine deaths that we're trying to get at.

Dr. Simmons: Did you save six out of ten patients?

Dr. Gliedman: Yes, I think that is correct. Six out of ten were retrieved in the original group and the retrieval rate is about the same with the others we have treated since.

Dr. Simmons: Forty percent mortality is another way of looking at that.

Dr. Howard: Again, we are assuming that there is a toxicity of acute pancreatitis. We went through this with burn patients for years and still we talk about the toxicity, the early toxicity, of thermal burns. Yet, there is mighty little hard data to back it up. I have a great deal of reservation about this underlying concept.

Dr. Eiseman: Didn't Galen start the whole business about bad humors causing disease? Dr. Gliedman, you are sort of a modern-day Galen!

Dr. Gliedman: Change is not necessarily progress!

The Zollinger-Ellison Syndrome

Robert M. Zollinger, M.D.

A direct relationship between non-beta islet cell tumors and a pancreatic phase of gastric hypersecretion, first advanced in 1955 [1], has been unequivocally established by experimental and clinical evidence (Fig. 1). Since 1960 it has been known that ulcerogenic tumors arising in the pancreas or duodenum, as well as their metastases, are capable of producing 35 times more gastrin than a similar weight of porcine gastric antrum [2]. The ability to measure elevated levels of circulating gastrin by sensitive and reliable radioimmunoassays in the past few years has made the diagnosis of the ulcerogenic syndrome almost commonplace. However, the symptoms of the ulcerogenic syndrome do tend to be variable and have a wide range of severity, depending upon the size and number of the adenomas, as well as the presence or absence of metastases. Surprisingly, there can be long delays in the diagnosis unless the symptoms are life-threatening, and patients still appear who have undergone multiple gastric resections for recurrent ulceration. Some of the current problems associated with the diagnosis and treatment of the ulcerogenic tumor syndrome will be presented.

The ulcerogenic syndrome presents classically as a fulminating ulcer diathesis, with or without diarrhea, in the presence of massive and intractable gastric hypersecretion. The patient will produce 100-200 ml of gastric juice per hour from an unobstructed stomach or very soon after a radical gastric resection, which may have included vagotomy. The free acid content will range from 100-300 mEq/L. Furthermore, Ruppert and others have found that the ratio of basal to maximal acid concentration is selective for an ulcerogenic tumor if it is greater than 0.6 [3]. Barium contrast studies are almost always abnormal with large gastric folds due to mucosal hyperplasia and large amounts of gastric juice. An ulcer in the duodenal bulb or the immediate postbulbar area will be seen in about 75%

Robert M. Zollinger, M.D., Department of Surgery, The Ohio State University College of Medicine, Columbus.

ULCEROGENIC SYNDROME

1955 Triad
Fulminating Ulcer Diathesis
Marked Gastric Hypersecretion
Non-Beta Islet Cell Tumor

Polyglandular Involvement

Diarrhea

Etiology – Gastrin **(1960)**

FIG. 1. The ulcerogenic tumor syndrome which was first suggested in 1955 has been unequivocally established by experimental and clinical evidence.

of the patients. The presence of a primary ulcer beyond the ligament of Treitz is considered pathognomonic of an ulcerogenic tumor and occurs in 20%-25% of the patients.

A challenging clinical problem arises when a patient demonstrates all or part of this presumptive evidence, in favor of an ulcerogenic tumor, but the fasting serum gastrin levels are repeatedly borderline (250-500 pg/ml). In the presence of an ulcerogenic tumor, the administration of calcium gluconate (15 mg/kg/hr) over a three hour period will result in a 300% or greater increase in the serum gastrin levels during the third hour [4]. The infusion of Jorpes secretin or glucagon will evoke similar responses. With these results in hand, surgical exploration of the pancreas is warranted. When both the fasting and the stimulated levels of gastrin are relatively low, the tumor may be quite small and difficult to find surgically, as in those cases of adenoma in the submucosa of the first portion of the duodenum.

Associated endocrine tumors occur in the ulcerogenic syndrome in about 25% of the cases. Hyperparathyroidism is the most common associated endocrine abnormality (28%), with adenoma or hyperplasia of the pituitary, thyroid and adrenal glands occurring in approximately 10%. A familial incidence of this syndrome was described by Wermer in 1954 [5], and it has been found to be present in about 5% of the reported cases. The unusually high incidence of associated hyperparathyroidism is of great current interest to many observers.

Kaplan, Peskin and colleagues recently emphasized the role of metabolic alkalosis in elevating the parathormone levels while depressing the calcium ion concentration [6]. They postulated that vomiting, nasogastric suction and/or ingestion of soluble antacids all contribute to this cycle of metabolic alkalosis. In addition, some patients with an ulcerogenic tumor have elevated levels of circulating parathormone with low or normal serum calcium values. Kaplan et al observed two such patients in whom the elevated PTH and low-normal preoperative serum calcium levels returned to normal after the ulcerogenic tumor was removed and the gastric hypersecretory state abolished [7]. The ulcerogenic tumors have also been shown to exert a direct effect on the parathyroid glands with an associated increase in the serum thyrocalcitonin levels [8], which may well depress the serum calcium levels and result in a secondary form of hyperparathyroidism.

The problem of evaluating the evidence of hyperparathyroidism in association with the ulcerogenic syndrome is a difficult one and often depends upon repeated measurements of both serum calcium and parathormone levels. In general, if *either* the serum calcium or the circulating parathormone level is not elevated, exploration of the parathyroid glands should be indefinitely delayed. If *both* of these values are elevated, exploration of the parathyroids may be warranted *unless* either the fasting or calcium-stimulated gastrin levels are diagnostic of an ulcerogenic tumor. Under these circumstances, it may be a difficult decision as to which should be explored first. The ultimate decision may depend upon the severity and risk involved from the marked gastric hypersecretion associated with an ulcerogenic tumor.

Since the introduction of the ulcerogenic syndrome, there has been a tendency to blame the islet cell tumor for all failures following standard operations for duodenal ulcer. The "iatrogenic" ulcerogenic syndrome, as it may be called, can occur in the presence of an overlooked vagus nerve, particularly the posterior one, antral distention from failure to place the gastrojejunostomy sufficiently near the pylorus (ie, 3-4 cm), a modest gastric resection without vagotomy, performance of a long-loop gastrojejunostomy after the Billroth II procedure and, more rarely, a retained gastric antrum. An ulcerogenic tumor can be overlooked at the time of surgery for ulcer with disastrous consequences from gastric hypersecretion, hemorrhage and perforation. The early persistence of large amounts of gastric juice with acid values in excess of 100 mEq/L should suggest the diagnosis of an overlooked tumor in postoperative patients. Furthermore, the serum gastrin levels will probably not be significantly elevated except in the presence of either an overlooked tumor or a retained gastric antrum.

The clinician should encounter little difficulty in diagnosing the patient with the "classical" ulcerogenic syndrome of either fulminating ulcer diathesis, diarrhea or steatorrhea, or a combination of both. The fasting serum gastrin concentration will generally be greater than 1,000 pg/ml and following calcium stimulation over a period of three to four hours will be augmented 10-11 times. The secretin or glucagon stimulation test carried out for one hour will likewise show marked elevations over the fasting gastrin levels. The patient should be prepared for total gastrectomy.

Patients suspected of harboring an ulcerogenic tumor must be fully informed prior to operation why it may be necessary to perform total gastrectomy along with splenectomy and partial resection of the pancreas. The surgeon should not be restricted at the operating table because the patient has not been well informed preoperatively.

Careful preoperative preparation is related to the patient's fluid and electrolyte balance. To ensure accurate laboratory values and to have the patient safely prepared for surgery, fluids and electrolytes should be administered day and night at rates equivalent to the losses by diarrhea and/or gastric aspiration. These patients should also have their weights monitored in the morning and in the evening, as a further check on their fluid needs. If dehydration or hypercalcemia has been a problem, the operation should be delayed, if possible, until the serum levels of blood-urea-nitrogen and creatinine nearly approach normal limits. The blood volume should be measured and restored to normal levels before the operation.

If the patient has undergone no previous operations on the upper abdomen, the preliminary exploration is performed through a midline incision which extends well over the xiphoid process and well below the umbilicus on the left side. The incision may need to be altered in the presence of one or more scars from previous operations on the upper abdomen. The xiphoid process should be removed as high as possible. Great care must be taken in opening the peritoneal cavity, especially in patients having had previous surgery, because of the frequent presence of penetration of a stomal ulceration up against the anterior parietes. Evidence of duodenal ulcerations may or may not be found; however, the finding of a primary ulcer beyond the ligament of Treitz is considered pathognomonic of an ulcerogenic tumor.

The type of definitive surgical procedure can only be determined after meticulous exploration of the entire pancreas, duodenum and gastric antrum. Regional lymph nodes and the liver are also carefully examined for evidence of metastases. However, these patients frequently present the surgeon with a variety of perplexing judgment problems that may challenge his surgical acumen. One of the biggest problems is what procedure should be carried out when no tumor is found at surgical exploration despite a firm preoperative diagnosis.

A thorough exploration for tumor should include mobilization of the head of the pancreas by a Kocher maneuver and complete mobilization of the spleen and body and tail of the pancreas for thorough inspection of the gland from both sides. The wall of the duodenum, particularly along the mesenteric border, is carefully palpated for tumor nodules arising from aberrant pancreas. The pylorus may be split and the lumen of the first and second portions of the duodenum explored for intramural adenomata. Lymph nodes in the gastroduodenal ligament should be excised for frozen section examination and the liver carefully inspected and palpated for evidence of metastases.

In the past, and before the widespread availability of the gastrin radioimmunoassay, it was common to mobilize the spleen and left side of the pancreas into the wound prior to ligation of the splenic vessels and division of the pancreas a short distance to the left of the portal vein. Such "blind" resections occasionally uncovered a small adenoma, grossly, or diffuse microadenomatosis, by pathologic examination. However, the incidence of complications was increased by this procedure which was carried out because microscopic proof of tumor was felt to be mandatory before total gastrectomy could be performed. Blind resections of the pancreas in a search for occult adenomas have been discontinued, and in the face of a negative exploration, the final decision for or against total gastrectomy may well depend upon the preoperative gastrin radioimmunoassay levels (Fig. 2).

If either the fasting or calcium-stimulated gastrin levels were diagnostic of an ulcerogenic tumor, total gastrectomy may be carried out. If the serum immunoassay values were borderline, even after calcium or secretin stimulation, the surgeon may prefer to do a routine ulcer operation which should include, however, resection of the antrum and as much of the first part of the duodenum as possible. The permanent pathologic sections

ULCEROGENIC TUMOR ?

Negative Exploration
- **Pancreas**
- **Duodenal & Antral Walls**
- **Lymph Nodes** – Frozen Section
- **Liver**

Borderline **Immunoassay – Ulcer Operation**

Positive " TOTAL GASTRECTOMY

FIG. 2. In the face of a negative exploration for an ulcerogenic tumor, the final decision for or against total gastrectomy may depend upon the preoperative gastrin radioimmunoassay levels.

should include evaluation of the entire circumference of the duodenal wall.

A second judgment problem facing the surgeon is the finding of an ulcerogenic tumor within the submucosa of the first portion of the duodenum. Duodenal wall tumors occur in more than 10% of the patients with the ulcerogenic syndrome. Wilson reviewed more than 100 such cases and found that they were solitary in less than one half of the series [9]. Oberhelman has long emphasized good long-term results following local or radical tumor excision; however, when there have been metastatic or multiple adenomas, total gastrectomy has generally been agreed upon [10]. Since these tumors are multiple or malignant in about one half of the cases, a recurrence rate of approximately 50% can be anticipated if total gastrectomy is not carried out.

In the recorded cases of ulcerogenic tumor, approximately 20 patients underwent an operation for peptic ulcer disease before their 16th birthdays. In reviewing these cases, Wilson and colleagues have found that those children who had total gastrectomy, even in the face of metastatic or multiple tumors, developed physically along essentially normal lines [11]. In contrast, an equal number of children who had less than total gastrectomy did not survive. The surgeon, therefore, should not hesitate to remove the entire stomach regardless of the young age of the patient.

At the other end of the spectrum are those elderly patients who develop a fulminating ulcer diathesis for the first time. This should strongly suggest the presence of an ulcerogenic tumor. Since these tumors produce such serious complications, the best interest of the patients would be served by removal of the acid-secreting surface by total gastrectomy, even in the presence of extensive liver metastases. While these tumors tend to grow slowly, it must not be forgotten that the metastases provide the same rich source of gastrin as the mother tumor. Wilson recently reported that patients with liver metastases who underwent total gastrectomy had survival rates of 42% and 30% at five and ten years, respectively [12]. In contrast, of the patients who had lesser gastric operations, only 7% survived at five years and none were alive at ten years.

Under rare circumstances, a solitary tumor which is of the size to be easily identified can be excised without total gastrectomy. This is especially tempting when the tumor occurs in the left half of the pancreas which is easily resectable. Evidence to support this conservative approach can be provided by a dramatic fall in the monitored nasogastric output of gastric juice from the nasogastric tube during the operation, suggesting that the major source of gastrin has been removed. Total gastrectomy would seem to be preferred in the great majority of instances to either local excision or resection of the involved head of the pancreas by the Whipple procedure.

In the classic ulcerogenic syndrome with one or more tumors found in the pancreas or microscopic proof of metastases to the adjacent lymph nodes or liver, there is general agreement that total gastrectomy is indicated. The type of reconstruction after total gastrectomy will vary according to the choice and experience of the individual surgeon; but, in general, the Roux-en-Y anastomosis has been preferred. The end of the jejunum is closed and an end-to-side esophagojejunostomy performed, with the end of the jejunum directed to the left side.

Since many of these patients will have had previous gastric operations, there may be dense adhesions about the esophagus. Great care must be taken to avoid fraying the nonperitonealized esophagus. Usually the esophageal wall has been carefully anchored to the crus of the diaphragm at four points to avoid retraction after it is divided. Furthermore, it seems advisable to ensure as large an anastomosis as possible by inserting a large Einhorn stomach tube along the Levin tube into the jejunum after the two-layer posterior anastomosis has been completed. The large tube serves as a stent which facilitates proper placement of the anterior row of sutures and, at the same time, ensures a larger anastomosis.

The long-term follow-up of these patients should include careful monitoring of caloric intake as well as weight trends. Vitamin B_{12} injections are given monthly. It is probably advisable to rehospitalize the patient at three and six month intervals for several years in order to re-survey dietary habits, the status of the esophagojejunal anastomosis and to scan the liver. When the serum alkaline phosphatase is elevated, or if liver metastases were found at the time of surgery, it may be advisable to perform an aortogram to monitor the rate of growth or regression of the tumor. To gain realistic information on the persistence of tumor tissue, a calcium infusion test should be carried out even though the fasting gastrin levels were within the normal range. Sanzenbacher et al reported that the calcium challenge will often reveal unexpectedly high elevations in serum gastrin, and the test should be useful in monitoring either the regression or progression of these tumors after total gastrectomy [13].

Nutritional difficulties have been observed in the late postoperative period; but, in general, these patients do better nutritionally than when total gastrectomy is carried out for carcinoma of the stomach. Neither chemotherapy nor irradiation has been routinely given to the patient, despite the presence of multiple metastases.

In a series of cases since 1953, 64% of the patients are living even though some had obvious extensive tumor involvement. Four of ten patients with malignant islet cell tumors, or 40%, lived longer than five years after total gastrectomy. Sufficient time has not elapsed to evaluate accurately the possible beneficial effects of total gastrectomy on the inhibition of growth of malignant tumors. Since 16, or more than 40% of the patients had preoperative symptoms for 5 to 14 years before total gastrectomy, it is logical to assume a very slow rate of growth of any retained tumor after removal of all acid-secreting surface of the stomach.

References

1. Zollinger, R. M. and Ellison, E. H.: Primary peptic ulcerations of the jejunum associated with islet cell tumors of the pancreas. Ann. Surg., 142:709, 1955.
2. Grossman, M. I., Tracy, H. J., Gregory, R. A.: II. Isolation of a gastrin-like substance from the primary and secondary tumors. Gastroenterology, 41:87, 1961.
3. Ruppert, R. D., Greenberger, N. J., Beman, F. M. et al: Gastric secretion in ulcerogenic tumors of the pancreas. Ann. Int. Med., 67:808, 1967.
4. Passaro, E. Jr., Basso, N., Walsh, J. H.: Calcium challenge in the Zollinger-Ellison syndrome. Surgery, 72:60, 1972.
5. Wermer, P.: Genetic aspects of adenomatosis of endocrine glands. Amer. J. Med., 16:363, 1954.
6. Kaplan, E. L., Peskin, G. W., Defeny, C. et al: Ulcer disease, metabolic alkalosis and hyperparathyroidism: A mechanism of interrelationship? Ann. Surg. (In press.)
7. Jaffe, B. M., Peskin, G. W., Kaplan, E. L.: Serum levels of parathormone in the Zollinger-Ellison syndrome. Surgery, 74:621, 1973.
8. Sizemore, G. W., Go, V. L. W., Kaplan, E. L. et al: Relationships of calcitonin and gastrin in the Zollinger-Ellison syndrome and medullary carcinoma of the thyroid. New Eng. J. Med., 228:641, 1973.
9. Hofmann, J. W., Fox, P. S. and Wilson, S. D.: Duodenal wall tumors and the Zollinger-Ellison syndrome. Surgical management. Arch. Surg., 107:334, 1973.
10. Oberhelman, H. A. Jr.: Excisional therapy for ulcerogenic tumors of the duodenum: Long term results. Arch. Surg., 104:447, 1972.
11. Wilson, S. D., Schulte, W. J. and Meade, R. C.: Longevity studies following total gastrectomy. In children with the Zollinger-Ellison syndrome. Arch. Surg., 103:108, 1971.
12. Fox, P. S., Hofmann, J. W., DeCosse, J. J. et al: The influence of total gastrectomy on survival in malignant Zollinger-Ellison tumors. Ann. Surg. (In press.)
13. Sanzenbacher, L. J., King, D. R. and Zollinger, R. M.: Prognostic implications of calcium-mediated gastrin levels in the ulcerogenic syndrome. Amer. J. Surg., 125:116, 1973

This work was supported by a grant from The John A. Hartford Foundation, Inc., New York, N.Y. and USPHS Grant RR-34.

Hypoglycemia in Infancy

Robert A. Ulstrom, M.D.

The spectrum of etiology of hypoglycemia in infants and children continues to expand and shift in emphasis. Twenty years ago, McQuarrie reviewed [1] his experience of the preceding decade at Minnesota and had not encountered an insulinoma in childhood. Boley et al [2] reviewed 17 reported cases of insulinoma in childhood in 1960 and found only two younger than 5 years of age. Sauls and Ulstrom [3] extended McQuarrie's experience, and by 1966 had observed two insulinomas: one in an infant female whose onset was in the second day of life and one in a 10-year-old boy. By 1969, the total number of childhood insulinomas reported had increased by 24 cases including 9 new cases in infants under 2 years [4]. Garces [5], Grant [6], Schwartz [7], Buist [8], Robinson [9] and Christiansen [10] have reported an additional eight cases in infants under 1 year of age since Mann's review [4]. Three additional cases have been treated during the first year of life at the University of Minnesota Hospitals (Table 1) and a fourth at the St. Paul Children's Hospital. A fifth case died in another local hospital, undiagnosed, on the third day of life. An insulinoma was found at autopsy.

The reason for this change of reported incidence of functioning islet cell adenoma in young infants is unclear. The accelerating rate of reporting as well as our own experience now requires that this diagnosis must be seriously considered in any infant whose serum glucose concentrations are repeatedly low, regardless of the age of onset.

Glucose homeostasis during the first day of postnatal life is unstable. Full-term infants may appear normal even when blood sugar is 30-40 mg/100 ml. Immature and low birthweight infants may be asymptomatic at concentrations between 20 and 30 mg/100 ml. That concentrations below 40 mg/100 ml are harmless to the developing brain has been questioned recently, however [11]. A delay in onset of feeding may prolong the period of low blood sugar in the normal infant. In the

Robert A. Ulstrom, M.D., Professor of Pediatrics, University of Minnesota, Minneapolis.

Table 1. University of Minnesota Hospitals (1974) Islet Cell Adenoma in Infants

Case	*B.W.*	*Age Onset*†	*Pre-Op Med Rx*	*Age Surg.*	*Response Surg.*	*Present Status*
A*	3900	36 hr. & 3 wk.	ACTH steroid Susphrine Zn Glucagon Diazoxide Growth Hormone Diet	8 mo.	Cure	M.R. seizures
B	3230	2 da. & 1 wk.	Diazoxide ACTH Diet	23 da. 33 da	None Cure	Normal (20 mo.)
C	2800	24 hr. & 7 wk.	Prednisone Diazoxide Diet	12 wk. 16 wk.	None ? Cure	M.R. (18 mo.)
D	3700	5 hr.	Steroid Diazoxide Phenobarb Dilantin	3 wk.	Cure	Seizures (6 mo.)

*Previously reported [3].

†Where a second "onset" is indicated, the infant had a short spontaneous remission preceding recurrence.

neonatal period, most hypoglycemia is in low birthweight infants and is transient. Symptomatic therapy beyond the first 48 hours is rarely required. Obese and high birthweight infants, frequently seen from diabetic mothers, also have a high incidence of transient hypoglycemia. Both of these varieties appear first within hours after birth and are frequently only one of many manifestations of the respective conditions. Infants born at term with normal birthweight rarely have hypoglycemia. When such cases occur, they demand, besides prompt symptomatic treatment, thorough investigation for underlying disorders, which are usually serious, prolonged and carry a grave prognosis for normal brain development. It is from this group of infants that cases of true hyperinsulinism will be frequently diagnosed; particularly when no physical abnormalities are present to suggest metabolic abnormalities of glycogen storage, galactosemia, amino acid dysmetabolism or hyperammonemic states. Jaundice, hepatomegaly and urinary reducing substances suggest the latter.

Convulsions or cyanotic attacks are the most frequent first symptoms of hypoglycemia in the young infant. Glucose determined at that time will frequently be below the lower limit of the method. For most laboratories, this will be 10 or 15 mg/100 ml. Our own experience with the bedside determination of glucose has been disappointing and has led to serious misinterpretations. In an infant experiencing symptoms compatible with hypoglycemia, attempted treatment should not be delayed until the laboratory report is in hand. Since most such infants will be unable to take a feeding, glucose should be given rapidly intravenously. Using solutions with 20%-50% concentrations of glucose, a dose of 0.5 gm/kg of body weight may be safely given over three to five minutes. Even in the presence of severe hypoglycemia, such therapy will raise the blood glucose over 100 mg%. If the symptoms were caused by hypoglycemia, improvement will be noted within a minute or two. If no change is forthcoming in the clinical condition, larger amounts of injected glucose will not help and are dangerous. The author has recently observed two fatal hyperosmolar reactions to amounts of hypertonic glucose that exceeded these recommendations.

Having established that an infant has hypoglycemic attacks, the etiology of the low blood glucose must then be found. Infants with hyperinsulinism must be distinguished from those with other causes. Although the availability of serum insulin determined by radioimmunoassay has improved the diagnostic potential, the long period between sampling and results adversely influences its clinical usefulness. Indirect assessment of glucose homeostatic mechanisms will also be necessary. Although no criteria are unique to infants with symptomatic hyperinsulinism, Table 2 lists characteristics commonly found.

Most infants with hyperinsulinism show a marked drop in blood glucose (> 15 mg%) after administration of l-leucine (150 mg/kg) or a feeding of whole milk. This may be very dramatic and require prompt administration of glucose to prevent a seizure. Unfortunately, it is common that the blood sugar levels are persistently low. In such cases, the results may be uninterpretable and the test dangerous. When a successful test is performed, serum insulin values usually rise greatly as glucose falls. In the infant whose low glucose values contraindicate this test, serial determinations of glucose and insulin are of value. Although a glucose-insulin ratio may be calculated, when glucose values are below 30 mg/100 ml, one should find insulin essentially absent from the serum. The presence of "normal" fasting values of serum insulin under these circumstances is highly abnormal since normal fasting glucose values are

Table 2. Hypoglycemia due to Hyperinsulinism in Infants

Normal weight at birth
Onset in first 48 hours
A short period of "apparent recovery"
Absence of physical abnormalities
Absence of other biochemical abnormalities
Characteristics of hypoglycemia
a) very low levels
b) worse after milk feedings
c) leucine sensitive
d) glucagon responsive
e) resistant to ACTH, steroids
f) resistant to diazoxide
g) medical management usually poor

not present. One need not observe marked elevations of serum insulin in the fasting state to make a diagnosis of hyperinsulinism. The presence of easily measured values of insulin when accompanied by very low levels of glucose is not physiological and represents a relative hyperinsulinemic state.

The infant with hyperinsulinism must have surgical exploration of his pancreas. The surgeon must be prepared to perform an excision biopsy even if no adenoma is found. Although one of the tumors in the author's experience was visible in situ, the other five were found only after multiple sections were made in the excised portion of the pancreas. Three of these were located in the head of the pancreas adjacent to the duodenum. One of these was found unexpectedly at autopsy. The other two were found by the surgical pathologist in tissue removed at a second operation. In each case, continued extreme difficulty with medical management following surgical removal of three fourths of the pancreas prompted re-exploration and 95% pancreatectomy. In every case, hyperglycemia occurred within eight hours of successful removal of the tumor. A diabetic state followed, requiring insulin therapy for only one and four weeks, respectively, even after the near-total pancreatectomy. No further medical therapy for hypoglycemia has been necessary in our cases, nor in other reported cases. Neurologic sequelae, however, continue to be a problem, including developmental retardation and nonhypoglycemia seizures. Our youngest surgical cure was at age 33 days. His subsequent course has been normal for 18 months, encouraging us in the direction of the earliest possible definitive therapy.

Even when no insulinoma is found, a 75%-80% subtotal pancreatectomy is indicated in infants with hypoglycemia due to hyperinsulinism [12]. Except for those unusual cases that are familial [3] or are easily managed by medical treatment with diazoxide (5-15 mg/kg), removal of a portion of the pancreas is essential both for diagnosis and satisfactory management. Pathology of the pancreas in these nontumorous cases may show no abnormality, islet hyperplasia or beta cell nesidioblastosis [13]. Only an adenoma or adenomatosis is subject to complete surgical cure, however. In most nontumorous cases, subsequent management with diazoxide administration and a limited leucine (protein) intake will be reasonably successful in the prevention of further hypoglycemia and its resultant brain damage. Most such infants require medical management for several years. Rarely, after a year the child will attain the ability to do well without further therapy. A period of three to six years is the usual duration of the hypoglycemic tendency. Regardless of the basic etiology, subsequent manifestation of brain damage is common, particularly if the hypoglycemia appeared during the first six months of life [14]. The urgency is great, therefore, to completely eradicate hypoglycemia as quickly as possible when it is found in a young infant. When hyperinsulinism is the probable cause and the hypoglycemia is persistent in an infant under 1 year of age, we recommend that a 75%-80% pancreatectomy be performed for diagnosis and therapy.

Summary

The incidence of islet cell adenoma as a cause of hyperinsulinism in infants appears to be increasing. Some of these adenomas are microscopic and may only be diagnosed after pancreatic excision. If 75%-80% pancreatectomy reveals neither an adenoma nor results in improved subsequent medical management, near-total pancreatectomy may be indicated. In two such cases, an adenoma of microscopic dimensions was present in the excised head of the pancreas. In most cases of hyperinsulinism not associated with tumor, 75%-80% excision of the pancreas, diazoxide administration and a diet low in the amino acid l-leucine will provide successful treatment of the hypoglycemia. Late brain damage from hypoglycemia in infancy may be thus favorably influenced.

References

1. McQuarrie, I.: Idiopathic spontaneously occurring hypoglycemia in infants. Amer. J. Dis. Child., 87:399, 1954.

2. Boley, S. J., Lin, J. and Schiffman, A.: Functioning pancreatic adenomas in infants and children. Surgery, 48:592, 1960.
3. Sauls, H. S., Jr. and Ulstrom, R. A.: Hypoglycemia. *In* Kelly, V. C. (ed.): Brennemann's Practice of Pediatrics, Vol. I. Hagerstown, Maryland:W. F. Prior Co., 1966.
4. Mann, J. R., Rayner, P. H. and Gourevitch, A.: Insulinoma in childhood. Arch. Dis. Child., 44:435, 1969.
5. Garces, L. Y., Drash, A. and Kenny, F. M.: Islet cell tumor in the neonate: Studies in carbohydrate metabolism and therapeutic response. Pediatrics, 41:789, 1968.
6. Grant, D. B. and Barbor, P. R. H.: Islet cell tumor causing hypoglycemia in a newborn infant. Arch. Dis. Child., 45:434, 1970.
7. Schwartz, J. F. and Zwiren, G. T.: Islet cell adenomatosis and adenoma in an infant. J. Pediatr., 79:232, 1971.
8. Buist, N. R., Campbell, J. R., Castro, A. et al: Congenital islet cell adenoma causing hypoglycemia in a newborn. Pediatrics, 47:605, 1971.
9. Robinson, M. J., Clarke, M. A., Gold H. et al: Islet cell adenoma in the newborn: Report of two patients. Pediatrics, 48:232, 1971.
10. Christiansen, R. O. and Johnson, J. D.: Studies of insulin secretion in hypoglycemia (abstract). Ped. Research, 8:431, 1974.
11. Pagliara, A. S. et al: Letter to the Editor. J. Ped., 83:695-697, 1973.
12. Hamilton, J. P., Baker, L., Kaye, R. et al: Subtotal pancreatectomy in the management of severe persistent idiopathic hypoglycemia in children. Pediatrics, 39:49, 1967.
13. Yakovac, W. C., Baker, L. and Hummeler, K.: Beta cell nesidioblastosis in idiopathic hypoglycemia of infancy. J. Pediatr., 79:226, 1971.
14. Haworth, J. C. and Coodin, F. J.: Idiopathic spontaneous hypoglycemia in children. Pediatrics, 25:748, 1960.

Islet Cell Transplantation

John S. Najarian, M.D., David E. R. Sutherland, M.D.
and Michael W. Steffes, M.D., Ph.D.

Although islet cell transplantation is still experimental in nature, it will have clinical application in the not too distant future.

Approximately one third of the 2 million insulin-dependent diabetics in the United States will die of renal failure. The other two thirds will probably die of cardiovascular complications. Surgeons at the University of Minnesota have had an interest in the treatment of the diabetic since the early explorations in pancreatic transplantation, first by Bill Kelly in 1966 and then by Richard Lillehei in 1967. The first ten pancreatic transplants on insulin-dependent diabetics, which were performed here, were combined with kidney transplants. All of these patients had renal failure secondary to juvenile onset diabetes. In this series, only one patient survived for an extended period of time with a functioning pancreas and kidney. He lived 12 months and was completely cured of his diabetes as far as carbohydrate metabolism was concerned. Unfortunately, he committed suicide by not taking his medication. As a result of this experience on ten patients, approximately four years ago, we decided that both a pancreaticoduodenal and renal transplant was too much of an operation for the diabetic patient. Complications of the operation, particularly sepsis, and the possibility of rejection of the pancreas and duodenum presented many problems. This series did prove that a transplanted pancreas could function normally.

The worldwide pancreatic transplant experience totals 34, and 13 of them were done at the University of Minnesota. As of March 1, 1974, only three pancreatic transplant recipients are living and only one has a functioning pancreatic graft.

John S. Najarian, M.D., Professor and Chairman, Department of Surgery; David E. R. Sutherland, M.D., Medical Fellow, Department of Surgery; and Michael W. Steffes, M.D., Ph.D., Medical Fellow, Department of Laboratory Medicine and Pathology, University of Minnesota Medical School, Minneapolis.

Since 1969 we have treated 75 diabetics with renal failure with kidney transplantation alone. The results of this series have been reported several times, most recently at a meeting on diabetic nephropathy held in Minneapolis. We have found that living related transplants in diabetic patients stand a 60% chance of being functional at the end of four years, a figure about 30% less than that achieved in nondiabetics who receive related grafts (90% survival in our series). If a diabetic receives a cadaveric transplant, the chances of having a functioning transplant at the end of four years is 40%, which again is 30% less than that which can be achieved in a nondiabetic recipient. Many diabetic patients are well rehabilitated by kidney transplantation, and we feel that this is a worthwhile procedure in this group of patients. Other institutions are now beginning to do kidney transplants in the diabetic, based upon the results of our series.

We have biopsied the transplant kidneys in these patients on a yearly basis, and after almost five years, we have not seen recurrence of the diabetic lesion in the kidney transplant. We suspect that it will recur eventually, however, because their diabetes has not been cured. By alleviating their uremia, we have improved their neuropathy, gastroenteropathy and eyesight, but they are still diabetic.

Shortly after we initiated our kidney transplant program for diabetics, we also started the investigation of isolating the islets of Langerhans from the pancreas. Our ultimate goal is correction of the carbohydrate metabolism defect in the diabetic by transplantation of isolated islets.

Our procedure for isolating islets is modified from those described originally by Moskalawski, Lacy, Lindall and others. Basically, the pancreas is distended with Hank's solution by cannulating the pancreatic duct. The pancreatic tissue is minced into small fragments and then incubated with collagenase in a shaking water bath for 10 to 30 minutes to break down the collagen and liberate islets. To obtain a relatively pure preparation of islets, the digested tissue is then placed on a discontinuous Ficoll gradient. The Ficoll gradient we use has specific densities of 1.085, 1.075, 1.060 and 1.045 from bottom to top. Acinar, ductal and vascular tissue remain in the bottom layer, while human islets usually localize at the 1.060-1.075 interphase. Pig islets seem to be less dense and rise to the upper layers. With this method we can achieve a reasonably pure preparation of islets. Figure 1 is an example of one of our best human islets isolated by this technique. It is completely free from all surrounding structures, and beta cells are readily identifiable within the islets when they are stained with aldehyde fuchsin.

Our laboratory model to study the effects that islet transplantation may have on diabetes and its secondary lesions is the rats made diabetic

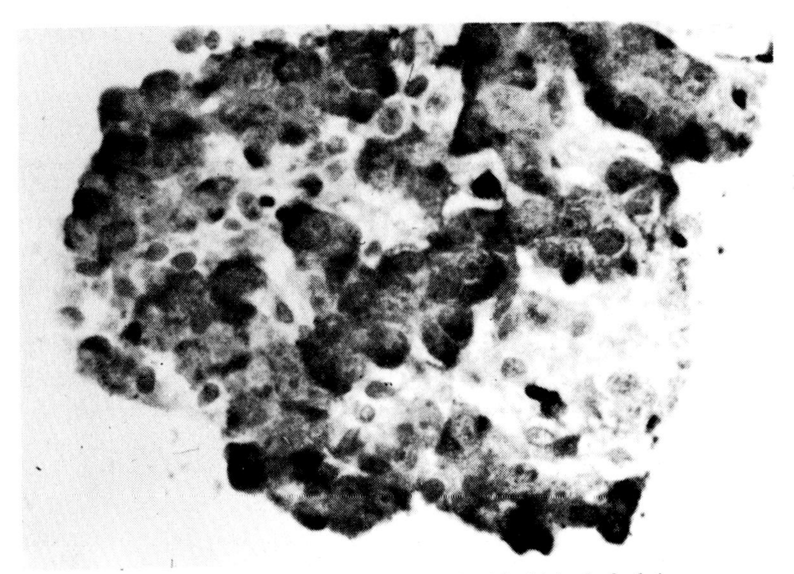

FIG. 1. Isolated human islet stained with aldehyde fuchsin.

with streptozotocin (an antibiotic specifically destructive to beta cells). Rats made diabetic by this technique have nonfasting blood sugars of greater than 600 mg/100 ml. Following islet transplantation, blood glucose levels begin to fall, and by two to three weeks they are normal. We transplant the islets intraperitoneally, although other investigators have had good success transplanting into the portal vein. The advantage of one route over another has not yet been completely resolved. We have maintained inbred rats, transplanted with syngenic islet tissue obtained from the same inbred strain, for over one year in the normoglycemic state.

All islet transplanted rats have normal intravenous glucose tolerance curves when blood glucoses are measured and compared to those of normal rats. Transplanted rats also have an insulin response to intravenous glucose testing; in some instances, the response is as vigorous, or more vigorous, than that seen in normal animals, while in other instances, the peripheral insulin levels are less than those of normal animals challenged with glucose. A response always occurs in the transplanted animals, compared to the lack of response in nontransplanted diabetic rats.

Our main interest in studying the rat model of diabetes was to determine what effect islet transplantation would have on the secondary lesions of diabetes. Diabetic rats develop lesions in their kidneys that are similar to those described by Kimmesteil and Wilson in the human diabetic. The lesions develop first by thickening of the glomerular mesangial matrix, followed by focal tuft sclerosis, and eventually hyaline nodules and glomerulosclerosis. We found that when an islet transplant is done during the early course of these lesions (six to nine months after induction of diabetes in the rat), the lesions are reversible and mesangial matrix thickening will actually regress or disappear. At the very least, the lesions will not continue to progress. More striking even than the light microscopic findings in these rats, however, is the glomerular pathology demonstrable by immunofluorescent microscopy. When stained for immunoglobulins IgG, and IgM, and for the B_1C component of complement, these macromolecules start to accumulate in large quantities within the glomerular mesangium six months after the onset of diabetes (Fig. 2). These deposits disappear if a diabetic rat receives an islet transplant. Figure 3A shows large deposits of IgG within the glomerular mesangium of a kidney biopsy from a diabetic rat prior to transplantation. Two months after reversal of the diabetes by islet transplantation the immunofluorescent positive material has disappeared (Fig. 3B). The dependency of both the light and immunofluorescent microscope renal lesions upon the diabetic state has been demonstrated by renal transplantation in the rat, by Dr. Chue Shue Lee in our laboratory. When Dr. Lee transplanted a diabetic kidney with secondary lesions to a normal rat, the lesions of that

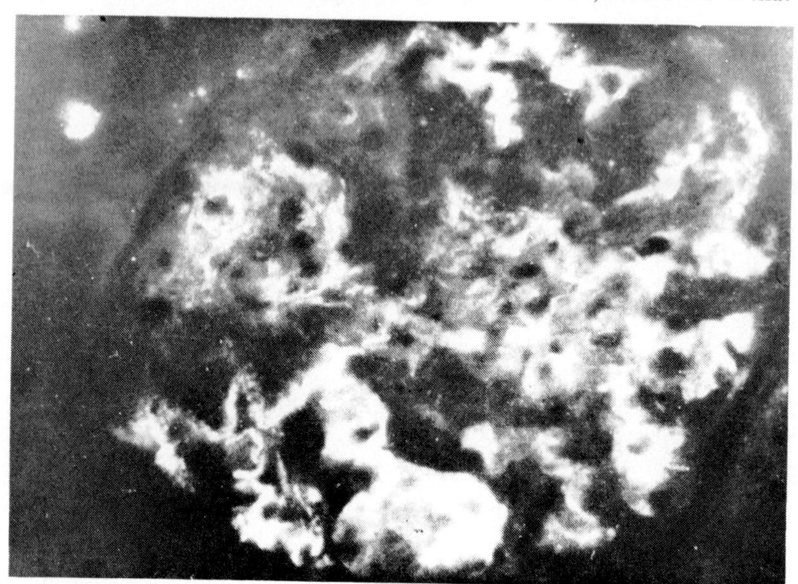

FIG. 2. Glomerulus of rat kidney six months after induction of diabetes showing large quantities of B_1C within the mesangium by immunofluorescent microscopy.

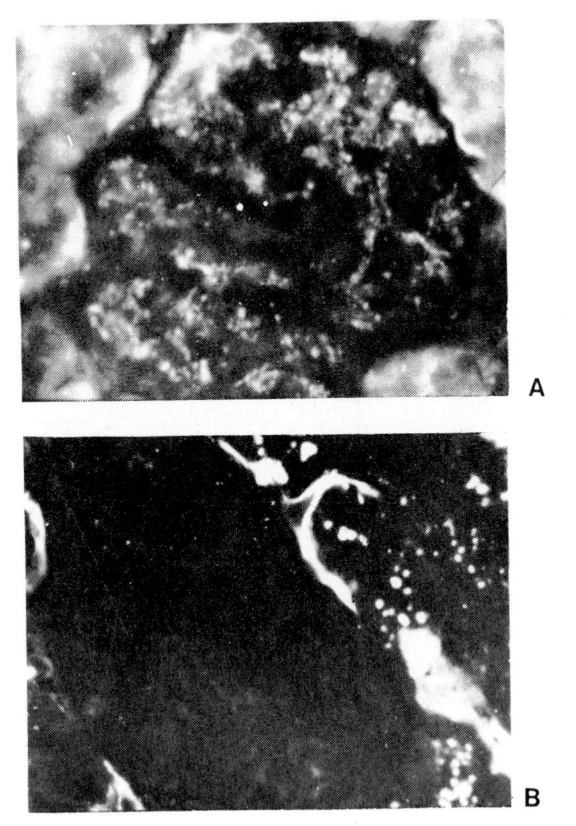

FIG. 3. Glomerulus of diabetic rat kidney stained for IgG before (*A*) and two months after (*B*) curative islet transplantation, demonstrating almost complete disappearance of the immunofluorescent pathology.

kidney disappeared or failed to progress. When he transplanted a normal kidney to a diabetic rat, the renal lesions developed in an accelerated fashion in the previously normal transplanted kidney.

These microscopic studies, which were carried out in conjunction with Dr. S. Michael Mauer of our Department of Pediatrics, show, in essence, that if the defect in carbohydrate metabolism of diabetic rats can be reversed, the secondary renal lesions can be stabilized or reversed. Whether this observation will hold true for humans remains to be seen.

The high mortality and morbidity associated with whole organ pancreatic transplants in humans stimulated us to explore the possibility of separating islets from the acinar pancreas. The acinar tissue's associated proteolytic and destructive enzymes precludes using unmodified pancreatic fragments for transplantation. If viable islets can be isolated in relatively pure form, clinical attempts to transplant the islets of Langerhans could be made.

We have also used the pig for experimental islet transplantation. We chose this large animal to mimic as closely as possible the human situation, in terms of pancreatic size, and to see if techniques could be developed to isolate an adequate number of islets from one pancreas for an effective transplantation. In the rat, multiple donors can be used for one transplant, but in the human, this circumstance would be difficult to duplicate. The pig pancreas is fairly similar to the human pancreas.

Our technique of islet isolation in the pig was similar to that used for the human. The islets were transplanted to pigs made diabetic by a complete pancreatectomy. Totally pancreatectomized pigs become diabetic immediately, have blood glucose levels of between 500 and 700 mg/100 ml and, if not treated with insulin, will die within ten days, with a mean survival of 6.0 ± 2.6 S.D. days in nontransplanted pigs. We performed autografts or allografts of islets, transplanted either intramuscularly or intraperitoneally; 11 totally pancreatectomized pigs transplanted with islet tissue had a mean survival of 15.3 ± 6.6 S.D. days. The number of islets transplanted, however, was small, and although blood glucose levels were lowered, the pigs did not become normoglycemic. One transplanted pig survived for 28 days. His blood sugar was lowered from over 600 mg/100 ml to close to 300 mg/100 ml where it was maintained for two weeks, when severe hyperglycemia (greater than 700 mg/100 ml) occurred. A second islet transplant was performed; the blood sugar again fell to 300 mg/100 ml, but within six days severe hyperglycemia recurred (suggesting a second set rejection phenomena) and the pig died 28 days after the initial transplant. Perhaps more intense immunosuppressive therapy would have allowed longer survival. The transplanted pigs had detectable circulating insulin (usually less than 14μU/ml), but we could not detect circulating insulin in the pancreatectomized pigs that did not receive an islet transplant. This finding indicates that isolated islets were able to synthesize and release insulin when transplanted.

We also have been procuring the pancreas from the human cadaver donors used in our renal transplant program. Following bilateral nephrectomy, the pancreas is removed fresh and either processed immediately in the laboratory or, if obtained at odd hours or from a distant source, placed on our Mox-100 hypothermic, pulsatile flow preservation machine for 4 to 16 hours. Islet isolation is then performed using variants of the basic collagenase digestion-Ficoll separation technique.

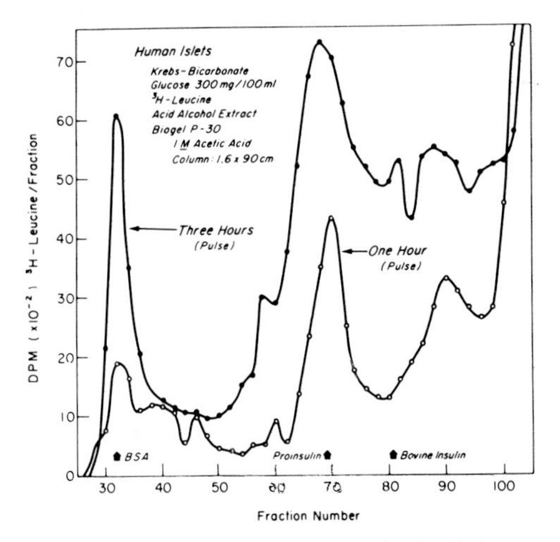

FIG. 4. Isolated human islets incubated at 300 mg/100 ml glucose with ^{3}H-leucine, acid-alcohol extraction performed on separate aliquots at one and three hours, extracted proteins subjected to gel filtration of a Bio-Gel P-30 column precalibrated with BSA, proinsulin and insulin, and fractions then assayed for radioactivity. Isolated islets incorporate ^{3}H-leucine into both proinsulin and insulin, in increasing amounts with time.

One of the questions we wanted to answer was whether isolated human islets are alive. Can they synthesize and release the islet hormones, insulin and glucagon? First we studied insulin synthesis of isolated islets in vitro. Figure 4 is an example of isolated islets incubated at high glucose concentration in the presence of ^{3}H-leucine, a radiolabeled amino acid precursor of insulin. Following incubation at one and three hours, respectively, the islets were homogenized, acid-alcohol extraction was performed and the extracted proteins were separated by gel filtration on a column of Bio-Gel P-30 precalibrated with BSA, proinsulin and insulin markers. Figure 4 illustrates that the radioactive leucine is incorporated into islet proteins that exactly correspond to insulin and proinsulin. At one hour there is incorporation into proinsulin, while at three hours a large amount of incorporation has occurred into the insulin area of the curve. The total amount of incorporation with time follows essentially a linear pattern with all islet proteins. Similar experiments have been carried out incubating islets in vitro at low glucose concentrations with radiolabeled ^{3}H-tryptophan, an amino acid precursor of glucagon. Again, specific concentration into a protein corresponding exactly to the area of glucagon elution on a Bio-Gel P-30 column occurs, and the incubated, extracted, filtered product of incorporation has glucagon immunoreactivity when subjected to radioimmunoassay. Our experiments that demonstrated incorporation of radiolabeled amino acid precursors into insulin and glucagon were carried out in conjunction with Drs. G. Eric Bauer and Bryan D. Noe. By showing protein synthesis capabilities we have provided evidence that isolated human islets are viable.

Another important question to answer in regard to islet isolation is: How pure are the preparations obtained? We attempted to answer this question of purity by measuring the amount of insulin in relation to amylase and protein in our final preparation. These ratios indicate the amount of islet tissue present, relative to the amount of acinar and other pancreatic tissue. In the normal, intact pancreas there are 1.2μg of insulin per milligram of tissue protein (I/P ratio) and 25μg of insulin per milligram of amylase (I/A ratio). Figure 5 shows examples of I/P and I/A ratios we have achieved from various human islet isolation procedures. In relation to total pancreatic tissue, as expressed by protein, up to a 27-fold purification of islet tissue has been achieved; in relation to acinar tissue, as expressed by amylase, over a 100-fold purification of islets has occasionally been achieved. The latter is probably the more important index of islet purity for ultimate transplantation use.

We also determined the total yield of islet tissue isolated from each pancreas by measuring the total amount of insulin present in each pancreas (directly proportional to the amount of islet tissue), and then measuring the total amount of insulin in our isolated islet preparation obtained from the same pancreas. Figure 6 shows the kind of results we have achieved on

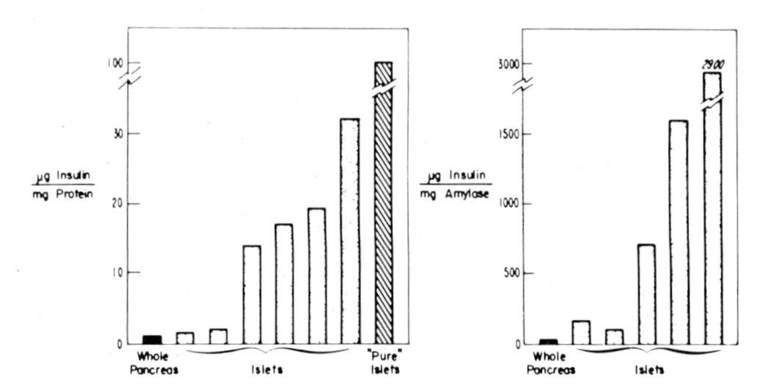

FIG. 5. Insulin/protein and insulin/amylase ratios in micrograms/milligram on various human islet isolations compared to the ratios for normal intact pancreas, indicating a significant purification of islet from acinar tissue in some preparations.

HUMAN ISLET ISOLATION YIELDS

Cadaver No.	Total Pancreatic Tissue Insulin (μgm)	Isolated Islet Tissue Insulin (μgm)	Yield
35	2,464	47	2%
37	2,296	26	1%
39	606	6	1%
40	360	61	17%
41	8,000	3	0.4%
42	4,570	2,391	51%
43	2,678	285	15%
44	3,019	180	6%
46	3,306	168	5%
47	10,500	21	0.2%
48	12,500	67	0.5%
49	15,100	32	0.6%
50	2,809	61	2%

FIG. 6. Yield of islets from various cadaver pancreata as calculated by measuring total pancreatic insulin and total insulin in the isolated tissue.

our last several islet isolation procedures. It is apparent that our yield of islets is usually less than 5%, but occasionally yields of 15% or 17% have been achieved and, on one occasion, over 50% of the islets were isolated. We have not been able to duplicate this one spectacular yield, but we feel that with continuing experience higher yields will be routine. Data from pancreatic resections indicate that up to 90% of the pancreas can be removed with sufficient islet reserve present to prevent overt diabetes. Thus, once we can consistently isolate 10% of pancreatic islets, we will have sufficient islet tissue to embark on a program of clinical islet transplantation.

We have also studied the ability of isolated human islets to secrete insulin when subjected to a hyperglycemic stimulus. Although we had previously demonstrated the protein synthesis capabilities of isolated islets, we wanted further evidence of their functional capabilities. Therefore, we now routinely perfuse isolated islets in a millipore chamber, first with a solution of low glucose concentration of 30 mg/100 ml until a stable baseline of insulin release is reached, and then with a hyperglycemic solution of 300 mg/100 ml. Figure 7 shows an example of such a perfusion where, after 60 minutes of hypoglycemic perfusion, a stable baseline of virtually zero insulin release was reached. Following hyperglycemic stimulation the islets responded with an immediate and sustained release of insulin, again indicating their viability and ability to withstand the isolation procedure.

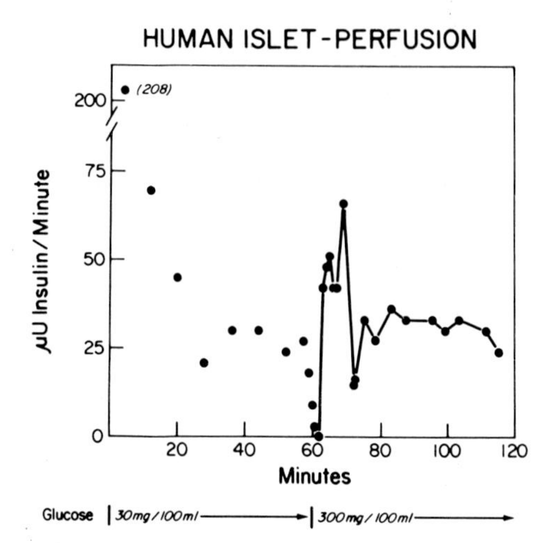

FIG. 7. Perfusion of isolated human islets. After stable baseline is reached, hyperglycemic stimulus with 300 mg glucose/100 ml results in immediate and sustained release of insulin.

In summary, we are still attempting to perfect the islet isolation technique in humans. We must be able to isolate islets in purified form, and we must consistently retrieve more than 10% of the islets from the pancreas. Then we can begin to attempt transplantation of islets to diabetic patients. It is our conviction that kidney transplantation alone is not enough for some of these patients, and that the diabetic state will ultimately adversely affect the transplanted kidney, as it does in diabetic rats. We feel that if we can obtain a preparation which will physiologically supply insulin to selected individuals, we will have provided an excellent treatment for insulin-dependent diabetes.

The Surgical Treatment of Chronic Pancreatitis

Rodney Smith, M.S.

In considering the place of surgery in the treatment of chronic pancreatitis, the first question must naturally be which patients require an operation. It is my opinion that there are only four indications for surgery:

1. *Pain*
2. Severe exacerbations of acute pancreatitis.
3. Complications, such as pancreatic cyst or fistula, obstruction of the duodenum, common bile duct or portal vein
4. Doubt as to the diagnosis and, in particular, a suspicion of malignancy.

Once it has been decided that an operation is necessary, what operation should be performed? Indirect operations upon the biliary tract have very little chance of success and, in my hands at least, the operation of sphincterotomy or sphincteroplasty has been a complete failure in the treatment of chronic pancreatitis. I do, however, acknowledge that this operation may play some part in the treatment of relapsing subacute pancreatitis, particularly in the presence of biliary tract disease. Similarly, operations to divide the splanchnic innervation of the pancreas have been of only transient success in my hands. If a patient with chronic pancreatitis is operated upon at all, my own view is that this must be a direct operation and, in fact, this in practice means that some form of resection must be carried out or some form of duct drainage or possibly some operation combining the two.

My own practice in these cases is to approach the pancreas through a bilateral subcostal incision and to expose the body of the gland widely by entering the lesser sac through the divided gastrocolic omentum. Incision

Rodney Smith, M.S., Senior Surgeon, St. George's Hospital, London, England.

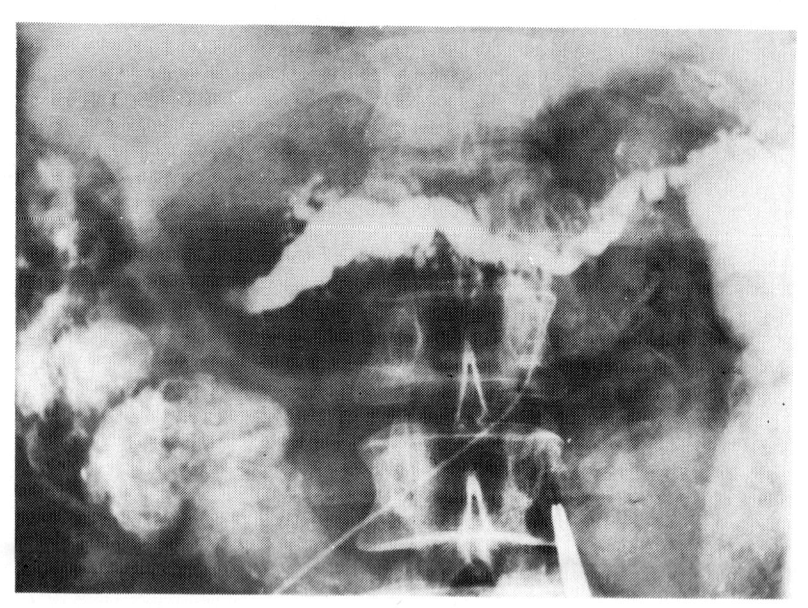

FIG. 1. Descending pancreatogram showing widely dilated pancreatic duct suitable for pancreatojejunostomy.

of the most accessible part of the body of the pancreas allows the duct to be identified and entered and pancreatography used in order to demonstrate the anatomy and pathological changes within the duct system. The type of operation selected depends upon the findings.

Pancreatojejunostomy

If it is found that the whole of the pancreatic duct, from end to end, is very widely dilated and without major strictures (Fig. 1), then anastomosis of this duct to the jejunum will give an excellent result, provided that this junction is made in such a way that the anastomosis will remain patent. In practice this means that there must be very careful apposition of the jejunal epithelium and the pancreatic ductal epithelium. A variety of techniques exist in order to secure this desirable result. My own practice is to employ a series of interrupted silk stitches and to splint the anastomosis with a temporary T-tube running through the lumen of the jejunum to the exterior, removed after 10 to 14 days when a postoperative pancreatogram has shown that there is no leakage and that the pancreatic duct can now empty freely through a broad anastomosis into the jejunum.

The Strictured Pancreatic Duct

If operative pancreatography demonstrates that the duct is dilated only in certain areas and that these areas are separated by multiple strictures (the appearances which Professor Puestow has likened to a "train of lakes"), then the mere anastomosis of a single dilated segment to the jejunum is unlikely to help materially. This is the situation which led Professor Puestow to devise his own "Puestow's operation," in which, after removal of the spleen, the tail of the pancreas is amputated, the duct system is laid open from tail to head and the split open pancreas is encased in a Roux loop of jejunum. Performed with meticulous care, this operation can give good results, though a high percentage of patients develop a recurrence of symptoms after a period of a year to 18 months. It is also an operation which has considerable hazard and many possible postoperative complications and for this reason my own preference in this group of patients is to perform a distal pancreatectomy, the body and tail of the gland being resected and the remaining duct system in the head anastomosed to the jejunum.

Chronic Pancreatic Sclerosis

Often, there is no dilated duct system to be found and the whole of the pancreas is firm and rubbery with a compressed and small duct system within it. Attempted anastomosis of a duct of this kind is technically nearly impossible and in any event is illogical and does not give good results. This type of pancreatitis will probably not be materially affected unless a major resection is carried out and this is a situation in which the so-called "Child" operation of 90% to 95% distal resection may be indicated. In this the whole of the body and tail and gland is removed and in addition a major part of the head, leaving just a small crescentic fragment of the gland in the curve of the duodenum, protecting the common bile duct.

Gross Pancreatitis Mainly Affecting the Head of the Gland

It is sometimes found that the head of the gland is much enlarged, irregular and very hard. Indeed, in circumstances of the kind it may be difficult to be sure whether the pathology is inflammatory or whether a carcinoma is present. Sometimes both may be present together. Not infrequently, obstruction of the common bile duct is also present, another feature suggesting the possibility of malignancy.

This type of chronic pancreatitis may very well require a pancreato-duodenectomy, the technique being precisely the same as that employed for a carcinoma and the operation, in fact, being a good deal more difficult for severe inflammatory disease than for a carcinoma. The results of pancreatoduodenectomy, assuming that the patient survives the operation, can be extremely good and this has led some surgeons to prefer this operation to others. It is my view, however, that although there may well be clear indications to perform this operation if the pathology is indeed mainly in the head of the gland, it is wrong to perform it in circumstances where less hazardous procedures may well give a good result. For instance, if there is a dilated pancreatic duct running throughout the whole length of the pancreas, while it is quite true that a successful pancreatoduodenectomy will give an excellent result, it probably gives a good result not because the head of the pancreas has been resected but because the obstructed pancreatic duct has been joined to the jejunum, and this could be achieved without resection.

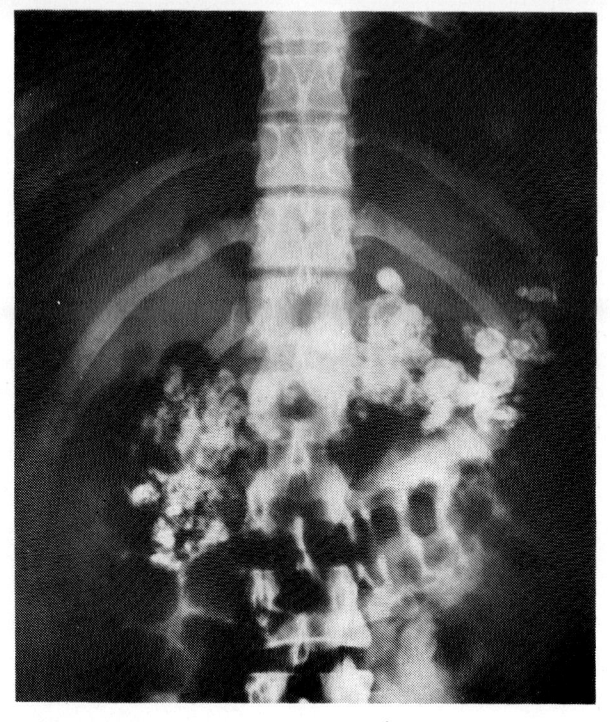

FIG. 2. Gross calcification in a severe case of chronic pancreatitis unlikely to be helped by any procedure short of total pancreatectomy.

Total Pancreatectomy

Total removal of the pancreas may be necessary in very gross cases of chronic pancreatitis (Fig. 2) or in cases of chronic pancreatitis and carcinoma. The indications are, however, infrequent and the metabolic problems that follow are not inconsiderable.

In selecting the operation most suitable in an individual case of chronic pancreatitis, one should rightly consider very carefully the pathology which is present. One should also consider carefully the patient, for while a patient of good moral fiber, not addicted to narcotics and willing to give up alcohol, may with intelligently applied surgery derive considerable benefit, the reverse is true and patients, who have acquired their chronic pancreatitis through alcohol and later become addicted to drugs which they cannot give up, are not likely to be improved by any treatment, medical or surgical.

Bibliography

Puestow, C. B.: Surgery of the Biliary Tract, Pancreas and Spleen. Chicago:Year Book Publishers, 1957.

Smith, R.: Progress in Clinical Surgery. London:J. & A. Churchill Ltd., 1969.

Pancreatic Pseudocysts and Ascites: Diagnosis and Treatment

W. Dean Warren, M.D.

As judged from published reports, there are certain principles for successful treatment of pancreatic pseudocysts that have not been clearly understood.

A canine pseudocyst model was developed in our laboratory. This animal does not have a lesser sac, so we placed an inflated polyethylene bag surrounded by omentum behind the stomach. The bag occupied a significant portion of the abdomen and many of the dogs did not survive the procedure. In those which did, a large cystlike structure composed only of fibrous tissue was formed; it had no mucosal lining and no submucosal or elastic fibers in the wall. Similarly, a human pseudocyst is comprised of fibrotic tissue and the tissues of adjacent organs and is formed in response to an inflammatory reaction. After two or three weeks, when the cyst wall was firmly in position, the pancreatic duct with a button of duodenal wall was implanted into the cystic space. It should be noted that in the dog the common bile duct enters the duodenum through a separate orifice. At the same time, the polyethylene bag was removed, and pure pancreatic juice poured into a cavity composed only of fibrous tissue with no mucosal lining.

One of the first things that we learned, and this is something that should be stressed, is that the fibrous wall cannot be relied upon to hold sutures and maintain water tight integrity. When lateral jejunal to cyst anastomoses were made, many of the dogs died from leakage at the suture line and development of extensive fatty necrosis and peritonitis.

The reason we did this experiment was to examine why patients in whom the stomach is opened directly into a big fibrous cavity in the lesser sac do so well. Theoretically, cyst-gastrostomy should be a horrendous operation.

W. Dean Warren, M.D., Joseph B. Whitehead Professor and Chairman, Department of Surgery, Emory University School of Medicine, Atlanta, Ga.

After opening the posterior stomach into the cyst wall of the dog, there was herniation of the gastric mucosa into the opening, so that a valvelike effect was created. Fluid injected into the cyst lifted the mucosal flaps and drained into the stomach. On the other hand, pressure built up in the gastric lumen further prolapsed the mucosa, and little or no gastric contents entered the cyst through the simple incision in the posterior wall of the stomach. This observation was quantitated by leaving a catheter in the cyst. When the animal drank milk shortly after the operation, none could be recovered from the cyst via the catheter. The obvious explanation was that the opening was sealed by a valvelike mechanism. Radiographic contrast media injected into the cyst flowed freely into the stomach. In other words, gross regurgitation from stomach to cyst was prevented but not the reverse.

Two technical points could obviate the function of the valve: (1) If the incision in the posterior wall of the stomach was 5 cm or longer, there was reflux of milk from the stomach into the cyst cavity. (2) If one excised a segment of the gastric wall, as most people recommend for a transgastric cyst-gastrostomy, there would also be free reflux of gastric contents into the cyst. These observations explain one mechanism by which the transgastric cyst-gastrostomy functions and why the results are quite satisfactory.

In a typical human case, the posterior wall of the stomach is ballooned up and fused with the anterior wall of the cyst. The content of these cysts is not pure pancreatic juice but is a mixture of blood and blood products with some pancreatic juice. In order to create a cyst-gastrostomy, an incision is made in the line of a Rugal fold on the posterior gastric wall. The cyst and gastric wall are firmly adherent. One could not dissect the two layers apart without getting into all sorts of problems and, of course, should not. The integrity of the opening does not depend upon sutures, because the two structures are already fused. The mucosal folds fall directly back against one another and, in fact, it is difficult to see where the incision has been made.

We began to perform this operation in 1956 in patients with pseudocysts of the pancreas and have since continued to do it in the same fashion. In a relatively small series of cases (approximately 20), we have not had major problems. Of course, the number is too small to be of great significance [1]. The principles we consider necessary in order to utilize the stomach for a drainage of a pancreatic pseudocyst are that the cyst be adherent and the incision be made through the posterior wall of the stomach. Some surgeons have recommended the use of an interlocking suture in an effort to prevent postoperative bleeding from the line of incision. Bleeding following a drainage of a pseudocyst by any technique is the most serious and most frequent complication. In the dog model, we found that if interlocking sutures were utilized, reflux from the stomach did occur. On the other hand, we noted that the suture does provide good hemostatis. At present we are uncertain whether such a suture has more advantages or disadvantages. In practice we do not use it but rather ligate each bleeding point individually and obtain careful hemostasis in order to prevent postoperative hemorrhage. Another relatively common problem is bleeding from multiple sites in the cyst wall. A further source of severe hemorrhage, too frequently encountered, is that of erosion of a major vessel in the base of the cyst.

To drain a pseudocyst of the pancreas, we utilize transgastric drainage and employ a small catheter or a small Penrose drain sutured to the end of a gastrostomy tube to prevent healing of the opening before collapse of the cyst is complete. We employ a simple incision, 3 or 4 cm in length, in the direction of the folds and concentrate on careful hemostasis at the cyst-gastrostomy site. We do not use a continuous suture for hemostasis nor do we excise a segment of the common wall to create free drainage. Regarding this last point, theoretical reasons suggest the reflux of gastric juice into the cyst might be disadvantageous from the standpoint of creating erosions and bleeding. I must admit, however, that in the recent series from the University of Illinois [2] a window was excised in 30-odd cases. There were no postoperative hemorrhages reported in any of these patients; so this technical point may be of more theoretical than practical importance.

Another question studied in the laboratory was that of utilizing a simple jejunal loop for drainage of the cyst. We explored this technique only because the Leahy Clinic recommended it. The suture line frequently gave way with leakage of intestinal contents, development of abdominal sepsis and death. We concluded, therefore, that one of the basic principles in the use of jejunum is that it must be defunctionalized. This fact has not been universally appreciated. There have been reports and we have had patients referred in whom a simple loop of jejunum has been sutured to the cyst with subsequent anastomotic breakdown and serious complications. We use a standard 18 inch Roux-Y loop which does prevent reflux of intestinal juices. The anastomosis should be large to avoid early closure. The most dependent, posterior and inferior, site for an anastomosis should be employed. One of the major theoretical advantages of the cyst-jejunostomy is that truly dependent drainage can be established with this procedure. Here also we employ a catheter through the jejunal loop and into the cyst. There have been several instances reported in the clinical literature in which the jejunal loop totally separated from the cyst wall; the only resulting complication was a simple recurrence of the pseudocyst, illustrating the importance of the Roux-Y principle.

Analyzing the literature we concluded that external drainage, which was then advocated by a number of people because it was the "safest" method of treatment, was, in fact, not the safest. Cyst-gastrostomy and the Roux-Y cyst-jejunostomy were just as safe and the reoperation rate was far less than after any other procedure. The reoperation rate for external drainage was so high as to make it an unsuitable operation, except when utilized in the desperately ill patient. The literature indicated further that attempted extirpation failed frequently and also carried a high mortality.

The most recent series by Balfour of the Strode Clinic in Hawaii [3] states essentially the same conclusions: internal drainage has as low a mortality and much lesser morbidity than does external drainage. Attempted excision has a prohibitive mortality. The treatment of choice, in stable pseudocysts, is an internal drainage procedure which does not rely on sutures for maintenance of gastrointestinal integrity. This means that if you operate through the stomach it must be a transgastric cyst-gastrostomy through an area of adherence of the cyst wall and the stomach. If you use a jejunal loop, it should be a defunctionalized Roux-Y loop.

A particularly difficult situation is that of a cyst collection following pancreatitis in the acute phase. One of the problems in this area is the decision whether or not to drain a clinically definable mass in the lesser sac in a patient who is septic. I want to call your attention to the extremely helpful use of ultrasound in identification of fluid filled masses. A typical example from our hospital was a patient with a palpable mass in the lesser sac which was thought to be a pseudocyst. Ultrasound showed this to be a solid mass. The surgeon operated anyway and found no fluid to drain. The operative procedure accomplished nothing and probably was harmful. Ultrasound can help prevent such mistakes.

The term pseudocyst is used only because there is not a better term. Acutely, the condition is not really a pseudocyst but rather a lesser sac accumulation of fluid or a peripancreatic abscess. In a septic patient, immediate external drainage of such an accumulation is followed by prompt resolution of the problem and may be life-saving.

A related clinical condition is that of pancreatic ascites. It is very similar in terms of etiology and pathogenesis to pseudocyst except that the pancreatic leakage is not confined to the lesser sac. By definition, ascites means fluid in the abdominal cavity. One must think of this entity in order to make the diagnosis. Once considered, the diagnosis is established simply by aspiration of the peritoneal fluid for amylase determinations. This problem may follow any pancreatic injury: blunt or penetrating trauma, familial pancreatitis in children, alcoholism or biliary tract disease. There have been a few cases reported with no definable cause. The major problem, of course, is that with ascites in an alcoholic adult, one thinks of cirrhosis. A number of patients have had portacaval shunts mistakenly performed for this form of "intractable ascites."

Ruptured pancreatic pseudocyst is the number one cause of pancreatic ascites. Another major cause is pancreatic duct disruption without a pseudocyst, in other words, a simple hole in the pancreatic duct, due to erosion by a pancreatic calculus or something of that sort. Pancreatitis without a demonstrable major duct injury has also been reported as a precursor of pancreatic ascites.

At the time of surgery, pancreatic ductograms are utilized to identify the site of leakage. External drainage in a desperately ill patient can be helpful. We have done this in one of our patients; he recovered and promptly developed a pseudocyst, which was then drained transgastrically. Partial pancreatectomy and/or Roux-Y drainage of the leaking site is the treatment of choice in the clinical situation of pancreatic ascites. The choice of procedure is dictated by the findings on ductogram of the site of the leak.

Summary

Pancreatic pseudocyst and pancreatic ascites are straightforward complications of pancreatitis or pancreatic injury. Apparently, there still is much confusion regarding the nature and treatment of these conditions. Pseudocysts are not suitable for suture because they are simply fibrous tissue. There are safer and better ways to treat these lesions. The treatment of pseudocysts should be transgastric drainage or Roux-Y cyst-jejunostomy. In the treatment of pancreatic ascites the stomach should not be used. A Roux-Y jejunal loop should be anastomosed either to the ruptured pseudocyst or to the disrupted duct.

References

1. Hutson, D. G., Zeppa, R. and Warren, W. D.: Prevention of postoperative hemorrhage after pancreatic cystogastrostomy. Ann. Surg., 177:689, 1973.
2. Schumer, W., McDonald, G. O., Nichols, R. L. et al: Transgastric cyst-gastrostomy. Surg. Gynec. Obstet., 137:48, 1973.
3. Balfour, J. F.: Pancreatic pseudocysts. Complications and their relation to the timing of treatment. Surg. Clin. N. Amer., 50:395, 1970.

Panel Discussion

Moderator:	**J. S. Najarian, M.D.**	
Panelists:	**R. M. Zollinger, M.D.**	**J. M. Howard, M.D.**
	R. Ulstrom, M.D.	**W. D. Warren, M.D.**
	R. Smith, M.D.	

Dr. Najarian: Dr. Zollinger, does the normal pancreas secrete gastrin?

Dr. Zollinger: Maybe a little. I don't really know. Dan Elliott said that you can extract gastrin from the pancreas in chronic calcific pancreatitis. On about three or four of our cases Dr. Handelbach, of the Mayo Clinic, didn't feel that that was true. But now, I think, when there has been a lot of fibrosis and so forth, gastrin can be extracted from the pancreas.

Dr. Najarian: How often does an insulinoma occur in the Z-E syndrome, Dr. Zollinger?

Dr. Zollinger: I think it is around 2% to 3%. I have seen one family with a series of ulcerogenic tumors and one patient's daughter had an insulinoma. It is very uncommon.

Dr. Najarian: Dr. Zollinger, you show several areas where the tumor could occur. Have you ever seen one or has anyone ever reported one in the stomach?

Dr. Zollinger: Yes, Dr. Scott, of Nashville, found one in the antrum of the stomach. He reported it as being made up of a variety of hormones, including ACTH, and MSH. There have been a couple in the wall of the antrum.

Dr. Najarian: There are some people who still don't do gastrins routinely, and they are wondering about gastric analysis. Dr. Zollinger, has this fallen by the wayside? There used to be a way of diagnosing a Z-E tumor by doing a gastric analysis for 12 hours. Is this still used? First, do you use gastric analysis at all? Second, while you are exploring the pancreas for a Z-E tumor, do you monitor the gastric analysis during the surgical procedure?

Dr. Zollinger: Doing gastric analysis is where you get your first clues, sometimes. But, as you know, if you quiz the young men on the American Board of Surgery, you ask them about gastric analysis and they don't know what it is all about. Even if they do gastric analysis, they don't know what the normal levels are. That is like saying that they do it for plain, clean fun to keep the patient in the hospital overnight. Actually, a volume of over 1000 cc of gastric contents in the unobstructed stomach, or milliequivalents over 100, and so forth, is supposed to be of value. I think that the availability of gastrin today at an economic level makes gastric analysis not nearly so important as it was previously. We used to monitor the gastric juice and cut the vagus and then, especially when we didn't find any tumor, keep hoping that we would see a reduction. When the tumor was enucleated, or when we did a blind resection, it would come down. But we didn't find it too useful. We formerly, too, monitored the gastric output with the same anesthetic preoperative preparation that the anesthesiologist was going to use – atropine, or whatever he was using the day before–so we had some idea of what the baseline would be. We have seen it decrease on occasion. But I think that if I didn't have any gastrin level and I couldn't find a tumor and I had such baselines, I would use it again.

Dr. Najarian: Dr. Warren, there are many reports in the literature of people who excise pieces of the stomach for pancreatic pseudocyst and sew the stomach to the cyst. You have made a great point of not doing it and, yet, others seem to get good results. How do you explain that?

Dr. Warren: One of the reasons is that you have to analyze your results critically. That is where the difficulty comes in, because no one, with few exceptions, has enough cases to make a really meaningful series. There are many people who excise. Let me make this point: We say that you shouldn't excise to prevent reflux. That is theory. But many people excise through an adherent area between the stomach and a cyst. I would wager that Mr. Smith does this, because it is just tradition – if you want to create drainage, create real good, free drainage. We cannot prove that is bad. Some people think it is definitely better. The thing that is bad is to excise a segment of the stomach that is not adherent and then do a suture anastomosis. You can get away with it, most of the time, but it is unphysiological to expect a fibrous sac to maintain a water-tight anastomosis enough of the time to prevent serious complications. As I have said, the results in both the pseudocyst and the pancreatic ascites cases have led to an unacceptably high morbidity and mortality.

Dr. Najarian: Mr. Smith, do you do as Dr. Warren does? Do you just make a slit in the stomach and get out?

Mr. Smith: No, I think that everything that he said about the anastomosis is correct. Apart from one thing which he didn't mention, that you must make a hole big enough not only to let the fluid escape but to put your finger in and see what is inside that cyst. A great many pseudocysts not only have a great deal of fluid, the character of which he showed in his slide presentation, but there is a great deal of solid necrotic debris inside that cyst. It is important to get all of that out. Unless you put your finger in, I think that you can miss it. You shouldn't put anything sharp in it, certainly don't curet that cavity. That is the road to disaster as sure as anything. Use a finger to gently detach the semi-solid necrotic debris. That is important. The other point that I would make about cysts is that many cysts are a legacy from a single attack of acute pancreatitis. By all means, treat these in this way, with internal anastomosis, and I agree that you must not open up a plane where there is no adherence. However, the cyst which is merely a part of the pathology in chronic pancreatitis is different. If you merely treat the cyst, you still have the chronic pancreatitis. You must treat the underlying disease. Another point, you may think that it is difficult to mistake a pseudocyst for a cystic tumor, but it is not, it is very easy to mistake a pseudocyst for cystadenoma. So, if you do extract some semi-solid tissue from a cyst, you ought to send it for frozen section, and you will find that one or two of them are cystadenomas and not a pseudocyst at all.

Dr. Najarian: I am glad you bought up that point, Mr. Smith. Someone asked the question, whether you shouldn't biopsy that cyst because occasionally it is a cystadenoma or even a cystadenocarcinoma.

Dr. Warren: I have never seen a cystadenoma present as a massive 14 or 15 cm cyst. You will recall my slide in which I showed the opening that we have in the posterior wall of the stomach. You can put three or four fingers through, and that way you can look in. If we biopsy the cyst wall, we biopsy it away from the stomach.

Dr. Najarian: But you do biopsy it?

Dr. Warren: If the patient has had obvious pancreatitis and the classic history, we do not biopsy. With regard to that ex resident of Emory University Hospital, who went to Philadelphia – I would like to say that had she stayed in Atlanta, we, at least, would have known what we were dealing with.

Dr. Zollinger: Panel members, how long do you wait before you explore these cysts? I get the impression that if they find the cyst they take it out immediately. I alluded to the timing of drainage very briefly because of time. I am doing this simply so you can put it in your book. But I shall change it tomorrow, that is the hell of it, you know.

Dr. Warren: This is a matter of semantics. I know that Dr. Howard gets upset about it, and rightly so. If you are talking about the immediate postpancreatitis acute collection of fluid, we really shouldn't call that a pseudocyst, rather, it is a peripancreatic collection of fluid, which may or may not be infected. If we demonstrate this by using ultrasound, and if it is cystic, and the patient is becoming asymptomatic and afebrile, we then wait and watch. If after four to six weeks there is still significant fluid collection, we probably would institute drainage. If, however, the patient is septic and not doing well, and has a demonstrable collection of fluid, then external drainage is the only safe thing to do. As has been pointed out by many people, one of the most lethal of all complications is a true peripancreatic abscess.

Mr. Smith: I largely agree with this. If the patient with a pseudocyst is asymptomatic, you are certainly justified in watching to see what happens. Very often, the cyst will get smaller and smaller and, finally, you cannot feel it at all. I have one patient in London, where the cyst got progressively smaller but, finally, it reached a stationary size. Because she was not inconvenienced by it, and she didn't want an operation, I did not press one on her. Over the years, the cyst became calcified and looked for all the world like a hydatid cyst with a rim of calcium around it. She certainly wouldn't part with this now, and for a variety of reasons: one of which is that every time that there is an examination for the final F.R.C.S. (Fellow Royal College of Surgeons) diploma in London, she trots up to the examination hall and collects a fee for presenting her symptoms to the assembled group.

Dr. Najarian: Dr. Howard, when do you decide to operate on a cyst?

Dr. Howard: I am not sure. I would like to reemphasize what Dr. Warren has said; if a patient comes in with an acute attack and develops a mass, this patient has either edematous pancreatitis or a rupture with a collection of pancreatic juice. If we call that a pseudocyst, and go ahead and drain it *internally*, we are going to have fatalities. It is going to be an anastomosis of *fibrinous* tissue to the intestine. That represents a collection of pancreatic juice; it is not a *fibrous*, lined cyst which by definition is a pseudocyst. Until one year or so ago, I said, "Wait for three or four months and if it is still there and hasn't resolved, go in and drain it internally." I had one patient with a persistently high amylase, but who was well, at home, within the three month period. He was completely asymptomatic, eating and doing well when he developed a thrombosis of his superior mesenteric vein and died. I have always felt that this patient was salvageable. I shall hedge and say that we would not operate on him early unless he was septic. If we did, we would drain him externally. We would try to wait three or four months. And yet, I have some reservations.

Dr. Najarian: Dr. Warren, suppose you have a big cyst in the head of the pancreas, what do you do? You can't get that in the stomach. Do you do a Roux-Y jejunostomy?

Dr. Warren: You can take the Roux-Y anywhere. That is why it should be the standard form of therapy. And, then, if you are lucky enough to have one retrogastric, densely adherent, you can use that with just as good results. When in doubt, make a Roux-Y loop.

Dr. Zollinger: Why would you do a Roux-en-Y? This is a big operation! You said the duodenum was no good to hook to it?

Dr. Warren: The duodenum is accompanied by many high complications in cyst-duodenostomies. We don't know why this is. But that has simply been an observation in our experience.

Dr. Zollinger: In your patients or the ones on whom you operated?

Dr. Warren: This has been the worldwide experience. I analyzed them.

Dr. Zollinger: Three cases!

Dr. Najarian: Is there a problem at Emory University Hospital about sutures, is there some reason why you don't like to use a suture?

Dr. Warren: This is what Dr. Zollinger has been telling me, that if I just knew how to put stitches in, this wouldn't happen!

Dr. Najarian: Has anyone on the panel followed these patients long enough to see that the cyst completely obliterates?

Dr. Warren: Yes, there is a good study which we did in the laboratory and they obliterate in a remarkably short period of time, within ten days. The cyst which was originally the size of a softball is down to the size of an egg or even smaller.

Dr. Howard: Did you start with a fibrous lined wall, or did you start with an acute process?

Dr. Warren: I started with a fibrous lined wall. You saw those big fibrous linings in my slide presentation. They were ¼ inch thick. But they heal by contraction and obliteration. It is not side-to-side granulation. We also did this recently in a patient at Emory University Hospital. We left the catheter in the cyst and drained it internally. I used the catheter to measure the decreasing size of the cyst. In ten days, it was all but obliterated. I think that this is the reason why cystogastrostomy patients do so remarkably well.

Dr. Najarian: Dr. Zollinger, do you have some clues about cysts?

Dr. Zollinger: I would like to ask Dr. Warren how he made these cysts. I would like to know what kind of rubberized material he used.

Dr. Warren: In the laboratory we used reactive polyethylene, which was used as a spray with the cleaning solution. It was very inflammatory and a lot of the dogs died. The dogs that survived had big fibrous cysts. Anastomosed, they would be full of active pancreatic juice, the only thing anywhere near to a true experimental model for pseudocysts which exists.

Dr. Najarian: Where did you publish your data?

Dr. Warren: It was published in *Surgery, Gynecology and Obstetrics, Annals of Surgery* and was presented at the Southern Surgical Association. It has not received the credit which is its due. It is a remarkable paper.

Dr. Najarian: How often does one see jaundice with pancreatitis that is not related to common duct stone or biliary pathology?

Mr. Smith: I think that the connection between biliary troubles and chronic pancreatitis has often been put the wrong way around. If you find that there are common duct stones, and if the patient has chronic pancreatitis, it is tacitly assumed that the stones and the biliary tract disease has caused the pancreatitis, whereas, it can be the other way around. Severe, chronic pancreatitis can often produce that rat-tailed deformity which was shown in one of Dr. Howard's x-rays in his slide presentation. The rat-tailed deformity was at the lower end, with a big, dilated choledochus above it. If you have a sufficient degree of stasis, jaundice and stones will develop as a secondary phenomenon, but I don't think that this happens too frequently. If this is the case, you may, in addition to treating the pancreatitis, have to add some form of lateral anastomosis to decompress the obstructed biliary apparatus. Even if you successfully treat the pancreatitis, it does not follow that all of that pathology is going to mysteriously and miraculously disappear. You often still have a chronic obstruction of the biliary apparatus. I don't think that it is rare to have jaundice and biliary tract troubles. You quite often have to do a secondary correction of this, as well as treating the pancreatitis.

Dr. Najarian: Dr. Warren, when you have a patient with acute pancreatitis, when do you operate on the biliary tree if you know that there is biliary pathology?

Dr. Warren: We do not operate on acute pancreatitis patients as a planned approach, unless complications ensue which demand it. In other words, we don't do the Massachusetts General Hospital type of approach of operating deliberately for biliary tract disease during the acute pancreatitis. I don't know whether they are right or not. We are watching the work being done in Massachusetts with interest. We would try to get the acute pancreatitis to subside and frequently even keep the patient in the hospital and operate seven to ten days later. In fact, some years ago Dr. Zollinger's group showed that that was a safe thing to do.

Dr. Najarian: Dr. Zollinger, do you agree or have you changed your approach?

Dr. Zollinger: No, I would agree with that. I would wait for one week to ten days.

Mr. Smith: I feel that prophylactic drainage of a normal common duct in acute pancreatitis is totally irrational and certainly should not be done.

On the other hand, there is a small group of patients who have histories suggestive of common duct stones, already, in that they have had recurring episodes of cholangitis and jaundice. If one of these gets acute pancreatitis, one should operate and explore the common duct. You will quite often find not only stones in the common duct, but also an impacted stone at the lower end, that it is important to get out.

Dr. Najarian: Dr. Zollinger, our French colleagues, whom you recently visited, operate on acute pancreatitis quite readily. Do they go in, find acute pancreatitis and immediately put a tube in the gallbladder or the stomach? Do you think that approach is of any rational use?

Dr. Zollinger: I think that it depends upon how bad the pancreatitis is and how many tubes you have available. I haven't done this often. I have always assumed that when you put tubes everywhere, in the lesser sac, in the gallbladder, in the jejunum, as the Massachusetts General Hospital description some time back, it meant that the patient had a fulminating type of hemorrhagic pancreatitis. It would have to be a life-and-death matter before I would get around to that sort of thing.

Mr. Smith: My old chief at St. George's Hospital in London, Gordon Taylor, used to say, if you open the abdomen because you have to, it is an acute abdomen, and if you haven't made a diagnosis, and if you find that it is, in fact, a case of acute pancreatitis, the best thing to do is close that abdomen and send the patient back to the ward, with a little note pinned to his pajamas, which says, "Opened in error. Return to sender."

Dr. Najarian: Dr. Howard, would you agree? How about draining these various regions if you were in there, and you didn't want to be?

Dr. Howard: We accomplish very little by operating during the early stage of acute pancreatitis. I would like to make one point – don't forget that a certain number of gallstones and a certain number of common duct stones are radiopaque. Look for them. You won't find many, but when you do you feel mighty smart.

Dr. Najarian: Dr. Howard, do you know of any drug-induced pancreatitis?

Dr. Howard: Certainly, cortisone-induced pancreatitis is found in the literature, also one of the diuretics has been associated with pancreatitis. I am not doing full justice to your question. There are several drugs that at least have been claimed to produce pancreatitis.

Dr. Najarian: Of course, the steroids are well known. Does any member of the panel have any idea about how to treat steroid-induced pancreatitis, besides stopping the steroids? Interestingly enough, we see it more frequently than we like in our transplant patients. By trying to reduce our steroids as rapidly as possible, most of these patients will lose their insulin-dependent diabetes. Thereafter, some of them can be controlled with either diet or tolbutamide. I would like to go now to insulinomas and hypoglycemia in children. Dr. Ulstrom, you showed around 100 cases, and you had only two cases of insulinoma. All of a sudden, now, you show us four or five cases that were operated upon, all less than 1 year old. Is your technique for pick-ups getting better? Or were these patients whom you missed previously? What this sudden increase?

Dr. Ulstrom: It is hard to say what the real reason is. This is not just a local phenomenon. I pointed out in my slide presentation that, since 1969, cases have appeared in the literature in increasing numbers from all over the United States. The size of these tumors and their location, frequently toward the head, make one think that they could have been missed in the past. But, unless we are dealing with a different type of adenoma that eventually obliterates itself, I doubt that we are missing them. There is a recent report of a 4-year-old child from Philadelphia, who was still having difficulty, even though the symptoms had gone back to the first year of life. So I doubt that these things disappear. In the other types of hyperinsulinism where we have declared them without adenoma, when 85% of the pancreas has been removed they get well, but are not cured. Their hyperinsulinism is gone by the time they are about 5 or 6 years old. They require no further treatment, and they don't become diabetic, but their whole pancreas is not working. At the moment I can only speculate that the spectrum of disease is changing. We don't really know whether it is drug-induced during pregnancy by some new drug or some other factor.

Dr. Howard: Dr. Ulstrom, are the early stages of diabetes represented by a functional hypoglycemia? We recently resected the tail of the pancreas in a female nurse, age 25 years. She had high blood insulin levels, but the blood sugars were never lower than 45, the blood insulin levels were never quite as high as we wanted them to be and an arteriogram was negative. We resected the tail of the pancreas and she was relieved. We found no tumor. Have we operated in the early stages of diabetes? Will she go on to diabetes mellitus? Have we made her worse?

Dr. Ulstrom: It can happen. It is less common in young children, but more common in the age group to which you refer. The young (30-40 years), adult obese male is the most likely person, statistically, to have clinical hypoglycemia preceding the onset of diabetes. We included two children in our slide presentation and I showed two slides of our own patients, who had preceding hypoglycemia. So it does happen. Among children who have hypoglycemia, subsequent diabetes mellitus represents less than 2%.

Dr. Zollinger: I had heard that many of the tests which one carries out on adults for insulinoma are not valid in children, including the insulin immunoassay.

Dr. Ulstrom: I don't think that the radioimmunoassay, itself, is of any less value.

Dr. Najarian: Dr. Ulstrom, when you can treat these patients with diazoxide therapy, or streptozotocin, or whatever, when do you decide to operate upon them? After you have made the diagnosis of insulinoma, should you go right in after you have them prepared, or should you treat them conservatively with agents that will control the hyperinsulin state?

Dr. Ulstrom: The case that I mentioned previously, which is 4 years old, is the only one about which I know anything. One month ago, at a meeting of pediatricians in Washington, this subject was discussed and this was the only case in childhood, where managment was at all effective in an adenoma with medical management, including diazoxide. So, for the most part, it isn't a real problem. The insulinoma patient reveals himself by being difficult to manage. If we have any inkling that there might be an adenoma, I think that exploration is warranted. However, if we are talking about an infant, under 6 months of age, excision biopsy of 75% to 80% of the pancreas is the procedure of choice. The reason being that these tumors are so small (1-2mm) that few of them are going to be seen, even at the time of removal. The pathologist finds them.

Dr. Najarian: Mr. Smith, you gave one of the nicest presentations I have ever heard on explaining the logic and therapy for treatment of chronic pancreatitis. The nicest part of it was that it wasn't cluttered with any data or results. What are your results with these various operations? How many of these people who get either resections or drainage, or whatever, get better?

Mr. Smith: The omission was entirely intentional. I try to avoid, whenever possible, doing a total pancreatectomy. I have somewhere between six and ten patients where I have done total pancreatectomies for chronic pancreatitis, nothing like the series that Dr. Thomas White has had. We had two deaths following the operation which is not good in this small series. They have been looked after very carefully by the medical unit at St. George's Hospital, with Professor Dornhorst. We are really rather depressed by the results. I think that most of their pain has been improved, but some pain is usually present in this group. They have not been quite so easy a metabolic problem as is being suggested. Perhaps we are not looking after them awfully well. Maybe we should ask Dr. Thomas

White about this. I am always surprised if the patients with a dilated pancreatic duct anastomosed to a loop of jejunum, if it is a great big duct, are not relieved of their symptoms. If we exclude that group, however, and work on the patients with dilated segments of duct, many of which are full of little stones, or the group with the pancreatic sclerosis who require a 95% resection, nearly up to the duodenum, you will improve better than one half of the patients. The rest of these patients are either not sufficiently improved to be glad that they have had the operation, or perhaps a little better than that but not much more. I regard this as a depressing disease. Perhaps it is because in so many of these patients the pathology is based on alcohol and the fundamental problem looms in the background, which you are never going to improve.

Dr. Najarian: Your most important indication was pain.

Mr. Smith: Yes, that is correct.

Dr. Najarian: We are equally discouraged with the variety of procedures as you are; I am sure that every member of the panel feels this way. It is a terrible disease to treat. But there have been some patients who respond to celiac block and, eventually, alcohol injection. Do you try that, at least initially, in the patient who is otherwise reasonably well, but his pain is his primary symptom?

Mr. Smith: No, we haven't. We had a relatively short series, about ten years ago, when we got a bit enthusiastic about celiac blocks. Perhaps we weren't good at it, but we didn't get good results. We got quite good results with splanchnic nerve section, but as I have already suggested, it was so temporary.

Dr. Najarian: Dr. Zollinger, would you ever do just a proximal gastric resection of parietal cell mass, if you had a negative exploration, rather than a full, total gastric resection?

Dr. Zollinger: It would depend upon the gastrin level. If the gastrin level was high and the calcium infusion was positive, I wouldn't do that. It would have to be relatively normal levels.

Dr. Najarian: Do you believe that you need a serial gastrin or is a single gastrin enough for you to make a diagnosis, if it is elevated?

Dr. Zollinger: I think that we generally get two or three. If somebody is going to take out all of my stomach or tell me that they were going to, I would want about 5,000 serial readings.

Dr. Najarian: One last question, Dr. Zollinger. If you had a negative laparotomy, would you do just a distal pancreatectomy?

Dr. Zollinger: No, I would not. Again, I would depend upon the gastrin levels. I used to do a blind resection, but I had collections and problems. I cut out that foolishness and I now go a lot by the gastrin levels. If the gastrin levels were high, I would take out the stomach; if they were borderline, I would do a vagotomy and hemigastrectomy with a part of the duodenum, to look for a little tumor that might be in the duodenum that I couldn't feel.

Dr. Najarian: Thank you, Dr. Zollinger.

Dr. Warren: We have a series of about 20 patients who had a 95% pancreatectomy for chronic pancreatitis. We have been impressed with our ability to control pain in the patient who is not actually addicted. As Mr. Smith said, when a patient is both a chronic alcoholic and a chronic drug addict, you are just fooling yourself to believe that you are going to accomplish something. But we have been very pleased with pain relief in our series. However, we already have had three late deaths from hypoglycemia induced by an overinjection of insulin. These patients had resumed drinking and were apparently giving themselves insulin while they were under the influence of alcohol. For that reason, I have become less enthusiastic about it than I was initially. Of the nonalcoholic patient, however, of which there are a few, it is still a very good operation.

Mr. Smith: Dr. Warren, would you tell us what percentage of these patients are in fact nonalcoholic?

Dr. Warren: We had about 25% of this group.

Mr. Smith: That means that you had 75% who were alcoholic. What sort of results do you get in them?

Dr. Warren: We get good pain relief in those we can get off of drugs in the hospital. It is amazing. We found that the patient in the hospital required far more medication than when outside. Just lying in the hospital, you have a tendency for drug ingestion as a habit because you can get it easily. Of those who did not require more drugs, we had excellent pain relief. They all have some residual symptoms, a cramping pain, or an ache, but each patient gained around 25 lb in body weight following this procedure. The gain was not caused by a change in digestion or absorption, it was due simply to the ability to eat while free from pain. We documented it on our metabolic unit. I think that a 95% pancreatectomy is a good operation for control of pain. If anything is going to help, that will, but, metabolically, it is just too risky in certain people.

Mr. Smith: I think that we are saying the same thing in rather a different way. In my practice, it is merely the patients who go out, stay off alcohol and off drugs who remain largely asymptomatic. It is a small percentage, around 50%, which is not high. Far too many of them are happy when they leave the hospital and during their first postoperative visit but, as the months go by, they go back on alcohol. The number who come back with renewed symptoms is to my mind depressingly large.

Dr. Warren: I agree.

Dr. Howard: I have become less and less impressed with the number of true narcotic addicts who have chronic pancreatitis. Obviously, there are such patients, and they are basically seen in the charity hospitals. We tell all the patients with chronic pancreatitis: "You have to stop all narcotics during your diagnostic phase. None, whatsoever. If you call us at home, you are not going to get any. You can go home, if you want to. But we are not going to give them to you. It interferes with gastric analysis, it interferes with gastric drainage, it interferes with stool collection, it interferes with assessment of pain, glucose tolerances, etc." Almost without exception, these patients will stop. They will pull a few fast ones the first day or so until they know that you really mean business. Postoperatively, some of the patients within the hour or two after operation will say, "Doctor, that pain is gone! That pancreatic pain is gone!" If they have advanced disease, narcotics per se is usually not as big a problem as I had thought. Alcohol, however, is a major problem.

Dr. Najarian: Mr. Smith, if you remove a piece of the pancreas and make an anastomosis, do you or do you not drain the bed of the pancreas?

Mr. Smith: Yes, I drain the pancreatic bed. I would use a very small vacuum drain and take it out as soon as there was nothing coming out of it.

Dr. Najarian: Do the other members of the panel drain after pancreatic resections?

Dr. Howard: I always drain after pancreatic resection, but I would leave it in longer than that. I want the patient to be afebrile. I want him to be eating and having gastrointestinal function, because I am afraid of a secondary leak.

Dr. Najarian: Dr. Howard, do you use a soft drain or a hard drain?

Dr. Howard: I have used soft, but I would be glad to accept the vacuum drain. I use several large, soft Penrose drains. When the residents tell me that I am increasing morbidity, I agree, but tell them that there is less threat to life.

Dr. Warren: Yes, we drain, largely because of the experience of others – we have never studied it. We use some suction or vacuum drains.

Dr. Najarian: Mr. Smith, do you use the same kind of t-tube in the pancreas that we put in the common bile duct?

Mr. Smith: Yes, it is a latex rubber t-tube. We leave it in until a later pancreatogram shows that the anastomosis is watertight, nothing is leaking. If we have a well, asymptomatic patient who is eating well, we pull the tube out. In practice, this takes about 12 or 14 days.

Dr. Najarian: Panel members, are pancreatic scans of any good whatsoever?

Dr. Warren: You have to go by your own experience and your own institution. We have done a fairly large number of 95% pancreatectomies, with scans on all of them. I think 14 of them were read as normal, 2 were read as mildly abnormal, and in only 3 did they suspect any pancreatic insufficiency. This is with no pancreas except that small rim. I haven't the courage to publish that but that is actually factual.

Mr. Smith: I don't feel as depressed about scans as that. If the scan is normal, we would reckon that we could usually rely on that as being a normal pancreas. On the other hand, if the report comes back, saying, "This is an abnormal pancreatic scan," it could mean almost anything. It could mean a carcinoma, a chronic pancreatitis, or a normal pancreas. We place a good deal of reliance on a normal scan, but hardly any reliance on an abnormal pancreatic scan.

Dr. Howard: We have quit using pancreas scans.

Dr. Warren: Something that is going to be extremely useful is the magnification radiology of the angiography of the pancreas. It is used now in Philadelphia and Boston. It is going to be a real diagnostic adjunct when you get it in your hospital. It can detect cysts and tumors that are only a couple of centimeters in size, far better than standard angiography. It is a new dimension altogether.

Dr. Zollinger: What is an ultrascan, or an ultrasound scan, and how does it work?

Dr. Warren: Well, it functions because the ultrasound waves travel through different tissues at different velocities and are reflected by fluids and solids. When you integrate those on a digital computer, it comes out with a picture. It is going to be a useful adjunct. Again, there is a certain amount of artistry in the utilization of these scans. In contrast to pancreatic scans, the ultrasound scans have been increasingly accurate as we have acquired more experience with it.

Dr. Najarian: It is a very useful tool in diagnostic radiology. We have several of them at the University of Minnesota that we have used for aneurysms, pseudocysts, for a variety of things.

Mr. Smith: I have had no experience with them but, quite obviously, it is of use in a great number of fields and I suppose that in obstetrics and gynecology it has proved of enormous value in a number of units.

Dr. Warren: Mr. Smith, may I ask you a very important question. When you do a Puestow or a so-called Puestow, do you or do you not suture it to the cut surface of the pancreas, to allow those secondarily divided radicals to drain, or do you attempt to get a mucosal-to-mucosal anastomosis, such as you showed in your slide presentation?

Mr. Smith: I don't ever do a Puestow operation. It is a Puestow type, in that it is an attempt to drain the main pancreatic duct into the jejunum. It is much more akin to the operation described by Dr. Thomas White, although the length is not quite as big. But the intent is the opposite of the Puestow. In the Puestow operation, he sutures the jejunum so that it largely encompasses the pancreas or, at least, the slit in the pancreas. My intent is to get an accurate mucosa-to-mucosa junction of the pancreatic epithelium and the jejunal epithelium.

Dr. Warren: Mr. Smith, I asked that question because I had two of Puestow's patients in this 95% pancreatectomy group and both of them had sealed completely. There was no communication between the pancreatic ductal system and the jejunal loop.

Mr. Smith: I think that the pancreas is often much too big to put itself inside the jejunum. But the reverse, to get the mucosa of the jejunum into the duct system, if you are doing it on the right case, with a big duct, that is not difficult. But you do have to cut a panel of thickened pancreatic tissue out of the front of the pancreas. Cut right through from the surface down to the duct which is guttered in the bottom of it. This provides the biopsy fragment. If you open the duct in that way, then it is not difficult at all to lay the epithelium in the base, with the intent of getting epithelium-to-epithelium junction. I may be a bore about this, but wherever you are trying to get two hollow systems to join together and to stay open permanently, this is something which you just have to have: epithelium-to-epithelium, otherwise you have a fistula which is lined by fibrous tissue or granulation tissue, and that will always close.

Dr. Najarian: It looks like that is an excellent method of handling a difficult problem. That was most impressive, as is your mucosal patch-up in the liver. Both of those are new, good additions to the surgical armamentarium, to make an operation simpler and perhaps a lot more anatomical.

Panel members, would you operate on a patient with nonalcoholic pancreatitis that occurs approximately two or three times a year and lasts for one to three days?

Mr. Smith: I don't know. You really have to see and talk to the patient before you can decide. You must decide whether you are dealing with a patient who has recurring attacks of either acute or subacute pancreatitis, or whether the patient has chronic pancreatitis with exacerbations. It is tacitly assumed that these two are the same things, but they are not; they are entirely different.

Dr. Warren: I agree with Mr. Smith. I have a patient like this with familial pancreatitis. There are two siblings in the family who both have recurrent bouts. The more bouts of pancreatitis, the less danger there is of nephrotizing hemorrhagic pancreatitis. If the patient begins to go into the chronic pancreatitis, as Mr. Smith has said, then you can undertake the appropriate therapy. These patients will get far better results than the patients with alcoholic pancreatitis.

Dr. Najarian: There are several questions from the audience that were addressed to me. One is: Has anyone ever transplanted an insulinoma? Yes, it has been done once, with marginal success. It is a good idea because it is obviously rich in beta cells.

The next question is: If the reason that diabetics get their nephropathies and vascular disease is from the use of insulin, why are you going to put in some islets and continue to give them insulin? Why is that going to make them better just by correcting their carbohydrate imbalance? Well, there is no such thing as a diabetic who stays on a normal keel. He goes through periods of hyperglycemia and hypoglycemia. It is pretty well accepted by diabetologists that the carefully controlled diabetic who really takes good care of himself by checking his urines frequently and using regular insulin frequently, when he needs it, has less complications. Many of you may know diabetics that stay at the baseline level. I know one physician approaching his late 50s, who is extremely famous, known to everyone in this room. He has had diabetes for 35 years; he has perfect eyesight, and he is doing perfectly well, but he manages his diabetes perfectly. There is no question but that, once you get out of that swing of carbohydrate imbalance you would be improved.

Another question is: What is the best site for transplantation of islets in animals? We think that the best site is probably in the intraperitoneal cavity. There are others who feel the portal vein is better. This question still needs to be answered in the laboratory, and we hope to have an answer in the not-too-distant future.

IV

Liver

Jaundice: Compelling Clinical Signs and Some Differential Laboratory Aids

C. J. Watson, M.D.

Jaundice is a pragmatic, always intriguing manifestation, one which demands early explanation. This may be defeated because of a too great reliance on laboratory tests, without sufficient primary attention to bedside phenomena, some of which, if sought and found, are compelling in diagnosis. I note that less and less attention is being given to this in teaching and practice, more and more to laboratory and x-ray. If in striving to deal with this inequity you find that I am telling you little that is new, please bear with me in my attempt to sort out relative values. I will omit discussion of the history, although as you know, it alone is often decisive in reaching an early diagnosis. As Louie Hamman used to say: "Let me take the history and I'll accept the physical examination of any intern."

Let me consider briefly some familiar, too oft neglected, but very compelling clinical signs (Fig. 1). First, and highly significant, the distended, smooth, nontender gallbladder. I shall speak of this as the "Courvoisier" gallbladder, although Courvoisier [1] did not describe a clinical sign or promulgate a law. He was a pathologist who gathered statistics at autopsy in patients having carcinomatous as contrasted with calculous biliary obstruction, noting the distended, thin walled gallbladder with the former, the thickened, often contracted gallbladder with the latter. I find that the Courvoisier gallbladder in jaundiced patients is often overlooked. For one thing, it may not be palpable when the patient is first examined in the outpatient, or shortly after admission to the hospital, probably because of apprehension and tenseness. With a more relaxed abdomen it may easily be felt and at times seen as a rounded eminence moving down with inspiration. Indeed, on occasion, it may be seen but not felt due to tensing of the recti on attempted palpation. It is thus of some

C. J. Watson, M.D., Regent's Professor of Medicine, Emeritus, and Senior Consultant, University of Minnesota Medical Unit, Northwestern Hospital, Minneapolis.

Jaundice: Compelling differential clinical signs

Obstructive (mechanical)	vs.	Parenchymal (hepatocellular)
The distended palp. GB		Foetor hepaticus
Supf. metastases		(porto-systemic shunt)
Neck - Virchow		Hepatic encephalopathy
Rectal shelf		Absence of liver enlargement
Umbilicus		Marked splenomegaly
Hepatic metastases		Outspoken estrogenic signs
Hepatic friction rub		
Hepatic tenderness		

not differential

Smooth hepatomegaly
Ascites
Biliverdin jaundice
Pruritus; xanthomata

FIG. 1. Jaundice – compelling clinical signs.

importance for the examiner, preferably seated at the bedside, to commence the palpation very gently in the left lower quadrant, with the patient's knees partly flexed, watching the right upper quadrant during inspiration, in preliminary fashion. On rare occasion, the Courvoisier gallbladder may be so large, even of grapefruit size, as to defy belief that the mass is indeed just a distended gallbladder due to carcinomatous biliary obstruction. The Courvoisier gallbladder is not invariably associated with complete biliary obstruction, though this is usual. I have encountered it rarely with incomplete obstructive jaundice due to carcinoma of the ampulla, or to chronic fibrous pancreatitis.

Little need be said about the tell-tale metastases, of such decisive significance when detected in cases of jaundice. The sole problem here is to remember to make a careful search for them on the first examination. I don't know how many times I have seen patients whose doctor has obviously neglected the old advice about "one finger in the neck and one in the rectum." The classical Virchow node must be very carefully sought and at times other cervical or even axillary nodes may be involved by retrograde lymph flow. To defend the rectal examination is scarcely necessary, but all too often when I ask house staff or students as to the rectal, the reply is that it was deferred, and when deferred, often forgotten. I don't have to tell you how serious an omission this can be. Careful palpation of the umbilicus, especially in patients with ascites, at times reveals small metastatic nodules. Also, nodules should be sought in the skin generally.

Even when hepatic metastases cannot be defined, the presence of "prodding" tenderness over the enlarged liver points to the need of listening carefully for an hepatic friction rub, in itself almost pathognomonic of tumor [2]. Alcoholic, hyaline sclerosing, hepatitis often causes marked hepatic tenderness, as well as pain, which may closely simulate cholecystitis, but I have not encountered friction rubs with either.

At the right of Figure 1 I have listed some of the more compelling signs of diffuse, especially chronic liver disease causing jaundice, but all of these may be noted with acute and subacute as well as chronic hepatitis, especially when liver atrophy follows extensive necrosis. I will presently return to this group.

At the bottom are a few important signs, not of themselves compelling in diagnosis. A smooth nontender hepatomegaly in a jaundiced patient may relate to one of many causes, especially chronic biliary obstruction, alcoholic fatty liver or cholangiolitic hepatitis-cirrhosis, to mention but a few. Ascites in itself is not of differential significance, unless accompanied by other compelling signs. Rapidly accumulating, bloody ascites is very likely due to tumor. Biliverdin or green jaundice [3, 4] in our experience has been encountered much more often with carcinomatous biliary obstruction, but it may rarely be seen with advanced cirrhosis, especially that of posthepatitic type. Pruritus is a nondifferential sign, but when accompanied by multiple xanthomata, it is most likely due to cholangiolitic or primary biliary cirrhosis, though a small overlap with biliary obstruction, stone or cancer must be recognized. A palpable spleen also belongs in the category of parenchymal jaundice, being fairly compelling in that direction.

The *foetor hepaticus* has been recognized for many years as a sign of diffuse and usually severe liver disease, not necessarily associated with jaundice (Fig. 2). If I am not mistaken, Sheila Sherlock first emphasized the relationships to bacterial activity in the colon and to portosystemic shunting. Recent gas chromatographic studies by Chen and Zieve in our Veterans Hospital have established that CH_3 mercaptan as earlier indicated by Challenger and Walshe [5] and dimethylsulphide are principal among the substances responsible for the foetor [6]. Unfortunately, in analogy with acetone, there are individual variations in perception and some individuals, like old bird dogs, lose their ability to detect it, as part of the ageing process. For those fortunate enough to have and retain this ability, the foetor is a valuable and compelling sign of diffuse liver disease, usually cirrhosis or diffuse necrosis, noted only rarely with extensive tumor. It often follows gastrointestinal bleeding and is commonly associated with hepatic encephalopathy and hyperammonemia. As a ıule, one is quickly

Foetor Hepaticus

Chemical basis: CH_3 mercaptans;
dimethyl sulphide
(Chen and Zieve)

Source: Bact. decomp. protein
in colon
Portal systemic shunting

FIG. 2. Foetor hepaticus.

made aware of this state by the early, characteristic disorientation often only slight at the outset, soon associated with asterixis, the "liver flap" or flapping tremor. Upper motor neurone signs such as clonus, rigidity, Babinski or Hoffman may soon appear. All of these signs disappear in stage IV (deep) coma.

Palmar erythema of outspoken degree, in a jaundiced patient, is generally pathognomonic of diffuse liver disease of chronic type, especially alcoholic cirrhosis. It is commonly associated with spider angiomata and gynecomastia, a triad of estrogenic signs, in the male, together with testicular atrophy. In the female the nevi and palmar erythema may occur in normal pregnancy and persist for years thereafter.

Let me now consider the jaundice itself and present a simple division of types which is quite helpful by way of preliminary sorting out (Fig. 3). In our experience, this has long involved use of a kinetic method based

Jaundice: A Chemical-Clinical Classification

Hyperbilirubinemia

Conjugated	Intermediate	Unconjugated
BR* > 40% (45-70) "Regurgita'ion" j. (A. Rich) Biliary obst. Cancer, stone, stricture Intrahepatic cholestasis Cholangiolitic disease (Cholangiolitic hepatitis cirrhosis - PBC) Acute or subacute hepatitis Diffuse hepatic necrosis Chemical toxicity Thorazine CH_3 testosterone D. J. & Rotor syndromes	15-40% (20-35 Liver disease with increased bilirubin production: Cirrhosis with "hypersplenism" Inc. Kupffer cell activity Hemolytic disease with liver injury: ex., malaria, also hepatitis with hemol. anemia (G_6PD defic.)	< 20% (5-15) "Retention" j. (A. Rich) Inc. bilirubin production: Cong. RBC or Hb abn. Kern icterus CN disease Acq. hemol. anemia

*BR (serum bilirubin ratio) = $\frac{1'PD}{Total} \times 100$

FIG. 3. Hyperbilirubinemia, chem.-clin. classification.

primarily on Van den Bergh's initial distinction of prompt direct and indirect reacting types [7]. This was described with Ducci [8] in our laboratory many years ago and more recently analyzed in some detail with Perelli [9]. In essence it determines the prompt direct (PD) or 1′ diazo reacting serum bilirubin and the total (T), the former representing conjugated and the difference, the unconjugated bilirubin. This is expressed simply as the bilirubin ratio (BR) = 1′PD/T × 100 [10, 11]. Parenthetically, the automated 12 channel battery of laboratory tests includes only the total bilirubin, not the 1′PD, hence this determination must be requested separately. Three main groups of jaundice are separated on this basis: (1) Conjugated or "regurgitation" jaundice, in accordance with the classification of Arnold Rich [12], which as you see does not differentiate between mechanical obstruction and intrahepatic "cholestasis" of various cause. The BR is $>$ 40%, range 40-70, usually 50-60%. (2) The "intermediate" group, in which the BR is in the range of 20-40. (3) "Unconjugated," BR $<$ 20%, usually 5-15. This group is synonymous with the "retention" jaundice of Rich's classification [12], related entirely to bilirubin production in excess, or failure of the liver cell to conjugate and excrete bilirubin, or both. The "intermediate" type is observed in cases of chronic hepatitis and cirrhosis or in alcoholic cirrhosis with portal hypertension and hypersplenism causing overproduction of bilirubin in the spleen. There is strong evidence [13, 14] that much of this splenic free bilirubin escapes conjugation in the liver by virtue of portosystemic shunting, thus lowering the serum bilirubin ratio in characteristic fashion as I shall presently illustrate. There are also pathologic states in the "intermediate" category in which increased red cell destruction in Kupffer cells is associated with hepatocellular injury, as for example in malaria, or in hepatitis plus G_6PD deficiency of the red cells or other causes of liver injury with hypersplenic hemolysis. The third or "unconjugated" category includes hemolytic jaundice in general, both congenital and acquired, often autoimmune. Lack of conjugating enzyme, with or without increased hemolytic activity, is also included, as is the mild, pure retention jaundice of Gilbert's disease. The "unconjugated" types are uniformly acholuric, which underlines the importance of testing the urine for bilirubin.

Alcoholic cirrhosis with marked "intermediate" jaundice, hepatic encephalopathy with outspoken portosystemic shunting, *bilirubin ratio 20-25%,* large increase of urobilinogen, increased reticulocytes. The hematinemia attests to the exhaustion of haptoglobin because of hemolytic activity (Fig. 4).

Hepatic cirrhosis with macrocytic hemolytic anemia

A. M. ♂ 54
#772214

Long standing chronic alcoholism;
jaundice, ascites, spider nevi;
recurrent somnolence, eventual coma
and death.
Macrocytic anemia;
Reticulocytes 15-20 per cent
Hematinemia;
Feces urobilinogen 950 mg./d.;
Urine urobilinogen 28-35 mg./d.
SB 1' 5.4 mg./100 cc.
SBT 20.5 mg./100 cc.

FIG. 4. Cirrhosis with 25% BR Alc.

Chronic hepatitis-cirrhosis transition with early portal hypertension and "intermediate" jaundice, BR 38% is illustrated in Figure 5.

It might be thought that in states of severe hepatocellular injury such as acute or subacute hepatitis proceeding to hepatic necrosis and even fatal outcome, the bilirubin conjugating ability of the liver would obviously be impaired, but it usually persists in remarkable degree.

In the case outlined in Figure 6 serial observations for the last month of life, in a case of subacute hepatitis, necrosis and atrophy, revealed a conjugated jaundice until the day before death. The cross hatched segments represent conjugated, the open segments the unconjugated, according to our kinetic method. The numbers in these two columns need not concern us. It is possible that in this last column we are seeing evidence of beginning failure of conjugation but you will note that the proportion of prompt direct fraction at least up to that point is of the

J.O. ♂ 32. Post-hepatitic cirrhosis (2)

Striking palmar erythema; many spider nevi.
Slight icterus; mod. hepatosplenomegaly.
SB 1' 0.8 T 2.3. Ceph. floc. 4+ TT 21.
Fasting B.S. 32 mg %; cholest. 146 mg %.
S-GOT 235; SGPT 734; LE clot neg.
A/G $\frac{3.0}{3.9}$ (2.0 = γ).

FIG. 5. Cirrhosis with 38% BR chronic hepatitis.

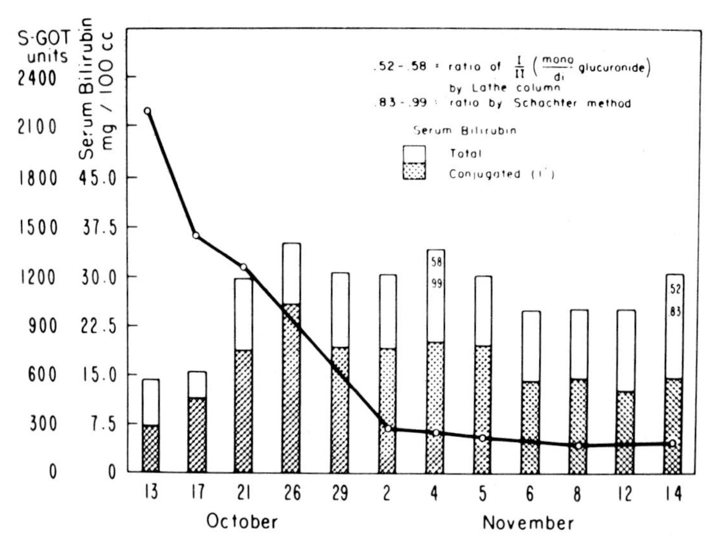

FIG. 6. Fatal hepatitis: SB and SGOT. (Reprinted from the *Journal of Laboratory and Clinical Medicine* by permission of publisher, C. V. Mosby Co.)

same magnitude as in extrahepatic obstructive jaundice, such as cancer of the head of the pancreas. You will also note, however, that the total serum bilirubin is much higher than is usual with mechanical obstructive jaundice of any cause, even with complete obstruction. Values of 30-40 or even higher, are often observed. The usually higher range with severe parenchymal liver disease is probably related to increased red cell destruction. Thus, it is all the more surprising that the proportion of conjugated bilirubin persists at such a high level. The large increase of SGOT at the outset of the study period, ie, 2100+ units, gave clear evidence of the severe diffuse hepatocellular injury, but it was probably much higher a few days earlier. Please note the importance of serial determinations of the SGOT and the SB. Here we see evidence of a rather rapid discharge of the enzyme from the injured or necrotic liver cells. If the patient had first been studied on November 5, the SGOT would not have been very impressive, and, as I shall mention later, values much higher than this are encountered in many cases of mechanical biliary obstruction. As this patient's SGOT fell, his liver became progressively smaller. This phenomenon of a persistently high bilirubin, a shrinking liver and falling hepatocellular enzymes is of decisive diagnostic and prognostic significance. The low plateau of the SGOT at the level of 250-300 units may be related to early regeneration of liver cells with continuing injury perhaps due to persistent antigen-antibody complex.

The patient seen in Figure 7 undoubtedly died of hepatitis B related to transfusions. On 12/13 he had been ill about ten days. The data antedate the availability of SGOT or other serum enzyme determinations in the University Hospital, but they are nevertheless decisive in their significance. The remarkably slow sedimentation velocity is quite ominous in a jaundiced patient, pointing to diffuse liver injury with a lack of fibrinogen. On 12/23 the contrast between sed rate and leukocyte count strongly indicates extensive hepatic necrosis. This is usually associated with severe prothrombin deficiency not corrected by vitamin K, also by a serious decline of factors 5 and 7, as emphasized by Koller [15]. In ordinary hepatitis the leukocyte count is generally normal or moderately reduced, not increased as seen here; the sed rate normal or mildly increased. The combination noted here is often seen with diffuse hepatic necrosis; also, the oliguria and developing uremia with rapid rise of creatinine are quite in accord. Again, note the very high serum bilirubin. One other point of interest in differential diagnosis is the observation that the exclusion of bile, though high grade, is not complete. When complete, as is usual with biliary tract cancer, excepting ampullary tumors, the feces contain less than 2 mg and the urine less than 0.3 mg of urobilinogen per day, in contrast with the higher values observed here, quite in accord with what we have often seen in acute hepatitis during peak suppression of bile flow.

One of the oldest and still one of the most useful procedures in the study of jaundice is the determination of urobilinogen in urine and feces [16]. An individual who is accustomed to the simple qualitative or semiquantitative test [17] can gain valuable information simply and cheaply and the value is often greatly enhanced by serial testing.

HOMOLOGOUS SERUM HEPATITIS →
ACUTE DIFFUSE NECROSIS

♂ 58 U.H. #838089

	12-13	12-23	12-25
SB 1'	6.8		30.9
SBT	10.9		39.3
Sed. 60'	0.5	1.0	
WBC		22,000	
U.U.		1.5	
F.U.	-	6.2	
BUN	18	Oliguria → & anuria	48.0
Creatinine		3.6	12.7

Death on 12-26

FIG. 7. Fatal hepatitis: various features.

This case (Fig. 8), studied nearly 40 years ago, was thought to have a common duct stone *except* for the complete biliary obstruction, highly exceptional with calculus. The colic was quite in accord with a stone, even to the disappearance of pain with the onset of jaundice. Nevertheless, at autopsy, a very small malignant stricture was found. This was in the days before we knew about vitamin K and prothrombin, and surgeons were not anxious to operate on jaundiced patients. Today there would have been an excellent chance of salvage.

The dynamic changes which urobilinogen studies may detect are often of great interest, as in this case (Fig. 9). First, high grade, but not complete obstruction, with marked oliguria as evidence of liver injury due to cholangitis above a common duct stone; then spontaneous improvement due to passage or more likely relocation of a stone, with striking evidence of release of the obstruction and residual liver injury, still later normal findings and the stone removed.

Carcinoma of the ampulla is an exception in that the biliary obstruction, unlike that with cancer of the pancreas, is often not complete, the jaundice only mild, and the anemia due to occult blood loss often prominent (Fig. 10). Note that the term "icteroanemia," commonly applied to hemolytic disease, was used to describe this patient on the preliminary examination and in fact it was at first thought that he had hemolytic jaundice. Fever is not infrequent due to cholangitis above the partial obstruction. As you see, this patient had only mild jaundice but of conjugated type with BR of 50%. Despite this and the presence of considerable fecal urobilinogen, the gallbladder was easily felt and of Courvoisier type.

Urobilinogen determinations may provide helpful information in respect to course and prognosis as well as diagnosis (Fig. 11). In a case of

Primary carcinoma of common bile duct
with painful attacks simulating gall stone colic

J.K. ♂ 60. Attacks of severe pain in R.U.Q. radiating through to back beneath right scapula. June - October, 1935. Onset of jaundice Oct. 3, 1935, no pain thereafter.

U. U. on 11-14-35 neg.
F. U. 11-11 to 11-15-35 1.4 mg. per day

Necropsy: Small scirrhus carcinoma at junction of cystic and common hepatic ducts, grossly resembling benign stricture.

FIG. 8. Small carcinoma stricture with biliary colic.

Common duct stone with cholangitis ♀ 37
Dynamic changes in UBG excretion

Previous R. U. Q. colics with jaundice
chills and fever (105°) with present attack

	SB	VdB	UBG Urine	UBG Feces
Deep jaundice	12.0	PD	4.2	12.8
Marked improvement	4.2	"	47.5	621.6
Jaundice fading	2.0	"		165.0
Op.: choledocholithotomy	2.5	"	2.3	100.0

FIG. 9. Common duct stone with cholangitis, etc.

painless jaundice with nearly but not complete exclusion of bile from the gut, values are more in accord with a viral hepatitis but unlike tumor [18]. After another two weeks he felt much better and free bile flow was now apparent, with large amounts of urobilinogen in both feces and urine. This, together with the patient's improvement of appetite and well-being, is so characteristic as to confirm the diagnosis of hepatitis if still in doubt. As a rule, in watching for the opening phase, which heralds recovery, one need only check the urine Ehrlich reaction serially, in qualitative or semiquantitative fashion.

The serum enzymes have not proven to be an unmixed blessing in differential diagnosis, though often of great help. The SGOT may at times reach levels unfortunately high in relation to diagnosis in cases of mechanical obstructive jaundice [19], even as high as 1200 units.

Characteristic Syndrome-Carcinoma of Ampulla of Vater

J. H. ♂ 57, U. H. #813659

Fever, anemia, mild jaundice ("icteroanemia");
Easily palpable, nontender, distended gall bladder
Occult GI bleeding; leukocytosis

Hb. 7.6 gm%, RBC 2.5 mill., WBC 22,000-31,000

Feces acholic in appearance, 4+ Guaiac

Feces urobilinogen 50.4 mg./100 gm.

SB 1' 1.0, T 2.0, bilirubin ratio 50%.

FIG. 10. Carcinoma of ampulla – incomplete biliary obstruction.

Acute hepatitis, ♂ 44
Dynamic changes in UBG excretion

		UBG	
		Urine mg/d	Feces mg/100 gm
11/14	Painless jaundice 2 weeks	3.8	10.2
12/7	Jaundice clearing, patient much improved	206.8	280.0

FIG. 11. Acute hepatitis – dynamic Ubg changes.

Figure 12 shows normal alkaline phosphatase (KA units) SGOT elevated in acute alcoholic hepatitis simulating acute cholecystitis; contrast with Thorazine-Valium jaundice.

The alkaline phosphatase and γ-GT (γ-glutamyl transpeptidase) are greatly elevated with intrahepatic cholestasis or cholangiolitic hepatitis-cirrhosis, as well as extrahepatic obstructive jaundice (Fig. 13). As you may surmise from this we have had quite a run on sclerosing cholangitis, a remarkably interesting disease. An advantage of the γ-GT is that unlike alkaline phosphatase none of it derives from bone, as evident in the case of osteogenic sarcoma with metastases. Otherwise, the values roughly parallel

Contrast in enzyme behavior in parenchymal jaundice of differing cause

	Alcoholic hepatitis A. P. ♀ 32	Thorazine-Valium jaundice M.S. ♀ 49
S. B. 1'	12.0	7.8
T	20.0	11.4
SGOT	350	184
AP	15	125
	? Cholecystitis Op: N. biliary tract Biopsy: Alc. hyal. hepatitis Stormy course, slow recovery	Rapid recovery

FIG. 12. AP and SGOT.

γ-GT and AP data

Case	γ-GT, units	AP, int'l units	S-GOT	Diagnosis
C.L.+	320	565	450	Sclerosing cholangitis
E.S.+	860	1075	86	" "
D.O.+	840	935	280	" "
O.M.*	19	5820	43	Osteogenic sarcoma with metastases to bone
R.J.*	546	2130	175	Alcoholic cirrhosis
n.	6-28	80	50	

+ jaundice (conjugated) * No jaundice

FIG. 13. AP and γ-GT.

those of the alkaline phosphatase in jaundice due to extra- or intrahepatic biliary tract disease. The γ-GT is a simpler procedure and appears to be highly useful.

In the foregoing I have tried to summarize for you some compelling clinical signs in the differential diagnosis of jaundice. When these are unequivocal there is generally very little need for extensive laboratory or x-ray studies, or liver biopsy. Given a man with jaundice and pruritus, a Courvoisier gallbladder and a Virchow node or a hard mass on the rectal shelf, I would simply recommend an early, palliative cholecystenterostomy. The palpable gallbladder alone, in such a case, fully warrants early operation.

In another case without any of the foregoing except jaundice, but with a bilirubin ratio of 25% (intermediate category) a more detailed study would be essential, leading to the probable need for liver biopsy, but if this patient also had a palpable spleen, outspoken estrogenic signs and ascites, the diagnosis of cirrhosis would be firm, requiring only those additional procedures essential in following treatment, such as serum electrolytes and albumin.

You may have judged that I happen to believe in a careful selection of laboratory and special procedures only after thorough consideration of the history and physical findings. I agree with that exemplary physician, Tinsley Harrison, who strongly advocates that the examiner should put down a diagnosis or alternative possibilities before he is aware of laboratory or x-ray reports, so that he will be more likely to select the right procedures in relation to this primary data base. In some respects I am unhappy about the 12 channel laboratory combine. Too often, I fear, it tends to give the impression that everything necessary has been done and that one only need, somehow, to fit the data to the patient.

References

1. Courvoisier, L. J.: Casuistisch-Statistische Beiträge zur Pathologie und Chirurgie der Gallenwege. Leipzig:Vogel Co. 57, 1890.
2. Fred, H. L. and Brown, G. R.: The hepatic friction rub. New Eng. J. Med., 266:554, 1962.
3. Larson, E. A., Evans, G. T. and Watson, C. J.: A study of the serum biliverdin concentration in various types of jaundice. J. Lab. Clin. Med., 32:481, 1947.
4. Greenberg, A. J., Bossenmaier, J. and Schwartz, S.: Green jaundice. Study of serum biliverdin, mesobiliverdin and other green pigments. Amer. J. Dig. Dis., 16:873, 1971.
5. Challenger, F. and Walshe, J. M.: Methyl mercaptan in relation to foetor hepaticus. Biochem. J., 59:372, 1955.
6. Chen, S., Zieve, L. and Mahadevan, V.: Mercaptans and dimethyl sulfide in the breath of patients with cirrhosis of the liver. J. Lab. Clin. Med., 75:628, 1970.
7. Hijmans van den bergh, A. A.: Der Gallenfarbstoff in Blute Leiden, van Doesburgh, 1918.
8. Ducci, H., and Watson, C. J.: The quantitative determination of the serum bilirubin with special reference to the prompt reacting and the chloroform soluble types. J. Lab. Clin. Med., 30:293, 1945.
9. Perelli, W. V. and Watson, C. J.: Comparison of the Weber-Schalm method with the Ducci-Watson modification of the Malloy-Evelyn method for serum bilirubin determination. Clin. Chem., 16:239, 1970.
10. Zieve, L., Hill, E., Hanson, M. et al: Normal and abnormal variations and clinical significance of the one minute and total serum bilirubin determinations. J. Lab. Clin. Med., 38:446, 1951.
11. Watson, C. J.: The importance of the fractional serum bilirubin determination in clinical medicine. Ann. Int. Med., 45:351, 1956.
12. Rich, A.: The pathogenesis of the forms of jaundice. Bull. Hopkins Hosp., 47:338, 1930.
13. Da Silva, L. D., Godoy, A., Mendes, F. T. et al: Indirect reacting hyperbilirubinemia after portosystemic shunt; its relation to other complications. Gastroenterology, 39:605, 1960.
14. Da Silva, L. D., Jamra, M. A., Maspes, V. et al: Pathogenesis of indirect reacting hyperbilirubinemia after portacaval anastomosis. Gastroenterology, 44:117, 1963.
15. Koller, F.: Theory and experience behind the use of coagulation tests in diagnosis and prognosis of liver disease. Scand. J. Gastroenterol., 8:51, 1973.
16. Schwartz, S., Sborov, V. and Watson, C. J.: Studies of urobilinogen IV. The quantitative determination of urobilinogen by means of the Evelyn photoelectric colormeter. Amer. J. Clin. Path., 14:598, 1944.
17. Watson, C. J. and Hawkinson, V.: Studies of urobilinogen VI. Further experience with the simple quantitative Ehrlich reaction. Amer. J. Clin. Path., 17:108, 1947.
18. Watson, C. J.: Studies of urobilinogen III. The per diem excretion of urobilinogen in the common forms of jaundice and disease of the liver. Arch. Int. Med., 59:206, 1937.
19. Ginsberg, A. Z.: Very high levels of SGOT and LDH in patients with extra hepatic biliary tract obstruction. Amer. J. Dig. Dis., 15:803, 1970.

Investigation of Chronic Cholestasis

Sheila Sherlock, M.D.

Definition [1]

Cholestasis is defined as failure of normal amounts of bile to reach the duodenum. It is jaundice associated with diminished or absent flow of bile. The term "obstructive jaundice" is not used, since in many instances no mechanical block can be shown in the biliary tract. Clinically, it is usually marked by jaundice and by predominant pruritus. The serum shows an increase in all the usual constituent bile, including conjugated bilirubin, trihydroxy bile acids, total cholesterol and alkaline phosphatase. The general effect of intestinal bile salt deficiency includes steatorrhea and failure to absorb calcium and fat soluble vitamins. Fecal urobilinogen is increased.

Morphologically, cholestasis is marked on light microscopy of the liver by visible evidence of stagnated or inspissated bile in the form of bile plugs.

Electronmicroscopy shows changes in all the organelles of the liver cell. The smooth endoplasmic reticulum is increased, the lysomes are full of pigment and the Golgi zone is enlarged and often vacuolated. The bile canaliculi are dilated and show blunting of their microvilli which are decreased in numbers. The pericanalicular zone is widened.

Causes

Prolonged or chronic cholestasis is defined when the clinical picture lasts more than six weeks. It can be due to mechanical obstruction to extrahepatic bile ducts as in ampullary sclerosing bile duct carcinoma, sclerosing cholangitis or choledocholithiasis. It may have an intrahepatic origin as in cholestatic viral hepatitis, cholestatic drug reactions, particularly to the promazine group and primary biliary cirrhosis. In the younger

---

Sheila Sherlock, M.D., Professor, Department of Medicine, University of London, Royal Free Hospital, London, England.

patients, particularly in the neonatal period and on into childhood, an increasing number of cholestatic syndromes are being recognized, often commencing as a neonatal hepatitis and proceeding to the clinical picture of intrahepatic bile duct atresia.

Clinical History

Aside from the general features of cholestasis, such as jaundice with relative well-being, pruritus and increasing skin pigmentation, dark urine and pale stools more specific points must be elicited. All drugs consumed within the last six months must be identified. Tranquilizers are particularly important. Many oral contraceptives are potentially cholestatic and can convert the clinical picture of hepatocellular jaundice, as in viral hepatitis, to a cholestatic one, so confusing the clinician. Associated ulcerative colitis is important both in sclerosing cholangitis and in bile duct carcinoma [2].

Slow onset with pruritus followed weeks, months or even years later by cholestatic jaundice suggests primary biliary cirrhosis [3]. An acute onset with general gastrointestinal symptoms and anorexia supports the diagnosis of cholestatic viral hepatitis.

Examination

The features of prolonged cholestasis such as xanthomas, deep skin pigmentation, clubbing of the fingers and bone thinning are so late and nonspecific that they are of little differential diagnostic assistance. Liver size is important for dilated bile ducts in the liver inevitably result in hepatomegaly. Therefore, if the liver is not enlarged the cholestasis is unlikely to be relieved by the surgeon.

General Tests

Routine biochemical methods should include the total serum bilirubin, the aspartate (oxalo-acetic) transaminase, total cholesterol, albumin and globulin levels and electrophoretic analysis of the plasma proteins. The serum 5-nucleotidase should be performed if the serum alkaline phosphatase is raised to confirm that the increase is of biliary origin. This is of particular importance in young people where the increased alkaline phosphatase can be of osseous origin.

The color of the feces must be recorded. Occult blood tests should be done; if positive in the absence of colitis this suggests neoplastic involvement of the biliary system.

A chest x-ray is always performed and a plain x-ray of the abdomen is useful in determining the liver size and showing the presence of any radiopaque calculi. In many instances a barium meal is indicated. Sigmoidoscopy with rectal biopsy, colonoscopy and barium enema may be needed if colitis is suspected.

Serum Mitochondrial Antibody [4, 5]

Serum from patients with primary biliary cirrhosis gives granular cytoplasmic staining in unfixed tissue sections, using a fluorescein-conjugate of antihuman gamma globulin and complement in the double layer immunofluorescent test (Fig. 1). The staining reactions are not organ or species specific, but they are known to be rich in mitochondria and are preferentially stained. The antigen is a component of the mitochondrial inner membrane. The antibody can in no sense be regarded as directed against bile ducts. Indeed, human renal tubular cells provide the best antigen. The mitochondrial antibody is present in 85%-95% of patients with primary biliary cirrhosis. Particular care has to be taken in making the diagnosis of primary biliary cirrhosis when the mitochondrial antibody test is negative. The test is usually negative in the cholestasis of ulcerative colitis and in cholestatic viral hepatitis. It is usually negative in drug related cholestasis and when positive is only in low titer.

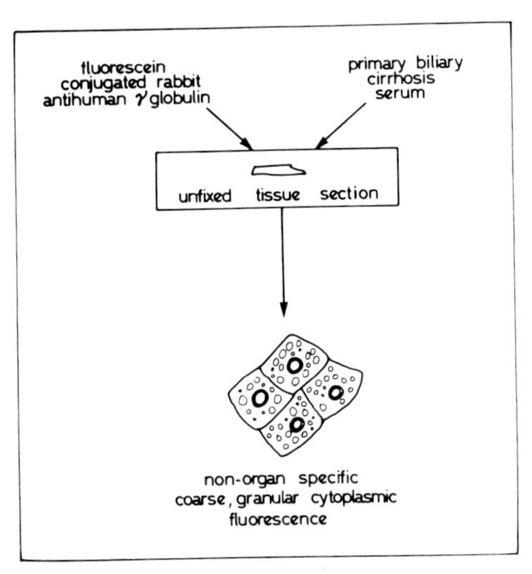

FIG. 1. The serum mitochondrial antibody test of primary biliary cirrhosis.

Hepatitic Scintiscanning

This technique is mandatory in any patient with chronic cholestasis. Dilated bile ducts at the hepatic hilum result in the filling defect (Fig. 2). Such an appearance often resembles the palm of a man's hand with the fingers outstretched. This confirms the presence of extrahepatic biliary obstruction. The usual cause is a bile duct carcinoma [6]. The hilum defect therefore is not due to a tumor mass itself.

In addition, hepatic scintiscanning reveals hepatocellular damage as a patchy uptake with increased splenic capture of isotope.

Endoscopic Retrograde Cannulation Pancreaticocholangiography (ERCP) [7-9]

With the development of side viewing fibro duodenoscopes the ampulla of Vater can be readily visualized and the common bile duct and pancreatic duct cannulated. The technique is not easy. Its performance

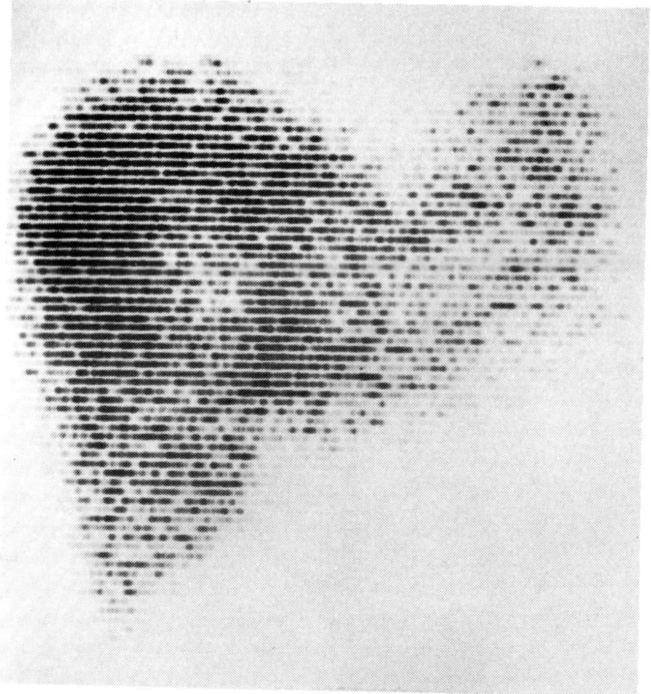

FIG. 2. Hepatic scintiscan using technetium in a patient with sclerosing hilar bile duct carcinoma. The filling defect at the hilum represents dilated bile ducts.

Table 1. Uses of Fibrotic Endoscopic Retrograde Cholangiography

1. To Demonstrate Bile Ducts Where IV Cholangiography Impossible eg, Primary Biliary Cirrhosis
2. Identify Bile Duct Obstructions Gallstones Stricture Carcinoma
3. Investigation Sclerosing Cholangitis
4. Investigation Postcholecystectomy Symptoms
5. Diagnosis (and Biopsy) of Ampullary Neoplasms

with regularity may be equated to acquiring perfection at playing the violin. It is not learned all at once. The technique is of inestimable value in the diagnosis of chronic cholestasis (Table 1).

The papillary region is reached easily, the stomach and duodenal bulb having been surveyed. Biopsy and cytology specimens and photographs are taken as necessary. The papilla is identified and any lesion in the area biopsied. The cannula is then introduced under direct vision into the papilla and bile ducts and contrast material injected under fluoroscopic control. The success rate is about 70% but much depends upon the experience of the operator and the underlying disease. The procedure is of inestimable value in the diagnosis of chronic cholestasis. The patency of the biliary system may be established in those with hepatocellular dysfunction where the usual intravenous cholangiographic procedures would fail to show contrast material in the biliary system. This applies, for instance, to early cases of primary biliary cirrhosis and to later ones where calculi in the bile ducts may be co-existent. Biliary duct obstructions due to such lesions as gallstones, stricture or carcinoma may be identified (Fig. 3). Sclerosing cholangitis produces a quite characteristic picture both in the common bile duct and in the intrahepatic ducts. Ampullary lesions may be diagnosed and, if necessary, biopsied. Postcholecystectomy symptoms can be investigated and any organic lesion in the bile ducts revealed.

Percutaneous Needle Biopsy of the Liver [10]

This procedure, even using the safe "one-second" Menghini technique [1], has been condemned in patients with deep cholestasis. It is, however, extremely safe and in a very large series at the Royal Free Hospital, complications, however deep the jaundice, have been very few

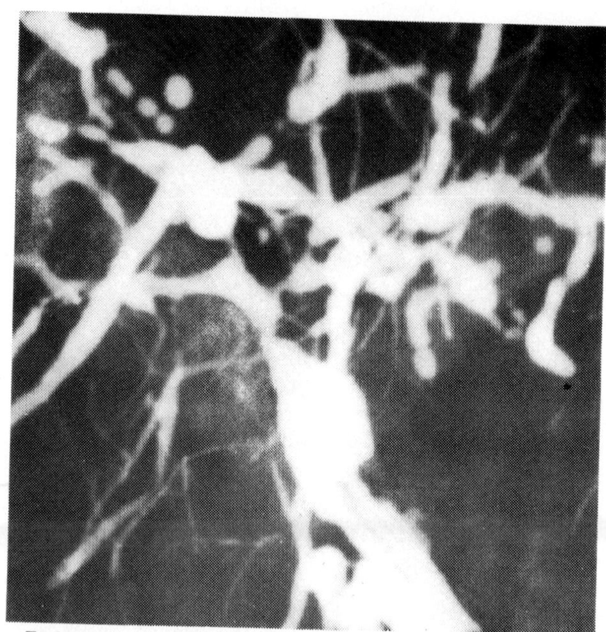

FIG. 3. Endoscopic retrograde cholangiogram shows irregularly dilated and constricted bile ducts in sclerosing cholangitis.

indeed (Table 2). If the prothrombin time is not more than two seconds prolonged after vitamin K_1 intramuscularly and the platelet count exceeds 60,000/cu mm, it is a safe procedure however deep the jaundice. The appearances of centrizonal cholestasis, stellate expansion of the portal zones with bile duct reduplication, polymorph infiltration and edema are characteristic of extrahepatic surgical cholestasis. If a pathologist experienced in reading liver biopsies is at hand, errors are surprisingly rare [10]. Careful observation for 24 hours after the biopsy is imperative. This must be done with the patient in hospital. A thousand biopsies may be done with no complications only for the 1001st to be fraught with disaster.

Table 2. Royal Free Hospital Needle Liver Biopsy in Surgical Cholestasis

S. Bilirubin (mg)	*No.*	*Complications*		
		Cholangitis	*Pleural Effusion*	*Pain*
>10	18	1	0	1
<10	39	1	1	0

The histopathological diagnosis of primary biliary cirrhosis is more confident with the larger operative wedge hepatic biopsy than with the smaller needle one, yet the number of such specimens is decreasing with the number of laparotomies. Greater importance is being placed on the reading of biopsy sections. The significance of focal portal zone lymphocyte accumulation, biliary type fibrosis and peripheral cholestasis is very suggestive of primary biliary cirrhosis. Diagnostic changes, which are destructive lesions of bile duct with granulomas, are infrequent but when they occur are absolutely specific for primary biliary cirrhosis (Fig. 4). The florid duct lesion must be distinguished from the peribiliary infiltration of long-standing bile duct obstruction. In the pericholangitis of ulcerative colitis the ducts are not destroyed, granulomas are absent and the infiltrate is predominantly lymphocytic with few or no plasma cells. A similar bile duct lesion, usually without granulomas, is found in a few patients with chronic viral hepatitis. Piecemeal necrosis in the later stages of primary biliary cirrhosis may lead to difficulty in distinction from chronic aggressive hepatitis and there are mixed forms. Features favoring primary biliary cirrhosis include intact lobules, slight piecemeal necrosis, periseptal cholestasis and lymphoid aggregates. When cirrhosis has developed and clinical features are atypical, cryptogenic cirrhosis may be wrongly diagnosed.

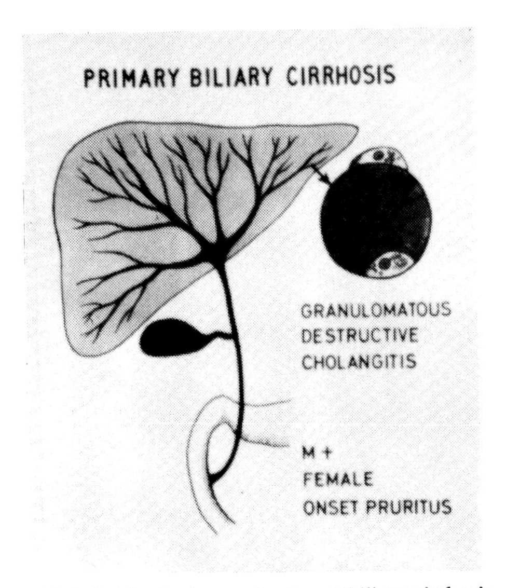

FIG. 4. The features of primary biliary cirrhosis.

Percutaneous, Transhepatic Cholangiography [11]

The main difference between extrahepatic and intrahepatic cholestasis is the presence of dilated bile ducts in the one group and not in the other. This suggests that attempts at puncture of ducts through the percutaneous route might be used to differentiate them, the bile duct being punctured readily in those who have a blockage to main duct but not in those with intrahepatic cholestasis [11]. The technique carries a small risk of biliary peritonitis and if a dilated duct is punctured, surgical exploration of the biliary tract should be performed within two to three hours. It is also important that a flexible plastic tube be used rather than a rigid needle for exploration as this lessens the risk of damage to the liver. If a dilated bile duct is not entered, bile duct exploration is not mandatory. The patient, however, must be followed carefully both by serial clinical observations of pulse and blood pressure and by observation of such symptoms as abdominal pain and distention. If a duct is not encountered easily, mechanical obstruction to major bile ducts is unlikely.

Summary

Knowledge of the possible causes, careful clinical history and examination with selected routine laboratory tests strongly suggest the nature and etiology of any patient with chronic cholestasis. The special techniques of serum mitochondrial antibodies, hepatic scintiscanning, retrograde endoscopic cholangiography and pancreatography, percutaneous needle biopsy using the Menghini technique and percutaneous transhepatic cholangiography usually put the site of the obstruction without doubt. The etiology of the block is also usually but not always determined.

References

1. Sherlock, S.: Diseases of the Liver and Biliary System, ed. 5. Philadelphia: F. A. Davis, 1974. (In press.)
2. Roberts-Thomson, I. C., Strickland, R. G. and Mackay, I. M.: Bile duct carcinoma in chronic ulcerative colitis. Aust. New Zeal. J. Med., 3: 264, 1973.
3. Sherlock, S. and Scheuer, P. J.: The presentation and diagnosis of 100 patients with primary biliary cirrhosis. New Eng. J. Med., 289:674, 1973.
4. Doniach, D., Roitt, I. M., Walker, J. G. et al: Tissue autoantibodies in primary biliary cirrhosis, active chronic "lupoid" hepatitis, cryptogenic cirrhosis and other liver diseases and their clinical implications. Clin. Exp. Immun., 1:237, 1966.

5. Klatskin, G. and Kantor, F. S.: Mitochondrial antibody in primary biliary cirrhosis and other diseases. Ann. Intern. Med., 77:533, 1972.
6. Whelton, M. J., Petrelli, M., George, P. et al: Carcinoma at the junction of the hepatic ducts. Quart. J. Med., 38:211, 1969.
7. Cotton, P. B.: Cannulation of the papilla of Vater by endoscopy and retrograde cholangiopancreatography (ERCP). Gut, 13:1014, 1972.
8. Okuda, K., Someya, N., Gotok, A. et al: Endoscopic pancreatocholangiography. Amer. J. Roentgen., 117:438, 1973.
9. Elias, E., Summerfield, J. A. S., Dick, R. et al: Endoscopic retrograde cholangiography (ERCP) in the diagnosis of jaundice associated with ulcerative colitis. Gastroenterology. (In press, 1974.)
10. Scheuer, P. J.: Liver Biopsy Interpretation, ed. 2. Baltimore:Williams and Wilkins Co., 1973.
11. George, P., Young, W. B., Walker, J. G. et al: The value of percutaneous cholangiography. Brit. J. Surg., 54:779, 1965.

Chronic Active Liver Disease

W. H. J. Summerskill, M.D.

Chronic Hepatitis

Chronic hepatitis conventionally encompasses certain related conditions within the more extensive framework of chronic inflammatory liver disease. These conditions comprise (a) *chronic persistent* (or inactive) hepatitis; (b) *subacute* hepatitis (with bridging or multilobular necrosis); and (c) *chronic active* – or "aggressive" hepatitis [1-4]. These morphologic features often identify separate, if not always readily distinguishable, clinical entities but can sometimes represent fluctuating degrees of hepatic inflammation during the course of chronic active liver disease [3]. All these patterns of hepatitis may be associated with *cirrhosis.* Chronicity of hepatitis is very probable if the clinical features and liver function tests associated with acute hepatitis fail to improve (or deteriorate) during the ten weeks following their onset.

Numerous eponyms or descriptive titles ("chronic viral," "lupoid," "autoimmune," etc.) were once applied to conditions which are now believed identical or very closely related [5].

Clinical, biochemical and morphologic features (Table 1) depend upon disease activity. *Biochemical indicators* of activity comprise particularly elevations of SGOT and gamma globulin together with positive serologic reactions caused by circulating nonhepatocyte specific antibodies [5]. *Liver biopsy* establishes a diagnosis of the type of hepatitis. When remission is induced by therapy or occurs spontaneously, features are similar to those in chronic persistent ("inactive") hepatitis. Histologic patterns of disease differ mainly with regard to their extent and severity (Fig. 1). Interpretation by an expert is often necessary.

Differential diagnosis between related conditions (unresolved or relapsing acute hepatitis, chronic persistent hepatitis and chronic active liver disease) may be difficult and often can only be made by recourse to

---

W. H. J. Summerskill, M.D., Professor, Department of Medicine, Mayo Graduate School of Medicine, Rochester, Minn.

Table 1. Classification and Common Features of Chronic Active Liver Disease

Disease Activity	*Clinical Features of Disease*	*Changes in Liver Function Tests*	*Immunoserologic Abnormalities*	*Histologic Characteristics*	*Prognosis*
Inactive Phase					
Inactive hepatitis	Non or non-specific	SGOT $< \times 2$ Others normal	None	Portal inflammation ± minimal piecemeal necrosis	Good without treatment
Inactive hepatitis with cirrhosis	± residual evidence of earlier activity	SGOT $< \times 2$ Others normal	None	Cirrhosis with minimal or absent inflammation and necrosis	Immediately good without treatment later?
Indeterminate Phase	Equivocal	SGOT $\times 2 - \times 10$	Perhaps	Portal inflammation; mild piecemeal necrosis	May be good, requires observation
Active Phases					
Chronic active hepatitis	Frequent	SGOT $> \times 3$ Others often abnormal	Frequent	Portal inflammation, moderate or severe piecemeal necrosis	Cautiously optimistic, may need treatment
Subacute hepatitis	Severe	Usually general and striking	Frequent	Bridging or multi-lobular necrosis with inflammatory changes	Guarded (good or poor), requires treatment
Active hepatitis with cirrhosis	Frequent	SGOT $> \times 3$ Others often abnormal	Frequent	Cirrhosis, cell necrosis and inflammatory changes	Fair only, even with treatment

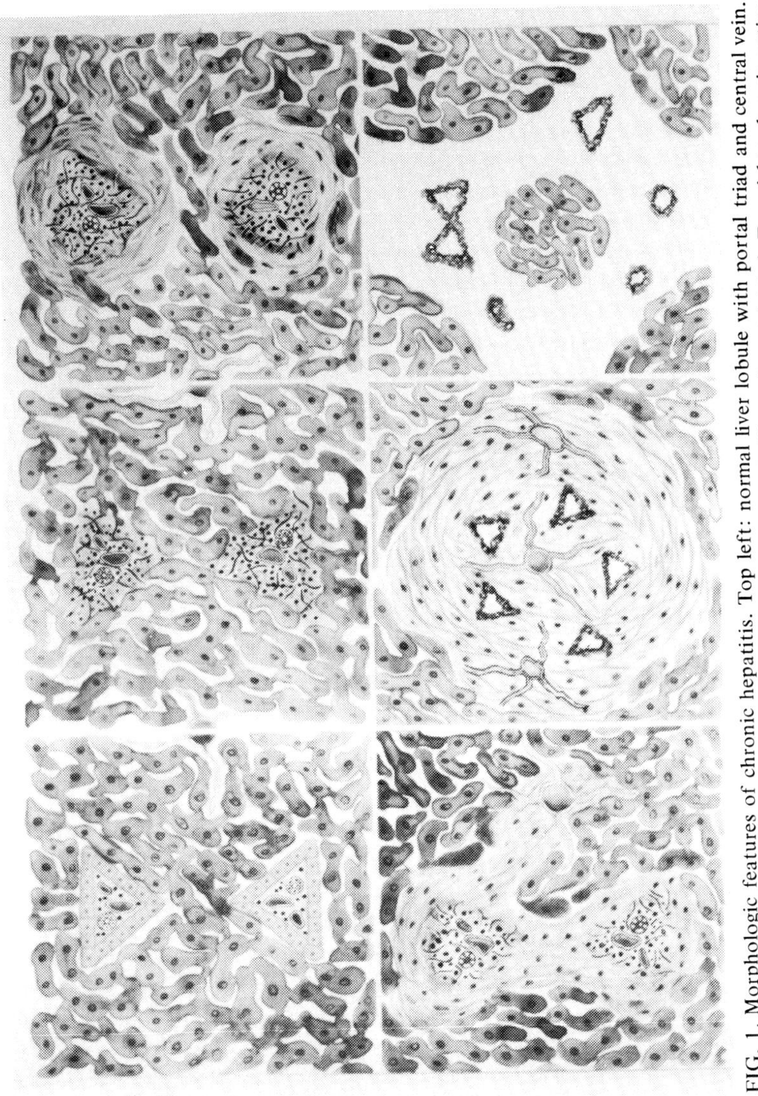

FIG. 1. Morphologic features of chronic hepatitis. Top left: normal liver lobule with portal triad and central vein. Top middle: chronic persistent hepatitis featuring inflammatory infiltrated portal triad. Top right: chronic active (aggressive) hepatitis with piecemeal necrosis extending outward from limiting plate. Bottom left: subacute hepatitis with bridging necrosis between portal tracts and central veins. Bottom middle: subacute hepatitis with multilobular necrosis characterized by collapse of adjacent liver lobules. Bottom right: macronodular (postnecrotic) cirrhosis as sequel in chronic active liver disease.

histology. In some unrelated conditions clinical, biochemical and histologic changes identical with those in chronic hepatitis may be found [6-8]. These comprise drug hepatitis (oxyphenisatin, methyl dopa, INH), primary biliary cirrhosis and Wilson's disease. Special measures establish the correct diagnosis.

The etiology of chronic hepatitis is unknown in the majority of instances. Patients (10%-30%) in U. S. also with hepatitis B antigen [9, 10] are assumed to have inflammation initiated, perpetuated or both by viral infection. Similar complications of infection with the hepatitis A virus [11] have not been confirmed. The mechanism of action of viruses (or other candidate mechanisms) on liver cells is undefined; delineation of circumstances predisposing a minority of those attacked by acute hepatitis to develop chronic disease also requires investigation. Host factors may include defects in the integrity of immunologic mechanisms, especially those mediated through T lymphocytes. Does CALD represent an "autoimmune" process? [12] – a debating point until organ (liver) specific antigens and antibodies are demonstrated.

Chronic Persistent Hepatitis [13, 14]

Often asymptomatic, usually no stigmata of chronic liver disease and elevations in SGOT ($< \times 3$ normal) but no other change in liver function tests. Approximately 10% of patients with acute viral hepatitis (HB Ag positive) may progress to chronic persistent hepatitis. Liver biopsy establishes diagnosis and prognosis thought to be benign, although fluctuations in activity may occur with the development of chronic active liver disease. No long-term follow-up has yet been published.

Chronic Active Liver Disease

Clinical Features

Until recently, CALD has been considered usually progressive and then ultimately fatal [15]. Revision of estimate depends upon newer modes of treatment [16, 17]. Findings depend upon extent and severity of hepatic inflammation and necrosis. Mild disease may be asymptomatic and difficult to distinguish from chronic persistent hepatitis. At the other extreme, severe cirrhosis or subacute hepatitis may be associated with a fulminant course rapidly leading to death [4].

Females are more commonly afflicted and the most frequent symptoms are nonspecific (fatigue, anorexia, etc.). Frequently, arthralgias, rashes and other complaints suggest multisystemic involvement. Indeed, 20% of patients may have associated inflammatory diseases of other organs (some of postulated "autoimmune" type) including ulcerative colitis, thyroiditis, sicca syndrome, etc.). Right upper quadrant pain is common and may be severe. In advanced cases, jaundice, ascites and other features of liver failure may be evident.

Etiology

Subacute hepatitis followed presumed acute viral hepatitis in 52 of 170 patients followed at Yale [4]. A prospective study in Copenhagen showed that eight of 112 patients with acute B hepatitis progressed to chronic active hepatitis [9]. The etiology and origin in other instances are uncertain (see earlier). "Lupoid" and other descriptive or eponymous titles have recently been shown to possess fallible scientific credentials [18] as independent disease entities.

Tests of liver function reflect the severity of the disease; all may be abnormal. Elevated SGOT and gamma globulin are the most sensitive indicators of disease activity. Rapid determination of serum bile acid concentrations by a highly sensitive radioimmunoassay technique may contribute greater precision over conventional tests for the diagnosis of ongoing activity of the disease [19]. A variety of immunoserologic tests may be positive, but only HB Ag has so far proved to be of practical importance. Reduction in serum albumin concentration and prolongation of the prothrombin time are factors indicating more severe disease and a poorer prognosis.

Histologic documentation is usually necessary for a diagnosis and to establish whether or not cirrhosis has developed (Fig. 1). Subacute hepatitis [20, 21] features necrosis extending between portal tracts or central veins ("bridging necrosis") or a more extensive hepatocyte damage with collapse of adjacent lobules (multilobular necrosis). Chronic active ("aggressive") hepatitis is characterized by piecemeal necrosis extending from the portal tracts beyond the limiting plate. All these conditions may be accompanied by fibrosis (septal formation) and focal lobular changes similar to those in acute viral hepatitis. In more advanced cases, cirrhosis has developed and may be accompanied by features of active hepatitis, including those specified [1-4].

Prognosis depends mainly upon two factors: (a) choice of the correct treatment and response to it and (b) the histologic appearances [22]. Subacute hepatitis and cirrhosis respond less well to therapy than chronic active hepatitis alone (see later).

Treatment of Chronic Hepatitis

Patients classified as having chronic persistent hepatitis require no treatment but should be carefully followed. The need for treatment in chronic active liver disease has been clarified recently.

Disagreement [5] concerning the efficacy or otherwise of prednisone, azathioprine and their derivatives in the treatment of CALD has been dispelled by three controlled studies. In London, Cook and his colleagues [17] showed that mortality in CAH was reduced by prednisolone (15 mg daily for a month, followed by variable maintenance doses, usually approximating 10 mg daily of prednisone). Treatment did not uniformly alter liver function tests; an effect on hepatic morphology was not sought. The Mayo study employed higher doses of medications, as well as additional methods [16]. Maintenance schedules with prednisone (20 mg daily) (Pred), or a combination of smaller doses of prednisone (10 mg) with azathioprine (50 mg) (Comb), were significantly more effective than azathioprine alone (100 mg) or placebo. Pred and Comb not only increased survival, but resulted in the resolution of jaundice, ascites and other clinical features of liver disease. Simultaneously, biochemical, immunochemical and histologic indicators of disease activity usually underwent remission. These points are illustrated (Fig. 2) and show that nearly all patients ultimately reach an end-point (remission or treatment failure). A later study [23] showed that prednisone (15 mg daily) was more likely to prolong survival than azathioprine (75 mg daily).

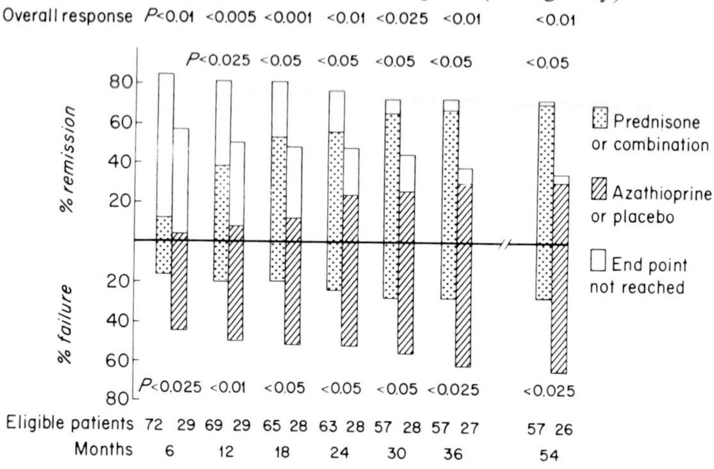

FIG. 2. Remissions and treatment failures compared in relation to treatment in a controlled trial involving 102 courses of therapy. Note that ultimately nearly all patients reach end-point.

More recently we have tested against our conventional programs the efficacy of giving prednisone on alternate days and in doses titrated to levels which keep liver function tests within the resolution range (biochemical resolution), since this method is extensively used [15, 17] and is thought to reduce the number of side effects. Our results show that such "Pred-Titrad" is as effective as other treatments in preventing treatment failures or the development of cirrhosis and in securing biochemical resolution. On the other hand, histologic resolution and, therefore, full remission of the disease, is found no more commonly than with less effective treatments (placebo and azathioprine). Pred-Titrad, therefore, secures disappearance of clinical and biochemical features of disease but does not suppress ongoing activity of the histologic lesion in the liver.

In all these studies, higher doses of medications were given initially and complications attributable to the drugs were far outweighed by the benefits of therapy.

Should all patients with chronic active hepatitis receive "immunosuppressive" therapy? The balance of benefit-risk factors includes the likelihood of severe side effects in 5%-10% of patients after more than a year of treatment. Patients with severe disease, specified by Mayo criteria [16], most urgently need treatment; there was otherwise a mortality of 40% within six months. By contrast, all patients with a diagnosis of chronic active hepatitis were included in the London trial [17]. In neither study was evidence presented that the postulated etiology of CALD greatly affects response to treatment. At present, the strongest indications for treatment of documented CALD are as follows: morphologic documentation; serious clinical deterioration or disability; all patients with subacute hepatitis; continued (ten weeks) SGOT $>\times 10$ or SGOT $>\times 5$ and gamma globulin $>\times 2$; and careful benefit-risk appraisal of other patients.

Remission is the aim of treatment and is characterized [24] by (a) absence of symptoms and return of the patient to all customary activity; (b) disappearance of biochemical and immunochemical abnormalities associated with active hepatitis; and (c) resolution of the histologic hallmarks of active hepatitis. The presence of cirrhosis does not preclude remission. Two thirds of patients become free from clinical features of disease by six months; previously abnormal liver function or immunologic tests revert to normal in three fourths after a year; by two years, when 90% of patients have no clinical or biochemical evidence of active disease, liver biopsy shows either inactive hepatitis or normal appearances in 70% (Fig. 3).

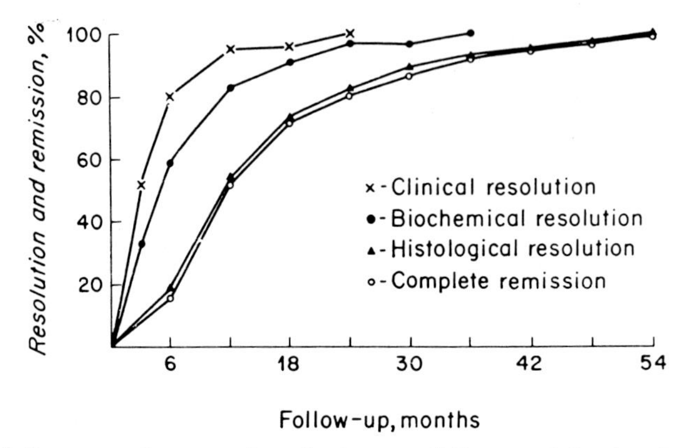

FIG. 3. Sequence of response in patients successfully treated for chronic active liver disease. Note clinical, biochemical and histologic resolution, all of which are necessary for remission, occur in sequence.

Relapse follows discontinuation of treatment in 50% of instances, nearly always within six months. Second or subsequent courses of treatment identical with the one initially procuring remission usually prove effective after relapse (Fig. 4). The majority of patients ultimately enter a sustained remission and one third of those followed under these circumstances for two years or longer have no residual evidence of hepatitis whatsoever on liver biopsy.

Treatment Failure

While approximately 80% of patients with CALD will enter remission with conventional treatment schedules, the remaining 20% will fail to respond by clinical or biochemical criteria; the majority die. Treatment failure seldom occurs in chronic active hepatitis, but involves 25% of

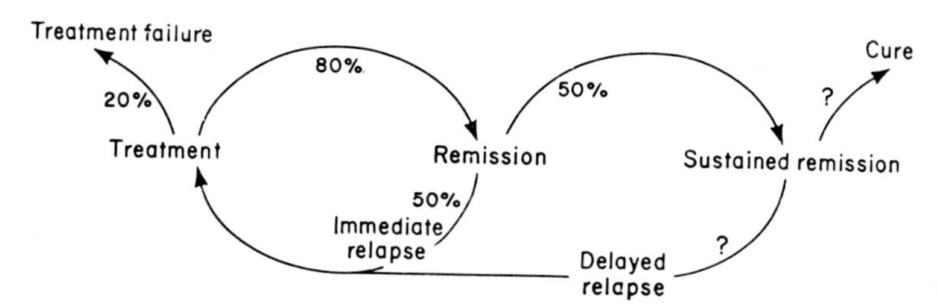

FIG. 4. Responses to initial and subsequent treatments in CALD. Approximately 50% of patients enter prolonged remission and after two years have no residual clinical, biochemical or histologic features of liver disease. The remaining 50% relapse within six months and require a further period of treatment.

patients with subacute hepatitis and 50% with cirrhosis. In fatal cases, death occurs early from fulminant hepatitis or as an end-point of slowly progressive chronic disease. When treatment is ineffective because of severe or fulminant disease, some patients respond to higher doses (usually 60 mg daily) of prednisone [25].

References

1. Summerskill, W. H. J.: Chronic active liver disease re-examined. Prognosis hopeful. Gastroenterology, 66:450-464, 1974.
2. DeGroote, J., Gedigk, P., Popper, H. et al: A classification of chronic hepatitis. Lancet, 2:626, 1968.
3. Baggenstoss, A. H., Soloway, R. D., Summerskill, W. H. J. et al: Chronic active liver disease: The range of histologic lesions, their response to treatment, and evolution. Hum. Path., 3:183, 1972.
4. Boyer, J. L. and Klatskin, G.: Pattern of necrosis in acute viral hepatitis: Prognostic value of bridging (subacute hepatic necrosis). New Eng. J. Med., 282:1063, 1970.
5. Geall, M. G., Schoenfield, L. J. and Summerskill, W. H. J.: Classification and treatment of chronic active liver disease. Gastroenterology, 55:724, 1968.
6. Goldstein, G. B., Lam, K. C. and Mistilis, S. P.: Drug induced active chronic hepatitis. Amer. J. Dig. Dis., 18:177, 1973.
7. Sternlieb, I. and Scheinberg, I. H.: Chronic hepatitis as a first manifestation of Wilson's disease. Ann. Int. Med., 76:59, 1972.
8. Cooksley, W. G., Powell, L. W., Kerr, J. F. et al: Cholestasis in active chronic hepatitis. Amer. J. Dig. Dis., 17:495, 1972.
9. Nielsen, J. O., Dietrichson, O., Elling, P. et al: Incidence and meaning of persistence of Australia antigen in patients with acute viral hepatitis: Development of chronic hepatitis. New Eng. J. Med., 285:1157, 1971.
10. Sherlock, S.: Long-incubation (virus B, HAA-associated) hepatitis. Gut, 13:297, 1972.
11. Doniach, D.: Autoimmune aspects of liver disease. Brit. Med. Bull., 28:145, 1972.
12. Galbraith, R. M., Smith, M. Mackenzie, R. M. et al: Familial seroimmunologic abnormalities in chronic hepatitis and biliary cirrhosis. New Eng. J. Med., 290:63, 1974.
13. Redeker, A. H.: Chronic viral hepatitis. *In* Vyas, G. N., Perkins, H. A. and Schmid, R. (eds.): Hepatitis and Blood Transfusion. New York:Grune & Stratton, 1972.
14. Vido, I., Selmair, H., Wildhirt, E. et al: Zur Prognose der chronischen Hepatitis. Deutsch. Med. Wschr., 94:2215, 1969.
15. Mistilis, S. P.: Active chronic hepatitis. *In* Schiff, L. (ed.): Diseases of the Liver, ed. 3., New York:J. B. Lippincott, 1969, p. 645.
16. Soloway, R. D., Summerskill, W. H. J., Baggenstoss, A. H. et al: Clinical, biochemical and histologic remission of severe chronic active liver disease: A controlled study of treatments and early prognosis. Gastroenterology, 63:820, 1972.
17. Cook, G. C., Mulligan, R. and Sherlock, S.: Controlled prospective trial of corticosteroid therapy in active chronic hepatitis. Quart. J. Med., 40:159, 1972.

18. Soloway, R. D., Summerskill, W. H. J., Baggenstoss, A. H. et al: "Lupoid" hepatitis, a nonentity in the spectrum of chronic active liver disease. Gastroenterology, 63:458, 1972.
19. Korman, M. G., Hofmann, A. F. and Summerskill, W. H. J.: Assessment of activity in chronic active liver disease: Serum bile acids compared with conventional tests and histology. New Eng. J. Med. (In press.)
20. Klatskin, G.: Subacute hepatic necrosis and postnecrotic cirrhosis due to anicteric infections with the hepatitis virus. Amer. J. Med., 25:333, 1958.
21. Tisdale, W. A.: Subacute hepatitis. New Eng. J. Med., 268:85, 1963.
22. Ammon, H. V., Summerskill, W. H. J. and Baggenstoss, A. H.: Initial morphologic appearances determine responses to treatment of chronic active liver disease (CALD); A prospective study, abstracted. Gastroenterology, 65:A-2/526, 1973.
23. Murray-Lyon, I. A., Stern, R. B. and Williams, R.: Controlled trial of prednisone and azathioprine in active chronic hepatitis. Lancet, 1:735, 1973.
24. Ammon, H. V., Baggenstoss, A. H. and Summerskill, W. H. J.: Characterization and incidence of remission and relapse in chronic active liver disease (CALD), abstracted. Gastroenterology, 62:173, 1972.
25. Summerskill, W. H. J., Ammon, H. V. and Baggenstoss, A. H.: Treatment of chronic hepatitis. *In* Schaffner, F., Sherlock, S. and Leevy, C. M. (eds.): The Liver and Its Diseases. New York:Intercontinental Medical Book Corp., 1974, pp. 216-226.

The Pathogenesis of Cholestasis

Hans Popper, M.D., Ph.D.

Cholestasis is defined by the morphologist as the visible stagnation of bile pigment in bile canaliculi, hepatocytes and in Kupffer cells [1, 2]. The clinician refers to it when biliary substances such as conjugated or direct reacting bilirubin, cholesterol, alkaline phosphatase activity and bile acids are increased in the blood, the elevation of the latter being associated with deposition of cholic acid [3] or chenodeoxycholic acid [4] in the skin causing itching. The physiologist, by contrast, considers cholestasis a disturbance of hepatocytic secretion of bile.

Extrahepatic Biliary Obstruction

Cholestasis may be produced by various factors, of which one is obstruction of the extrahepatic biliary passages in an axis from the papilla of Vater to the bifurcation of the main hepatic duct at the hilus of the liver. Obstruction not compromising this axis, for instance in the cystic duct, does not produce cholestasis. The various factors producing extrahepatic obstruction are well known to include biliary calculi or tumors, primarily carcinomas which either originate from the duct or encroach from the outside upon it and fix it, like a carcinoma of the pancreas or the stomach. Lymph node enlargement, even from leukemias or metastases, as a rule does not obstruct the extrahepatic ducts because they may move away in the delicate connective tissue of the lesser omentum. Of the lymphomas, only reticulum cell sarcoma or Hodgkin's disease invades the duct sufficiently to obstruct it, while jaundice associated with other lymphomas or leukemia is not on an extrahepatic obstructive basis. Infiltration of the hilar connective tissue of the liver, however, by metastatic tumor tissue may produce obstructive jaundice. Inflammation

Hans Popper, M.D., Ph.D., The Stratton Laboratory for the Study of Liver Diseases, Mount Sinai School of Medicine of The City University of New York. At present Fogarty Scholar-in-Residence, Fogarty International Center, National Institutes of Health, Bethesda, Md.

including stricture following surgery on the duct or primary sclerosing cholangitis [5] produces jaundice, as do a variety of rare circumstances such as an occasional abscess, including amebic pseudoabscess, parasites within the duct or some developmental alterations such as choledochus cysts or extrahepatic biliary atresia or an exceptional duodenal diverticulum. Extrahepatic mechanical obstruction causes, depending upon the duration, dilatation of the bile ducts above the obstacle and throughout the liver, hydrohepatosis.

Intrahepatic cholestasis may be the result of mechanical obstruction demonstrable radiologically, at operation, or at autopsy or may fail to exhibit such an obstruction on these examinations.

Intrahepatic Mechanical Biliary Obstruction

It leads only exceptionally to jaundice, because obstruction of only one part of the biliary duct system, even including one main branch of the duct, causes hydrohepatosis in the involved portion of the liver and biochemical alterations referable to obstruction, such as elevated serum activity of alkaline phosphatase, but does not cause jaundice as long as the nonobstructed liver functions normally and excretes the excess bilirubin in a compensatory fashion. Extrahepatic biliary obstruction with jaundice is found in the following rare conditions:

Carcinoma at the bifurcation of the common duct. This lesion, more frequently found in older people, is technically intrahepatic but practically has all the features of an extrahepatic mechanical obstruction, particularly if both ducts are equally involved.

Suppurative cholangitis. Previously purulent infections of the intrahepatic bile ducts were a frequent cause of jaundice. They result from both ascending intraductal processes as well as biliary excretion of bacteria reaching the liver by the hematogenous route. Today, because of successful therapy with antibiotics readily excreted in the bile this condition has become rare.

Intrahepatic sclerosing cholangitis. Sometimes the process in the extrahepatic bile ducts may extend into the liver, particularly if associated with chronic ulcerative colitis [6] or antimigraine therapy. Histologically, portal inflammation is associated with centrolobular cholestasis.

Intrahepatic biliary atresia. Previously, this condition was considered a developmental defect. It is now recognized that few instances are associated with chromosomal abnormalities, but most seem to derive from intrauterine virus infections, such as with rubella, causing a destruction of the intrahepatic bile ducts in prenatal life [7]. Usually, portal inflammation persists after birth. It is often associated with extrahepatic atresia or with giant-cell hepatitis.

Carcinoma metastases. Cholestatic jaundice associated with hepatomegaly is sometimes the first indication of a metastatic malignancy. More frequently, it is seen in late stages when widespread hepatic metastases are thought to compromise the lumen of sufficient bile ducts throughout the liver to create cholestatic jaundice. However, significant discrepancy between the extent of the metastases and the severity of cholestasis incriminates other factors similar to those found in the absence of demonstrable cholestasis.

The Problem of Intrahepatic Primary Cholestasis

Cholestasis without obstruction demonstrable on surgical exploration or on cholangiography [8], or on autopsy, but with all the clinical, laboratory and often also histologic characteristics of extrahepatic biliary obstruction, has been one of the main problems in the differential diagnosis of jaundice.

"Cholangiolitis." Sometimes, jaundice with increased direct-reacting serum bilirubin is observed which cannot be explained by alteration of hepatocytes or by changes of the bile ducts in the portal tracts on the basis of histologic and functional studies. Then the assumption was made that the link between the bile canaliculi, formed by a specially adapted portion of the cell membrane of the hepatocytes, and the bile ducts, a link called originally cholangiole, may be the site of an obstruction by an inflammatory exudate compressing or amputating it. This concept was presented both in Germany by Roessle [9] and here in Minneapolis by Watson and Hoffbauer [10], who coined the term "cholangiolitic" hepatitis and cirrhosis. Today, the structure then called a cholangiole is designated as a ductule since the term cholangiole has different meaning in various languages. Such a portal or "cholangiolitic" inflammation was also incriminated as the cause of jaundice when Hanger and Gutman [11] described what was probably the first record of drug-induced cholestasis resulting from administration of organic arsenicals.

Subsequent clinical pathological correlations [12] revealed that the characteristic picture of severe cholestatic jaundice may be observed in the absence of any portal inflammation, for instance after administration of anabolic steroids as well as in later, sometimes even fatal, stages of cholestatic hepatitis, produced by such drugs as chlorpromazine. On the other side, severe inflammatory reaction, presumably on hypersensitivity basis, was noted in the liver [13], eg, after antibiotic therapy, revealing the classic picture of a cholangitis in the absence of jaundice.

Lesions of bile-secretory apparatus. The subsequent development of electron microscopy moved the site of the lesion from the biliary passages to the hepatocytes [14-16]. A characteristic alteration of not only the bile canaliculi but also of the hepatocellular organelles surrounding them was demonstrated in all forms of cholestasis, namely, widening of the bile-canalicular lumen associated with swelling or stunting or disappearance of their microvilli, which on scanning microscopy appear contracted [17, 18], widening of the pericanalicular zone, and changes in the neighboring Golgi zone, lysosomes and in the smooth endoplasmic reticulum. The junctional complexes sealing the bile-canalicular lumen from the intercellular and the pericellular tissue space, however, remain intact as long as the hepatocytes are viable and secrete bile. This militates against another previous assumption that rupture of bile canaliculi accounts for jaundice by regurgitation of bile into the blood [19].

This hepatocytic alteration is seen throughout the lobule in cholestasis from whatever cause, but the stagnation of bile, including electron-microscopically characteristic cytoplasmic deposits of either bile pigment or phospholipids, is in early cholestasis conspicuous in the centrolobular zone. The lesion is brought upon by pressure in mechanical obstruction, primarily extrahepatic and rarely intrahepatic, and by primary, presumably metabolic, processes in the other conditions without obstruction [1]. In the latter group, it may be the only alteration as it is produced regularly by anabolic steroids both in rodents and in man [20, 21], or it may be associated with alterations of other groups of organelles conventionally designated as hepatitis as it is seen in the various forms of viral, alcoholic and drug or chemical-induced hepatitis, as well as in cirrhosis. Electron microscopy does not detect a difference between the lesions produced by mechanical obstruction and the primary form of cholestasis. Also, liver function tests do not separate the two groups. The differential diagnosis is therefore not based on the functional or structural evaluation of the cholestasis, but rather on appreciation of accompanying features such as infections or type of liver cell damage, on etiology, or on the empiric knowledge of the evolution [22].

The Mechanism of Primary Intrahepatic Cholestasis

The mechanism or the metabolic basis of primary cholestasis, conventionally called the intrahepatic form, is not really established at this time and has been the subject of many hypotheses.

Dysfunction of smooth endoplasmic reticulum. Electron-microscopically, in all earlier forms of cholestasis the smooth endoplasmic reticulum of the hepatocytes is increased [23, 24]. This organelle is the site of microsomal biotransformation of many exogenous or endogenous substances, including the synthesis of cholesterol and its transformation to bile acids. Specifically, the 7-alpha-hydroxylation is required for the formation of the dihydroxy chenodeoxycholic acid (which depends upon the mixed function oxidase cytochrome P-450) [25, 26] and the 7-alpha, 12-alpha-hydroxylation in the synthesis of the trihydroxy cholic acid. Mitochondria also participate by cleaving side chains. The augmented endoplasmic reticulum in cholestasis may be related to the demonstrated increased lipoprotein and cholesterol synthesis [27] reflected in the cholesterol-rich abnormal lipoprotein X, which is of diagnostic significance in cholestasis in general [28].

Increase of the membranes of the smooth endoplasmic reticulum, as morphologically demonstrated, is, however, not necessarily associated with an increase of all biotransformation functions. Rather, in many instances, particularly under abnormal circumstances, the hypertrophic endoplasmic reticulum may be hypoactive in one or many enzymatic activities, as demonstrated in the dieldrin intoxication of the rat as well as in other models, including cholestasis [29]. It is therefore possible that the hydroxylation of cholesterol or bile acid precursors may be incomplete, to result in an excess of underhydroxylated bile acids, namely, monohydroxy bile acids, of which lithocholate is an example. This bile acid is formed as a secondary bile acid in the intestines by dehydroxylation by bacteria of the physiologic chenodeoxycholic acid. Several forms of monohydroxy bile acids, namely, lithocholic acid and 5-beta-cholenic acid [30, 31], have been found in excess in cholestasis. The possible damage from lithocholate acid has been emphasized already many years ago by Carey here in Minneapolis [32]. Indeed, experimental administration of lithocholate to experimental animals rapidly produces cholestasis both by functional [33] parameters and on ultrastructural appearance [34]. Di- and trihydroxy bile acids are essential in the formation of the polyionic aggregates of mixed micelles in which the bile acids are combined with cholesterol and phospholipids. These substances are thus carried in the bile and probably excreted into it. Monohydroxy bile acids, however, are poor micelle formers, which might result in liquid crystals. Therefore, it is possible that faulty hydroxylation of bile acids may lead to inadequate micelles in cholestasis, with resulting precipitation of bile in the form of plugs associated with structures looking like liquid crystals, composed of phospholipids, seen under the electron microscope both in the plugs and in the cytoplasm. This assumes that interference with the secretion of the bile acid-dependent fraction (which is the bile flow following meals amounting to approximately 1000 ml/day) is the initiating event in primary cholestasis. There is, however, in addition a much larger bile acid-independent fraction, approximately 5000 ml/day, of which the bulk is reabsorbed in the ductular system. Secretion of the bile acid-independent fraction depends upon a magnesium-requiring ATPase-dependent ion (sodium and potassium) pump. This is most probably located in the microvilli of the bile canaliculi, in analogy to the localization of ion pumps in other organs. Interference with the bile acid-independent fraction may lead to inspissation of bile in the canaliculus and in turn to precipitation. Both bile acid-independent and dependent fraction are inhibited by lithocholate, by sex and anabolic steroids, by dyes and drugs, particularly those inhibiting transport [36, 37]. It is today not decided which is the more important process in initiating cholestasis although it is established that at least in experimental circumstances hyperbilirubinemia will only result from interference with the bile acid-dependent fraction.

Mitochondrial and canalicular membrane injury. Hepatocellular mitochondria reveal in cholestasis a characteristic curling of their cristae and functional alteration, particularly the oxidative phosphorylation, is inhibited [27], and mitochondrial cytochrome activity is decreased [38]. Impaired energy release from excess of either bile acids or bilirubin in the mitochondria may affect all cytoplasmic processes but also the canalicular membrane, which as the site of the rate limitation of bile secretion [39] shows the morphologic expression of the disturbed function in cholestasis. This alteration is histochemically reflected in a loss of the characteristic ATPase reaction of the dilated canaliculi [40]. Chemical examination of biliary plasma membrane fractions shows a reduction of ATPase and 5-nucleotidase activity and increase in sialic acid, with the synthesis and breakdown rate of other components barely altered [41]. This membrane change is associated with disturbed micelle formation and with a shedding of canalicular membranes of different fatty acid content and reflected in the presence of the plugs containing granular bile pigment and phospholipid whorls mixed with each other.

The "vicious circle" in cholestasis. Thus, the centrolobular primary cholestatic process may be initiated by an altered bile acid metabolism from defective biotransformation in the smooth endoplasmic reticulum, or by a faulty bile acid-independent secretion in the microvilli, or in the mitochondria, or in the pericanalicular ectoplasm, or in the canalicular membrane itself, where prosthetic groups of steroids are known to disturb micelle formation, or in the lumen, where drugs like chlorpromazine may form insoluble complexes with bile salts. Thus, wherever the cholestatic process is initiated, it will induce secondary alterations in other organelles, for instance, the bile acid-dependent and independent secretion are coupled since the presence of ions in the lumen is probably required for secretion [36]. Moreover, intracellular accumulation of bilirubin and of bile acid has by itself a secondary cholestatic effect [42, 43] which is readily explained in the case of bile acids by their known detergent ability which damages all cellular organelles. This additional damage, particularly of the smooth endoplasmic reticulum, aggravates cholestasis with mutual reenforcement of the injury to set up a vicious circle [2] (Fig. 1). Thus, whatever the initial cause of the cholestasis, whether extrahepatic or intrahepatic, whether mechanical or metabolic, a secondary intrahepatic cholestasis is produced which in turn leads to a common pathway. The latter has the same functional manifestations and may terminate in the same type of hepatic failure; that particularly creates problems in the differential diagnosis by laboratory and histologic techniques.

Consequences of Cholestasis

While the initiation of the cholestasis remains problematic, the evolution of the common pathway, based on the detergent action of bile acids on organelle membranes and particularly on the endoplasmic

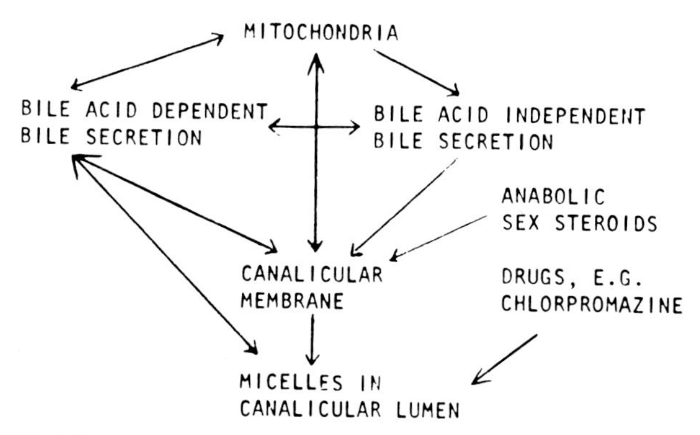

FIG. 1. Potential initial locations of centrolobular primary cholestasis.

reticulum, has been well worked out in in vitro studies as well as in investigations on experimental animals and man in both mechanical extrahepatic and drug-induced intrahepatic cholestasis [24, 44]. The P-450-dependent microsomal transformation system is especially vulnerable in that its synthesis is inhibited while degradation is only partially altered [45, 46]. In this detergent activity, dihydroxy bile acids have far greater effect than trihydroxy ones, and conjugated acids are more active than free ones in both inhibition of drug metabolism and in detergent activity. In rodents the detergent action is temporarily reduced by an alternate pathway of bile acid formation resulting in accumulation of less detergent bile acids [47].

In man, by contrast, initially trihydroxy cholic acid predominates in the liver, but eventually sufficient dihydroxy bile acids, primarily chenodeoxy cholic acid, accumulate to result not only in the inhibition of drug metabolism but also in hepatocellular injury expressed as reduction of specific enzyme activity [48]. The morphologic reflection of this detergent action is a vacuolization of the cytoplasm seen under the conventional microscopy and designated as feathery degeneration [49] and accumulation of characteristic whorls consisting of phospholipids in small cavities within the cytoplasm under the electron microscope. These changes of feathery degeneration correlate well with the dihydroxy bile acid concentration in human liver tissue obtained at operation [48]. This hepatocellular degeneration proceeding to biliary necrosis induces a reactive intralobular inflammation, again in both mechanical and primary cholestasis. This biliary hepatitis differs from other forms of hepatitis by the topographic relation to the cholestatic zone.

Prolonged cholestasis of any type is followed by inflammatory reaction in the portal tracts. The bile ductules proliferate, show alteration of cytoplasm and are surrounded by inflammatory infiltrate [50]. Lithocholic acid administration to animals, both in acute experiments as well as in chronic feedings, produces a bile-ductular reaction [51] which is electron-microscopically characterized by alteration of the ductular epithelial cells with morphologic evidence of reabsorption of irritating material into the periductular tissue. Persistence of this inflammatory exudate is followed by fibrosis and scarring resulting in compression with atrophy and eventually amputation of bile ductules. The periductular inflammation and particularly fibrosis thus interfere eventually with the bile flow and produce mechanical cholestasis on the periphery of the lobules which, in view of different degrees of inflammation, varies in intensity throughout the liver. Perilobular fibrosis resulting in septa formation may eventually lead to secondary biliary cirrhosis from prolonged mechanical obstruction, usually extrahepatic. There is little evidence that pure cholestasis without initial mechanical features leads to cirrhosis in adults, although apparently it does so in children. This peripheral inflammatory reaction just described is not necessarily relieved by surgical correction of prolonged extrahepatic biliary obstruction and is thus the reason why a sustained defect in biliary secretion often follows surgical restoration of the bile flow. It appears, in contrast to previous belief, that the "cholangiolitis" with periductular inflammation is not the mechanical initiating cause of centrolobular cholestasis. Rather, it is a late consequence of intrahepatic obstructive features.

The peripheral parenchymal cholestasis differs from the one seen in bile ductules and ducts, particularly at autopsy, in patients with liver disease with or without jaundice. This ductal cholestasis is sometimes associated with impressive biliary microcalculi and is the result of a terminal inspissation of bile in ductules and ducts by excessive reabsorption in stages of electrolyte imbalance without any correlation to the severity of jaundice.

Pure cholestasis. The described primary intrahepatic cholestasis on a metabolic basis may be the only lesion present [1, 2] as it is found in the neonatal period, particularly with pyloric stenosis [52] and hyperalimentation [53], in some infections in children especially involving the urinary tract, in recurrent benign familial cholestasis, in recurrent jaundice of pregnancy, and in pure drug cholestasis following, for instance, administration of steroids and exceptionally, contraceptive drugs. In many of the last mentioned instances genetic differences in sex steroid metabolism are assumed. Pure cholestasis is also exceptionally seen in viral hepatitis and has been observed in Hodgkin's disease without cellular infiltration of the liver, and even in metastatic carcinoma.

Cholestatic hepatitis. Pure cholestasis must be contrasted to the one in which it is associated with a mild degree of hepatitis which clinically and in laboratory findings may not be conspicuous but is recognized readily on liver biopsy. Examples of conditions best designated as cholestatic hepatitis are found in the vast majority of drug-induced forms of jaundice, for instance, the one following chlorpromazine, in some forms of viral hepatitis and even alcoholic hepatitis.

Hepatitis with cholestasis. Most instances of cholestasis, of course, are associated with various types of hepatitis in which lesions of organelle groups not related to biliary secretion are also present, that means the typical hepatitis and cirrhosis.

Cholestasis of unknown pathogenesis. There remains a group of conditions in which today the mechanism and even the etiology of cholestasis are unknown. This includes besides the recurrent benign cholestasis in adolescents and adults some hereditary forms in children (eg, Byler's disease) [54] which have a tendency to cirrhosis formation. Possibly genetic alterations of bile acid metabolisms are important. They include also the occasional postoperative, not mechanically explained, cholestasis, which is usually a multifactorial process in which shock, renal failure and hemolysis from blood transfusions may play a role.

Elevated Direct Reacting Bilirubin Without Cholestasis

Finally, brief reference should be made to the conditions in which elevated direct reacting bilirubin is present, although morphologically and biochemically, cholestasis is not demonstrable. One example is pure bile duct disease as it is found in early primary biliary cirrhosis, the stage of chronic nonsuppurative destructive cholangitis [55, 56]. Then, bile regurgitates through the destroyed bile duct walls without significant cholestasis. Initially, the bilirubin retention may be compensated for by increased excretion, and then, conspicuous itching and elevation of serum cholesterol as well as activities of alkaline phosphatase may be found in the absence of jaundice. Eventually, icterus may develop before histologic cholestasis is seen. Administration of cholestatic drugs in this early stage with or without jaundice leads regularly to centrolobular cholestasis with either appearance or deepening of jaundice. Only in later stages of primary biliary cirrhosis when significant, apparently reactive, inflammation and fibrosis of the portal tracts have developed, peripheral cholestasis sets in on a mechanical basis and is characteristically of different degree throughout the liver. In early bile duct disease the biochemical findings do not necessarily differ from that of real cholestasis.

Another group of conditions with elevated direct reacting bilirubin without cholestasis is represented by the Dubin-Johnson syndrome associated with pigmentation, and also the Rotor syndrome without pigment. The biliary secretion of organic anions with the exception of bile acid is specifically disturbed resulting in elevation of bilirubin and impaired excretion of test dyes, but not in elevation of alkaline phosphatase activities, of serum cholesterol, or of serum bile acids [57].

Summary

Contrary to the previous belief that cholestasis is a mechanical process in the biliary passages, its initial centrolobular stage is today considered a defect of specific hepatocellular organelles produced by pressure in mechanical obstruction and by metabolic processes in primary cholestasis and resulting in faulty hepatocellular bile secretion. The initial organelle site is not established, with the lesions of the smooth endoplasmic reticulum altering bile acid-dependent secretion a candidate and the membrane of the bile canaliculi a definite target. The interaction of the various organelle lesions results in a vicious cycle aggravated by the detergent action of bile acid retained in hepatocytes which in any type of cholestasis leads to a common pathway with the same functional features. It starts with hepatocellular injury and necrosis, continues with parenchymal and subsequently portal inflammation which eventually interferes mechanically with ductular bile flow and thus creates peripheral mechanical intrahepatic cholestasis. "Cholangiolitis" is a consequence rather than a cause of centrolobular cholestasis. Cholestasis thus resembles cholesterol gallstone disease, which was also previously considered a mechanical process and now is thought to be caused by altered hepatocellular function. These considerations have implications in prognosis and therapy, but less in differential diagnosis of cholestasis, which probably is today best established by physical devices, such as intrahepatic cholangiography or by endoscopic bile duct cannulation rather than by biochemical and histological techniques.

References

1. Popper, H.: Cholestasis. Ann. Rev. Med., 19:39-56, 1968.
2. Popper, H. and Schaffner, F.: Pathophysiology of cholestasis. Hum. Path., 1:1-24, 1970.
3. Herndon, J. H., Jr.: Pathophysiology of pruritus associated with elevated bile acid in serum. Arch. Int. Med., 130:632-637, 1972.
4. Stiehl, A.: Gallensaeuren und Gallensaeurensulfate in der Haut von Patienten mit Cholestase und Juckreiz. Z. Gastroent., 12:121-124, 1974.
5. Warren, K. W., Athaniassiades, S. and Monge, J. J.: Primary sclerosing cholangitis. A study of forty-two cases. Amer. J. Surg., 111:23, 1966.
6. Thorpe, M. E. G., Scheuer, P. H. and Sherlock, S.: Primary sclerosing cholangitis, the biliary tract and ulcerative colitis. Gut, 8:435, 1967.
7. Strauss, L. and Bernstein, J.: Neonatal hepatitis in congenital rubella. A histopathological study. Arch. Path., 86:317-327, 1968.
8. Cotton, P. B.: Cannulation of the papilla of Vater by endoscopy and retrograde cholangio-pancreatography. Gut, 13:1014, 1972.
9. Roessle, R.: Entzuendungen der Leber. *In* Henke, F. and Lubarsch, O. (eds.): Handbuch der Speziellen Pathologischen Anatomie und Histologie. Berlin: Springer Verlag, 1930, Vol. 5, Part 1, pp. 243-250.
10. Watson, W. J. and Hoffbauer, F. W.: Problem of prolonged hepatitis with particular reference to cholangiolitic type and to development of cholangiolitic cirrhosis of liver. Ann. Int. Med., 25:195-227, 1946.

11. Hanger, F. M. and Gutman, A. B.: Postarsphenamine jaundice apparently due to obstruction of intrahepatic biliary tract. JAMA, 115:263-271, 1940.
12. Popper, H. and Szanto, P. B.: Intrahepatic cholestasis ("cholangiolitis"). Gastroenterology, 31:683-699, 1956.
13. Herrold, K. M., Rabson, A. S. and Smith, R.: Involvement of the liver in generalized hypersensitivity reaction. Arch. Path., 66:306-310, 1958.
14. Schaffner, F. and Popper, H.: Morphologic studies of cholestasis. Gastroenterology, 37:565-573, 1959.
15. Steiner, J. W., Jezequel, A. M., Phillips, M. J. et al: Some aspects of the ultrastructural pathology of the liver. *In* Popper, H. and Schaffner, F. (eds.): Progress in Liver Diseases. New York:Grune & Stratton, Inc., 1965, Vol. II, pp. 307-372.
16. Biava, C. G.: Studies on cholestasis. A re-evaluation of the fine structure of normal human bile canaliculi. Lab. Invest., 13:840-864, 1964.
17. Miyai, K., Mayr, W. and Richardson, A.: Freeze fracture study of bile canalicular changes induced by lithocholic acid. Lab. Invest., 30:384, 1974.
18. Compagno, J. and Grisham, J. W.: Scanning electron microscopy of extrahepatic biliary obstruction. Arch. Path., 97:348, 1974.
19. Rouiller, C.: Les canalicules biliares: Etude au microscope electronique. Acta Anat., 26:94-109, 1956.
20. Schaffner, F., Popper, H. and Chesrow, E.: Cholestasis produced by the administration of norethandrolone. Amer. J. Med., 26:249, 1959.
21. Schaffner, F. and Kniffen, J. C.: Electron microscopy as related to hepatotoxicity. Ann. NY Acad. Sci., 104:847, 1963.
22. Desmet, V. J.: Morphologic and histochemical aspects of cholestasis. *In* Popper, H. and Schaffner, F. (eds.): Progress in Liver Diseases. New York:Grune & Stratton, 1972, Vol. IV, pp. 97-137.
23. Schaffner, F. and Popper, H.: Hypothesis. Cholestasis is the result of hypoactive hypertrophic smooth endoplasmic reticulum in the hepatocyte. Lancet, 2:355-359, 1969.
24. Schaffner, F., Bacchin, P. G., Hutterer, F. et al: Mechanism of cholestasis. 4. Structural and biochemical changes in the liver and serum in rats after bile duct ligation. Gastroenterology, 60:888-897, 1971.
25. Boyd, G. S., Grimwade, A. M. and Lawson, M. E.: Studies on rat-liver microsomal cholesterol 7-alpha-hydroxylase. Eur. J. Biochem., 37:334-340, 1973.
26. Boyd, G. S. and Percy-Robb, I. W.: Enzymatic regulation of bile acid synthesis. Amer. J. Med., 51:580, 1971.
27. Schersten, T.: Metabolic differences between hepatitis and cholestasis in human liver. *In* Popper, H. and Schaffner, F. (eds.): Progress in Liver Diseases. New York:Grune & Stratton, 1972, Vol. IV, pp. 133-150.
28. Seidel, D., Alaupovic, P. and Furman, R. H.: A lipoprotein characterizing obstructive jaundice. 1. Method for quantitative separation and identification of lipoproteins in jaundiced subjects. J. Clin. Invest., 48:1211, 1969.
29. Hutterer, F., Klion, F. M., Wengraf, A. et al: Hepatocellular adaptation and injury. Structural and biochemical changes following dieldrin and methyl butter yellow. Lab. Invest., 20:455-464, 1969.
30. Mankinio, I., Sjovall, J., Norman, A. et al: Excretion of 3-beta-hydroxy-5-cholenic and 3-alpha-hydroxy-5-alpha-cholanoic acids in urine of infants with

biliary atresia. FEBS Letters, 15:161, 1971.
31. Back, P.: Die primaere hepatische Synthese von Mono-Hydroxy-Gallensaeuren bei extrahepatischer Gallengangsatresie. Klin. Wschr., 51:926-932, 1973.
32. Carey, J. B., Jr., Wilson, I. D., Zaki, F. C. et al: The metabolism of bile acids with special reference to liver injury. Medicine, 45:461, 1966.
33. Javitt, N. B. and Emerman, S.: Effect of sodium taurolithocholate. J. Clin. Invest., 47:1002-1014, 1968.
34. Schaffner, F. and Javitt, N. B.: Morphologic changes in hamster liver during intrahepatic cholestasis induced by taurolithocholate. Lab. Invest., 15:1783-1792, 1966.
35. Erlinger, S.: Physiology of bile flow. *In* Popper, H. and Schaffner, F. (eds.): Progress in Liver Diseases. New York:Grune & Stratton, 1972, Vol. IV, pp. 63-82.
36. Erlinger, S. and Dhumean, D.: Mechanism and control of secretion of bile water and electrolytes. Gastroenterology, 66:281, 1974.
37. Horak, W., Grabner, G. and Paumgartner, G.: Inhibition of bile salt-independent bile formation by indocyanine green. Gastroenterology, 64:1005-1012, 1973.
38. Ozawa, K., Takasan, H., Kitamora, O. et al: Alteration in liver mitochondrial metabolism in a patient with biliary obstruction due to liver carcinoma. Amer. J. Surg., 126:653, 1973.
39. Mulder, J. G.: The rate limiting step in the biliary elimination of some substrates of uridine-diphosphate glucuronyl transferase in the rat. Biochem. Pharmacol., 22:1751, 1973.
40. Ronchi, G. and Desmet, V.: Histochemical study of so-called "marker enzymes of cholestasis" during extrahepatic bile duct obstruction in the rat. Beitr. Path. Anat., 149:213-226, 1973.
41. Simon, F. R. and Arias, I. M.: Alteration of bile canalicular enzymes in cholestasis. A possible cause of bile secretory failure. J. Clin. Invest., 52:765-775, 1973.
42. Boyce, W. and Witzleben, C. L.: Bilirubin as a cholestatic agent. II. Effect of variable doses of bilirubin on the severity of manganese-bilirubin cholestasis. Amer. J. Path., 72:427, 1973.
43. Ronchi, G. and Desmet, V. J.: Histochemical study of gamma glutamyl transpeptidase (GGT) in experimental intrahepatic and extrahepatic cholestasis. Beitr. Path. Anat., 150:316-321, 1973.
44. Denk, H., Schenkman, J. B., Bacchin, P. G. et al: Mechanism of cholestasis. 3. Interaction of synthetic detergents with the microsomal cytochrome P-450 dependent biotransformation system in vitro. A comparison between the effects of detergents, the effects of bile acids, and the findings in bile duct ligated rats. Exp. Molec. Path., 14:263-276, 1971.
45. Denk, H., Greim, H., Hutterer, F. et al: Turnover of hepatic cytochrome P-450 in experimental cholestasis. Exp. Molec. Path., 19:241-247, 1973.
46. Mackinnon, A. M. and Simon, F. R.: Reduced synthesis of hepatic microsomal cytochrome P-450 in the bile duct ligated rat. Biochem. Biophys. Res. Commun., 56:437, 1974.
47. Greim, H., Trulzsch, D., Roboz, J. et al: Mechanism of cholestasis. 5. Bile acids in normal rat livers and in those after bile duct ligation. Gastroenterology, 63:837-845, 1972.
48. Greim, H., Trulzsch, D., Czygan, P. et al: Mechanism of cholestasis. 6. Bile acids

in human livers with or without biliary obstruction. Gastroenterology, 63:846-850, 1972.

49. Gall, E. A. and Dabrogorski, O.: Hepatic alterations in obstructive jaundice. Amer. J. Clin. Path., 41:126-139, 1964.
50. Sasaki, H., Schaffner, F. and Popper, H.: Bile ductules in cholestasis: Morphologic evidence for secretion and absorption in man. Lab. Invest., 16:84-95, 1967.
51. Hunt, F. D. and Leveille, G. A.: Dietary bile acids and lipid metabolism. III. Effects of lithocholic acid in mammalian species. Proc. Soc. Exp. Biol. Med., 115:277-280, 1964.
52. Levine, G., Favara, B. E., Mierau, G. et al: Jaundice, liver structure and congenital pyloric studies. Arch. Path., 95:267, 1973.
53. Touloukian, R. J. and Downing, S. E.: Cholestasis associated with long term parenteral hyperalimentation. Arch. Surg., 106:58, 1973.
54. Clayton, R. J., Iber, S. L., Reubner, B. H. et al: Byler disease. Fatal familial intrahepatic cholestasis in an Amish kindred. Amer. J. Dis. Child., 117:112-124, 1969.
55. Rubin, E., Schaffner, F. and Popper, H.: Primary biliary cirrhosis. Chronic nonsuppurative destructive cholangitis. Amer. J. Path., 46:387-407, 1965.
56. Sherlock, S. and Scheuer, P. J.: The presentation and diagnosis of 100 patients with primary biliary cirrhosis. New Eng. J. Med., 289:674-678, 1973.
57. Gartner, L. and Arias, I. M.: Formation, transport, metabolism and excretion of bilirubin. New Eng. J. Med., 280:1339-1345, 1969.

Alcoholic Hepatitis in the Context of Alcoholic Liver Disease

Leslie Zieve, M.D.

The association of alcohol and liver disease is common knowledge. The occurrence of the liver damage is dependent upon three factors: the total dose of alcohol ingested over a specific time interval, the susceptibility of the individual to the toxic effects of alcohol and, to some extent, the type of beverage ingested. The correlation between the death rate from cirrhosis and the population's consumption of alcoholic beverages is approximately 0.70. During prohibition from 1916 to 1932, the death rate from cirrhosis dropped precipitously in this country from 12 to 7 per 100,000. Following repeal, the death rate has climbed steadily and at present is approaching 15 per 100,000. The importance of individual susceptibility to the effects of alcohol is indicated by the fact that only 1 of 12 heavy alcoholics develops cirrhosis. The exact reason for this low incidence is unknown. Intermittence of drinking may play a significant role.

The three types of alcoholic liver disease are fatty liver, alcoholic hepatitis and cirrhosis, usually portal or Laennec's cirrhosis. Though listed as distinct types of abnormalities, all three lesions may be, and in fact are often, present at the same time in a given patient. The kinds of mixtures one expects and finds are shown in the diagram of Figure 1. One or another of these lesions may predominate in any given patient or may be present alone. Usually more than one lesion is present in biopsy or autopsy specimens, and all three lesions may be present in a given liver specimen quite frequently.

Since portal cirrhosis resulting from chronic alcoholism is a familiar entity, I will focus in this paper primarily on fatty liver and alcoholic hepatitis, with particular emphasis on the latter.

Leslie Zieve, M.D., Department of Medicine, Minneapolis Veterans Hospital; University of Minnesota School of Medicine, Minneapolis.

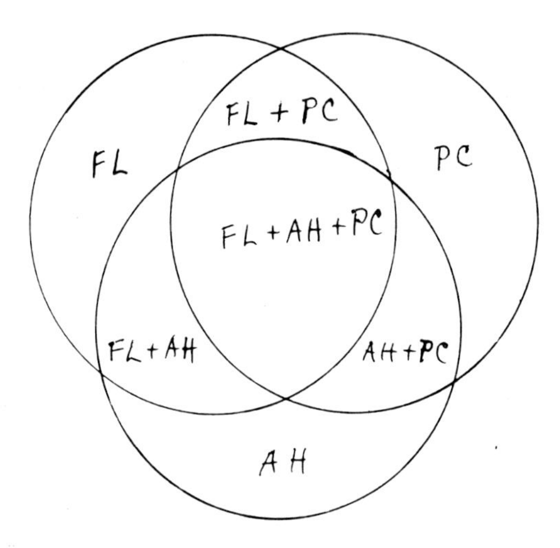

FIG. 1. Diagrammatic representation of the interlocking nature of fatty liver, alcoholic hepatitis and portal cirrhosis.

Fatty Liver as a Base of Reference

All cases of fatty metamorphosis may be subdivided into those related to alcoholism and those not related to alcoholism. In the latter category would be included patients with malnutrition, burns, diabetes, obesity, toxic hepatitis, etc. Of the two broad groups, the alcoholic fatty liver cases are most abundant in this country [1-5].

Alcoholic fatty liver may be classified as in Table 1. Before characterizing each of the categories listed, it will be useful to briefly summarize a composite picture of the manifestations of acute alcoholic liver disease in which fatty infiltration predominates. The *general clinical* symptoms are malaise, weakness, weight loss, fever, anorexia, nausea, vomiting and sometimes diarrhea. Occasionally, chilliness and cough will be associated with the fever. Pain in the upper abdomen, either in the epigastrium or the right upper quadrant, is often prominent. It may be severe. The patient is tremulous if drinking has persisted to the day or two before hospitalization, and signs of vitamin deficiency may be apparent. Tissue or blood levels of vitamins are usually reduced.

The more *specific clinical* findings are an enlarged liver, which is often tender, and jaundice, which is quite variable. It may be prominent and is sometimes absent. Splenomegaly is infrequent unless cirrhosis coexists. When it is present, it is not prominent. Edema may be present and often develops insidiously. Ascites is infrequent. Portal pressure is often increased and esophageal varices are occasionally present. The varices,

Table 1. Classification of Alcoholic Fatty Liver (F. L.)

1. Simple F. L. with hyperlipidemia or anemia.
2. Simple F. L. without hyperlipidemia or anemia.
3. F. L. with sudden death.
4. F. L. with concurrent severe alcoholic hepatitis.
5. F. L. with concurrent mild or moderate alcoholic hepatitis.
6. F. L. with concurrent cirrhosis, the fatty liver predominating.
7. F. L. with concurrent cirrhosis, the cirrhosis predominating.

when present, characteristically recede as the fat is mobilized. Rarely, bleeding from varices will occur with severe fatty liver in the absence of cirrhosis. Spider naevi are seen infrequently. As a rule once these patients are hospitalized improvement is rapid.

Certain *nonspecific laboratory* abnormalities are commonly seen in these patients. Anemia is frequent. It may be nutritional or hemolytic in origin. Often both factors are involved. Folic acid deficiency is common. Hemolysis is not due to hypersplenism. Leukocytosis and an increased sedimentation rate are the rule. The platelets are low at first, but then increase sharply in numbers so that supernormal values are temporarily seen within a few days. The serum lipids are generally increased to some extent and are sometimes very high. Serum protein concentration is often abnormal, albumin being reduced and the globulins elevated. The blood urea nitrogen is commonly low because of poor protein intake during the alcoholic episodes. The blood sugar is often increased, but on rare occasions may be decreased. Albuminuria is transient.

More *specific laboratory* abnormalities are observed with liver function tests. The most sensitive index of abnormality is the sulfobromophthalein (BSP) retention test. Its abnormality reflects a decrease in hepatic blood flow. The serum bilirubin concentration is commonly but variably abnormal. The serum transaminase activity is generally abnormal but rarely in proportion to the hepatic cell abnormality. Values are usually less than 200 units/100 ml. Serum alkaline phosphatase activity is often increased and occasionally high. The prothrombin concentration may be transiently reduced.

Variations in the Clinical Syndromes Associated With Fatty Liver

F. L. With Hyperlipidemia and Anemia [6]

This syndrome probably occurs in individuals having an intense alcoholic episode following a period of relative abstinence. The general symptoms, previously described, are prominent. Abdominal pain is also a prominent complaint. The liver is usually very much enlarged, and jaundice is often present. Fluid retention is probably common. The bone marrow shows normoblastic hyperplasia and the blood its associated peripheral changes. Frank lipemia is common, and all the serum lipids are elevated. The serum proteins are often normal, but at times the serum albumin is low. The BUN is usually low. Liver function is only slightly and transiently deranged; however, the alkaline phosphatase is typically elevated. Improvement after the cessation of drinking is rapid.

Detailed illustrative examples of this entity will be found in the literature [6]. The following four very brief sketches indicate some of the variations that may be seen. The biopsy of Figure 2A was obtained during the second week of hospitalization. The patient was a 26-year-old man with severe abdominal pain, malaise, weakness, chilliness, cough and pleural pain. Chest x-ray was normal. His serum bilirubin was 16.8 and cholesterol 720 mg/100 ml. The alkaline phosphatase was 24 KA units.

The biopsy of Figure 2B was obtained from a 35-year-old man during the third week after hospitalization. He was very tremulous and had a serum bilirubin of 43 mg/100 ml. His cholesterol was 530 mg/100 ml and alkaline phosphatase 25 KA units. Figure 2C shows a biopsy obtained from a 35-year-old man during the second week after admission to the hospital. He was not jaundiced, but had edema and ascites. His serum albumin was 2.1 gm, serum bilirubin 1.5 mg, cholesterol 984 mg and BUN 3 mg/100 ml. A serum alkaline phosphatase was 34 KA units. Improvement was very rapid.

The biopsy of Figure 2D was obtained from a 42-year-old man during the first week after admission to the hospital. He was relatively asymptomatic by the time of hospitalization. He was not jaundiced and his serum alkaline phosphatase was normal. However, his serum was milky, the total lipids exceeding 8000, triglycerides 5000, phospholipids 2100 and cholesterol 1100 mg/100 ml. His improvement was rapid, and within three weeks the serum lipid concentrations were normal.

F. L. Without Hyperlipidemia or Anemia

This is an illness of more gradual onset and less prominent manifestations. Vague upper abdominal distress and unexplained hepatomegaly focus attention on the liver. Jaundice is slight or absent. Improvement is rapid.

F. L. With Sudden Death

This complication is very rare if one excludes patients with delirium tremens who die suddenly. The reason for the unexpected and sudden

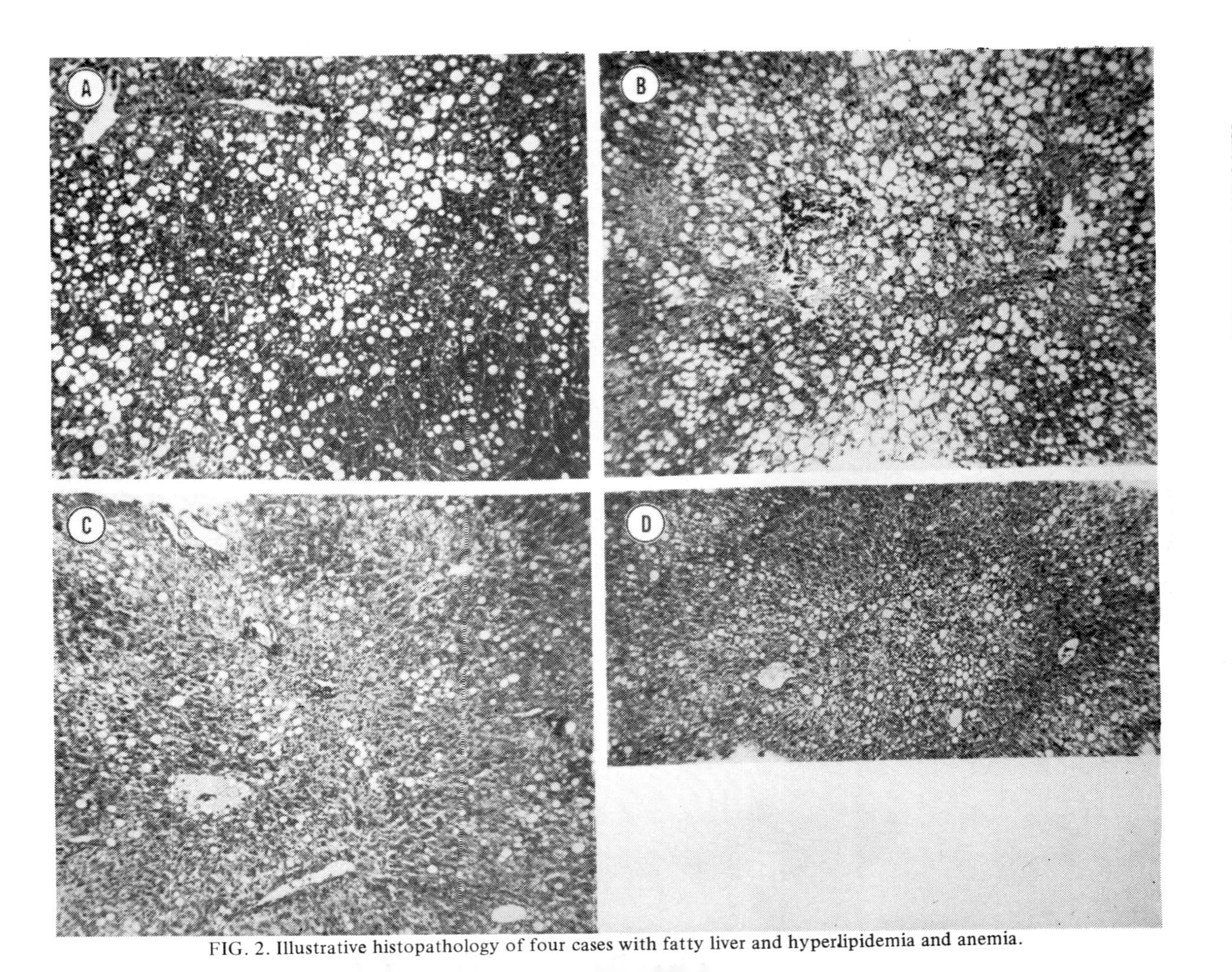

FIG. 2. Illustrative histopathology of four cases with fatty liver and hyperlipidemia and anemia.

death is unknown, though possibly, as in delirium tremens, a cardiac arrhythmia is the cause. Fat embolism has been suspected, however typical fat emboli are not found in the brain.

F. L. With Concurrent Severe Alcoholic Hepatitis and Acute Hepatic Insufficiency [7-9]

One sees a rapidly progressive course in an alcoholic with a large fatty liver. Hepatic coma and death usually ensue within one to two weeks. A few may recover slowly. Characteristically these patients show widespread lesions of alcoholic hepatitis. Coexisting cirrhosis is common but not necessary. Complicating illness, particularly infection with bacteremia, often precipitates the terminal event.

Persistent fever and leukocytosis are striking. Sometimes a leukemoid blood picture is seen. Jaundice is usually prominent and may appear obstructive in nature. It may however be absent. The patients complain of abdominal pain and tenderness. The liver is enlarged in almost all cases, the spleen in about one half. Liver function is severely deranged. Transaminase elevations are not consistent with the degree of liver cell necrosis. Serum values are usually under 250 units/100 ml, though occasionally they may exceed 1000. Ascites, gastrointestinal bleeding and azotemia are frequent. Hepatic coma is the usual terminal event. An example of the histopathology observed in a subacute case that died in hepatic coma after several weeks of hospitalization is shown in Figure 3. A few patients may recover, but slowly. Those that recover usually show a rapid transition to cirrhosis if it does not already exist [10, 11].

F. L. With Concurrent Mild or Moderate Alcoholic Hepatitis [7-9, 12-15]

These patients have fatty infiltration, focal hepatic cell necrosis with polymorphonuclear infiltration and Mallory's hyaline degeneration. Bile duct stasis and bile duct proliferation are also often seen. The extent of each of these abnormalities is highly variable. Cirrhosis may also be present. The acute process subsides gradually, usually over a period of one to three months. Thus the improvement is not so dramatic as with simple fatty liver. After hospitalization, the patient may show no improvement, or may appear to get worse for a month or two, before improvement begins. Sometimes the course is prolonged.

The primary complaints of the patients are anorexia, weakness, weight loss, nausea, vomiting and abdominal pain. Less frequently they will have fever and chills, diarrhea and paresthesias. Occasionally they will present

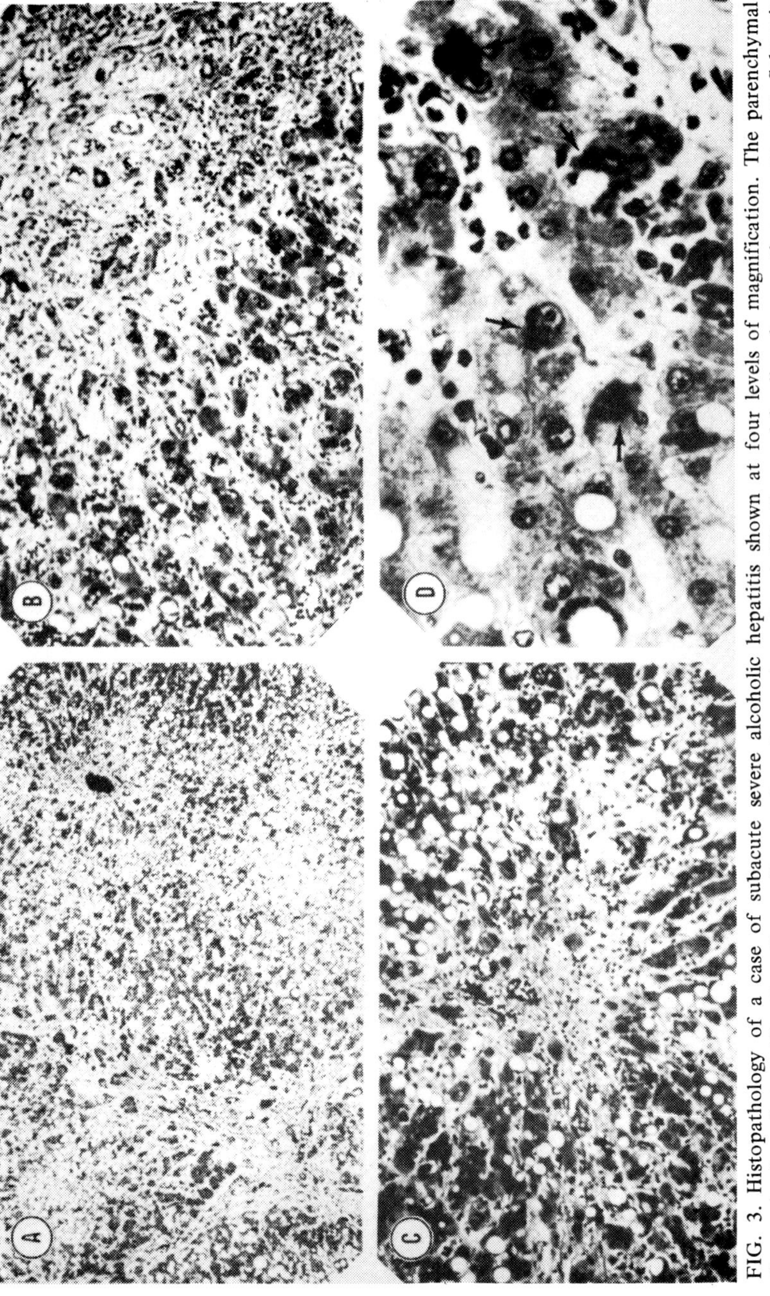

FIG. 3. Histopathology of a case of subacute severe alcoholic hepatitis shown at four levels of magnification. The parenchymal disorganization, fatty infiltration, liver cell necrosis, polymorphonuclear infiltration and hyaline degeneration are apparent. Sclerosis about a central vein is apparent in section C. A few of the many Mallory bodies are marked by small arrows in the high-power section D.

with hematemesis or melena. A persistent low grade fever and leukocytosis in the range of 10-30 thousand are common. Jaundice is frequent but variable in intensity. It may appear obstructive in type, and often gets worse after hospitalization before improvement begins. The liver is uniformly enlarged, but the spleen is generally not prominent and often not palpable. Ascites and edema are seen in about one half of the cases, usually those in whom cirrhosis coexists. One or more peripheral signs of liver disease such as vascular spiders, palmer erythema, gynecomastia, parotid gland enlargement or Dupuytren's contractures occur in about one half of the cases. Peripheral neuropathy and mental confusion may each be seen about 20% of the time. Liver function is abnormal but highly variable in the degree of abnormality. The serum lipids are normal or elevated. Pancreatitis occurs in about one fourth the cases. Anemia is common because of gastrointestinal bleeding, folic acid deficiency or hemolysis. The combination of jaundice, hyperlipidemia and hemolytic anemia may be seen in as many as one fourth of the cases if looked for.

This category may be illustrated briefly by two moderately severe cases. Though of approximately equivalent severity one died after 21 days of hospitalization and the other improved slowly. The patient who recovered was a 48-year-old man hospitalized with chills and fever and upper abdominal pain. His nutrition was poor. He was weak and anorexic and had recurrent nausea and vomiting. His liver was large, but the spleen tip was just palpable. His hemoglobin dropped from 11.8 to 7.7 gm/100 ml, but stool guaiacs were negative. The white count was 15,000 cells/mm^3. His serum albumin at its lowest was 1.5 gm/100 ml. Serum cholesterol was 276 mg/100 ml and alkaline phosphatase 80 KA units. The first serum bilirubin was approximately 24 mg/100 ml and transaminase (SGOT) 80 units/100 ml. A prothrombin time was 19 seconds and was not corrected with vitamin K. The earliest that a liver biopsy could be attempted was 80 days after admission. The histopathology at that time is shown in Figure 4A and B. The patient was febrile for 40 days, the highest temperature being 101°F. His white cell count rose to a peak of 23,000 cells/mm^3 and was not yet normal by the 100th day. The serum bilirubin rose to a peak of 31 mg/100 ml by the 15th day and was still over 10 mg/100 ml at the 40th day. At that time the alkaline phosphatase still exceeded 80 KA units. The transaminase was normal by the 20th day and never exceeded 240 units/100 ml. The patient was discharged after 100 days, markedly improved but still quite ill.

The second patient deteriorated progressively and died after 21 days of hospitalization, with liver damage (Fig. 4C and D) similar in extent to that

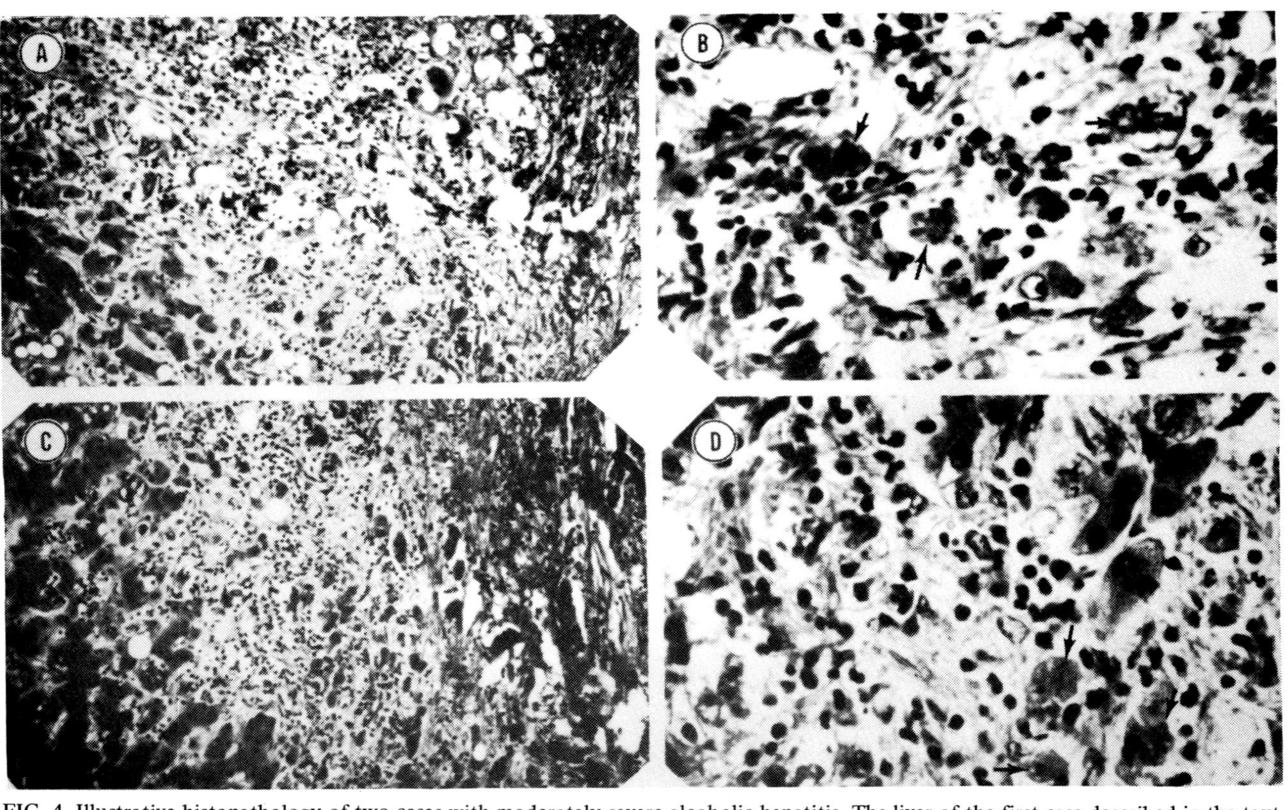

FIG. 4. Illustrative histopathology of two cases with moderately severe alcoholic hepatitis. The liver of the first case described in the text is shown in sections A and B, the second case in C and D. The lesions are similar to that shown in Figure 3. In B and D some of the Mallory bodies are indicated by arrows.

of the first case. This patient was an obese 50-year-old man who complained of chills, fever and severe itching. He was markedly jaundiced and his liver was very large. A foot drop was apparent. His hemoglobin was 12 gm/100 ml and white cell count 12,500 cells/mm^3. The serum bilirubin was 24 mg/100 ml, alkaline phosphatase 40 KA units and transaminase 82 units/100 ml. A urine amylase was normal. The serum albumin was 1.8 and globulin 6.7 gm/100 ml. The prothrombin time was 17.2 seconds. Surgery for obstructive jaundice was contemplated on the sixth day but deferred. The patient's temperature dropped to normal from an initial value of 102°F. The white count peaked at 21,000 and was approximately 14,000 cells/mm^3 by the 20th day. Over the 20-day period that the patient lived, the serum bilirubin rose to 31 mg/100 ml, the alkaline phosphatase rose to 60 KA units and the transaminase dropped to 30 units/100 ml. The patient died in hepatic coma on the 21st day. Despite this short clinical course his hepatic damage at autopsy was similar in extent to the group of cases that usually recover. He thus exemplifies the borderline between the severe and moderately severe cases.

F. L. With Concurrent Cirrhosis,
the Fatty Infiltration Predominating [4]

Such cases are commonly seen in general hospitals. Fatty liver is no longer believed to be causally related to cirrhosis though the two abnormalities often coexist and fatty infiltration usually precedes the development of cirrhosis in the alcoholic. On the basis of chemical analyses, Galambos and Shapira [16] found significantly increased fibroblast activity in alcoholic hepatitis but not in simple fatty liver.

The development and progression of the cirrhosis is usually gradual over a period of years. The manifestations of the illness are similar to those outlined earlier in the composite picture, except that the onset and recovery are slower, the functional abnormalities are more severe and persistent, and the signs of portal hypertension become more prominent. The more severe the cirrhosis, the less the lipogenic response in the liver and the less frequently the serum lipids will be found increased.

F. L. With Concurrent Cirrhosis,
the Cirrhosis Predominating [4]

These patients have well-developed cirrhosis, but fatty infiltration recurs as they persist with their drinking. The clinical and laboratory findings reflect the cirrhotic process primarily. Such cases comprise a large segment of the patients with liver disease who come to autopsy in our city hospitals.

Alcoholic Hepatitis as the Base of Reference

Though the base of reference until now has been the fatty liver, discussion has been unavoidably involved with alcoholic hepatitis and cirrhosis. Similarly when alcoholic hepatitis is the base of reference, the same sort of involvement with fatty liver and cirrhosis is unavoidable. The concept of alcoholic hepatitis as an entity is still evolving despite the fact that as long ago as 1911 Mallory delineated a specific hepatic lesion as a toxic effect of alcohol [17]. The concept has different meanings to different students of the subject, as one can judge from the variety of names that have been used to refer to the same phenomenon. The essential lesion of alcoholic hepatitis, steatonecrosis, florid cirrhosis, progressive alcoholic cirrhosis, acute hepatic insufficiency of the chronic alcoholic, fatty liver with hepatic failure in alcoholics and sclerosing hyaline necrosis [18] are one and the same. The differences among patients described under these various names have been due to (1) the acuteness or chronicity of the injury to the hepatic cell, (2) the severity and extent of the injury, (3) the nature of a preexisting hepatic abnormality and (4) the nature of concurrent hepatic changes not due to this specific injury.

All of these entities have in common certain hepatic changes that may be considered the *defining characteristics of alcoholic hepatitis:*

1. Hepatic cell necrosis, usually focal but may be diffuse.
2. Reactive inflammation with polymorphonuclear cell infiltration.
3. Hyaline degeneration with formation of Mallory bodies.
4. Parenchymal disorganization.

No information as to the specific cause of this lesion in man is available, except that alcoholism is important. Rubin and Lieber [19] have recently shown that alcoholic hepatitis and cirrhosis may be produced in baboons fed a nutritious diet containing 18% of calories as protein and 50% of calories as alcohol. The lesions, including Mallory bodies, developed over periods of nine months to four years.

The Mallory body is an insoluble protein complex that appears to be made up of cytoplasmic debris. It is usually found in association with alcoholism, however occasionally, perhaps 5% of the time, it is seen in a context other than alcoholic hepatitis.

Some Generalizations About Alcoholic Hepatitis

This is an entity that cuts across the spectrums of fatty liver and cirrhosis (Fig. 1). Though seen most often in a fatty or cirrhotic liver, it

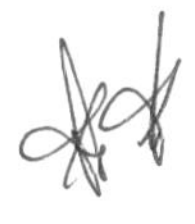

may be present alone. It is important to recognize as a distinct entity, even when seen in fatty or cirrhotic livers, because it is the lesion that largely accounts for the severity, duration and outcome of the patient's illness during its acute phases. It is much more important than fatty infiltration in the development of cirrhosis. Had we paid more attention to Mallory's observations recorded in 1911 and focused less on whether the Mallory body was or was not due to alcohol alone, we would not have waited until the 1960s to put this lesion in its proper perspective.

Most published reports have suggested that alcoholic hepatitis is a grave, rapidly progressive entity. This is undoubtedly a matter of selection [20]. Since there is no pathognomonic basis for a clinical diagnosis, liver tissue must be examined to establish the diagnosis. Therefore, two views of the entity may be seen, depending upon the source of the histologic material, biopsy or autopsy. Both must be studied, as was done by Zimmerman and his colleagues [9], in order to understand all the variations to be seen. The biopsied cases can never be severe, because of the risk of the biopsy in such patients. The converse is generally true of the autopsied cases. Thus, it is important to look at both. There is surprisingly little difference between the biopsied and autopsied groups with respect to the severity of a given focal lesion. However, the extent and diffuseness of the lesions are greater in the autopsied cases. Mallory bodies are more profuse, fatty infiltration more extensive, necrosis and surrounding inflammation more widespread and cholestasis more prominent.

The clinical course of patients with alcoholic hepatitis is highly variable, so it is important to think of this entity as a spectrum of changes of varying severity having in common a specific histologic alteration. The Mallory body, which occurs almost exclusively in alcoholics, is a handle on which to hinge the entity. As with alcoholic fatty liver and cirrhosis, there is no specific therapy for these cases. Steroids have been tried, but their effectiveness is doubtful [20-22]. Careful nutritional support and patience are essentially what the doctor has to offer, and the latter is most important.

References

1. Goldberg, M. and Thompson, C. M.: Acute fatty metamorphosis of the liver. Ann. Intern. Med., 55:416-432, 1961.
2. Leevy, C. M.: Fatty liver: A study of 270 patients with biopsy proven fatty liver and a review of the literature. Medicine, 41:249-276, 1962.
3. Isselbacher, K. J. and Alpers, D. H.: Fatty liver: Biochemical and clinical aspects. *In* Schiff, L. (ed.): Diseases of the Liver. Philadelphia: J. B. Lippincott Co., 1969, pp. 672-688.

4. Popper, H. and Schaffner, F.: Liver: Structure and Function, New York: McGraw-Hill Book Co., 1957, pp. 503-519.
5. Brodus, S., Korn, R. J., Chomet, B. et al: Hepatic function and serum enzyme levels in association with fatty metamorphosis of the liver. Amer. J. Med. Sci., 246:35-41, 1963.
6. Zieve, L.: Jaundice, hyperlipemia, and hemolytic anemia. A heretofore unrecognized syndrome associated with alcoholic fatty liver and cirrhosis. Ann. Intern. Med., 48:471-496, 1958.
7. Phillips, G. B. and Davidson, C. S.: Acute hepatic insufficiency of the chronic alcoholic. Arch. Intern. Med., 94:585-603, 1954.
8. Zimmerman, H. J.: The evolution of alcoholic cirrhosis. Clinical, biochemical and histologic correlations. Med. Clin. N. Amer., 39:241-259, 1955.
9. Harinasuta, U., Chomet, B., Ishak, K. et al: Steatonecrosis – Mallory body type. Medicine, 46:141-162, 1966.
10. Popper, H., Szanto, P. B. and Parthasarathy, M.: Florid cirrhosis. A review of 35 cases. Amer. J. Clin. Path., 25:889-901, 1955.
11. Popper, H., Szanto, P. B. and Elias, H.: Transition of fatty liver to cirrhosis. Gastroenterology, 28:183-192, 1955.
12. Green, J., Mistilis, S. and Schiff, L.: Acute alcoholic hepatitis. A clinical study of fifty cases. Arch. Intern. Med., 112:67-78, 1963.
13. Lischner, M. W., Alexander, J. F. and Galambos, J. T.: Natural history of alcoholic hepatitis. I. The acute disease. Amer. J. Dig. Dis., 16:481-494, 1971.
14. Alexander, J. F., Lischner, M. W. and Galambos, J. T.: Natural history of alcoholic hepatitis. II. The long-term prognosis. Amer. J. Gastroent., 56:515-525, 1971.
15. Galambos, J. T.: Natural history of alcoholic hepatitis. III. Histological changes. Gastroenterology, 63:1026-1035, 1972.
16. Galambos, J. T. and Shapira, R.: Natural history of alcoholic hepatitis. IV. Glycosaminoglycuronans and collagen in the hepatic connective tissue. J. Clin. Invest., 52:2952-2962, 1973.
17. Mallory, F. B.: Cirrhosis of the liver: Five different types of lesions from which it may arise. Bull. Hopkins Hosp., 22:69-75, 1911.
18. Edmondson, H. A., Peters, R. L., Reynolds, T. B. et al: Sclerosing hyaline necrosis of the liver in the chronic alcoholic. Ann. Intern. Med., 59:646-673, 1963.
19. Rubin, E. and Lieber, C. S.: Fatty liver, alcoholic hepatitis and cirrhosis produced by alcohol in primates. New Eng. J. Med., 290:128-135, 1974.
20. Galambos, J. T.: Alcoholic hepatitis: Its therapy and prognosis. Progr. Liver Dis., 4:567-588, 1972.
21. Helman, R. A., Temko, M. H., Nye, S. W. et al: Alcoholic hepatitis. Natural history and evaluation of prednisolone therapy. Ann. Intern. Med., 74:311-321, 1971.
22. Porter, H. P., Simon, F. R., Pope, C. E. et al: Corticosteroid therapy in severe alcoholic hepatitis. A double-blind drug trial. New Eng. J. Med., 284:1350-1355, 1971.

Hepatic Changes Associated With Obesity and Jejuno-Ileal Bypass

Henry Buchwald, M.D.

Liver failure following jejuno-ileal bypass surgery for management of marked morbid exogenous obesity has recently been given considerable attention in the medical literature. Some of these reports have been sensationalistic in intent and not erudite in effort. I will present a compilation of the available scientific data in this field. These data demonstrate that obesity per se is associated with fatty metamorphosis of the liver and that only about 5% of post jejuno-ileal bypass operation patients progress to liver failure.

At the outset, the jejuno-ileal bypass operation for obesity must be clearly differentiated from the partial ileal bypass procedure for the hyperlipidemias. The jejuno-ileal bypass operation, in which the most proximal jejunum is anastomosed to a small segment of terminal ileum, attempts alleviation of morbid exogenous obesity. With better than 90% of the small intestine bypassed, the therapeutic goal is weight loss. Lipid reduction is a valuable and accompanying benefit. The partial ileal bypass operation short-circuits only the distal 200 cm, or one-third the small intestinal length, whichever is longer. The partial ileal bypass procedure does not cause significant weight reduction nor is it ever associated with fatty infiltration of the liver.

An understanding of the post jejuno-ileal bypass liver changes can best be gained by examining the liver changes associated with obesity. Fatty liver changes have characteristically been associated with malnutrition and protein deficiency syndromes, eg, Kwashiorkor and alcoholism. Ironically, morbidly obese animals and humans have fatty livers as well. Brobeck [1] has shown that the obesity produced by hypothalamic ablation, in various animal species, causes fatty liver degeneration. Fenton and Chase [2] inbred congenitally obese mice and produced an hereditary form of fatty

---

Henry Buchwald, M.D., Associate Professor, Department of Surgery, University of Minnesota Medical School, Minneapolis.

liver damage. The relationship of a weight 100 pounds, or greater, above age and sex norms and the existence of fatty liver infiltration has been examined in several series of individuals who were not considered for jejuno-ileal bypass. Berkowitz [3] studied 100 patients, 20 of whom underwent liver biopsy: 76% of the total number had an abnormal BSP test and 18% had an elevated alkaline phosphatase level; all of the patients who underwent liver biopsy had fatty livers and occasionally evidence of cirrhosis was seen. Westwater and Fainer [4] found that 11 of their 12 patients who underwent liver biopsy had fatty livers and 13 of the total 14 patients in their series had abnormal BSP tests. All of Zellman's [5] 20 individuals had abnormal BSP tests; of the 19 who underwent liver biopsy, 53% demonstrated fatty degeneration, 47% pigment retention and 47% fibrosis. Finally, Rozental and associates [6] did not demonstrate abnormal BSP tests in five individuals; all five, however, had fatty livers on biopsy. It is interesting to note that after starvation management, four of these five patients developed fibrosis and three of the five developed focal necrosis of the liver. Thus, 50% to 100% of the obese patients in these studies had fatty hepatic changes, and subsequent to starvation for weight reduction, further histological deterioration occurred.

The cause of fatty metamorphosis of the liver in obese individuals is not well understood. Paradoxically, the hepatotoxicity may be related to a relative protein deficiency. Within the confines of this hypothesis, it would be logical to assume that a further reduction in protein intake or absorption would accentuate the fatty changes and, possibly, induce additional pathological findings.

The relationship of further fatty metamorphosis of the liver to the jejuno-ileal bypass operation for morbid obesity was first described by Payne [7] in 1963. Subsequent workers in the field (Scott [8] and others) have repeatedly published similar observations. Of urgent concern to the medical community, at a time when jejuno-ileal bypass surgery is becoming more common, are the answers to the following questions: (1) What is the type and extent of liver damage in morbidly obese patients at the time of bypass? (2) How are the histological characteristics of the liver affected during the period of rapid weight reduction (the first year or so after operation)? (3) How does bypass-induced weight reduction affect hepatic architecture after weight stabilization (two years or so after bypass)? These questions can be answered properly only by the performance of serial liver biopsies in a sufficient number of patients after initial intra-operative biopsies in all patients.

Let me address myself to the first question – liver pathology at the time of jejuno-ileal bypass, ie, prior to any associated effects of the bypass procedure itself. Our current jejuno-ileal bypass series includes 300 patients, and in 1973 we reported on the intra-operative liver biopsies in 77 consecutive patients [9]. The liver biopsy specimen from each patient was graded in the following manner: I = normal architecture, II = minimal fatty metamorphosis (less than 25%), III = moderate fatty metamorphosis (25%-50%), IV = severe fatty metamorphosis (greater than 50%) and V = the presence of fibrosis. Twenty-eight of the patients (36%) had normal liver architecture (grade I), 24 (31%) were graded II, 9 (12%) grade III, 16 (21%) grade IV, and no patient exhibited fibrosis (grade V). There were only 11 males in this series of 77 patients; yet, of the 16 patients with severe changes (grade IV), five were males. This represents 46% of the total males in the series, in comparison to the 17% of females (11 of 66) with severe fatty changes. To this time, we have yet to perform a jejuno-ileal bypass operation on a man with normal hepatic architecture. We also demonstrated a linear correlation of the degree of overweight with the severity of the liver findings. Representative photographs of the morphologic aspects of the livers graded as I, II, III and IV are illustrated in Figures 1 to 4.

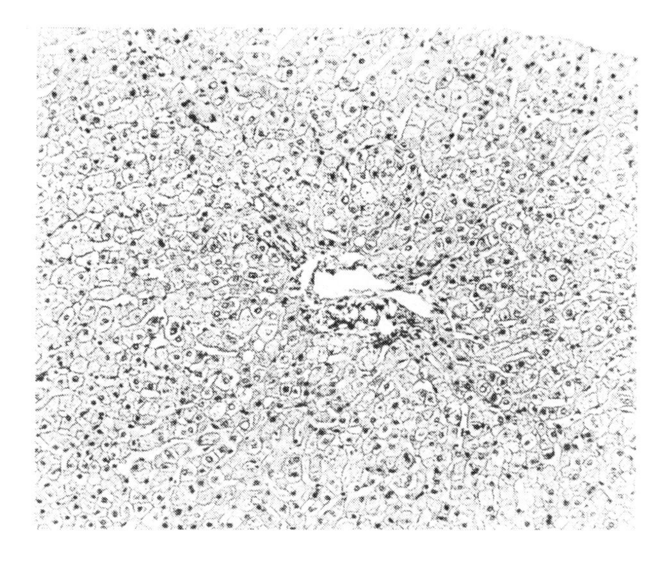

FIG. 1. Low power view (original magnification × 100) of hepatic structure in a grade I patient (normal histology).

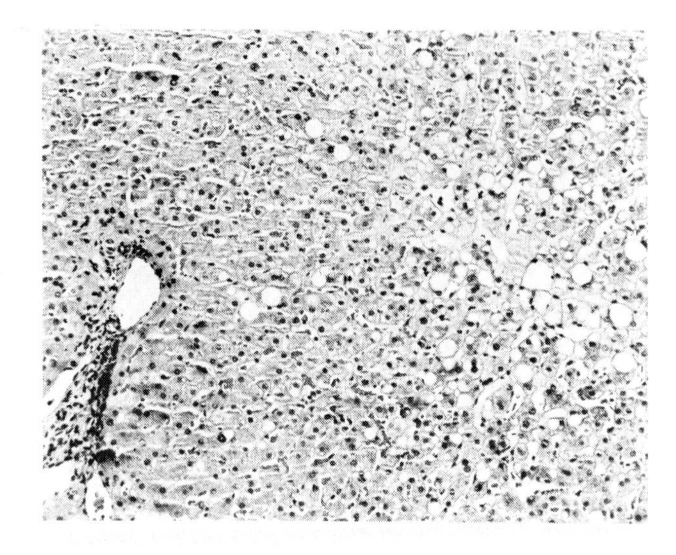

FIG. 2. Low power view (original magnification × 100) of hepatic structure in a grade II patient (less than 25% fatty infiltration).

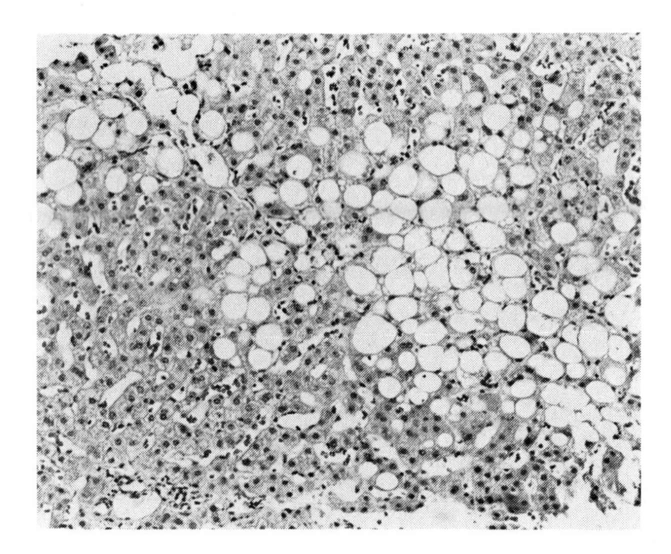

FIG. 3. Low power view (original magnification × 100) of hepatic structure in a grade III patient (25%-50% fatty infiltration).

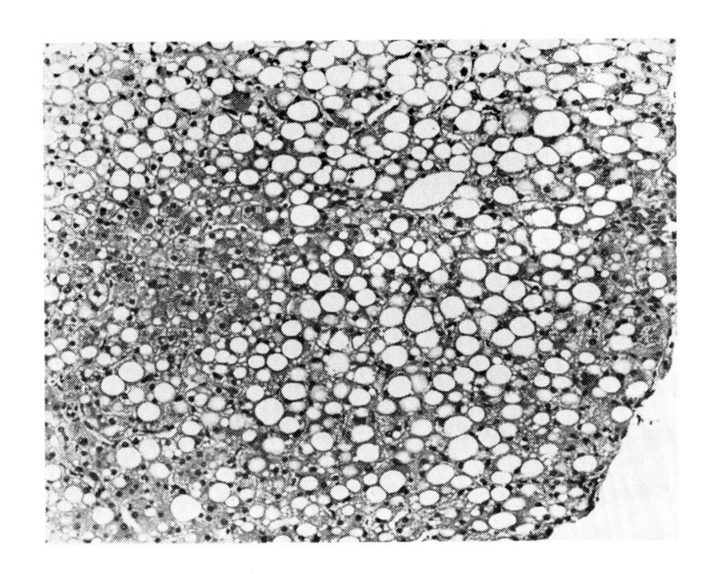

FIG. 4. Low power view (original magnification × 100) of hepatic structure in a grade IV patient (greater than 50% fatty infiltration).

Other investigators have reported similar biopsy findings at the time of jejuno-ileal bypass. The incidence of fatty metamorphosis was shown to be 71% (5 of 7) by Juhl and co-workers [10], 96% (70 of 73) by Payne and DeWind [11], 61% (20 of 33) by Salmon [12], 98% (28 of 29) by Thompson and Meyerowitz [13] and 65% (88 of 123) by Weismann [14]. Thus, I believe we can conclude that obese individuals have fatty livers prior to therapeutic intervention, operative or otherwise.

Let us now turn to the next, possibly the most crucial, question – what happens to these livers and these patients after jejuno-ileal bypass. Here, the available information is quite sketchy. A review of the literature allows us to make the following general statements: (1) The majority of patients undergo a progression of liver changes away from the histologic normal over the first year or so following jejuno-ileal bypass. (2) A limited number of patient biopsies several years after the procedure have been reported and they indicate a return toward normal architecture and, possibly, a histological pattern of improvement relative to the original intra- or preoperative biopsy. Dr. Salmon [12] has reported upon this and Dr. Shibata [15] of Montreal has reported on liver biopsy findings up to

Table 1. Preliminary Sequential Liver Biopsy Data

	Intra-operative	*One Year Postoperative*
Grade I = Normal	5	0
Grade II = < 25% fat	11	7
Grade III = 25-50% fat	4	10
Grade IV = > 50% fat	10	13
Grade V = Fibrosis	0	0
Total	30	30
Grade±S.D.	2.63±1.13	3.20±0.81

ten years after jejuno-ileal bypass. (3) A certain number of individuals following jejuno-ileal bypass, on the average of 5% to 8%, show manifestations of clinical liver failure and in the absence of, or a delay in, remedial measures have died.

Our own preliminary sequential liver biopsy data are based on only 30 individuals. Nevertheless, it may be helpful to review this material (Table 1). Five of these individuals were graded as having normal hepatic architecture at the time of their bypass operation; one year after the procedure, none of these patients had a normal histological pattern; there were 11 grade II patients at the time of bypass, seven at one year; there were four grade III patients at the time of bypass, ten at one year; and the grade IV group had increased to 13 one year following jejuno-ileal bypass from ten at the time of the procedure. No patient exhibited fibrosis either at bypass or one year thereafter. The average grade score of this 30 patient cohort was 2.63 ± S.D. 1.13 at the time of their operative intervention and 3.20 ± S.D. 0.81 one year thereafter. Thus, there was a shift in fatty infiltration, on the average, from somewhat below 50% to somewhat above 50%. We have, at this time, only a handful of individuals rebiopsied two years after their bypass procedure. As previously stated, in these patients there has been a shift toward a more normal architecture in comparison to the sections obtained one year following the operation.

Possibly, fatty infiltration is not the histological key to impending liver failure. What other changes have we noted in our one year follow-up biopsy data? Certain individuals have shown, as either a new finding or as an increase in a pre-existing condition, the presence of fibrous strands in the periportal or pericentral areas (this is not true fibrosis of the liver), bile ductual proliferation, portal mononuclear cell infiltration, periportal necrosis, or spotty parenchymal necrosis. On the other hand, there have been patients, albeit a small number, who have exhibited a decrease in bile ductual proliferation, periportal necrosis and parenchymal necrosis one year after the jejuno-ileal bypass procedure in comparison to the intra-operative biopsy specimen.

If hepatic pathology is common in obesity and an increase in fatty infiltration and other abnormal changes are seen, at least temporarily, in the majority of patients after jejuno-ileal bypass, why do 5% of these patients go on to liver failure? Various theories have been advanced to explain this liver failure: critical protein depletion [16], fatty acid deficiency [17], vitamin E deficiency [18] and a relative choline deficit [19]. In addition to the deficiency theories, the absorption of toxic substances from the gut has also been postulated. Notably among the absorption of toxins theories are the postulates of Drenick and associates [20] and O'Leary and Woodward [21]. Drenick et al believe that toxic quantities of lithocholic acid are absorbed from the colon. Lithocholic acid is a secondary bile acid formed by the action of colonic bacteria on the primary bile acid chenodeoxycholic. This theory is logically untenable. In our 11 year study of the partial ileal bypass operation for hyperlipidemia, we have never seen post bypass hepatic toxicity though this procedure allows increased concentrations of chenodeoxycholic acid to reach the colon. In addition, in an experiment utilizing the rabbit, we have clearly shown that excision of the distal half of the small intestine induces no weight loss and no chemical or histological evidence of hepatotoxicity [22]. At the recent meeting of the AGA, O'Leary and Woodward related hepatic toxicity in dogs to the absorption of bacterial toxins from the bypassed segment. Their work is similar to a previous report by Bondar and Pisesky [16].

The above hypotheses are theories, at times based on some experimental evidence, but not proven causative mechanisms. It seems clear to my associates and me that in order to have liver failure after intestinal bypass, there must be weight loss; the presence of a bypassed intestinal segment is not enough. Furthermore, the mechanism of liver failure must be such as to spare 95% of obese patients with a bypassed segment and losing weight. It may well be that a single explanation cannot account for the hepatic failures seen following jejuno-ileal bypass procedures.

Do we have any help from the clinical laboratory in selecting out the individuals who will develop hepatic complications following jejuno-ileal bypass operation? Table 2 reviews the liver chemistry findings in our series one year after jejuno-ileal bypass. As a rule, the liver chemistry data were within the normal range prior to bypass and again one year thereafter. There were several trends that were statistically significant (eg, an increase

Table 2. Preliminary Sequential Liver Chemistries Data

Parameter & Lab Norm	*Preop $\bar{x}$ ± SD*	*1 Yr Postop $\bar{x}$ ± SD*	*Paired t Analysis*
Alk. Phosph. 30-160	41.5±60.1	149.6±68.1	$p < 0.001$ (N1 R Δ)
SGOT 7.1-26.0	20.3±14.0	22.2±9.9	$0.50 > p > 0.40$ (NS), (N1 R Δ)
Total Protein 6.0-7.5	6.9±0.4	6.1±0.6	$p < 0.001$ (N1 R Δ)
Albumin 3.5-4.8	3.9±0.5	3.4±0.4	$p < 0.001$ (Borderline ↓)
Bilirubin < 0.1-1.6	0.6±0.3	0.5±0.3	$0.40 > p > 0.30$ (NS) (↓)
Pro Time 10-13	10.8±0.6	11.6±0.4	$p > 0.90$ (NS), (N1 R Δ)
Cholesterol	218.6±77.3	115.6±26.7	$p < 0.001$
Triglyceride	268.5±411.7	120.8±89.9	$0.025 > p > 0.02$

Analysis of the pertinence of these data is provided in the text ($\bar{X}$±S.D. = mean ±1 standard deviation, t = Student's "t" test, p = derived statistical significance, N1 = normal, R = range, Δ = change, NS = nonsignificant).

in the alkaline phosphatase and a decrease in the total proteins) and one deviation (a decrease in the serum albumin) from the normal to the borderline. Clinically, the only liver function parameter that we have found to be truly indicative of impending liver failure has been the serum albumin concentration. Incidentally, Table 2 also shows the marked decrease that occurred in the average serum cholesterol and serum triglyceride levels following jejuno-ileal bypass; an additional benefit of this operation.

Finally, how have we handled the 5% who have developed frank liver failure? Better than half of these patients can be restored to good health by a high protein diet, elemental amino-acid supplementation and, at times, a short course of intravenous hyperalimentation. We have resorted to a feeding jejunostomy into the proximal end of the bypassed segment in two individuals. By the frequent daily infusion of amino acid solutions via the jejunostomy, we have been able to restore the hepatic architecture of these patients toward normal and to bring them out of liver failure.

Failures of these remedial nutritional approaches, and those individuals judged to be insufficiently reliable to adhere to a program of protein supplementation, must be subjected to reoperation and take-down of the intestinal shunt. Our incidence rate for shunt take-down has been less than 2% of our total number of jejuno-ileal bypass patients. We have not lost any of our patients from liver failure.

In conclusion: (1) Obesity per se is associated with fatty metamorphosis of the liver. (2) During the first year following jejuno-ileal bypass, there is, as a rule, progression in liver architecture away from normal; commonly, the changes are in the opposite direction – toward normal – in ensuing years. (3) Only about 5% of jejuno-ileal bypass patients will have any overt problems associated with their liver changes and only about half of these individuals will have to be subjected to intestinal shunt take-down. (4) To this time, we have not determined a liver histological finding indicative of impending clinical failure. (5) To this time, the serum albumin appears to be the best laboratory indicator of potential clinical failure. (6) Finally, the diagnosis of clinical liver failure following jejuno-ileal bypass operation is currently based on the overall clinical picture, ie, edema, weakness, etc. Certainly, one should not have to wait for the presence of jaundice to make the diagnosis of early or impending liver failure.

I have saved this point to emphasize at the end of this presentation. Due to the possibility of liver failure, among many other equally pertinent considerations, jejuno-ileal bypass procedures should not be undertaken in a casual manner. These operations should only be performed in a setting of interested physicians equipped to follow these individuals adequately over many years' duration.

References

1. Brobeck, J. R.: Mechanism of the development of obesity in animals with hypothalamic lesions. Physiol. Rev., 26:541, 1946.
2. Fenton, P. F. and Chase, H. B.: Effect of diet on obesity of yellow mice in inbred lines. Proc. Soc. Exp. Biol. Med., 77:420, 1951.
3. Berkowitz, D.: Metabolic changes associated with obesity before and after weight reduction. JAMA, 187:103, 1964.
4. Westwater, J. O. and Fainer, D.: Liver impairment in the obese. Gastroenterology, 34:686, 1958.
5. Zellman, S.: The liver in obesity. Arch. Intern. Med., 90:141, 1952.
6. Rozental, P., Biava, C., Spencer, H. et al: Liver morphology and function tests in obesity and during total starvation. Amer. J. Dig. Dis., 12:198, 1967.
7. Payne, J. H., DeWind, L. T. and Commons, R. R.: Metabolic observations in patients with jejunocolic shunts. Amer. J. Surg., 106:273, 1963.

8. Scott, H. W., Jr., Sandstead, H. H., Brill A. B. et al: Experience with a new technic of intestinal bypass in the treatment of morbid obesity. Ann. Surg., 174:560, 1971.
9. Buchwald, H., Lober, P. H. and Varco, R. L.: Liver biopsy findings in seventy-seven consecutive patients undergoing jejuno-ileal bypass for morbid obesity. Amer. J. Surg., 127:48, 1974.
10. Juhl, E., Christoffersen, P., Baden, H. et al: Liver morphology and biochemistry in eight obese patients treated with jejuno-ileal anastomosis. New Eng. J. Med., 285:543, 1971.
11. Payne, J. H. and DeWind, L. T.: Surgical treatment of obesity. Amer. J. Surg., 118:141, 1969.
12. Salmon, P. A.: The results of small intestinal bypass operations for the treatment of obesity. Surg. Gynec. Obstet., 132:965, 1971.
13. Thompson, R. H., Jr. and Meyerowitz, B. R.: Liver changes after jejuno-ileal shunting for massive obesity. Surg. Forum, 21:366, 1970.
14. Weismann, R. E.: Surgical palliation of massive and severe obesity. Amer. J. Surg., 125:437, 1973.
15. Shibata, H. R.: Personal communication.
16. Bondar, G. F. and Pisesky, W.: Complications of small intestinal short circuiting for obesity. Arch. Surg., 94:707, 1967.
17. Moore, J. L., Richardson, T. and Deluca, H. F.: Lysosomes and essential fatty acid deficiency. Lipids, 2:8, 1967.
18. Schwartz, K. H.: S. Z. F. Physiol. Chem., 281:101, 1944.
19. De La Huenga, J. and Popper, H.: Urinary excretion of choline metabolites following choline administration in normals and patients with hepatobiliary disease. J. Clin. Invest., 30:463, 1951.
20. Drenick, E. J., Simmons, F. and Murphy, J. F.: Effect on hepatic morphology of treatment of obesity by fasting, reducing diets and small bowel bypass. New Eng. J. Med., 282:829, 1970.
21. O'Leary, J. P., Maher, J. W., Hollenbeck, J. I. et al: Hepatic failure following jejuno-ileal bypass. Prog. AGA:A236, May 1974.
22. Schwartz, M. Z., Varco, R. L. and Buchwald, H.: Liver function and morphology following distal ileal excision in the rabbit. Surg. Forum, 22:355, 1971.

Figures 1-4 are reproduced with permission from *American Journal of Surgery* (127:48, 1974).

The Present State of Halothane Hepatic Toxicity

Joseph J. Buckley, M.D.

There has been much dispute about whether a clear-cut cause-and-effect relationship is established between halothane anesthesia and liver damage. Arguments in favor of the existence of "halothane hepatitis" have often been based on concepts which are unproved or not justified by present knowledge. Since many physicians wonder whether they should permit halothane to be used on their patients, I will review the current information on this problem and provide an assessment of the present status of this controversial subject.

Let's review for a moment the history of the problem. When halothane was introduced in 1956, its chemical similarity to chloroform and carbon tetrachloride suggested that it might be apt to cause liver damage. But the basic animal studies and the early trials in man dispelled this worry. Nevertheless, scattered clinical reports of liver damage thought to be due to halothane began to appear in 1958, the first year the agent was used in clinical anesthesia in the United States. But it was not until 1963 that widespread alarm was aroused by publication of several reports [1-3] of 15 new cases of hepatic necrosis which followed the administration of halothane. This general concern spread even to the lay press where *Time* [4] and the *Wall Street Journal* [5] discussed it. Because halothane was already in wide use, the implications of these reports were serious enough that the National Academy of Science – National Research Council that year launched a massive retrospective survey of hepatic damage following anesthesia and surgery which has come to be known as the National Halothane Study [6].

The National Halothane Study reviewed retrospectively the incidence of fatal hepatic necrosis occurring within six weeks of anesthesia in 850,000 surgical patients (Table 1); about one third of these patients had received halothane. Among the 850,000 cases, 82 cases of fatal massive

---

Joseph J. Buckley, M.D., Professor, Department of Anesthesiology, University of Minnesota Health Sciences Center, Minneapolis.

Table 1. Raw Incidence of Fatal Postsurgical Hepatic Necrosis (Data from the National Halothane Study)

	No. of Patients	*No. of Deaths*	*Incidence*
After all general anesthetics	850,000	82 [9]	1:10,000
After halothane	250,000	7	1:35,000

hepatic necrosis were discovered. In all but nine of the 82 cases, the liver damage was explainable as due to either the patient's primary disease or the surgical procedure, or on the basis of a recognized postoperative complication *other than* damage by the anesthetic agent. Hence, nine cases were finally attributed to the anesthetic agent and seven of these nine cases had received halothane within six weeks of the final operative procedure.

Thus, the overall incidence of massive hepatic necrosis after surgery, *regardless of the anesthetic used,* was approximately 1 in 10,000; I emphasize that this incidence includes *all* cases of liver necrosis or injury from *all* causes, both surgical and anesthetic. In only nine of these patients could hepatic necrosis be attributed to the anesthetic agent itself. Hepatic necrosis occurred seven times among the 250,000 patients who received halothane, an incidence of about 1 in 35,000, and not, as is widely quoted, 1 in 10,000. Thus, fatal postoperative hepatic damage due directly to anesthetic agents proved to be a relatively rare entity and this seems to be so in the case of halothane also.

But mortality is too gross a criterion by which to assess the toxicity of a drug. We must look also at other studies [7-12] undertaken to identify not only *fatal* cases of posthalothane hepatitis, but also the sublethal reactions. These studies provide interesting information. Among approximately 150,000 administrations of halothane anesthesia that these studies encompassed, the incidence of postanesthetic hepatitis, both nonfatal and fatal, from *all* causes, was found to be about 1 in 2,500; the mortality rate was slightly more than 1 in 11,000. If those figures are corrected by allowing for the more common and likely causes of hepatic dysfunction which the experts of the NHS found were operative, then the incidence of "unexplained" fatal and nonfatal hepatitis following halothane becomes about 1 in 9,000 and mortality occurs in 1 in 40,000 cases. These figures are strikingly similar to the National Halothane Study findings.

But to gain a clearer perspective of the problem, we must also compare the incidence of hepatitis after halothane with the incidence of hepatic complications after nonhalogenated anesthetics. The National Halothane Study found that massive hepatic necrosis occurred after use of *every* type of general anesthetic agent; the *highest* rate of hepatic damage followed cyclopropane and it was seen after local anesthesia and with the intravenous agents. Another large study [13], which examined 15 years of autopsy material, uncovered three cases of postoperative massive hepatic necrosis; a local anesthetic had been used in one case, cyclopropane in the second and a combination of pentothal sodium and nisentil in the third. Six other retrospective studies [10-12, 14-16] also found that hepatitis followed the use of nonhalogenated anesthetic agents. Among the 175,000 anesthetics which did *not* involve halothane, the incidence of fatal hepatitis from all causes was 1 in 12,000. Thus, the raw death rate from hepatitis following use of *non*halogenated anesthetics was about the same as the rate which followed all anesthetics, including halothane.

Another important fact that we must recognize is that the overall incidence of postoperative jaundice has increased substantially in the past two decades; this is due to a multitude of factors such as the increased prevalence of viral hepatitis, the increased use of blood transfusions, the increased complexity of operative procedures and the large variety of drugs used in medical practice today. Table 2 compares the incidence of postoperative jaundice among patients operated in the 1950s with the rate seen in the 1960s at Toronto General Hospital [11]; in the earlier decade, the incidence of jaundice was 1.1 per 1,000 patients; in the 1960s it was 4.2 cases per 1,000 patients, almost a fourfold increase. One might be tempted to conclude that the increase was related to the fact that halothane came into use during the second period; *but*, if we examine the incidence (Table 3) of postoperative jaundice within this later 1960s series, broken down into those which occurred after *non*halogenated anesthetics and those after *halothane*, the incidence of jaundice is *identical* in each group; thus, jaundice after surgery *is* significantly more common now, but the increase cannot be related to a particular anesthetic.

Table 2. Postoperative Jaundice After General Anesthesia (Data from Henderson and Gordon [11])

	No. of Anesthetics	*Cases of Jaundice*	*Incidence Per 1,000*
1953-56	44,609	49	1.1
1960-63	48,311	201	4.2

Table 3. Postoperative Jaundice After General Anesthesia 1960 - 1963 (Data from Henderson and Gordon [11])

Agents	*No. of Anesthetics*	*Cases of Jaundice*	*Incidence Per 1,000*
Halothane	21,461	88	4.1
Other agents	26,850	113	4.2

From these studies we are left with the inescapable conclusion that in modern surgical and anesthetic practice, hepatic damage attributable to or at least associated with anesthetic agents *does* occur, but its incidence is small indeed. I think, viewed in that light, halothane hepatitis is now recognized as a real but a *rare* entity. But let's not forget the important fact that *all* anesthetics, even local and spinal anesthesia, are at one time or another followed by hepatic dysfunction. On the basis of substantial statistical data, halothane appears to be no *more* likely to produce postoperative hepatic dysfunction than any other agent, and it is better in this regard than some.

Now a word about diagnosis of halothane hepatitis.

Several investigators [17, 18] have attempted to identify a specific clinical course which typifies halothane hepatitis. The first abnormal event is said to be the development of fever, usually about seven days after the anesthetic. The fever is accompanied by malaise, loss of appetite, nausea and vomiting, and pain in the right upper quadrant. After repeated halothane anesthesia, the fever may develop earlier, from 1 to 11 days postoperatively. Jaundice appears soon after the fever. The white blood cell count is usually normal, but sometimes an eosinophilia is present. The serum bilirubin may rise to very high levels in fulminant cases but usually remains below 10 mg%; serum transaminases are in the range usually found in viral hepatitis.

Although, at first glance, this description appears diagnostic, at best it represents only circumstantial evidence and does not reliably differentiate halothane hepatitis from other causes of postoperative liver damage. Dykes [19] has determined that postoperative fever is as common after the use of other anesthetics as it is after halothane. Likewise, postoperative jaundice is of limited diagnostic value, since it can result from a variety of other causes, including blood transfusions, various drugs used today in modern clinical medicine, operative procedures, septicemia, shock and coincident viral hepatitis. In regard to the probability that postoperative jaundice may indeed be due to viral hepatitis, we should realize that more than 50,000 cases of infectious hepatitis are reported annually [20]; and at least another 50,000 additional cases go *un*reported for a variety of reasons; an even greater number of cases of serum hepatitis occur each year after the administration of blood and blood products. Dykes and Bunker [21] estimate from Public Health Service figures that as many as 300 patients each year are unwittingly subjected to anesthesia during the incubation period of coincident viral hepatitis.

These difficulties of diagnosis are compounded by the fact that identification of a typical morphologic hepatic lesion has been difficult. The six-man Pathology Panel of the National Halothane Study, made up of leading hepatic pathologists, examined the slides without knowledge of the anesthetic and was not able to identify a histologic pattern attributable to halothane. Other pathologists, even when they *were* aware of the anesthetic administered, were also hard pressed to delineate a pattern characteristic of "halothane hepatitis."

The histologic changes are virtually indistinguishable by ordinary light microscopy from those of acute viral hepatitis, although leukocyte infiltration, granuloma formation and fatty changes in the hepatocytes favor a toxic hepatitis. There is also some evidence to suggest that stromal injury with the deposition of significant amounts of collagen occurs in halothane hepatitis, while the viral lesion is limited to the parenchymal cells. Popper's group [22] claim that electron microscopy also reveals differences between halothane hepatitis and acute viral hepatitis. Where halothane is the cause, the mitochondria show segmental loss of the outer membrane and infolding of the inner one; these changes are not seen in viral hepatitis. Halothane seems also to leave the rough endoplasmic reticulum intact, while the viral infection fragments the endoplasmic reticulum and the lysosomes become prominent and vacuolated. But as Sherlock [23] has pointed out recently, detection of these subtle differences largely depends on the experience of the pathologist and in the individual case there is no absolute diagnostic difference between the two conditions.

Thus, the diagnosis of halothane hepatitis must usually be reached by excluding the more likely causes. Very often it is not possible to rule out a coincident viral hepatitis which was exacerbated by illness, surgery and drugs.

But, since there *are* cases on record in which no other cause than halothane can be offered to explain an untoward hepatic reaction, most reasonable physicians recognize that halothane may, in rare instances, damage the liver. If this is so, what mechanism(s) provoke this damage in some patients and not in most? This is *more* than an academic question. The answer is crucial to reaching sensible clinical decisions in this dilemma.

There are three ways in which halothane could cause an adverse effect on liver structure and function (Table 4). First, it could be a true hepatotoxin like chloroform or carbon tetrachloride, which, when given in a sufficient dose, consistently produces toxic necrosis of the liver parenchyma. Halothane does *not* satisfy the established criteria of an hepatotoxin. But possibly a byproduct of the parent anesthetic *could* damage the liver. We have learned recently that about 20% of an administered dose of halothane undergoes metabolic change in the liver and we know that the final metabolic product, trifluoroacetic acid, is not hepatotoxic. It has been suggested, though in no way proven, that some as yet unidentified intermediate metabolite could be far more reactive and damaging to the liver cell than the halothane molecule or its end products and thus might impair liver cell function by a direct toxic action.

A second postulate is that halothane somehow facilitates the development of viral hepatitis. There is no direct evidence to support or refute this possibility either, chiefly because we have no animal model of human viral hepatitis in which to study the halothane effect. The precise incidence of viral hepatitis in the world is unknown, but it *is* known that the disease is more prevalent today than in the past and is affecting an older age group. Unfortunately, no fully satisfactory diagnostic test for viral hepatitis exists either; the discovery of the hepatitis-associated-antigen (Australian antigen) initially led to the expectation that this would make it possible to positively identify viral hepatitis. It is now clear that hepatitis-associated-antigen occurs only in serum hepatitis and even in confirmed cases the test for it may be positive for only a relatively short period of time. Furthermore, other viruses than those responsible for infectious and serum hepatitis may give rise to jaundice – for example, the cytomegalic virus, for which there is also no satisfactory or easy test. Therefore, when

Table 4. Possible Causative Mechanisms in Halothane Hepatitis

1. Direct hepatotoxicity
   a) by halothane molecule?
   b) by halothane metabolites?
2. Exacerbation of viral hepatitis
3. Hypersensitivity reaction
   a) to the halothane molecule? hapten?
   b) to a halothane metabolite?

postoperative jaundice or liver failure appear, a negative Australian antigen test does not unequivocally rule out viral infection.

The importance of this infectious hepatitis factor was cited earlier when I stated that about 300 patients each year are subjected to anesthesia while incubating viral hepatitis. The potential effects of anesthesia on such patients, or on those with chronic active hepatitis, are not fully known. Recently, it has been suggested that carriers of viral infection, who are normally symptom-free, may develop an active form of the disease postoperatively as a result of nonspecific depression of their normal immunological mechanisms by surgery and anesthesia. Most anesthetics, among them halothane, do indeed depress cellular defense mechanisms against *bacterial* pathogens; whether a similar influence occurs in *viral* disease is unknown. It may be that halothane paralyzes the immunological system which normally holds the hepatitis virus in check and thus exacerbates that disease.

Finally, a hypersensitivity phenomenon may explain posthalothane hepatitis. The presence of hypersensitivity to halothane in an anesthetist has been nicely documented recently by Klatskin [24], but the mechanism of its production has not yet been established. Halothane is a heavily halogenated, two-carbon molecule which would not be expected to provoke antibody formation. A sensitivity response of the antigen-antibody type *could* occur if halothane or one of its metabolites conjugated to a liver protein in the form of a hapten. This protein hapten combination might then cause antibody production against the basic liver protein carrier molecule and thus provoke an autoimmune hepatitis. If this is what happens, then it must occur only under very special circumstances, otherwise hepatic dysfunction should not be so unusual. The extreme rarity of liver dysfunction among children who have received halothane is also difficult to explain on this basis, since children are certainly competent immunologically. One possibility is that it is not the halothane molecule itself which provokes the sensitivity reaction but rather an atypical metabolite produced perhaps in a genetically unusual individual. This could explain the rarity of the hepatitis while emphasizing the futility of trying to predict its occurrence with the diagnostic techniques presently available. This hypersensitivity explanation enjoys the most favor at the present time among hepatologists, who point to other sensitivity phenomena in these patients such as activation of their lymphocytes in culture when they are exposed to halothane and the presence in these "sensitized" patients of antibodies to rat liver mitochondria. The validity or significance of these tests is by no means clear and the hypersensitivity theory remains just that, a theory still unproven.

The strongest clinical evidence to support the hypersensitivity theory is those isolated reports of several operating room personnel and one worker manufacturing halothane who developed hepatic dysfunction each time they were re-exposed to halothane. One patient [24], an anesthesiologist, had recurrent attacks of hepatitis whenever he resumed occupational contact with halothane; an attack of hepatitis was deliberately provoked in this anesthetist by a direct challenge with halothane, a technique which virtually proves the existence of hypersensitivity to the compound, in this patient at least.

The evidence *against* the hypersensitivity theory must also be considered. Halothane is present in the atmosphere of every operating room; and halothane has been detected in the blood and expired air of operating room personnel and its metabolites have been found in their urine; yet only a handful of reactions have occurred among the many thousands of anesthetists, operating room nurses and surgeons so exposed; a recent survey of the causes of death of 441 American anesthesiologists provided no evidence of a higher incidence of liver disorders in this group than was seen in a general population sample. In view of the large number of operating room personnel exposed to halothane throughout the world, it is indeed surprising that so few reactions to halothane have been reported among that group.

Another controversial aspect of the halothane hepatitis problem concerns the apparent hazard of repeated administrations (Table 5). As indicated earlier, the National Halothane Study revealed that hepatic necrosis occurred after halothane in 1 in 35,000 cases. But among the 14,000 patients who received halothane two or more times, the incidence of hepatic necrosis was about 1:3,500 – a tenfold increase in the complication!! Carney and Van Dyke [25] have recently re-examined all the published reports of hepatitis following exposure to halothane and found that 50% of the cases had received repeated halothane anesthetics

Table 5. Incidence of Fatal Postsurgical Hepatic Necrosis Following Multiple Operations Under Halothane (Data from the National Halothane Study)

	No. of Patients	*No. of Deaths*	*Incidence*
Single halothane exposure	250,000	7	1:35,000
Multiple halothane exposure	14,000	4	1: 3,500

within three months. Thus, it would appear that there is a problem with repeated administrations of halothane and, of course, this finding fits nicely with the hypersensitivity causation theory.

However, a large series of cases which refutes the alleged hazard of multiple halothane administrations comes from the Brooke Army Burn Center [26], where over 400 patients received multiple halothane anesthetics (about four repeats per patient) at short intervals; no instances of hepatic damage due to the anesthetic were seen; one of these patients was given halothane 22 times. Numerous other anecdotal reports [7, 27, 28] of the safety of repeated halothane administrations have been made, one involving 89 separate anesthesias.

It is *my* judgment that all of these data on the question of increased hazard of repeated halothane permit two general and rather obvious conclusions – first, that a small percentage of patients who receive two halothane anesthetics within a short interval of time *will* develop an untoward, sometimes fatal hepatic reaction; the risk of liver damage *does* appear to be significantly greater under this circumstance than when a single administration of halothane is involved; the *reason* this is so has not been fully determined. Second, the many individuals to whom halothane has been administered repeatedly *without* the development of hepatic damage indicates that multiple administrations of halothane do not *necessarily* damage the liver.

It may be useful to reflect for a moment on who receives multiple anesthetics.

An example of the type of patient who requires repeated anesthetic administration is the burned patient who must be anesthetized every other day or so for dressing changes and debridement. Another is the patient who requires staged reconstructive surgery following trauma. Others are those who have chronic infectious processes such as osteomyelitis or wound infections. Are these patients drawn from the same general population as those having a single elective procedure? One way in which they differ, which is generally not discussed, is the state of their nutrition. Patients requiring multiple surgical procedures are often seriously malnourished. It is well known that starvation increases the content of neutral fat in liver cells. Since halothane is highly fat-soluble, such an increase in liver fat content favors the accumulation of large quantities of halothane or its byproducts in the liver. Irrespective of how halothane may produce liver toxicity, be it toxic damage by metabolites or hypersensitivity, if more halothane is present in hepatocytes, the likelihood of damage would be increased.

A patient receiving multiple anesthesias is frequently a very sick patient who has experienced a stormy course following the initial surgery. Under these circumstances, he generally is receiving a number of other drugs concurrently. If any of these medications cause induction of microsomal drug-metabolizing enzyme activity, the production of toxic halothane metabolites could be increased. Until more is known about the normal and the unusual metabolic pathways of halothane degradation in man, we can only speculate about this.

So much for the statistical and hypothetical aspects of the halothane hepatitis problem. Let's now come to grips with some of the more pragmatic questions which arise out of the problem and which demand at least temporary answers – I hasten to add that when better information about the cause and the nature of postoperative hepatitis becomes available, these presently tenuous conclusions may require substantial revision.

The first question that usually arises as a result of this hepatitis problem is, should halothane be abandoned? The answer to this question must take into account the substantial advantages which halothane provides and the alternatives for successful anesthetic management of patients, if halothane were abandoned. First of all, halothane's safety record is impressive. In the National Halothane Study, the overall mortality rate was 1.87% with halothane, compared to 1.93% for all general anesthetics.

Another major advantage of inhalation anesthesia with halothane is the breath-by-breath control that the skillful anesthetist can exercise with it. Such control is difficult to achieve with most of the other popular anesthetic techniques.

There are other explanations for the widespread popularity of halothane. It is a pleasant anesthetic from the patient's point of view and it is an easy anesthetic to administer. A smooth anesthetic course is more consistently achieved than with other agents. There is no question that halothane anesthesia is a more precise, controllable, predictable and uncomplicated technique than the older ones which it has replaced. Its use is also relatively easy to teach, a fact we must not lose sight of, for in this country nearly half the anesthesias are given by nurse anesthetists and by physicians without formal training in anesthesia.

Halothane can be used in the presence of electrocautery, and its replacement would have to be found among those agents in the nonexplosive category since electrocautery has become virtually indispensable.

For these reasons I believe it would not be in the overall best interest of surgical patients to abandon the use of halothane, since problems from it are rare and there is no fully acceptable substitute for it at this time.

The second question is, can the drug be used more than once, and if so, what "safe" interval between uses seems reasonable?

Yes, halothane *can* be repeated with safety if the previous anesthetic was well tolerated. In order to determine this point, it is important that the patient's previous hospital course be reviewed carefully for clinical and laboratory evidence of an untoward hepatic reaction. It has been suggested that a patient who develops an unexplained fever following halothane anesthesia is not a candidate for a second administration. While this has been generally accepted, Dykes [19] has shown that fever is not a very useful diagnostic aid. He found, in a study of a large number of consecutive patients who received general anesthesia of all types, that virtually *every* patient had a temperature elevation of some degree during the first postoperative week; 55% of the fevers could *not* be explained as due to usual causes such as atelectasis, wound sepsis or urinary infection.

My colleagues and I have come to discount *pyrexia alone* as a useful indicator in deciding whether or not to repeat halothane. However, any patient who, in addition, has not been feeling well, has been eating poorly or is in a substandard nutritional state, probably should not receive halothane soon again. Obviously, if dark urine or jaundice followed the first anesthetic with halothane, it should *not* be repeated.

Is there an appropriate waiting period or safe interval between halothane administrations? I think the answer to this depends upon whether you subscribe to the toxic metabolite or the hypersensitivity theory to explain halothane hepatitis. If the hepatic reaction is due to the accumulation of toxic metabolites, then some interval should probably pass before halothane is administered again to forestall the accumulation within the hepatocytes of a greater amount of metabolite than can be coped with by the microsomal enzymes and to allow complete elimination of halothane and its metabolites. We presently try not to repeat halothane within a three month span; I readily admit that there is no really solid scientific data to support the three month safe-interval philosophy but since the majority of the hepatic dysfunctions following multiple halothane administrations occurred when the drug was repeated within a three month period, this conservative approach seems to us to be appropriate.

On the other hand, if halothane hepatitis is due to hypersensitivity, as some claim, then it is not likely that any arbitrary waiting period is going to lessen the likelihood of an allergic response upon re-exposure; in fact, there are cases on record in which hepatic dysfunction occurred when halothane was repeated after a five year interval. There is at present no practical method of predicting such a response other than by identifying a previous intolerance to the drug.

I should point out here that it is generally agreed that children seem almost immune to halothane hepatitis. The previous recommendations therefore need not apply to children. We have no hesitation at all to repeat halothane frequently in children.

What about using halothane when pre-existing hepatic disease such as cirrhosis or biliary tract obstruction is present? Although several important studies [6, 8, 29] failed to show any increased incidence of mortality or liver damage when halothane was given to these patients, we prefer *not* to use halothane here simply to avoid "muddying the waters" should the hepatic process worsen after surgery. A current example of the wisdom of this approach has revealed itself recently with the jejunal-ileal bypass operation for morbid obesity – liver biopsy reveals that most of these patients have substantial fatty infiltration of the liver and several of our recent patients have developed serious postoperative liver dysfunction; it is likely that halothane would have been blamed had it been used in these patients. On the other hand if, in an individual case, halothane offers clear advantages over other anesthetic methods, it should be used despite the presence of hepatic disease.

To summarize, it is now reasonably clear that halothane hepatitis is a real, though rare entity, whose precise cause is still unknown. No specific pathological features or diagnostic tests reliably differentiate it from viral hepatitis. Until a routine specific test for either disease is available, the apparent incidence of halothane hepatitis will probably remain higher than its actual incidence.

Because "halothane hepatitis" cannot yet be diagnosed with certainty, we recommend strongly to our physician colleagues that when a patient develops jaundice after surgery, the specific diagnosis, halothane hepatitis, *not* be entered in the patient's hospital record unless a complete investigation has ruled out the more common and likely causes. A diagnosis such as "unexplained postoperative hepatitis following halothane" would be a better reflection of current knowledge. Such a patient, however, should be warned not to receive halothane again.

References

1. Brody, G. L. and Sweet, R. B.: Halothane anesthesia as a possible cause of massive hepatic necrosis. Anesthesiology, 24:29, 1963.

2. Bunker, J. P. and Blumenfeld, C. M.: Liver necrosis after halothane anesthesia. Cause or coincidence? New Eng. J. Med., 268:531, 1963.
3. Lindenbaum, J. and Leifer, E.: Hepatic necrosis associated with halothane anesthesia. New Eng. J. Med., 268:525, 1963.
4. Anesthetics. A gas and the liver. Time, March 22, 1963.
5. Lawson, H. G.: Doctors debate use of anesthetic linked to liver disorders. Wall Street Journal, March 20, 1963.
6. Bunker, J. P., Forrest, W. H., Mosteller, F. et al (eds.): The National Halothane Study. A Study of the Possible Association Between Halothane Anesthesia and Postoperative Hepatic Necrosis. Washington:U. S. Government Printing Office, 1969.
7. Wilson, R. D., Tarrow, A. B. and Garvin, S.: Hepatic effects of halothane. A clinical and laboratory evaluation of 10,129 administrations. Anesth. Analg., 43:40, 1964.
8. Dawson, B., Jones, R. R., Schnelle, N. et al: Halothane and ether anesthesia in gallbladder and bile duct surgery. A retrospective study into mortality and hepatobiliary complications. Anesth. Analg., 42:759, 1963.
9. Allen, H. L. and Metcalf, D. W.: A search for halothane liver complications. Anesth. Analg., 43:159, 1964.
10. Mushin, W. W., Rosen, M., Bowen, D. J. et al: Halothane and liver dysfunction. A retrospective study. Brit. Med. J., 2:329, 1964.
11. Henderson, J. C. and Gordon, R. A.: The incidence of postoperative jaundice with special reference to halothane. Canad. Anaesth. Soc. J., 11:453, 1964.
12. Dykes, M. H. M., Walzer, S. G., Slater, E. M. et al: Acute parenchymatous hepatic disease following general anesthesia. Clinical appraisal of hepatotoxicity following administration of halothane. JAMA, 193:339, 1965.
13. Caravati, C. M. and Wootton, P.: Acute massive hepatic necrosis with fatal liver failure. Southern Med. J., 55:1268, 1962.
14. Gingrich, T. F. and Virtue, R. W.: Postoperative liver damage. Is anesthesia involved? Surgery, 57:241, 1965.
15. Keeri-Szanto, M. and Lafleur, F.: Postanaesthetic liver complications in a general hospital. A statistical study. Canad. Anaesth. Soc. J., 10:531, 1963.
16. Perry, L. B. and Jenicek, J. A.: Massive hepatic necrosis associated with general anesthesia. Milit. Med., 129:1148, 1964.
17. Trey, C., Lipworth, L., Chalmers, T. C. et al: Fulminant hepatic failure. Presumable contribution of halothane. New Eng. J. Med., 279:798, 1968.
18. Tygstrup, N.: Halothane hepatitis. Lancet, 2:466, 1963.
19. Dykes, M. H. M.: Unexplained postoperative fever. Its value as a sign of halothane sensitization. JAMA, 216:641, 1971.
20. Hepatitis on rise (edit). JAMA, 210:1686, 1969.
21. Dykes, M. H. M. and Bunker, J. P.: Hepatotoxicity and anesthetics. Pharm. for Physicians 4:1, 1970.
22. Klion, F. M., Schaffner, F. and Popper, H.: Hepatitis after exposure to halothane. Ann. Intern. Med., 71:467, 1969.
23. Sherlock, S.: Halothane hepatitis. Gut, 12:324, 1971.
24. Klatskin, G. and Kimberg, D. V.: Recurrent hepatitis attributable to halothane in an anesthetist. New Eng. J. Med., 280:515, 1969.
25. Carney, F. M. and Van Dyke, R. A.: Halothane hepatitis: A critical review. Anesth. Analg., 51:135, 1972.

26. Gronert, G. A., Schaner, P. J. and Gunther, R. C.: Multiple halothane anesthesia in the burn patient. JAMA, 205:878, 1968.
27. Visser, E. R. and Tarrow, A. B.: Fluothane for multiple burn dressing anesthetics. Anesth. Analg., 38:301, 1959.
28. Galvin, H. J.: Liver damage and Fluothane. Lancet, 1:1164, 1964.
29. Jones, R. R., Dawson, B., Adson, M. A. et al: Halothane and non-halogenated anesthetic agents in patients with cirrhosis of the liver: Mortality and morbidity following portal-systemic venous anastomoses. Surg. Clin. N. Amer., 45:983, 1965.

Medical Management of Cirrhosis

Sheila Sherlock, M.D.

Etiological Factors

Cirrhosis is an irreversible chronic disease of the liver characterized by widespread fibrosis and nodule formation. Certain etiological factors have been clearly defined and their control is all-important in management. Accurate diagnosis is therefore mandatory and investigations usually include needle biopsy of the liver if the patient's condition permits.

The most important etiological factor in the Western world is alcoholic excess (Fig. 1). If this factor can be controlled the clinical improvement in the patient, even if the liver failure is advanced, is quite remarkable. The prognosis is so much better than in cryptogenic cirrhotic or in those where immunological factors seem at fault. The resilience of the alcoholic with liver disease is quite amazing.

If Wilson's disease can be diagnosed, then penicillamine treatment usually enables the patient to live to a normal age and have a normal life. If hemochromatosis is present, then venesection treatment is of undoubted benefit. Patients with active chronic liver disease, whether of the lupoid variety or associated with the presence of hepatitis B antigen, benefit from prednisolone treatment [1, 2]. Deaths during the first two years are much reduced, but progression to cirrhosis is not prevented.

Factors Precipitating Hepatic Failure

The cirrhotic patient is particularly vulnerable to any factor decreasing hepatocellular function. A careful search must therefore be made for any such factor in a patient with known cirrhosis developing liver failure. The cirrhotic nodule depends largely upon blood supply by the hepatic artery, hence any reduction in hepatic arterial flow will lead to necrosis of the nodule center and hepatocellular failure. Hemorrhage and surgical shock

---

Sheila Sherlock, M.D., Professor, Department of Medicine, University of London, Royal Free Hospital, London, England.

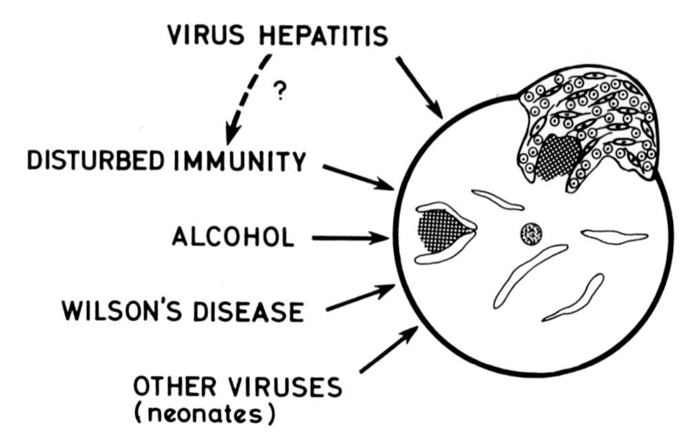

FIG. 1. Etiological factors in cirrhosis formation. These must be controlled whenever possible.

are therefore poorly tolerated. Repeated hemorrhages result in a vicious circle. Each hemorrhage is followed by increasing hepatic failure and blood clotting is further reduced with a greater tendency to bleed again.

The commonest precipitant of coma in cirrhosis today is probably electrolyte imbalance induced by too vigorous diuretic therapy. Hypokalemia per se cannot be incriminated and the picture seems to be induced by any factor disturbing electrolyte balance. Other precipitating factors include infections, alcohol excess and injudicious use of tranquilizers and sedatives generally. In the patient with chronic hepatic encephalopathy, for instance, that developing after portacaval anastomosis, a high protein intake (large steak meal), particularly if combined with constipation, is important in leading to stupor and coma.

General Measures

The management of the well-compensated cirrhotic is that of the early detection of hepatocellular failure, the diagnosis and treatment of any etiological factor and avoidance and treatment of anything that would precipitate hepatocellular failure. The principles of an adequate mixed diet and avoidance of alcohol must be explained. A diet of 1 gm protein/kg body weight is adequate unless the patient is an obviously malnourished alcoholic. Additional choline or methionine or various liver "tonics" are unnecessary. Avoidance of fat, eggs, coffee or chocolate is not of proven benefit.

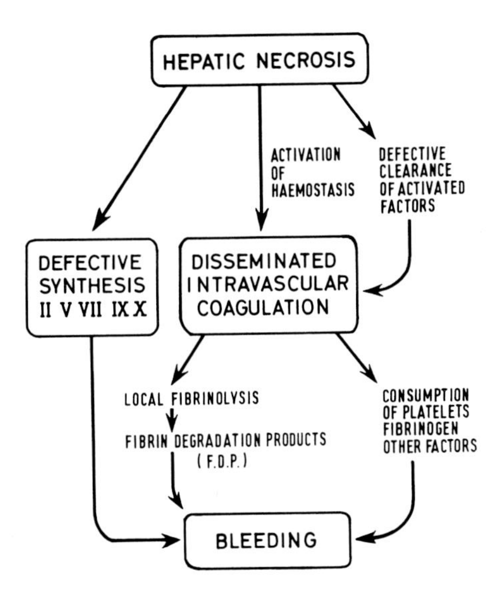

FIG. 2. The effect of hepatic necrosis on blood coagulation.

Hepatocellular Failure

This is a syndrome marked by failure of all the functions of the liver cell.

Failure of hepatic protein synthesis is particularly shown by reduction in clotting factors, particularly V, VII, IX, X and prothrombin (Fig. 2). These proteins have a particularly short half-life and levels provide a sensitive index of hepatocellular function (Fig. 3).

Failure of hepatic albumin synthesis is reflected in the low serum albumin level, edema and muscle wasting generally. Serum albumin levels are of critical importance in ascites formation. In the later stages, renal failure accompanies fluid retention and the renal cortical blood profusion is reduced. Hypotension is a feature. The peripheral resistance is reduced but the cardiac output is increased.

Hepatic encephalopathy is multifactorial. Deficiency of hepatic Krebs cycle enzymes results in retention of ammonia and amines and blood urea levels fall. Protein and bacterial action in the large and small bowel and the portal systemic collateral circulation contribute. Hypoglycemia is occasionally present but is more frequent in acute hepatocellular failure (fulminant viral hepatitis) rather than cirrhosis.

Jaundice per se is not harmful except in the neonate and does not require treatment.

THROMBOTEST and PROGNOSIS in ACUTE HEPATIC FAILURE

● SURVIVED
† DIED

THROMBOTEST	OUTCOME
> 25%	● ● ● ●
21 – 25%	●
16 – 20%	●
11 – 15%	● ● † † † † †
5 – 10%	● ● ● ● † † † † †
< 5%	† † † † † † †

FIG. 3. The prognosis of acute hepatic failure is closely reflected by the blood coagulation as measured by the thrombotest.

Control of Ascites (Table 1) [3]

The control of ascites in patients with cirrhosis is more difficult than in other forms of fluid retention, for diuretic therapy is particularly liable to be followed by electrolyte disturbances, encephalopathy and renal failure. The patient is put to bed. Daily measurement of weight and urine output give adequate indication of response to treatment.

Table 1. General Management of Ascites

1. Bed rest, 22 mEq Na diet. Restrict fluids to 1 liter.
   Check serum (if possible urinary) electrolytes.
   Weigh daily. Measure urinary volume.
   Add KCl 100 mEq daily.
2. After four days if weight loss less than 1 kg start spironolactone 100 mg *or* amiloride 10 mg daily
   Reduce KCl to 50 mEq daily.
3. After one more day check serum electrolytes.
   Add frusemide 80 mg daily as required.
4. After four more days check serum electrolytes. If weight loss less than 2 kg, amiloride 10 mg twice daily or spironolactone 200 mg daily.
5. If necessary increase frusemide to 120 mg daily.
   Stop diuretic drugs if precoma ("flap") hypokalemia, azotemia or alkalosis or weight loss more than 0.5 kg daily.

The daily intake of sodium must be restricted to less than 22 mEq (0.5 gm) daily, and even to less than 10 mEq daily. Fluid intake is restricted to 1 liter daily. Most protein-containing foods such as meat, eggs and dairy produce have a high sodium content. Salt-free bread and butter is used and cooking is done without added salt. Many low sodium foods are now available including soup, ketchups and crackers.

Diuretics should be given only if the weight loss is less than 2 lb after four days on the dietetic and fluid restriction regime alone. The dose and frequency of administration must be calculated for each individual patient. Diuretics can be divided into two groups (Table 2). The first comprises the thiazides, frusemide, and ethacrynic acid. These are powerful natriuretic agents but also powerful kaliuretics. Potassium chloride supplements are always necessary when these diuretics are given alone. The second group comprises spironolactone, triamterene and amiloride. These are weakly natriuretic but conserve potassium. When they are combined with a diuretic of the first group, the potassium chloride supplements are reduced and may become unnecessary. In general, it is advisable to start with one of these diuretics and then add a first group diuretic as required. Using this regime, a diuresis with ultimate control of ascites can be anticipated in over 90% of patients with cirrhosis. Failures are usually in those with poor hepatocellular function.

Electrolyte disturbances are frequent. Hypokalemia is reduced by using a potassium-sparing diuretic and giving potassium chloride supplements. Hyponatremia is a frequent electrolyte disturbance. It is treated by stopping the diuretic and restricting fluid intake to 500 ml a day. Alternatively, mannitol may be used as an osmotic diuretic. The clinician may be tempted to give sodium supplements, in fact, body stores of sodium and water are excessive, and giving more sodium will only lead to weight gain and pulmonary edema. Azotemia is particularly important for, if progressive, it leads to a picture of renal failure in the cirrhotic.

Table 2. Diuretics for Ascites

Urine Loss		
Group 1		
Na ++	K ++	Thiazides Frusemide Ethacrynic acid
Group 2		
Na +	K –	Spironolactone Triamterene Amiloride

Portacaval Anastomosis

A side-to-side shunt will relieve ascites. This procedure not only decompresses the splanchnic veins but also relieves the hepatic venous outflow block. The mortality for this procedure when performed for ascites is as high as 35% [4]. Hypoalbuminemia persists postoperatively. Neuropsychiatric complications are extremely frequent in these patients. The operation should be reserved for those whose remoteness from medical supervision makes a low sodium diet and adequate diuretic therapy impossible.

Ascites Ultrafiltration and Reinfusion [5]

This procedure removes ascitic fluid at a constant rate, filters it through a disposable filter which removes fluid and crystalloids with the molecular weight of less than 50,000 and reinjects it back to the patient by the intravenous route. The concentrate contains two to four times as much protein as the ascitic fluid. About 5 liters of ascites can be removed in about ten hours. Mild pyrexia is the only consistent side effect. The method is unsuitable for removing high protein fluids, for instance those due to malignant disease, as the membrane becomes clogged and carcinoma may be disseminated. This approach may be of particular value in patients with cirrhosis who develop renal failure.

Functional Renal Failure (Hepatorenal Syndrome) [6, 7]

Renal failure in cirrhosis may be related to primary kidney disease, but more often occurs spontaneously or in response to changes in blood volume or shifts of fluid within body compartments [8]. The renal failure is enhanced by over-vigorous diuretic therapy, paracentesis or diarrhea but may develop without a precipitant. The classic clinical features of uremia are usually absent.

The renal failure seems to be related essentially to reduction of the effective renal circulation. Blood flow is diverted away from the renal cortex and this change can be shown even in well-compensated cirrhotic patients. This may explain their susceptibility to develop oliguric failure after hemorrhage not sufficiently large to reduce the blood pressure or after minor shifts of fluid within blood compartments, such as happens with vigorous diuretic therapy or with abdominal paracentesis.

The etiology is unknown. Circulating vaso-active substances released or not metabolized by a diseased liver could be responsible but have not been identified. Another possibility is that false sympathetic neurotransmitter

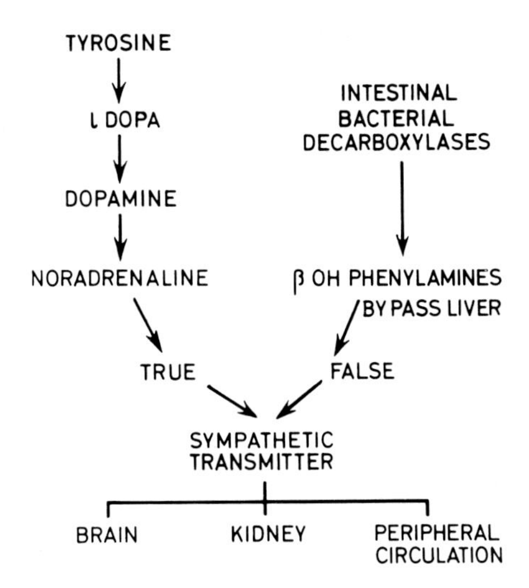

FIG. 4. The hypothesis that false sympathetic transmitters, produced by bacterial decarboxylation in the gut compete with the true transmitter and lead to a cerebral disturbance with interference with renal and peripheral circulations.

amines produced in the gastrointestinal tract are involved [9] (Fig. 4). These would lead to depletion of sympathetic transmitter stores. A temporary favorable response to a direct sympathomimetic amine (metaraminol) observed in eight patients would favor this view.

The syndrome is prevented by avoiding electrolyte imbalance hemorrhage or infection in patients with cirrhosis. The conservative management is that of renal and hepatic failure whatever the cause. Hepatic failure holds the key to the problem and must be treated. Volume expansion and such drugs as octapressin, metaraminol or angiotensin are not of sustained benefit. Hepatic transplantation has even been used with delayed resumption of renal function [10].

Hepatic Encephalopathy

Hepatic coma is of multiple causation and the factors acting in the individual patient must be defined and treated. The major ones are toxic nitrogenous substances formed in the intestine by bacterial action on proteins.

All dietary protein is stopped and adequate calories are supplied as carbohydrate orally or intravenously. In acute cases, a few days' deprivation of protein is usual, but long-term reduced intake of protein is indicated in those with chronic hepatic encephalopathy. Other patients with liver disease may benefit by high protein feeding, particularly if alcoholic or if ascites is forming.

Neomycin given orally is very effective in decreasing gastrointestinal ammonium formation. In the acute case, 4 gm are given daily in divided doses. This antibiotic, however, should be avoided long term, because of the development of impaired hearing.

Lactulose [11] is a disaccharide which does not occur naturally. The human intestinal mucosa does not produce a lactulase to split it. When given by mouth the bulk reaches the cecum where it produces a fall in fecal pH. The growth of lactose-fermenting organisms is favored and organisms such as bacteroids, which are ammonia-formers, are suppressed. The aim of therapy is to produce acid stools without diarrhea. The usual dose is 10-30 ml three times a day and is adjusted to produce two semisolid stools daily. It should not be given at the same time as neomycin. It should not be given in acute hepatic coma where nitrogenous intoxication is best controlled by neomycin. Its greatest use is in the long-term management of the hepatic encephalopathy following portacaval shunting.

Other Precipitating Factors

Care should be taken concerning the use of sedatives and tranquilizers and diuretics in these patients. Potassium deficiency must be assessed. The possibility of delirium tremens should not tempt the clinician to give alcohol to an alcoholic patient in impending hepatic coma.

Some of the clinical features of hepatic encephalopathy resemble parkinsonism and dopamine depletion in the brain has been postulated (Fig. 4). Dopamine cannot be administered as it does not pass the blood/brain barrier, but its precursor levodopa is readily available. It may cause temporary arousal in acute hepatic encephalopathy and is also sometimes of benefit in the chronic case [12]. However, the side effects, particularly nausea and psychiatric disturbance, often prevent its continued use.

Hepatic transplantation may be the ultimate answer to the problem of chronic hepatic encephalopathy. However, the chances of long-term survival in this situation have not been established.

Jaundice

Corticosteroids will usually effect a whitewash in patients with hepatocellular jaundice and have proved of benefit in active chronic hepatitis with or without a positive hepatitis B antigen disease [1, 2]. In partial cholestasis, cholestyramine or phenobarbital increase bile flow and may reduce the serum bilirubin and bile acid level. Phenobarbital also acts as a potent microsomal enzyme inducer.

Summary

Hepatic cirrhosis is a complex condition of multiple etiology. Once established, hepatic architecture is destroyed and the condition is irreversible. Attention to etiological factors, however, produces considerable improvement. Such factors include alcoholism, chronic liver disease, hemochromatosis and Wilson's disease.

Attention must be paid to any precipitating factor which would reduce hepatocellular function. These include shock, infection, drugs, particularly sedatives and diuretics, constipation and dietary protein indiscretion in those with chronic hepatic encephalopathy.

Failure of hepatocellular function has many effects. Blood clotting failure is an early feature.

Failure of albumin synthesis is a major contribution to ascites formation. The importance of a low sodium diet and chronic use of diuretics alone or in combination is emphasized. The ultrafiltration reinfusion technique for ascites control may be useful in those with massive ascites. Diuretic overdose may precipitate renal failure; this has an ominous outlook.

Hepatic encephalopathy is managed by dietary protein restriction, wide spectrum antibiotics and lactulose.

Jaundice, if hepatocellular, may merit corticosteroid therapy; in partial cholestasis, cholestyramine or phenobarbital may be of value.

References

1. Cook, G. C., Mulligan, R. and Sherlock, S.: Controlled prospective trial of corticosteroid therapy in active chronic hepatitis. Quart. J. Med., 40:159, 1971.
2. Soloway, R. D., Summerskill, W. H. J., Baggenstoss, A. H. et al: Clinical, biochemical, and histological remission of severe chronic active liver disease: A controlled study of treatments and early prognosis. Gastroenterology, 63:820, 1972.
3. Sherlock, S.: Ascites formation in cirrhosis and its management. Scand. J. Gastroent., 5, (suppl.), 1970.
4. Welch, H. F., Welch, C. S. and Carter, J. H.: Prognosis after surgical treatment of ascites: Results of side-to-side shunt in 40 patients. Surgery, 56:75, 1964.
5. Parbhoo, S. P., Ajdukiewicz, A. and Sherlock, S.: Treatment of ascites by continuous ultrafiltration and reinfusion of protein concentrate. Lancet, 1:949, 1974.

6. Kew, M. C., Brunt, P. W., Varma, R. R. et al: Renal and intrarenal blood-flow in cirrhosis of the liver. Lancet, 2:504, 1971.
7. Kew, M.: Renal changes in cirrhosis. Gut, 13:748, 1972.
8. Shear, L., Ching, S. and Gabuzda, G. J.: Compartmentalization of ascites and edema in patients with hepatic cirrhosis. New Eng. J. Med., 282:1391, 1970.
9. Fischer, J. E. and James, J. H.: Treatment of hepatic coma and hepatorenal syndrome: Mechanism of action of l-dopa and Aromine. Amer. J. Surg., 123:222, 1972.
10. Iwatsuki, S., Popovtzer, M. M., Corman, J. L. et al: Recovery from "hepatorenal syndrome" after orthotopic liver transplantation. New Eng. J. Med., 289:1155, 1973.
11. Fessel, J. M. and Conn, H. O.: Lactulose in the treatment of acute hepatic encephalopathy. Amer. J. Med. Sci., 266:103, 1973.
12. Lunzer, M., James, I. M., Weinman, J. et al: The treatment of chronic hepatic encephalopathy with levodopa. Gut, 15:555, 1974.

Panel Discussion

Moderator: **W. H. J. Summerskill, M.D.**

Panelists:

H. J. Burhenne, M.D.	**C. J. Watson, M.D.**
S. Sherlock, M.D.	**H. Popper, M.D.**
L. Zieve, M.D.	**H. Buchwald, M.D.**
J. Buckley, M.D.	

Dr. McQuarrie: Just for those of you who are statisticians, I added up the bibliographies of all the panel members. This panel represents the output of over 1,800 scientific articles, so I hope that you take the opportunity to ask questions of this panel.

Dr. Summerskill: The first question is directed to Dr. Sherlock: How do you treat or investigate a patient with a positive Australia antigen found on "routine" check-up?

Dr. Sherlock: First, try to find out why the patient acquired the antigens. A distinction must be made between three different circumstances: (1) the patient who is developing acute HBAG hepatitis and who is probably very infectious; (2) the patient who has been a chronic carrier for many years and who has normal liver function tests; and (3) the patient with chronic liver disease who harbors the antigen. All merit slightly different treatment. The one developing the disease should have some symptoms. The chronic carrier, with normal liver function tests, should be warned about hygiene. The patient who has abnormal function tests and a positive HB antigen should have a liver biopsy and be treated on the basis of the results.

Dr. Summerskill: We will also probably delve further into this subject in a later session of this symposium. Meanwhile, there is an important question here for all of us: How do you determine when a patient with acute viral hepatitis is no longer contagious; in other words, need no longer be isolated?

Dr. Zieve: I think we should be careful about the use of the term "contagious." I don't think of viral hepatitis as a contagious disease in the sense of childhood diseases. Nevertheless, for some months after recovering from viral hepatitis patients should take sanitary precautions to avoid contamination of the immediate environment. But I think that is all that is needed. By and large, except for the factor of blood transfusions (which should be checked before donors should be considered) no special attention need be considered after recovery.

Dr. Summerskill: Dr. Watson, do you have anything to add?

Dr. Watson: I have little to add. What Dr. Zieve has said is entirely right. We don't know, in any given case, whether the virus is there; and there are no practical means of finding out. Earlier studies indicated that in most instances the infectious agent had disappeared after one month to six weeks following recovery. That by no means excludes the chronic carrier state, which is hard to detect even under present circumstances. I think that patients should be indoctrinated from the start concerning good hygiene for several months.

Dr. Summerskill: We in Rochester do not follow the enteric precautions of the Public Health Service totally rigorously. But none of us can find the real truth yet in the answer to the question. Dr. Buchwald, I have two questions for you. These may occasion ventilation of viewpoints among the members of the panel. First, considering known complications of small intestinal bypass operations for obesity, which are the hardest to control? Second, what types of bypass are you using for obesity?

Dr. Buchwald: Answering the second question, we employ a bypass between the proximal 40 cm of jejunum (measured from the ligament of Treitz) to the terminal 4 cm of ileum, measured from the ileocecal valve. These pieces of bowel are joined by an end-to-end anastomosis. The 90% of bowel that is bypassed is closed proximally, with that end being attached to adjacent viscera to prevent intussusception; the distal end is anastomosed, end-to-side, to the cecum. This is the standard procedure we employ at the University of Minnesota for the "obesity shunt" in contradistinction to the one-third "hypercholesterolemic" shunt. As for complications after the procedure, the potential for liver failure is the most difficult to control because we cannot predict which patients will develop this postoperatively. Some patients enter the operating room with normal livers, whereas others have already developed severe fatty degeneration. Some of the first group proceed to liver failure, whereas some in the second group apparently improve and have no clinical problems relating to liver failure. Lacking a predictive base is the toughest thing to deal with. Other problems, such as electrolyte losses, can be anticipated. We give supplemental calcium, potassium and vitamin B_{12}. Immediate pre-, intra- and postoperative care can be given in such a manner that the actual complications associated with the operative procedure are held to a minimum.

Dr. Summerskill: There are maybe two follow-ups on these operations: First, Dr. Woodward's group, from Gainesville, Florida, presented some persuasive data from dogs. Following such procedures one group received antibiotics and all survived. The second group of dogs received no antibiotics; all died with liver disease. This raises the question, of course, of bacterial overgrowth and bacterial exotoxin (or maybe endotoxin) contributing to this particular hepatic disease syndrome. The second report was also presented this year by the group at the Cleveland Clinic. They have given up these operations for patients with morbid obesity, often because of hepatic complications. Parenthetically, I would mention that at Mayo we haven't started them. We are still just evaluating the results of others. What are you doing in London, Dr. Sherlock?

Dr. Sherlock: We don't do any at the Royal Free Hospital Medical School, but St. George's Hospital does them.

Dr. Summerskill: It seems that several dilemmas related to these operations remain to be ironed out. They probably are not yet appropriate for general use. Dr. Buchwald, would you like to comment?

Dr. Buchwald: That was to be my closing statement: The operation, I think, can be done with relative safety as a procedure in the operating room and with respect to postoperative care. I think that we have shown this at the University of Minnesota. We have a 2% wound infection rate and about a 1% or 2% pulmonary embolization rate. And so on. The operation can be conducted safely relative to other major abdominal surgery. What happens afterwards needs critical testing, follow-up and careful documentation. I fully agree that the procedure should be done only by people willing to make a commitment to these patients and their welfare for many years. It should not be done as a casual procedure.

Dr. Summerskill: Thank you, Dr. Buchwald. Dr. Burhenne, would you comment on the risks of intravenous cholangiography? Would you also comment on the approaches to be taken in patients who may be sensitive to any given dye and have reactions to it?

Dr. Burhenne: The figures show that one out of 50,000 dies from intravenous cholangiography. Some of this material comes from Dr. Ansel in Great Britain. Of the five patients who died in his series, three had intravenous cholangiography directly following a double dose oral cholecystography. I recommend that you wait at least two or three days, if you follow a single or double dose cholecystogram with intravenous cholangiography. We in California are in the predicament that we have to explain possible complications to the patient before intravenous cholangiography is done. We have difficulty persuading some of these patients to go through with the procedure.

Dr. Summerskill: In terms of hypersensitivity reactions in patients for whom this procedure is strongly indicated, are there alternative dyes, reliable results of skin testing, and so forth that are helpful?

Dr. Burhenne: We have more experience with intravenous urography and, with it, testing is of no use whatsoever. A history of asthma may indicate some patients who will have allergic reactions. We are most concerned about anaphylactic (vascular) reactions. We do not do intravenous urography or cholangiography as an office procedure, but only in the hospital where we know that we have help nearby. An additional consideration is that if you combine two contrast media, liver and kidney function studies are more likely to become abnormal than if you stick to one. You can even take telepaque, which we all use, and see minor functional changes in a significant number of patients. The same is true for other media, which are more frequently used in Europe. Nephrotoxic effects are not that uncommon. There are at least six or seven fatalities reported in patients with underlying kidney disease.

Dr. Summerskill: Dr. Popper, this is a "one-two punch" question for you: First, are the cystic duct and gallbladder ever involved in sclerosing cholangitis? Second, if not, why not?

Dr. Popper: I have seen an instance in which the cystic duct clearly was involved. The reason why duct and gallbladder are not more often involved, I cannot give you, but we see in some instances extension into the liver, and, in other instances not, without a known reason.

Dr. Summerskill: I would imagine that you would agree that sometimes the differential diagnosis between sclerosing cholangitis and carcinoma of the biliary system can be very difficult and that some patients with sclerosing cholangitis may develop carcinomas of the gallbladder or the cystic duct, Dr. Popper?

Dr. Popper: They may. The differential diagnosis is difficult. I have been guilty of making a wrong diagnosis – of having diagnosed sclerosing cholangitis histologically when, subsequently, it turned out to be a carcinoma. So one can be wrong even if one takes a biopsy.

Dr. Summerskill: Dr. Sherlock, have you anything to add?

Dr. Sherlock: I have seen a patient with sclerosing cholangitis in whom the gallbladder was involved. The association of sclerosing cholangitis with carcinoma of the hepatic duct is a very real one. I have seen two such patients this very year both with longstanding ulcerative colitis, complicated by bile duct carcinoma and with the typical intrahepatic lesions of sclerosing cholangitis.

Dr. Summerskill: Dr. Buckley, there are two questions for you. The first I think is a "non-question" because it impinges upon "union" and other principles. If you have trouble with halothane, why not try acupuncture? We won't put you on the spot there just yet. The second question, to which Dr. Popper might also contribute is: What evidence is there that halothane hepatitis may, in fact, be an inherited sensitivity phenomenon?

Dr. Buckley: First, with regard to acupuncture, postoperative hepatitis is still a possibility – "dirty" needles! I don't think that there are data which indicate that halothane hepatitis is an inherited phenomenon, unless you can infer that from the fact that cases that have been proven by direct challenge indicate an inherent sensitivity in that individual rather than a sensitivity acquired through a previous exposure. Perhaps another point that might bear on this would be the fact that there are cases on record in which hepatic dysfunction occurred after the first administration of halothane. This might indicate some inherited tendency although it is more likely that these were viral hepatitis infections which were activated by the stress of the surgical illness and therapy.

Dr. Summerskill: There are some interesting data in terms of the antimitochondrial antibody test which sometimes is positive in such patients. These data originate from Great Britain and indicate that relatives of patients with a positive test will sometimes have a positive test themselves.

Dr. Popper: I would like to raise three points: First, in halothane hepatitis the mitochondrial antibody test, this is only positive if rat stomach and not if human kidney is used as test organ. So, apparently this antibody is different from the antibody in primary biliary cirrhosis. Second, a theory which may or may not be true holds that halothane may be metabolized to short lived hydroxylated compounds which may bind covalently proteins. Their life span is usually too short for this. In some persons this life span is prolonged and this may lead to a binding resulting in liver cell necrosis and hepatitis. Third, we believe that in patients with liver diseases the tendency for halothane hepatitis is lower than in patients without liver diseases. This is important because many surgeons favor halothane for portacaval shunts or other operations on the liver. Apparently, halothane liver injury which resembles viral hepatitis is rare in patients with pre-existing liver disease. I have yet to see this type of hepatitis occur in a patient with cirrhosis. I think this is an important question which I would direct to Dr. Buckley. What do you consider the anesthetic of choice for patients with liver diseases?

Dr. Buckley: As I indicated in my presentation, from the data gathered to date on this point there appears to be no increased incidence of hepatitis, either fatal or nonfatal, when halothane is used in patients with established hepatic disease. However, most anesthetists feel that they already have enough trouble sorting out the various postoperative hepatic injury problems. They expect an increased incidence of hepatic complications in patients with hepatic disease from other causes. Therefore, since there are acceptable anesthetic alternatives, they frequently take the conservative route and avoid halothane. But I think that the few studies that are available, which are good in terms of volume of cases and design, indicate that patients with hepatic disease are not particularly vulnerable.

Dr. Summerskill: That is certainly our viewpoint at the Mayo Clinic. The next question is replete with human implications. Dr. Watson, what instructions do you give a patient, after recovery from acute viral hepatitis, with regard to the use of alcohol?

Dr. Watson: I am afraid I am variable on that. I cannot say that I give the same advice to each patient. I don't believe that alcohol in moderation is harmful after hepatitis. But one has to be somewhat arbitrary in terms of the interval of time after apparent recovery. As long as patients still have jaundice or a definitely elevated serum bilirubin or other positive tests, I don't think that they should drink anything. But when they have returned to normal, clinically and chemically; then I don't believe that there is any reason at all why they should not live like anyone else.

Dr. Summerskill: Dr. Zieve, please comment on current viewpoints concerning the use of gamma globulin in the prevention of hepatitis due to both the putative A and the B virus types.

Dr. Zieve: First, it is not useful unless given in advance of disease features. If somebody has been exposed prominently, there is good evidence that hepatitis-A can be prevented if gamma globulin is given in advance. The evidence that hepatitis-B can be prevented is equivocal.

Dr. Summerskill: You might want to modify your stance about prevention in relation to the latest Veterans Administration study which, as I understand it, showed that "A-type" hepatitis was attenuated rather than prevented. In other words, gamma globulin usually resulted in a milder attack.

Dr. Zieve: Yes, that is correct. I didn't mean to say that you never get hepatitis after gamma globulin. But one can either prevent or attenuate it.

Dr. Summerskill: It should be emphasized that there at present is no proof that gamma globulin is of help in B-type hepatitis. But there is also a "hyperimmune B-type" of globulin which has been used in a national trial with suitable control. All the data so far indicate that it hasn't helped patients in hepatic coma due to acute hepatic necrosis. The only question I have about this trial is whether or not enough of the immune globulin was always given.

Liver Failure and Liver Support in the Surgical Patient

B. Eiseman, M.D. and L. Norton, M.D.

This is a review of liver failure as it occurs in the surgical patient, the current status of its treatment and a brief report on the status of extracorporeal liver support systems. Previous analyses of clinical series of liver failure have been written largely by internists. As this review will demonstrate, their well-documented experience differs basically from surgeons who see liver failure in the postoperative period.

Clinical Experience

Consecutive cases of liver failure occurring in the immediate post-operative period were reviewed from four of the University of Colorado Medical School Hospitals; Denver General Hospital, Colorado General Hospital, Denver Veteran's Hospital and General Rose Hospital. Charts of patients coded as suffering hepatic failure were retrospectively analyzed. Only those patients dying from metastic carcinoma were excluded from the study.

A total of 73 cases were available for retrospective study during a three year period ending August 1, 1973. Criteria for diagnosing liver failure were those of the Boston Liver Study Group, class III and IV [1]. All patients were comatose on the basis of liver disease as well as being jaundiced and having grossly abnormal liver function tests characteristic of liver failure. The causes are outlined in Table 1.

Etiology

Sepsis

Intraperitoneal bacterial sepsis was a major contributing factor in precipitating liver failure in 27 of the 73 patients, or 37%. Thirteen of

---

B. Eiseman, M.D. and L. Norton, M.D., Department of Surgery, Denver General Hospital and University of Colorado Medical Center.

Table 1. 73 Surgical Patients in Hepatic Coma

73 SURGICAL PATIENTS IN HEPATIC COMA		
27	Sepsis	37%
14	Blood loss	19%
25	Portal Hypertension and Cirrhosis	34%
3	Halothane	4%

these 27 patients with sepsis died, a mortality of 48%. Most such patients in this unique hospital population had varying degrees of pre-existing alcoholic cirrhosis, but bacterial infection precipitated the coma. This is obviously in contradistinction to the usual incidence of sepsis causing liver failure as documented by internists.

Klatskin [2] has recently reviewed the association of hepatitis and infection. Although jaundice following systemic infection is an occasional clinical observation, its exact pathogenesis remains obscure in most cases. Cirrhotics are liable to infection due to the violence of their life styles and perhaps to depressed immunologic responses [3]. Once established, sepsis can more easily overwhelm the metabolic reserve of the hepatocytes and precipitates liver failure. The frequency with which infection precipitates hepatic failure in the postoperative period has not previously been emphasized due, no doubt, to the infrequency of intraperitoneal sepsis in the patients seen by internists, who have been the main contributors to the literature in this field.

Hypotension

Massive blood loss and prolonged hypotension, not associated with portal hypertension or varices, were the precipitating cause of liver failure in 14 patients (19%). Many bled from peptic ulcer associated with pre-existing liver disease [4]. Hepatic necrosis is particularly prone to occur following hypotension in a cirrhotic liver where viability depends inordinately upon hepatic arterial blood supply [5].

Portal Hypertension and Underlying Liver Disease

Postoperative liver failure associated with portal hypertension was present in 25 of these surgical patients. A dismal prognosis was observed; 23 of these 25 patients (92%) died.

Serum Hepatitis

Four patients (6%) had serum hepatitis of which two died.

Anesthesia

There were three cases where no specific cause could be identified for liver failure in the postoperative period and the toxic effects of anesthesia, therefore, were suspect. Halothane had been one of the several drugs used by the anesthetists, but was of doubtful significance since this agent is used in half of all operations in these four hospitals and other halogenerated hydrocarbons used in an additional 14% of cases. Two of these three patients died.

The exact relationship of halothane and postoperative toxic hepatitis is still violently debated [6]. It occurs once in approximately 10,000 halothane administrations, causes death in hepatic necrosis at a rate of approximately one in 35,000 [7]. Hepatitis is apparently more likely to occur when the agent is readministered within a short period of time to those sensitive to the drug. So-called halothane hepatitis is not so common as once suspected. This very effective drug is probably no more toxic than most other anesthetic, narcotic and tranquilizing agents. It is used so commonly that the true incidence of its hepatotoxicity is undoubtedly magnified. It certainly is an uncommon cause of postoperative hepatic coma.

Therapy

Next, let me review the current status of treatment of liver failure in the postsurgical patient.

Drain Pus

Sepsis was responsible for precipitating liver failure in 37% of the patients in this study. The obvious prophylactic corollary is to avoid intraperitoneal sepsis and when it does occur, treat it vigorously! Such advocacy cannot rank as controversial, but the frequency of sepsis as a precipitating cause of liver failure has not been heretofore emphasized.

The clinical surgical corollary remains as it was when Hannibal served in this city – "Ubi Pus ibi Evacua." Aggressive re-exploration should be employed in a patient where an occult septic focus might be the inciting factor for liver failure in a patient with marginal hepatic reserve. Reliance cannot be placed on antibiotics.

General Medical Support

The metabolic complexity of the liver precludes any one drug from specifically reversing the biochemical deficit of hepatic failure – yet the list of drugs advocated for treatment continues to lengthen. Most provide no more than occupational therapy for the surgeon and his consultants while they await the patient's spontaneous outcome from hepatic failure.

Early enthusiasm for drugs such as sodium glutamate or arginine designed specifically to lower blood ammonia has not withstood the inexorable test of time. Liver coma is not caused simply by ammonia toxicity.

L-dopa

One new drug, L-dopa, however, deserves special mention. Parkes [8] in England and Fischer in Boston [9] report moderate success using L-dopa to temporarily reverse the neurologic deficit of heaptic failure. This drug had been used with benefit in Parkinson's disease. It is based on the hypothesis that a false neurotransmitter such as octopamine that blocks normal response of the brain to norepinephrine is released in hepatic failure. L-dopa is a precursor of norepinephrine. It is hypothesized that L-dopa or norepinephrine competes with the false neurotransmitter and thereby allows normal neurologic transmission (Fig. 1). Recent experimental evidence documented depletion of norepinephrine in the brains of animals in experimental hepatic coma and thereby supports this hypothesis.

Fischer, in his latest personal communication [10], reports neurologic improvement in 13 of the 22 patients in hepatic coma given L-dopa. He advised pulsing the drug administration for 24 hours once a week.

Exchange Transfusion

Total exchange blood transfusion continues to be of occasional value in the treatment of hepatic coma. Rationale for its use is based on removing some theoretic circulating toxin. The latest worldwide collected figures report 24% reversal of coma in 152 trials [11]. Dr. Charles Trey in Boston is the International Liver Coma Scorekeeper.

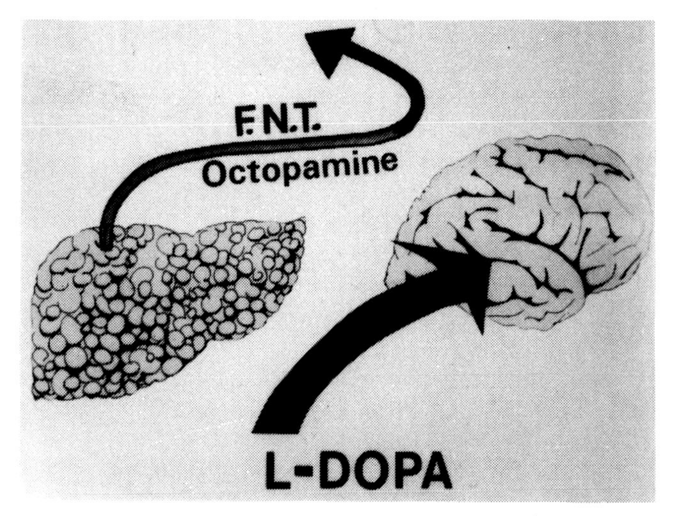

FIGURE 1.

Colonel Klebanoff of the United States Air Force in San Antonio, Texas, has used a spectacular variant of the technique achieving instant exchange with a pump-oxygenator and hypothermia. Dr. Klebanoff reports 11 temporary reversals of coma and nine long-term survivors out of 27 patients thus treated [12].

Exchange transfusion in one of its forms is effective sufficiently often to be worth trying in a patient with potential reversible hepatic failure. It occasionally can provide temporary reversal of the neurologic syndrome.

Enzymes in an Extracorporeal System

Roger Williams at King's College, London, has revived and refined the idea of using pure enzymes in an extracorporeal unit for hepatic assist. Kimoto in Japan had previously explored this idea in 1959 using both dogs and humans. The current King's College experience has not yet been reported in the scientific press but apparently has been associated with clinical improvement when used in patients with acute drug overdose toxicity. The clinical experience of the King's College group under Williams may make a place for using extracorporeal units containing charcoal impregnated with enzymes. If so, it will be vastly simpler than extracorporeal units containing living liver cells.

Hepatic Assist

Our own efforts for over ten years have rested on the hypothesis that functioning liver cells are the only effective means to provide the many complex metabolic functions of the liver for a patient in hepatic failure. Short of an orthotopic substitute or an auxiliary liver such an end can only be achieved by vascular connection between the comatose patient and (a) a normal human or subhuman compatible primate, or (b) a mechanical device containing hepatocytes.

Support by another human involves the generally unacceptable risk of passing viral hepatitis to the normal donor.

It is appropriate to record that support by a subhuman primate was pioneered by our late good friend and colleague Professor David Hume of Richmond in 1969 [13].

For ten years we have been seeking a simple, effective method for hepatic support utilizing extracorporeal perfusion of compatible heterograft whole liver [14]. During the past decade, variants of our technique have been used many times but unfortunately there have been only occasional clinical recoveries. Herculean efforts have kept essentially anhepatic patients alive for several weeks [15], but the technique is complex and does not invite repetitive use (Fig. 2).

Our experimental efforts for the past few years have been to provide a technique for extracorporeal support that will be more suitable for repetitive long-term use; we seek a technique for liver failure analogous to renal hemodialysis. We use extracorporeal chambers containing perfused (a) liver slices, or (b) liver cell suspensions.

Units containing liver slices sufficiently thin to maintain viability of hepatocytes by diffusion have the advantage of permitting perfusion with

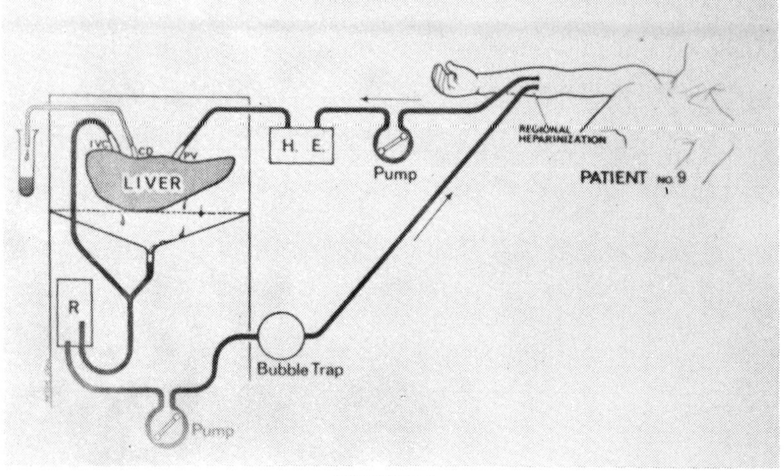

FIGURE 2.

the comatose patient's whole blood. We have recently reviewed the design of our several perfusion units using such liver slices [16]. In general, they are about 10% as effective metabolically as an equal volume of whole liver and provide significant, but far from total, metabolic support to anhepatic animals [17]. These devices do not yet warrant clinical trial.

Simultaneously we developed chambers that use suspensions of individual hepatocytes for support of the anhepatic experimental animal. The design of such chambers is complex, requiring a flow-through of the comatose subject's blood or plasma while keeping the liver cells within the device.

We have come to the conclusion that the specific gravity of liver cells and erythrocytes is so similar that no ordinary filtration system can be devised to use whole blood. Arterialized plasma must therefore be employed. Fortunately, cell-plasma separators exist that perform this function on a continuous basis.

Previous chamber designs have been described [18].

For the past year we have been using various types of centrifuge systems wherein hepatocytes are kept in rotating bags while perfused with arterialized plasma. The AMINCO unit designed for washing erythrocytes has the advantage of a continuous flow-through system. The IBM cell centrifuge works in computerized phases of inflow of perfusate (plasma), agitation of cells with plasma, centrifugation and expulsion of plasma while hepatocytes remain in the centrifuge unit. Each phase can be controlled by computer.

Currently we employ 200 gm of pig hepatocytes in each of two centrifuge bags. The cells are obtained by 1% trypsin infusion into the portal vein and subsequent passage through a brass screen filter. Viability (trypan blue exclusion) is 95% or better.

The device is mechanically sound for our purposes. For the first time in five years we have a reliable filtration method that will contain hepatocyte suspensions.

At the moment we keep the plasma in contact with hepatocytes during 15 minute cycles.

Clinical use of this device will require a cell separator to provide oxygenated plasma for hepatocyte perfusion while the erythrocytes are kept in a holding pattern prior to reintroduction into the experimental animal or patient in coma. Such continuous cell separators are commercially available from IBM.

It is too early to predict whether this, our latest unit, is going to be the answer. I am convinced of its mechanical suitability. It remains to be shown that it will give total support to the anhepatic animal or man for many days or weeks. This is the only valid test for an extracorporeal hepatic support unit.

Conclusions

A review of 73 patients who lapsed into hepatic failure following operation disclosed a clinical spectrum far different from that previously documented on medical services.

Intraperitoneal sepsis precipitated coma in 37% of our cases. Patients with cirrhosis tolerate infection poorly and the added metabolic burden of sepsis can decompensate a diseased liver. Intraperitoneal pus must be attacked aggressively in the patient with liver disease.

The rarity of anesthetic toxicity has been confirmed (three in 73 cases of coma).

Treatment of hepatic failure remains inefficient. No single antitoxin has proven consistently beneficial. L-dopa is worthy of critical clinical trial. Exchange transfusion is relatively simple to perform and can be anticipated to provide temporary neurologic improvement in 24% of cases.

Extracorporeal hepatic assist at the moment appears to be of very limited clinical value. Whole liver perfusion as we first demonstrated is metabolically effective but is so complex of performance that it is not suitable for repeated long-term use as is needed clinically for a patient in hepatic failure.

I have briefly reviewed our efforts to construct an effective yet simple extracorporeal unit using liver slices and liver cell suspensions for liver assist. The most promising uses hepatocytes suspended in arterialized plasma within a special IBM centrifuge unit.

The only valid criterion for a clinical technique is ability to support an anhepatic subject for many days or weeks. No such technique yet exists.

References

1. Child, C. C. III: Controversial Post-operative Jaundice. Critical Surgical Illness. J. D. Hardy. W. B. Saunders (ed.): Phila. p. 362, 1971.
2. Klatskin, G.: *In* Schiff, L. (ed.): Diseases of the Liver. Phila.:Lippincott, 1969.
3. Trige, D. R. and Wright, R.: Hyperglobulinemia in liver disease. Lancet, 1:1493, 1973.
4. Silen, W. and Eiseman, B.: The nature and cause of gastric hypersecretion following portocaval shunts. Surgery, 46:38, 1959.
5. Nunes, G., Blaisdell, F. W. and Margaretten, W.: Mechanism of hepatic dysfunction following shock and trauma. Arch. Surg., 100:546, 1970.

6. Simpson, B. R., Strunin, L. and Walton, B.: The halothane dilemma: A case for the defence. Brit. Med. J., 4:96, 1971.
7. Committee on Anesthesia, National Academy of Science, National Research Council. Summary of the National Halothane Study. JAMA, 197:775, 1966.
8. Parkes, J. D., Sharpstone, P. and Williams, R.: Levodopa in hepatic coma. Lancet, 2:1341, 1970.
9. Fischer, J. E., James, J. H. and Bladessarini, R. J.: Treatment of hepatic coma and hepatorenal syndrome: Mechanism of action of L-dopa and aramine. Amer. J. Surg., 123:222, 1970.
10. Fischer, J. E.: Personal communication.
11. Trey, C., Burns, D. G. and Saunders, S. J.: Treatment of hepatic coma by exchange blood transfusions. New Eng. J. Med., 274:473, 1966.
12. Klebanoff, G., Hollander, A. D., Cosimi, A. B. et al: Asanguinous hypothermic total body perfusion in the treatment of stage IV hepatic coma. J. Surg. Res., 12: January, 1972.
13. Hume, D., Gayle, W. E., Jr. and Williams, G. M.: Cross circulation of patients in hepatic coma with baboon partners having human blood. Surg. Gynec. Obstet., 128:495, 1969.
14. Eiseman, B., Liem, D. S. and Raffucci, F.: Heterologous liver perfusion in treatment of hepatic failure. Amer. Surg., 162:329, 1965.
15. Abouna, G. M., Serrou, B., Bohmig, H. G. et al: Long term hepatic support by intermittent multi-specific liver perfusion. Lancet, 2:391, 1970.
16. Eiseman, B. and Soyer, T.: Prosthetics in hepatic assistance. Transp. Proc. III (4):1519, 1971.
17. Soyer, T., Lempinen, M., Walker, J. E. et al: Extracorporeal assist of anhepatic animals with liver slice perfusion. Amer. J. Surg., 126:20, 1973.
18. Soyer, T., Lempinen, M. and Eiseman, B.: In vitro extracorporeal liver slices and cell suspensions for temporary hepatic support. Ann. Surg., 177:393, 1973.

Supported by NIH Grant No. 7 R017022-01. U. S. Public Health Service.

Current Status of Hepatitis B Antigen

Sheila Sherlock, M.D.

During the 1940s and 1950s, the epidemics of hepatitis of the major World Wars were intensively investigated and the biochemical and hepatic-histological changes associated with hepatitis were recorded. In the 1960s, such projects had been largely completed and interest in viral hepatitis was at a low ebb. The discovery of Australia antigen therefore came at a most opportune moment and provided a great impetus for research. In 1965, Blumberg, a geneticist, and his colleagues were working in Philadelphia on the development of antibodies against human serum lipoproteins in multiply transfused subjects (Fig. 1). They found that in two hemophiliac patients there was an antibody which reacted with an antigen in a single serum in their panel and this came from an Australian aborigine. The antibody, an immunoglobulin G, was found in patients who had been multiply transfused. Later, it was detected in some 20% of patients with viral hepatitis. Because of its discovery in an aboriginal serum, the antigen was called Australia antigen. Later, the term hepatitis-associated antigen (HAA) was employed, but the currently accepted term is hepatitis B antigen (HBAg). The antigen is present in about 82% of sera of patients suffering from long incubation (type B serum) hepatitis if tested within 12 days of the onset of symptoms (Fig. 2). It is usually cleared from the serum by three to four weeks. If it persists more than three months, the patient is very likely to develop a carrier state either without the features of chronic liver disease or with some form of chronic hepatitis [2].

Originally, Australia antigen was reported in association with both types of hepatitis, ie, the short incubation type now called type A hepatitis, but formerly referred to as infectious, and the long incubation period type, formerly called serum or posttransfusion but now termed type B. Later, it became apparent that a clear distinction could be made and that hepatitis B antigen was found only in the long incubation type.

Sheila Sherlock, M.D., Professor, Department of Medicine, University of London, Royal Free Hospital, London, England.

BLUMBERGS DISCOVERY OF AUSTRALIA ANTIGEN

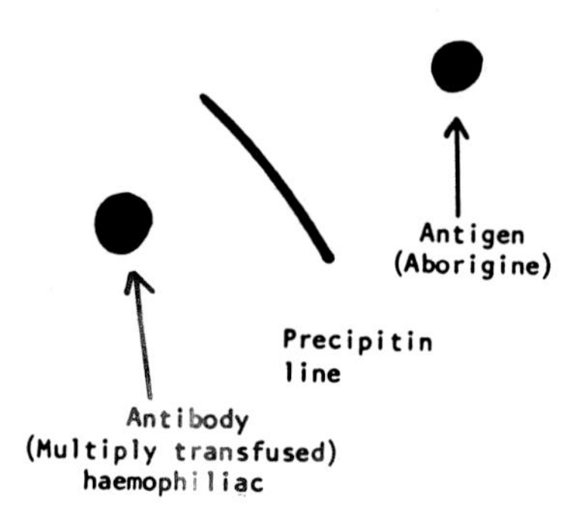

Ouchterlony's Immuno-diffusion plate

FIG. 1. Blumberg's discovery of Australia antigen.

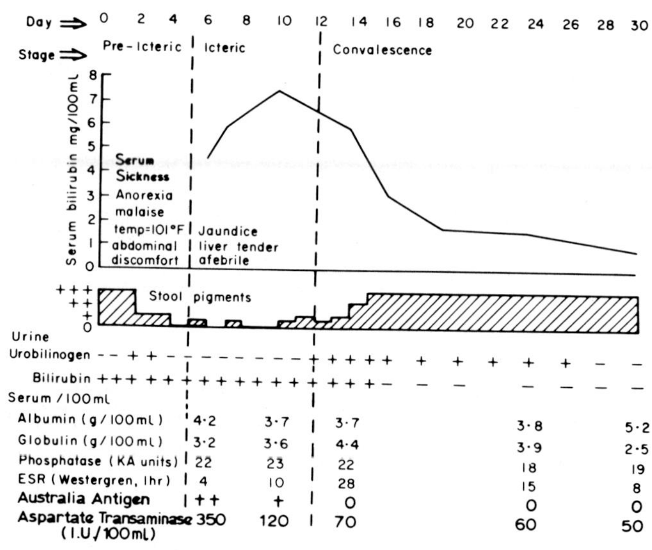

FIG. 2. The course of an adult patient with type B hepatitis. Note serum sickness-like syndrome at the onset and the disappearance of Australia antigen (HBAg) after the 12th day of illness.

Persons transfused with blood containing the antigen will either develop icteric or anicteric hepatitis or will remain asymptomatic.

Nature

The exact relationship of the antigen to the causative agent of virus B hepatitis remains uncertain. Unfortunately, the agent has not been propagated in tissue culture. Chimpanzees are susceptible to the infection but for obvious reasons this preparation is unlikely to be useful for routine testing. The relation of the antigen to virus B hepatitis rests on the close association between its presence in the blood and acute hepatitis and the infectious nature of blood containing it when transfused into a susceptible human being.

Under the electron microscope (Fig. 3), three types of particles can be seen in the serum of patients with antigen positive type B hepatitis: small, 20 nm spheres; tubules 20 nm in diameter and 100 nm long; and the more complex 42 nm Dane particle [3]. The Dane particle consists of a core and an outer surface component, each having specific antigenic properties. The surface component is antigenically similar to the 20 nm particles. The 20

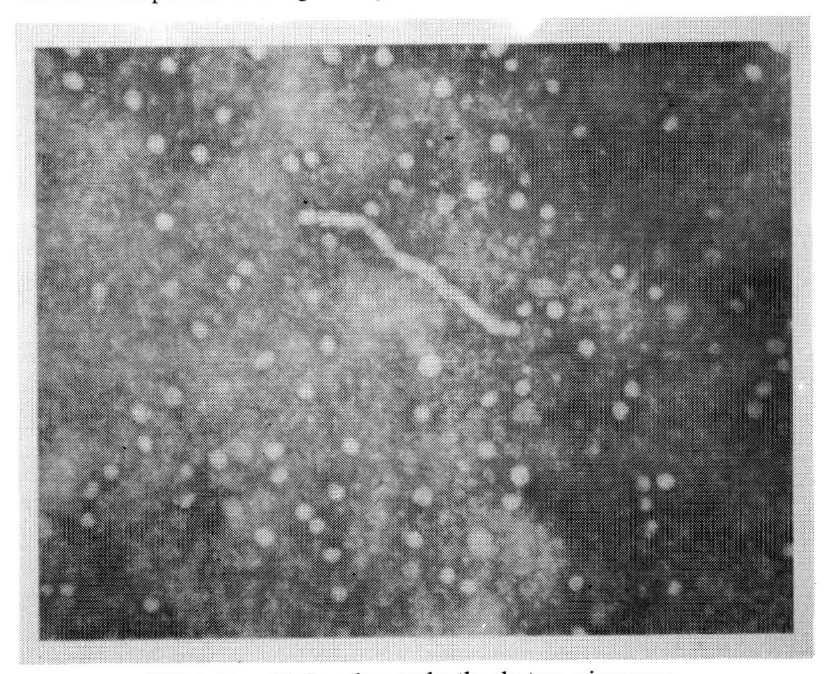

FIG. 3. Hepatitis-B antigen under the electron microscope.

nm particles appear to be formed as a result of the overproduction of the surface component of a Dane particle. The Dane particle may represent the actual *virion* of type B hepatitis and be produced in the liver cell nucleus. The smaller particles are hepatitis B antigen and may be produced by multiplication in the cytoplasm of the liver cells. The inner core bears some resemblance to a rhino virus. The inner spherical core remaining after detergent treatment of the Dane particle has its own antibody which may persist in the blood in convalescent sera of patients who have had type B hepatitis and who are now HBAg negative. Persistence of the core antibody may be useful in the late diagnosis of those who have recovered from type B hepatitis [4].

The surface antigen manifests other antigenic determinants. One is a group specific designated "a" and there are also subtype specific determinants "d" or "y" and "w" or "r." [5]. These viral subtypes appear to breed true and the epidemiologically consistent behavior of their putative gene products, the HBAg subtype determinants, have now been amply verified. These antigenic subtypes are important epidemiologically. They allow the mode of spread of infection in a community to be assessed. They are also interesting geographically. As things now stand there are distinct zones, within which one subtype predominates among patients and healthy carriers. At the same time other zones exist in which the subtypes either "d" and "y" or "d" and "r" show varying degrees of mixing. Presently, the "y" zone extends throughout most of the Mediterranean and Middle East and probably includes Western and Northern Africa, but the "d" zone seems to be more diffuse than the "y" and it may indeed at this point in evolution be multifocal. The finding of "d" among the remote and almost "untouched" peoples both in Southern Africa and in South America suggests that this is the "ancient subtype." In the Far East, both "d" and "r" are common often to the virtual exclusion of "y." The nearly complete restriction of the "r" subtype to the Far East and Oceania suggests that it may well have originated there, perhaps by mutation in a strain of "d" virus. North America and Northern Europe are mixed zones where "d" and "y" subtypes co-exist but where their relative prevalence may even now be changing. The powerful liaison between "y" and drug addiction is the most likely reason for its encroachment into areas previously dominated by "d." In Greece, for instance, the prevailing subtype is "y" and this is associated with all categories of acute and chronic hepatitis with asymptomatic carriage and with other conditions that are often accompanied by persistent HB antigenemia such as leukemia and hepatocellular carcinoma. The "d" zone lands show exactly the opposite of the rule. In mixed zone populations one sees hints of a vague but recurrent pattern, HB-type "d" predominates among blood donors, volunteers and healthy carriers and among patients with the chronic active hepatitis and cirrhosis, whereas "y" is more often encountered in hemodialysis units and most characteristically among drug abusers and their contacts [5]. A new "e" antigenic complex has been described [6]; the specificities are physically distinct from the particles of HBAg. This has been linked with the presence of chronic liver disease and the formation of anti-"e" antibody by an absence of liver disease. Further work needs to be done on this new antigenic subtype.

Spread of Infection (Fig. 4)

The classic infection by virus B is parenteral through infective blood transfusions, for instance, or the use of contaminated syringes and needles. In urban areas, the increasing incidence of drug abuse exposes larger numbers to syringe-borne infection. Infection from patients carrying the antigen is an obvious risk for hospital staff. The attendant may be infected by pricking while treating the blood of a HBAg antigen positive patient (a "prickie"). Surgeons are particularly at risk. Gloves are frequently punctured after a major operation. Steel sutures add to the risk of lacerating the glove and the skin. A minor epidemic of hepatitis occurred among a group of surgeons and attendants operating on a HB antigen positive patient. Patients who are hippies or drug abusers or suffering from chronic liver disease must always be suspected as carrying HBAg. Those tattooed should also be regarded with suspicion for the procedure has often been

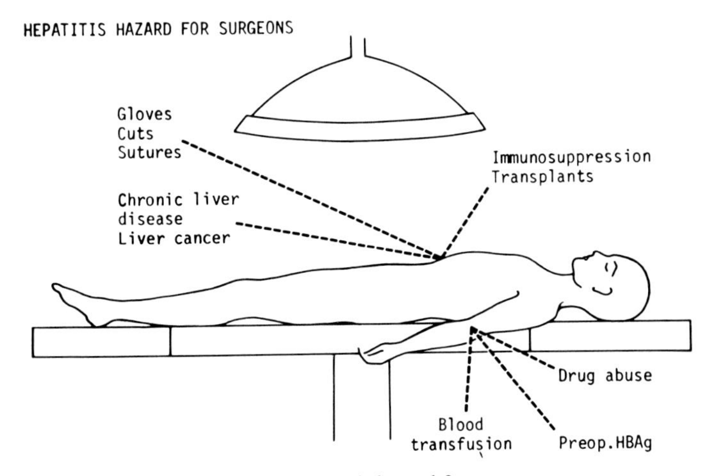

FIG. 4. The hepatitis hazard for surgeons.

performed under unsterile conditions. Positive donors of blood are more frequently found in those paid for the blood and these include alcoholics, narcotic addicts and convicts rather than the Red Cross-type volunteer.

Patients who have defective cell-based immunity are particularly liable when they come in contact with HBAg to have a minor acute attack but to harbor the hepatitis B antigen long term [7]. This applies to patients on transplant services, especially renal, and particularly if receiving immunosuppressive therapy. Patients suffering from leukemias or reticuloses are also liable to spread infection.

It is surprising that obstetricians do not acquire more HBAg positive disease. The mother is frequently antigen-positive and blood is spilled lavishly.

Nonparenteral spread must also be considered. Blood is probably infectious by swallowing and possibly by sexual transmission [8]. Saliva and semen of HBAg patients have been shown by sensitive methods to contain the antigen [9]. This opens up methods of spread by kissing, menstrual discharge, contaminated tooth and shaving brushes, dental instruments and infected scratches. In one study, 67 patients admitted to two London hospitals were surveyed to find the source of HBAg antigen [8]. Only 16 had likely parenteral exposure to the HBAg in the six months before they became ill. Of the remaining 51 patients, 13 had had sexual contact and another 12 nonsexual contact with individuals who were either jaundiced or HBAg positive. No definite source of infection was identified in 24 patients, but nine of the 20 males in this group were either homosexual or bisexual. On the whole, sexual or domestic contact was the definite or most likely source of infection in 27 patients. Hepatitis B is one of the most important venereal diseases at the present time, particularly among homosexuals.

Blood-sucking insects probably spread infection in tropical areas. Mosquitoes feeding on HBAg positive patients have been shown to contain HBAg.

Prevention

Blood Transfusion

An obvious method of control is to restrict blood transfusion and to make sure that all blood is free of hepatitis antigen. Blood products should not be administered unless really indicated (1 unit blood transfusions are never necessary). Commercial donors are avoided as far as possible.

All blood used must be screened for hepatitis B antigen. Methods of detection vary in their sensitivity and specificity. Counter immunoelectrophoresis is generally employed, although less sensitive than radioimmunoassay. However, a positive radioimmunoassay must always be checked as nonspecific results are found. Hemagglutination is a new rapid method which is simple and inexpensive but slightly less sensitive than radioimmunoassay [11]. Screening by the most sensitive method will reduce posttransfusion hepatitis only by about one quarter. Some of the hepatitis developing in recipients of HBAg negative blood could be of type A. Older studies show that the blood of patients with type A hepatitis is capable of producing the disease in volunteers. There is, as yet, no satisfactory marker for type A disease.

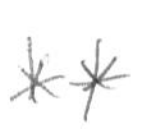

Sterilization of Equipment

Where possible, sterile, disposable equipment should be used for medical, dental and public health procedures and nondisposable equipment should be thoroughly washed and sterilized before use. This implies boiling for at least ten minutes or subjecting to steam under pressure or to dry heat. Surgeons and dental surgeons should always wear gloves when treating patients, particular care should be taken with steel sutures and special care taken when operating on HBAg positive patients.

Control of HBAg Carriers

Persons found to be hepatitis B carriers should be warned that their blood is infectious and if in the Health Services should take precautions, such as wearing gloves when carrying out any procedure in which the skin is broken. There is no evidence that they are infectious without blood being spilled or without very close contact. Studies of hospital patients and staff exposed to carriers of HBAg over a long period have shown no hepatitis B developing in the contacts.

In the domestic environment, hepatitis B carriers are probably infectious to their close family, particularly sexual contacts. There is evidence that hepatitis B carriers who have chronic liver disease, rather than being "healthy," are more infectious [11] (Table 1). Such contacts

Table 1. HBAg and HBAb in Contacts of HBAg Carriers and Controls (From Heathcote et al[11].)

Contacts of:	*No.*	*HBAg*	*HBAb*
Healthy carriers	19	0	1
Carriers with liver disease	35	3	13
Controls	61	0	1

have high hepatitis B antibody levels but a history of an acute attack of HBAg hepatitis is unusual.

Hepatitis B Immune Globulin

Although currently available gamma globulin is of value in the prophylaxis of type A hepatitis, its place in type B is in some doubt. In a prospective double-blind study on soldiers assigned to Korea, 5 ml gamma globulin intramuscularly reduced the instance of hepatitis both type A and type B for about six months. The preparation used had a high anti-HBAg titer. If an immunoglobulin is to be used in prevention, its antibody potency must be established. Hyperimmune globulin is now being assessed but is only available on a controlled-trial basis. It should be used for infants of HBAg positive mothers and for medical and other personnel who accidentally suffer exposure to HBAg blood, particularly by pricking. It is essential that the HBAg status of the recipient be examined before the gamma globulin is given for there is a small and uncertain risk of an HBAg antibody-antigen reaction being precipitated. Active immunization is under investigation using a heat inactivated HBAg containing preparation. However, such protection would require at least four months to confer immunity and would not solve thc problem of hepatitis in susceptible unimmunized persons requiring transfusion or being accidentally inoculated with contaminated materials.

Summary

Hepatitis B antigen is associated with long incubation period hepatitis. If it persists in the blood for longer than three months, a carrier state ensues.

Under the electron microscope, hepatitis B antigen (HBAg) appears as spheres, tubules and the larger Dane particles, which probably represent complete virions. Antigenically distinct surface subtypes are of interest epidemiologically and geographically.

Infection is spread by blood through transfusion or skin puncture. Nonparenteral spread by blood, possibly by urine and saliva and semen, is to close contacts, usually in the domestic environment. Sexual transmission is undoubted and in an urban situation is often homosexual.

Spread by biting insects is likely.

Patients with defective cell-based immunity (eg, on renal units) are liable to become chronic carriers.

Prevention is by control of blood donors and testing all blood used for transfusion for HBAg. Equipment used for parenteral use must be sterilized and preferably be disposable.

Hepatitis B immune globulin may be useful if given to those exposed, for instance by pricking, but is in short supply and not currently available.

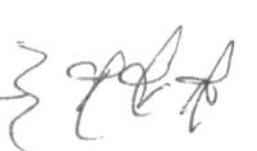

References

1. Sherlock, S.: Long-incubation (virus B, HAA-associated) hepatitis. Gut, 13:297, 1972.
2. Nielsen, J. O., Dietrichson, O., Elling, P. et al: Incidence and meaning of persistence of Australia antigen in patients with acute viral hepatitis: Development of chronic hepatitis. New Eng. J. Med., 285:1157, 1971.
3. Dane, D. S., Cameron, C. H. and Briggs, M.: Virus-like particles in serum of patients with Australia antigen associated hepatitis. Lancet, 1:695, 1970.
4. Almeida, J. D., Rubenstein, D. and Stott, E. J.: New antigen-antibody system in Australia-antigen-positive hepatitis. Lancet, 2:1225, 1971.
5. Le Bouvier, G. L.: Subtypes of hepatitis B antigen: Clinical relevance? Ann. Intern. Med.. 79:894. 1973.
6. Magnius, L. O. and Espmark, J. A.: New specificities in Australia antigen positive sera distinct from the Le Bouvier determinants. J. Immun., 109:1017, 1972.
7. Dudley, F. J., Fox, R. A. and Sherlock, S.: Cellular immunity and hepatitis associated Australia antigen liver disease. Lancet, 1:723, 1972.
8. Heathcote, J. and Sherlock, S.: Spread of acute type-B hepatitis in London. Lancet, 1:1468, 1973.
9. Heathcote, J., Cameron, C. H. and Dane, D. S.: Hepatitis-B antigen in saliva and semen. Lancet, 1:71, 1974.
10. Cayzer, I., Dane, D. S., Cameron, C. H. et al: A rapid haemagglutination test for hepatitis-B antigen. Lancet, 1:947, 1974.
11. Heathcote, J., Gateau, Ph. and Sherlock, S.: Spread of hepatitis B from carriers to their contacts. Lancet, 1974.

Fetal Antigens and Autoimmunity in Liver Disease

Charles F. McKhann, M.D. and Richard B. Helgerson, M.D.

Introduction

Antigens peculiar to liver disease have become important diagnostic tools. Of these, two major categories are of significance. The fetal antigen, alpha-feto-protein, is frequently associated with primary carcinoma of the liver and its presence in the circulation is highly significant in making the diagnosis of this disease. The antigens associated with hepatitis and cirrhosis may not only be diagnostic but have also been postulated to play a role in the pathogenesis of some of these disorders, as forms of autoimmunity. The following paragraphs will outline the current status of our knowledge in both of these areas.

Alpha-Feto-Proteins

The globulin alpha-feto-protein has been detected in the serum of normal subjects as well as a variety of pathological conditions. This protein was originally thought to be quite specific for primary hepatocellular carcinoma. However, as further screening and, particularly, as sensitivity of assays has increased, it has been found in other conditions. In this way it is similar to our experience with carcinoembryonic antigen (CEA) which was also thought to be very specific at one time, but is now known to be much less so. Alpha-feto-protein is the first globulin to appear in mammalian serum and is the dominant serum protein in embryonic life. Its electrophoretic mobility is close to that of albumin and its molecular weight is about 70,000.

Our current thinking about the origin of embryonic antigens is that the normal embryonic cell has a gene responsible for the production of a normal embryonic material – in this case, alpha-feto-protein. As the

Charles F. McKhann, M.D. and Richard B. Helgerson, M.D., Department of Surgery, University of Minnesota, Minneapolis.

individual and his cells mature, this gene is repressed and stops making this material, not making it again in any quantity in normal adult life. However when the cell becomes malignant or undergoes other changes, this gene becomes derepressed and the antigen is again expressed in adult life. The relative levels of alpha-feto-protein are high in embryonic life, dropping very rapidly at the time of birth and then rising again in conditions involving liver regeneration and, particularly, in hepatocellular carcinoma. The antigens are also found in the circulation in certain teratocarcinomas. In early ontogenesis, the yolk sac and the hepatocyte secrete large quantities of alpha-feto-protein into the blood stream. The maternal level rises early in gestation, but falls during the last trimester, rising again transiently at the time of placental disruption. The fetal level remains high until just prior to birth and then falls rapidly to adult levels between two and four weeks postpartum. This material can exist in normal adults, but at a level which is a small fraction of the fetal level. The liver, however, retains the ability to produce alpha-feto-protein as well as the ability to regenerate on a large scale, the latter being a property that is quite unique to liver tissue. It is not known whether one of these processes can occur without the other; but it is known that regenerating and neoplastic hepatocytes are the sites of synthesis of alpha-feto-protein.

The incidence of elevated levels of alpha-feto-protein in primary liver carcinoma is difficult to determine because of differing sensitivities of the various assays used. At this time, at least 70% of patients with primary liver carcinoma have elevated levels. With more sensitive assays the numbers can be much higher. In some cases, the circulating level of alpha-feto-protein has dropped following successful treatment with chemotherapy or irradiation and it can be expected to drop dramatically following resection of the tumor. Cholangiocellular and metastatic tumors to the liver are usually not associated with elevated alpha-feto-protein levels although metastatic carcinoma from the stomach is occasionally. As the sensitivity of tests for alpha-feto-protein has increased, it has been discovered to exist in a variety of benign liver diseases. These include a high percent of patients with fulminant hepatitis and a smaller percent of patients with mild hepatitis. It has been suggested that the level of alpha-feto-protein in these patients may be a measure of the ability of the liver to regenerate and that elevated levels may be an early and favorable prognostic sign.

The effect of cirrhosis of the liver on levels of alpha-feto-protein is not yet clear. Some reports indicate elevated levels when regenerating nodules are present while others using radioimmunoassays have been unable to confirm this. Other benign conditions associated with elevated levels of alpha-feto-protein include prolonged obstructive jaundice, embryonic tumors of ovarian and testicular origin and the congenital anomaly of ataxia telangiectasia.

Autoimmunity and Liver Disease

It is now clear that the immune interaction with liver disease is a complex one operating at several levels, including an autoimmune response which has been postulated to be responsible for some types of liver disease. The immune mechanism with which we are endowed is capable of responding to myriads of foreign antigens. However, it is essential that it *not* respond to what have been termed "self" antigens. On the other hand, these very same "self" antigens are strong antigens and are the materials which are responsible for the rejection of transplanted tissues. Among the antigens with which most of our tissues are endowed are those which are specific for individual tissues within the species and sometimes even across two different species. These antigens are involved primarily with autoimmune diseases and include those which are specific for kidney, thyroid, or in this case, perhaps, liver. These must be distinguished from individual specific antigens which are responsible for transplantation reactions that result when one transfers tissues from one individual to another within the species.

Of importance in autoimmunity is the location of the antigen: Is it on the cell surface or inside the cell? The immune response can react with surface antigens and utilize them to destroy the cell. Most cell destruction appears to be mediated by immunity against surface antigens. If the immune response is to internal cellular antigens, it probably cannot damage the living cell, since the mediators of this response, regardless of whether they are lymphocytes or antibody, do not appear to be able to get inside the target cell and do much damage if the target cell is intact and viable.

Of importance in a consideration of autoimmunity and liver disease is the situation where the cell is disrupted by some other mechanism, releasing internal antigens which may then come in contact with the immune response. Immunity against internal cellular antigens can very definitely be detected in a variety of liver diseases. The systems in which these internal antigens are identified are highly artificial and strongly indicate that the internal cellular antigens being studied are probably not directly related to the destruction of liver cells.

The normal immune response against transplanted foreign tissues is prompt and vigorous. The paradox is why we do not exercise this destructive capacity against our own cells. As early as 1949, Burnet and Fenner postulated that the immune machinery with which each of us is endowed had deleted from it in ontogeny the particular clones of lymphoid cells that could lead to "self" destruction. The result of this is that the "forbidden" clones are gone and that we do not have an immune response capable of reacting against our own "self" materials.

Autoimmune diseases do exist; therefore, there must be exceptions to this "clonal deletion" theory of immunity. One possibility is that the forbidden clone reappears, probably by means of a mutation within the immune system itself. The result of this is that the individual would have a clone of cells endowing him with an immune competence which he should not have and with which he was not originally endowed, but which now is capable of reacting against normal tissue antigen, providing a mechanism for autoimmune disease. An alternative mechanism is that some of our normal cells, with their tissue-specific antigens, are normally hidden from the immune response. In such cases, the antigen which is present in these cells at all times does not ordinarily come in contact with the normal immune response. This would be the situation where the normal cells exist in a privileged location where it is shielded from the immune response. We know of two or three such locations: the meninges, the anterior chamber of the eye, and more recent studies suggest that the prostate gland may also be a privileged site. There almost certainly are others. The privileged site remains a sanctuary for the cells only so long as the cells remain inside the confines of the sanctuary and the sanctuary itself remains intact. Any breakdown in the system would expose the cells to a normal immune response, resulting in an autoimmune disease directed against that particular tissue.

Another obvious mechanism for autoimmune disease is where the cell surface undergoes a change so that the normal antigen on the cell surface becomes abnormal. In this way, the antigen itself changes so that it can now arouse the immune response in a normal fashion. This mechanism has particular importance in a consideration of liver disease because it implies that any mechanism that can alter the normal antigens of the cell may cause the cell to induce an autoimmune response against liver tissue. Mechanisms that we know of that can cause such antigenic changes include some drugs which may interact with the normal antigens on the cell surface, virus infections which may add new antigen or alter old antigens on the surface of normal cells and malignancy which can alter cell surface antigens.

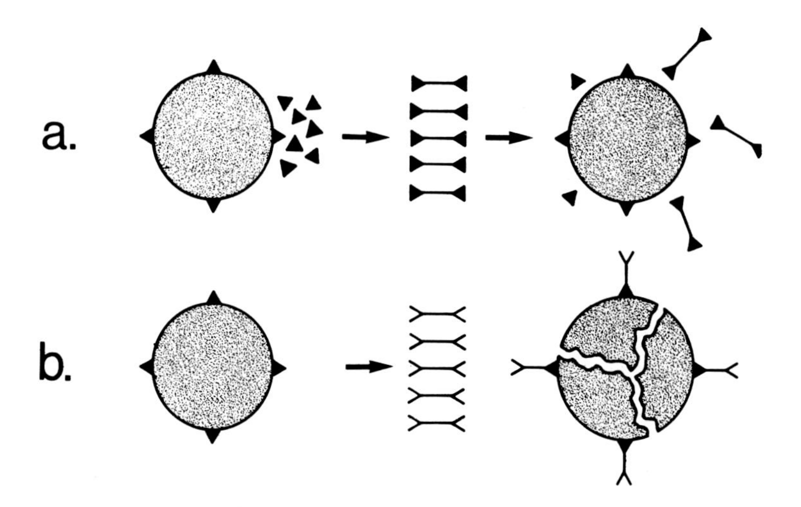

FIG. 1. Self-recognition and autoimmunity. (*A*) Normal "self" cells, present in large numbers, release quantities of antigens that block and suppress the potential immune response against one's own tissues. (*B*) Tissue releasing insufficient amounts of antigen fails to block or suppress immune response and is damaged by "autoimmunity."

An entirely different mechanism for "self" recognition and autoimmunity can be proposed on the basis of recent studies (Fig. 1). In this case, the individual has a perfectly normal immune response, capable of reacting against himself and perhaps doing so at a very reduced level all of the time. Self destruction is avoided by the fact that normal cells are present in large numbers and are producing antigen in very substantial quantities all of the time. This antigen is not only in the cell surface but is exported into the circulation where it literally binds up the immune response in situ and in that way blocks or prevents the immune response from damaging the normal, antigen-producing cells. In this way, the production of large amounts of antigen by the large mass of one's own cells acts as a feedback mechanism, inhibiting the immune response against those very cells. The abnormality resulting in autoimmunity would occur when certain cells or tissues stop making normal antigen in the quantity required to saturate the immune response. As the quantity goes down, the price goes up. The immune response would no longer be overwhelmed

Table 1. (Auto)-Immune Responses in Liver Disease

Immune Response	*Primary Biliary Cirrhosis*	*Chronic Active Hepatitis*	*Cryptogen. Cirrhosis*	*Acute Viral B Hepatitis*	*Persistent Viral B Hepatitis*	*Drug Jaundice*	*Extra Hep. Biliary Obstruction*	*Normal*	*Other Diseases*
	% of Patients Showing Positive Assays								
Mitochondrial Ab	96	25	25	rare	0	few	3	0	Thyroiditis, pern. anemia, Addison's d., myesthenia, collagen d.
Nuclear Ab	24	70-80		rare				elderly	Drugs, virus inf., collagen d.
Sm Muscle Ab	49(low titer)	25-60		60, trace	0			0	Infect. mono., tumors
Liver Prot. Ab		85		20, trace			3	0	
Cell. Imm./ liver Ag.	64	53	29			5/7			
Australia Ag.	13	10-30 (low titer)	30	100, transient	80	0		0	

with antigen and would then be able to go after the cells or tissue itself. One could expect to see this occur in the following situations: (a) abnormal growth of the cell where almost all materials are being used for production of new cells with little or none being released into the circulation, as might be the case in some forms of continuous liver regeneration; (b) loss of cell mass below a critical level as might be seen in some forms of liver destruction; (c) decreased production of surface antigen material by the cell, even though the cell remains intact; (d) inhibition of release of antigen by the cell; (e) breakdown or autolysis of antigen.

Immune responses have been associated with many liver diseases. In addition to those directed against viral materials and associated with acute hepatitis are several diseases in which autoimmunity may play a role. Of these, three have received special attention: primary biliary cirrhosis, chronic active hepatitis and cryptogenic cirrhosis. An outline of the immune responses associated with liver diseases is shown in Table 1. The immune responses which have been most carefully studied include antimitochondrial antibody, antinuclear antibody and antibody against smooth muscle. These three antigens have much in common in that they are nonspecific. Two of the three are certainly internal cellular antigens and therefore carry with them the implication that any immunity against them is probably the result of prior destruction of liver cells by some other mechanism with the release of internal materials which then cause an immune response. In this way, they reflect cell destruction rather than being directly responsible for it. All of these antigens are seen in this particular constellation of diseases thought to have autoimmune implications. They are rarely seen in viral hepatitis, be it acute or persistent. They have also been seen in rather few cases of drug jaundice. They are rarely seen in extrahepatic biliary obstruction except when the obstruction lasts longer than three months, by which time one can visualize destruction and abnormalities of the liver cells that are secondary to the obstruction itself. The other important component is that these same three types of antigens, or more particularly the antibody directed against them, are found in other diseases, most of which have autoimmune implications. These include thyroiditis, pernicious anemia, Addison's disease, myasthenia gravis, collagen disease, some drug diseases and virus infection.

In addition to these three nonspecific antigens, there are two more against which the immune response appears to be much more specific for liver disease. Antibody has been detected in some patients which is directed against liver proteins which are not shared with a variety of other cells. Similarly, cellular immunity has been found in some patients to be directed against liver antigens. Both of these immune responses seem to have their highest incidence in the same three diseases which are thought to be autoimmune diseases of the liver, occurring much less frequently in other diseases. The problem with these two more recently studied antigens is that their specificity has not been worked out completely satisfactorily yet.

There is some evidence that there may be a familial genetic disorder that underlies some autoimmune diseases, including those involved with the liver. Relatives of patients with active chronic hepatitis and primary biliary cirrhosis have been found to have a very much higher percent of positive antibody directed against mitochondrial antigen, smooth muscle antigen, nuclear antigen, thyroid antigen and gastric mucosal antigen than do age-matched controls. The relatives sampled here did not have any signs of liver disease. A similar and possibly related finding is that two particular HL-A types, HL-A1 and HL-A8, are associated with a higher than ordinary incidence of chronic active hepatitis. In the normal population, the frequencies of these two HLA types are 31% and 18%, respectively. In patients with chronic active hepatitis, they are 60% and 68%, respectively. Both of these studies suggest that some predisposition for liver disease may be hereditary and even associated with known genetic markers.

Summary

Under circumstances of disease, adult cells may revert back to producing materials which they normally produced in embryonic life but not as adults.

Autoimmunity is implicated in some liver disease. It is probably not a direct mechanism of cell destruction but rather a byproduct of it.

The mechanism of autoimmunity is not well understood but may have some relationship to the capacity of cells to produce "self" antigens which serve as a source of their protection against immune destruction.

Technical Aspects of Hepatic Resection

Seymour I. Schwartz, M.D.

The liver has long been an organ which was destined to be divided. It was, in fact, the first organ of divination, and the Babylonians in the 2nd Century B.C. used it to portend the future. A sheep's liver was divided into squares with holes in it. The subject, or patient, blindfolded, inserted a stick in a hole, and depending upon the hole selected, the future was determined. The liver was the first seat of the soul, antedating the heart and the brain.

Surgically, hepatic resection has represented an evolution from imprecise removal of parts of the liver, frequently accompanied by extensive hemorrhage, through a phase of true controlled vascular inflow and outflow, and anatomic segmental resection, to its present state. The era of anatomic resection was an outgrowth of the work of Healey and Shroy, in 1953.

It is now appreciated that the liver is divided into two lobes, along a line extending antero-inferior from the bed of the gallbladder posterior-superior to the bed of the inferior vena cava. This line and segmental lines are based on the pattern of efferent hepatovenous circulation. The left lobe is divided into a medial segment and a lateral segment by the falciform ligament.

Thus, there are established (Fig. 1) a series of lines of resection. The interlobar plane is the line for standard right or left lobectomy, extending from the gallbladder bed to the inferior vena cava. The so-called extended right lobectomy, which incorporates in the specimen a segment of the medial aspect of the left lobe, is performed approximately 2 cm to the right of the falciform ligament. The left lateral segmentectomy, which had been classified in the old literature as a left lobectomy, is performed approximately 2 cm to the left of the falciform ligament. All approaches to hepatic resection are directed at two major problems. The first is the

Seymour I. Schwartz, M.D., Department of Surgery, University of Rochester School of Medicine, N. Y.

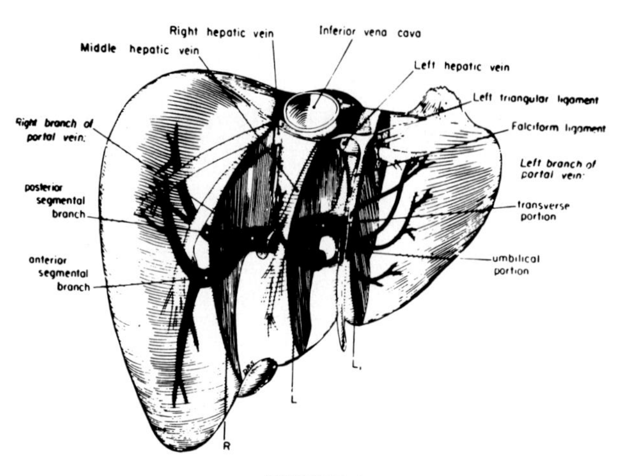

FIGURE 1.

prevention of an inordinate amount of bleeding from major vessels and the raw surface. The second is the avoidance of compromise of the vascular supply, especially the hepatic venous drainage of the remaining liver segments.

Resection of the left lateral segment and the left lobe can generally be accomplished through an upper midline incision. While planned resection of the right lobe for tumor in the dome is usually facilitated by a thoraco-abdominal incision, either using a transverse right upper quadrant incision, which is T'd into the right pleural space, or extending a midline incision, through the midline of the sternum, and T-ing that to the right pleural space.

Regardless of the type of resection employed, the first step is transection of the ligamentum teres and the triangular and coronary ligaments on the side to be removed. Without these maneuvers, mobilization of the liver cannot be accomplished. It had generally been my policy to perform hepatic resection, particularly in patients with hepatic tumors, by isolating the vascular inflow and efferent channels before progressing to the liver parenchyma itself. This is accomplished by isolating the appropriate vessels in the hepatoduodenal ligament, doubly ligating and transecting the vessels and ducts to the portion to be removed and then rotating the liver parenchyma to ligate the hepatic veins as they enter the inferior vena cava. After vascular isolation of the segment to be removed, Glisson's capsule is then incised and the parenchyma is transected along one of the anatomic planes. The advantages of these techniques are that bleeding is reduced and lines of demarcation are readily appreciated. The disadvantages are the time expended plus the unpredictable course of the middle hepatic vein, which must be precisely defined, particularly in performing either a standard right, as contrasted with an extended right lobectomy, or a standard left lobectomy.

Professor Lin suggested what has come to be known as the finger fracture technique. This technique is the preferred approach to resection of the liver in a patient with trauma. It is also my preferred approach for the management of liver tumors. Glisson's capsule is incised, and beginning antero-inferior, the parenchyma is divided between the thumb and index finger. Vessels and ducts, as they traverse the line of dissection, are doubly clamped and divided. It is to be emphasized that the afferent vessels, ie, the major branches of the hepatic artery and portal vein, plus the hepatic duct to that lobe, are divided within the liver parenchyma and not within the porta hepatis. Bleeding can be reduced to some extent by performing the Pringle maneuver, cross clamping the hepatoduodenal ligament. This maneuver can be carried out with safety in the normothermic patient for periods of 20 minutes, after which time the fingers or clamps are released to permit temporary perfusion of the liver. The maneuver can then be repeated. The dissection is continued down through the parenchyma, posterior-superior, at which point the major hepatic veins are ligated within the hepatic parenchyma. This obviates the problem of inappropriately ligating an hepatic vein, which drains a segment remaining in the patient. The dissection is carried down to the vena cava, which is bared, and the specimen is removed. The raw surface is then covered either with the falciform ligament or with a free graft of omentum.

The entire procedure has recently been facilitated by the application of a large compressing clamp, parallel to the line of incision on the segment of remaining liver.

Drainage is an important requirement of the procedure. Drains are placed in the subphrenic space and in the region of the raw liver bed. Drainage of the biliary tract is not carried out as a routine. Using this technique, Professor Lin, in the *Annals of Surgery* of April 1973, reported on 107 resections with a surgical mortality of 11%.

In regard to general management, we have felt it important to place all patients on preoperative antibiotics, utilizing those which attain a high level in bile. Postoperatively, all patients undergoing significant hepatic resections are placed on 10% glucose or fructose solution and receive 50 gm of albumin a day for a period of seven to ten days, at which time the albumin is tapered.

Bibliography

Healey, J. E., Jr. and Schroy, P. C.: Anatomy of the biliary ducts within the human liver: Analysis of the prevailing pattern of branching and the major variations of the biliary ducts. Arch. Surg. 66:599, 1953.

Lin, T.-Y.: Results in 107 hepatic lobectomies with a preliminary report on the use of a clamp to reduce blood loss. Ann. Surg., 177:413, 1973.

Schwartz, S. I.: Surgical Diseases of the liver. New York:McGraw-Hill Book Company, 1964.

Introduction to

Judd Lecture

One of the highlights of this course has always been the Judd Lecture, one of the oldest and most prestigious surgical lectureships in the United States. It is named after E. Starr Judd, born in 1878, who became a very prominent surgeon on the gastrointestinal tract.

E. Starr Judd was the first assistant to Dr. Charles Mayo, at the Mayo Clinic in Rochester, Minn., and I believe he became the number 3 surgeon there after the two Mayo brothers. In 1934, a year before he died, he endowed this lectureship.

The list of E. Starr Judd Lecturers reads like the surgical history of the United States and Great Britain. It is interesting that out of this group of lecturers, five have confined themselves to the liver, just as Dr. Thomas E. Starzl does today. The liver and the biliary tract were of special interest to Dr. Judd, as evidenced by the clinical and experimental papers he wrote on the subjects.

In 1934 Dean Louis, from Johns Hopkins University, gave the first Judd Lecture, followed by Elliot Cutler the next year. Frank Mann, in 1936, discussed "The Hepatic Physiology and Pathology from the Surgical Viewpoint." Evarts Graham, Wilder Penfield, Dallas Phemister, Edward Churchill, A. C. Ivy, Fred Coller, Al Blalock, Norman Kirk, Allan Whipple, Sam Harvey, I. S. Ravdin, Alfred Adson, Alton Ochsner, Henry Beecher, Emile Holman, Thomas Orr, Charles Huggins, Warren Cole, and E. Dahl Iverson followed as Judd Lecturers. Then in 1956, 18 years ago, Robert Zollinger, one of the speakers at this year's symposium, gave the Judd Lecture entitled "Clinical and Experimental Observations on the Pancreas." Since 1956 the E. Starr Judd Lecturers have been Philip Allison, Lester Dragstedt, Charles Illingworth, J. Engelbert Dunphy, Norman Barrett, Michael DeBakey, and both Charles Mayo and Philip Sandblom in 1963. From 1964 through 1972 the lecturers were Henry Harkins, Gardner Child, Edward Judd, Jr., Francis Moore, Owen Wangensteen, Clarence Dennis, William Longmire, Cushman Haagensen and Edwin

Wiley. Last year, John Goligher gave an excellent lecture on "The Surgical Treatment of Peptic Ulcer: A Retrospect and a Prospect."

Dr. Starzl, our 41st Judd Lecturer, complements this list of past lecturers very well. He has made major contributions in surgery and has advanced our knowledge in neurophysiology, transplantation surgery and the physiology of the liver and the biliary tract. Dr. Starzl is not a stranger to the Midwest. He was born in Iowa, where he received most of his education. He subsequently went to Missouri, and he obtained his medical education at Northwestern University. He received his Ph.D. in neurophysiology, and the first 20 papers that he published were on the subject of neurophysiology.

He obtained his surgical training at Johns Hopkins University, at Miami University and at the Veterans Hospital of Chicago, in thoracic surgery. He was on the staff at Northwestern University and subsequently he was brought to the University of Colorado, wisely so, by Dr. William Waddell. Dr. Starzl started the transplant program at Colorado in 1961, which was one of the initial and premier transplant programs in this country. While he has maintained his interest in renal transplantation, he has had a long and continued interest in the difficult problem of liver transplantation. The University of Colorado Medical Center is one of the few in the world where liver transplantation is done successfully, primarily because of his assiduous efforts. He has had too many honors to mention; he is on many editorial boards, and he has authored over 350 publications. I am very pleased to present to you Dr. Thomas E. Starzl to give the E. Starr Judd Lectureship for 1974, "Portal Hepatotrophic Factors: A Century of Controversy."

J. S. Najarian
Professor and Chairman
Department of Surgery
University of Minnesota Medical School

Judd Lecture

Portal Hepatotrophic Factors: A Century of Controversy

Thomas E. Starzl, M.D., Ph.D.

For this Judd Lecture, I would like to emphasize some of our work that has broad implications in physiology as well as in medicine and surgery. It is not a talk on transplantation. But what I will have to say should be of interest to liver transplanters and to those employing shunt procedures to decompress esophageal varices. It should also provide insight into some really important advances in the treatment of certain inborn errors of metabolism, as well as probably having some application to liver regeneration. This will be a review of one of the most persistently controversial problems in experimental surgery and hepatic physiology, namely, whether or not there are specific factors in the venous blood flowing up through the portal vein that are of any importance in the maintenance of liver structure and function.

Anatomical Notes

There may be some for whom a brief anatomical review is in order. The double blood supply of the liver consists of a hepatic artery which, of course, transmits completely mixed blood from the heart, and the portal vein which contains less completely mixed blood from the various splanchnic viscera. About 20% or 25% of the blood coming to the liver is brought by the hepatic artery and the other three-quarters to four-fifths comes in the portal blood supply. The double blood supply is retained down to the smallest structural unit of the liver, the lobule.

The capillary circulation of the liver and the means by which the two aforementioned separate sources of blood are brought to bear on the same

Thomas E. Starzl, M.D., Ph.D., Department of Surgery, University of Colorado Medical Center and the Denver Veterans Administration Hospital, Denver.

capillary bed has been clarified in recent years. Both the arterial and portal venous branches perfuse the hepatic sinusoids lined with Kupffer cells, drain into the lobular central veins, and then into the larger hepatic veins and on to the heart. The portal blood supply is intimately related to the hepatocytes of the so-called limiting plate. These hepatocytes are rich in pentose nucleic acids, and they are the most active centers of regeneration. Variations in the relative quantity of blood from the portal vein and the hepatic artery can be imposed by vascular sphincters.

Historical Vignettes

From some of the anatomical features I have just described, most old-time biologists concluded that there was a special reason for the interposition of the liver between the splanchnic viscera and the heart. It is obvious that the special ingredients could include alimentary nutriments (mainly from the intestines) or hormones (from both the pancreas and bowel). A teleologist of the old days might also have concluded, and most did, that diversion of the portal venous blood around the liver should have been incompatible with life.

It was at this point that the famous paper of Nicholas Eck arrived on the scene and thoroughly upset the apple cart. Eck's article was published in the *Military Medical Journal, Moscow,* of 1877 [1]. It consisted of about one page. First, it described the technique of the operation by which the portal vein and vena cava could be anastomosed, thereby diverting the portal blood past the liver. Second, it described eight dog experiments. Seven of the animals died within one week, leaving a single chronic survivor.

This sole experimental subject lived for about 2½ months and ran away from the dog farm. Doctor Eck obviously envisioned the possible clinical use of his venous fistula, since he discussed its possible application for the treatment of ascites in humans. He said, "I consider the main reason to doubt that such an operation can be carried out on human beings has been removed because it was established that the blood of the portal vein, without any danger to the body, could be diverted directly into the general circulation and this by means of a perfectly safe operation," a not atypical surgical exaggeration since the mortality had been 88%. Doctor Eck was never heard from again in scientific circles, but the ripples from his innocent manuscript have continued to agitate surgical and physiologic waters for almost a century, involving many scientific great names in the process.

Eck's disarming conclusion of the safety of Eck fistula was challenged in 1893 by Hahn and his co-workers, including the famous Pavlov of St. Petersburg, Russia [2]. Hahn and Pavlov described the syndrome in dogs which soon came to be called meat intoxication because it could be caused or made worse by eating meat. Animals affected by this disorder developed lethargy, ataxia, convulsions and death.

The essential technical feature of Eck's fistula was the coaptation of the portal vein and vena cava with two rows of interrupted sutures. Then, the tissue between the anterior and posterior rows of sutures was either ripped out or cut out by a pull-out suture inserted with a special instrument. The crude nature of the anastomotic technique made it difficult or impossible to consistently ensure a wide open anastomosis as can be routinely achieved with vascular suture techniques today. The inconsistency of results by different workers with Eck fistula probably was, therefore, partly explained by variations in the size of the resulting hole created between the vessels.

The work of Pavlov and Hahn tilted the balance back slightly toward the concept that there *were* factors in the portal blood that were at least important, if not vital, for the support of liver structure and function, as did also the publications of Rous and Larimore [3] who were fascinated with the atrophy affecting the liver after the performance of Eck fistula. In a statement made in 1920, Rous and Larimore said: "If so, its completeness (that is, the atrophy) would indicate that the liver has no essential activity – none on which its maintenance depends – that is not intimately connected with substances derived from organs drained by the portal system."

The somewhat mystical concept of Rous and Larimore was neither supported nor denied by the works and writings of Dr. F. C. Mann of the Mayo Clinic, who in a summary of his work presented at the Mount Sinai Hospital, New York, in 1944, said, "We have made several investigations for the purpose of determining if a specific physiologic stimulus is responsible for hepatic restoration. None has been found to date. The results of all of our experiments appear to indicate that the restoration of the liver after partial removal is dependent upon the *flow* of portal blood through the organ. It appears that the restoration of hepatic tissue occurs primarily in order to maintain the portal pathways and the restoration of functioning hepatic tissue is secondary" [4]. In many ways this hypothesis of Mann has dominated all thinking about hepatic physiology until very recently. To put it more clearly, it seemed to state that the important factor in portal blood flow was not the qualitative characteristics of the blood but rather its quantity.

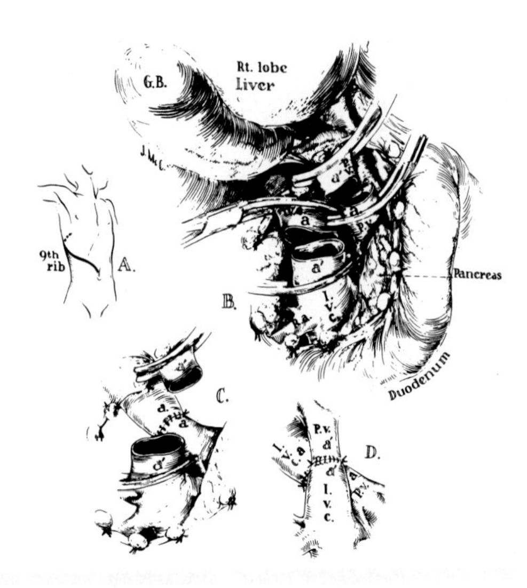

FIG. 1. Technique of portacaval transposition performed on a child in October 1963, in an effort to alleviate the symptoms of glycogen storage disease. Note that all the portal blood is diverted around the liver but that vena caval blood is used to replace this loss. (By permission of *Surgery,* 57:687, 1965.)

The flow theory seemed to derive crucial or even incontrovertible support from a paper which is truly a classic, authored by C. Gardner Child who retired last June as Chairman of the Department of Surgery at the University of Michigan. The paper was published in 1953 [5].

With this operation which, incidentally, is shown in Figure 1 as carried out in a human, the splanchnic venous blood is diverted by an end-to-end anastomosis to the vena cava flowing behind the liver, but the lost portal blood is replaced with an inflow to the hilar portal vein from the inferior vena cava. With the blood flow replacement, Child avoided in dogs most of the adverse effects of Eck fistula. The concept became completely accepted that the *quality* of portal venous inflow was *not* a prime determinant for good hepatic function, structure or the capacity for regeneration. Instead, it now became the fashionable dogma that the *quantity* of total blood flow was the main consideration.

The numerous publications of Dr. Bernie Fisher, today a Professor of Surgery at the University of Pittsburgh, were particularly persuasive in support of the flow hypothesis. In one of Fisher's publications from 1954, data appeared to show that the capacity of regeneration of a partially resected dog liver was, if anything, greater than normal when splanchnic

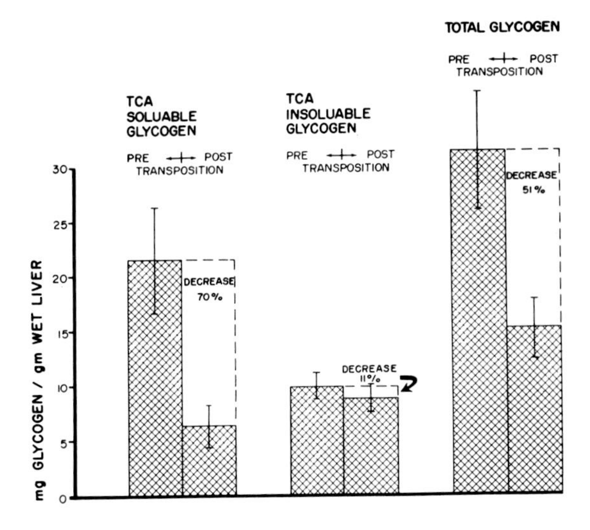

FIG. 2. Mean changes in liver glycogen concentration in 17 dogs following portacaval transposition. Vertical lines represent ±1 standard error. (By permission of *Surgery*, 57:687, 1965.

venous blood was diverted and replaced by arterial blood [6]. For reasons still not understood, it is now my opinion that these observations, as well as other later ones by Fisher, were either incorrect or else misinterpreted by him.

I found it hard to believe the flow hypothesis and in 1958 I submitted a research application from Northwestern University (Chicago) for $28,000. The application proposed to determine if subtle changes were not brought about by portal diversion, specifically affecting carbohydrate and insulin metabolism. It was suggested that portal diversion procedures might help disease states of carbohydrate metabolism such as diabetes mellitus (and also glycogen storage disease). It alluded to an interplay between the liver and incoming blood-borne endocrine factors. And, as a bonus, it promised to deliver a new method of creating cirrhosis in dogs.

Actually, the grant contributed little to the subject of hepatotrophic factors except for the kinds of data shown in Figure 2. The dogs which provided this information [7] underwent Child's portacaval transposition and afterwards were perfectly healthy. Nevertheless, the total and labile liver glycogen within approximately a month fell to about half of its previous value. In many of these animals the total hepatic blood flow was measured and found to be essentially normal. Thus, there were easily demonstrable major changes in these livers effected by the loss of portal blood even though there was replacement with vena caval blood, a vital clue pointing to the existence of portal blood factors.

The Challenge to the Flow Hypothesis

However, the most significant step in reopening the hepatotrophic issue was taken during laboratory efforts to evaluate auxiliary liver homotransplantation for the treatment of patients with non-neoplastic hepatic disease such as cirrhosis. The auxiliary operation was that originally described by C. Stuart Welch of Albany [8]. It involved the transplantation of an extra canine liver in the right paravertebral gutter or the pelvis of a nonrelated mongrel recipient. The hepatic arterial supply was derived from the iliac artery. Portal venous inflow was reconstituted by anastomosing the distal inferior vena cava to the homograft portal vein, providing a blood supply for this extra liver much the same as with Child's transposition (Fig. 3). Outflow was into the vena cava. In our laboratory in 1963, auxiliary transplantation in *immunosuppressed canine recipients* (using Imuran) was attempted for the first time and with very curious results [9]. It was soon found that these auxiliary homografts underwent rapid shrinkage which was usually evident within two weeks and which was very advanced at all times after one month (Fig. 4). The gross appearance and lobar proportions of the now diminutive homografts remained relatively unaltered except for size. The duct system was spared from the shrinkage. But within the parenchyma, there was massive loss of hepatocytes from focal or widespread necrosis, reticulum collapse and the consequent crowding together of intrahepatic portal tracts. The blood flow in these auxiliary transplants was shown by Daloze, one of our Canadian Fellows, to be actually greater than in the native liver [10]. Thus, the remarkable atrophy was not compatible with the blood flow hypothesis of Child and Fisher. Instead, it was speculated from the beginning "that competition of the homograft with the dog's own liver for nutritional or some other portal substrate may have been an unfavorable condition" [9].

We supported the hypothesis of competition between co-existing livers the following year in a paper by Marchioro in 1965 [11]. In these experiments canine homografts were placed in the right paravertebral gutter the same way as with the classical Welch procedure *except* that the portal vein of the homograft was connected to the superior mesenteric vein of the recipient (Fig. 3B). Splanchnic flow through the auxiliary liver was then promoted by ligating the portal vein at the hilum of the host liver.

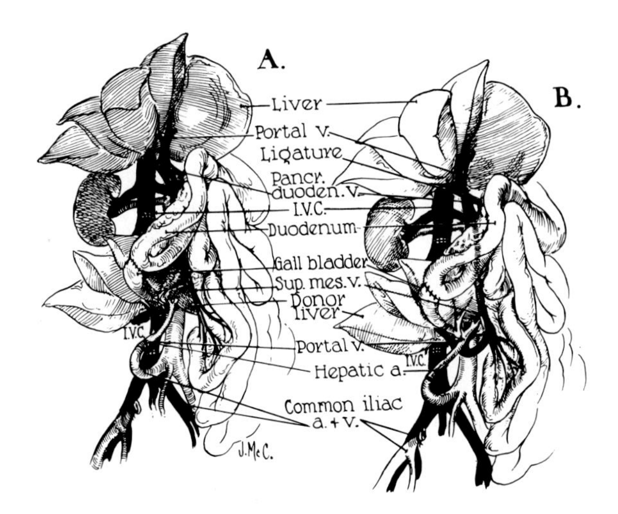

FIG. 3. Auxiliary liver homotransplantation. (*A*) Modification of Welch technique. Homograft undergoes rapid atrophy. Portal blood flow is from the systemic venous system. (*B*) Modification whereby splanchnic venous flow is diverted to the homograft. With this preparation, the homograft retains its size and the animal's own liver undergoes shrinkage. It is usually more convenient to bring the hepatic artery behind rather than in front of the portal vein as depicted. (By permission of *Surgery*, 121:17, 1965.)

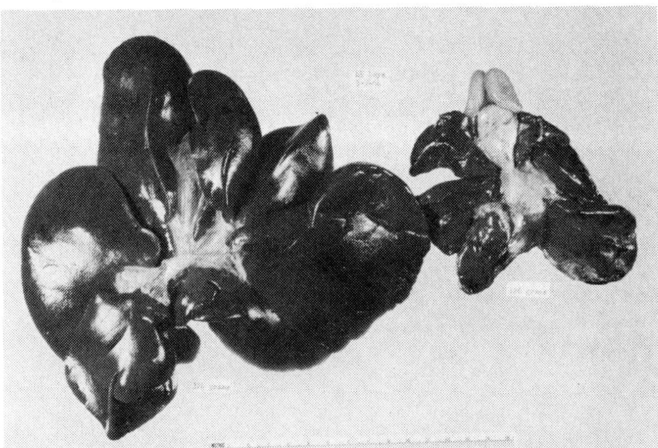

FIG. 4. The auxiliary homograft (*right*) and the recipient dog's own liver (*left*), after the kind of transplantation shown in Figure 3A. The donor and recipient were of approximately the same size at the time of the original operation. Note the well-preserved but dimensionally reduced general structure of the homograft. The gallbladder did not shrink proportionately. The specimens were obtained 45 days after transplantation. (By permission of *Annals of Surgery*, 160:411, 1964.)

These animals, which were also treated with azathioprine, now usually had atrophy of their own livers but not of the homografts. These donors and recipients had been of approximately the same size before operation but afterwards in most cases the donor liver or homograft outweighed the native organ.

Histopathologically, the characteristic injury suffered by the native liver which was starved of splanchnic blood consisted of centrilobular atrophy or variable cell necrosis, and collapse of the reticulin-supporting framework of the liver.

I will not bore you with the details of confirmation of these findings except to say that important supporting studies in the auxiliary transplant model were made from our laboratories by Halgrimson [12] and Faris [13] and by Thomford [14] of the Mayo Clinic and Tretbar [15] of the Cleveland Clinic all by 1966. However, the transplant preparations which had made apparent the foregoing physiologic effects had two serious flaws which prevented the hepatotrophic concept from being accepted by many observers. First, the total flows delivered to the two co-existing livers were often different. Second, there was by definition an additional inherent inequality of the two organs, since the homograft was often under immunologic attack *despite* host immunosuppression, whereas the animal's own liver was not. Consequently, we undertook other experiments which were designed to circumvent one or both deficiencies.

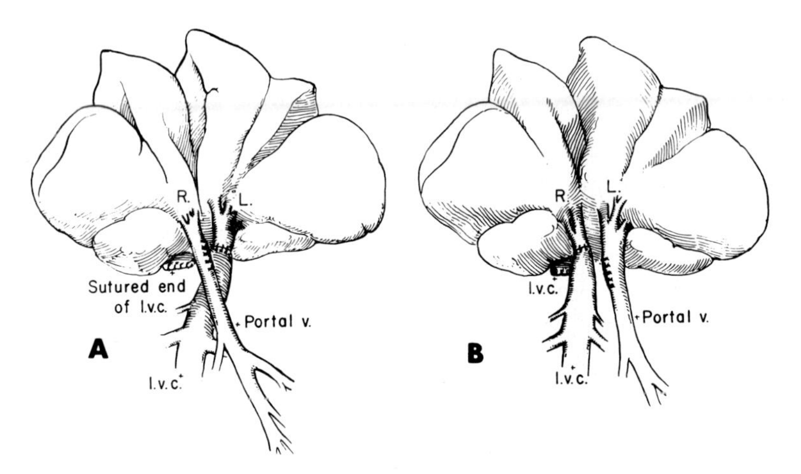

FIG. 5. Partial (split) portacaval transposition. Note that the entire vena caval flow is directed into either the left or right portal venous branch. (By permission of *Surgery, Gynecology and Obstetrics,* 137:179, 1973.)

Partial Portacaval Transposition

The key paper introduced what has been since termed a split or partial transposition [16]. With this operation, splanchnic venous blood is provided for one portal branch of the liver, whereas the other portal branch is detached and supplied with blood from the inferior vena cava (Fig. 5). The *quantity* of flow was measured in many of these experiments and found to be invariably greater on the side perfused by vena caval blood.

The results from this work were extremely clear cut and in morphologic terms are summarized in Figure 6. In these experiments the right liver lobes which normally constitute about 30% of the total liver mass had vena caval inflow. These lobes were smaller than the anticipated 30%, indicating atrophy. The left lobes receiving splanchnic blood were larger than the expected 70% normal contribution to total liver mass, indicating hypertrophy.

In mirror image experiments, the right lobes received *portal* venous inflow and now had become much larger than their normal 30% during the 30- to 60-day period of observation. The left lobes which received systemic venous input from the vena cava underwent atrophy down from the expected 70%. Histopathologic and biochemical analyses of these liver

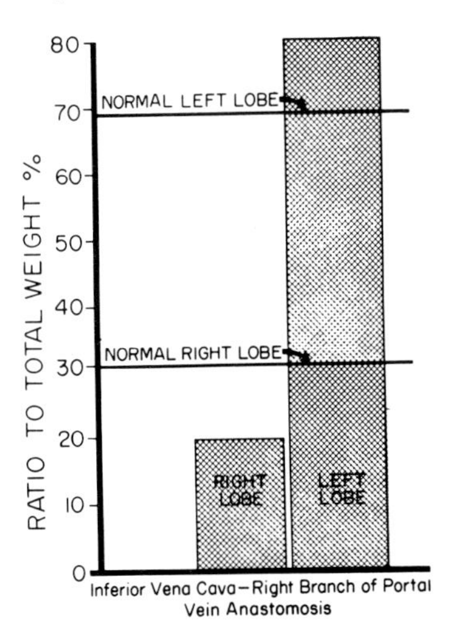

FIG. 6. Results with the kind of partial portacaval transposition depicted in Figure 5B. Note the atrophy of the right lobes supplied with vena caval blood and the hypertrophy of the left lobes which were receiving splanchnic venous blood. The results were abstracted from the original article by Marchioro et al [16].

fragments showed that the advantaged lobe complexes which were receiving splanchnic venous blood had hypertrophy of the individual hepatocytes, that these hepatocytes were also undergoing hyperplasia and that the hepatocytes were glycogen-rich.

Findings of Other Authors

These original papers describing split transposition were published in 1965 and 1967. Within a year or two, J. B. Price of Columbia [17], Sun Lee and James Chandler of San Diego [18, 19] and ther associates performed analogous experiments exploiting the qualities of the double liver fragment model. Price used canine partial hepatic autografts and Lee and Chandler used isografts of inbred rat livers. All of these experiments showed hypertrophy in the hepatic tissue which was perfused with splanchnic blood and atrophy of the other hepatic fragments. In addition, with quantitative studies of DNA synthesis, Lee and Chandler provided further evidence that the hepatotrophic effects of splanchnic venous blood upon the liver included hyperplasia as well as hypertrophy [19]. By this time, it had become increasingly accepted that portal hepatotrophic factors were probably not just artifacts of transplantation and other experimental maneuvers, but were prime determinants of the initiation and control of liver hypertrophy and hyperplasia in many circumstances, presumably including regeneration.

However, claims of the hepatotrophic factor concept were not received by the surgical community with unmitigated joy. The most vigorous resistance came from Dr. Bernie Fisher of Pittsburgh who, in a widely quoted paper published in 1967, vigorously criticized the hepatotrophic hypothesis [20]. He presented data purporting to indicate that his previous position about the primacy of flow had been once more vindicated. The summary of this article began, "Studies of auxiliary liver transplantation have revived the concept that portal blood contains specific nutrients essential for the maintenance of the morphologic and functional integrity of hepatic tissue. Prior investigations from this and other laboratories provided *no support* to such a contention. It was concluded from these studies that the volume of flow via the portal system was the essential factor." Since the perpetrators of this controversy were identified as being from our Colorado group, we had all begun to feel more than a little nervous at our apparent adversary relationship to such a distinguished surgical scientist.

Consequently, it was with no small relief, to say nothing of amazement when scarcely three years later, Fisher published the first of two papers [21] in support of that very concept to which he had been previously implacably opposed. In rats, he had exploited the double liver fragment model originally developed with auxiliary liver transplantation and then carried out partial resections of one or the other of these co-existing livers. The critical observation was that the liver remnant receiving systemic blood did not regenerate well at all. In discussing these results, Fisher conceded that . . . "The conclusion from this study that there is a portal blood factor which is capable of stimulating hepatic parenchymal cell replication *might* seem to be in conflict with other findings previously reported from this laboratory."

I hope I will not be accused of small-mindedness in making the Fisher saga a subplot to the larger story of hepatotrophic substances which I am attempting to tell. I have mentioned Fisher only to indicate that sometimes the most outspoken critics of an idea became its most ardent advocates. When that occurred, thanks to the clever exploitation of the double liver fragment model, opposition to the hepatotrophic concept markedly diminished. Most students of hepatology began to concede the qualitative specialness of portal venous blood. But, now, I would like to look to three additional questions concerning the source, the nature and the mechanism of action of these special hepatotrophic substances.

Recent Experiments With Partial Portacaval Transposition

One approach was simply to do biochemical analyses of the regional liver tissues that were receiving different kinds of portal venous input, using again the split transposition model (Fig. 5). The differences in glycogen I mentioned earlier were highly quantifiable, as summarized in Table 1, from a batch of experiments in which the splanchnic venous blood went to the right lobes.* In addition to having higher glycogen concentration, the right or splanchnic-fed lobes had more glucokinase and lower concentrations of cyclic AMP and active phosphorylase. Of course, the glycogen, cyclic AMP and glucokinase findings all suggested that the right or hypertrophic lobes were being affected by endogenous insulin. It could be equally well suggested that the increased cyclic AMP and active phosphorylase in the left lobes were attributable to the adrenal epinephrine content of the insulin-poor vena caval blood supplying these lobes. In any event, a reasonable generalization would be that these two liver sides were living in different metabolic environments in which hormone control played a significant role [22].

*The full data from these experiments have been published [22].

Table 1. Biochemical Dissociation Following the Kind of Split Transposition Depicted in Figure 5A*

	Right	*Left*
Glycogen	3.7 mg/gm	2.2 mg/gm
Glucokinase	3 micromoles/gm/min	1.7 micromoles/gm/min
Cyclic AMP	1100 picomoles/gm	1700 picomoles/gm
Active Phosphorylase	55 millimicromoles/min/mg	76 millimicromoles/min/mg

*The data and statistical analyses are fully documented elsewhere [22].

Cyclic AMP concentration as an isolated measure gives a very limited view of the rate of cyclic AMP synthesis. Studies in which aminophylline was used to block the phosphodiesterase degradation of cyclic AMP demonstrated a greater synthetic rate in the vena caval lobes. However, the differences were not great and they were not obvious for several minutes [22].

Consequently, another dynamic study was devised to demonstrate the biochemical dissociation under special pharmacologic conditions [22]. In the preliminary experiment shown in Figure 7, intravenous tolbutamide was given to induce the release of endogenous insulin. Using a radioimmunoassay technique, the insulin was found to rise sharply in the portal venous blood but with almost no detectable systemic increase. Thus, in these normal controls the background of endogenous insulin was standardized. It is well known that insulin suppresses cyclic AMP formation.

Then in dogs with the split transposition, an exogenous agent which acts by *elevation* of cyclic AMP, namely glucagon, was added to the tolbutamide challenge. The side which was receiving endogenous insulin from the splanchnic bed, whether this be on the right or left, had very minor cyclic AMP increases. In contrast, the liver tissue in which the infused glucagon could act in an uninhibited manner had unrestrained and colossal increases in cyclic AMP (Fig. 8).

It is obvious that the foregoing circumstantial evidence again pointed at hormones, particularly pancreatic hormones, as the most important hepatotrophic factors. To further examine the hypothesis, dogs with the split transposition model shown in Figure 5A were made diabetic either with alloxan or with total pancreatectomy and then treated with 15 to 20 units NPH insulin for a two-month period of observation. The presence of either kind of treated diabetes slightly reduced the magnitude of hypertrophy of the right lobes (Fig. 9), but the hypertrophy was still significant compared to that in unoperated dogs. To put it differently, the removal of endogenous insulin or even the whole pancreas did not

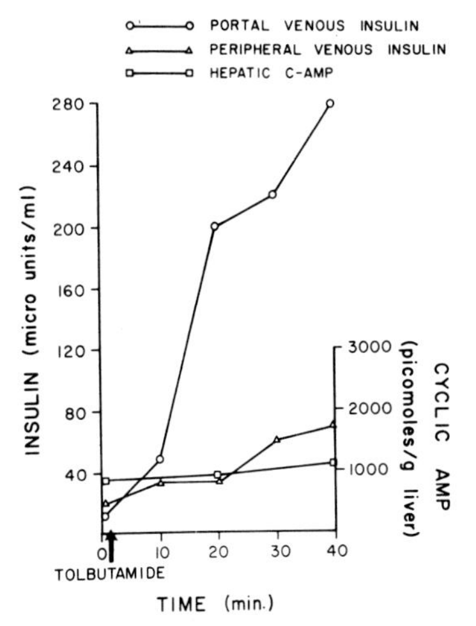

FIG. 7. Changes in peripheral and portal venous insulin and hepatic cyclic 3′,5′-adenosine monophosphate (cyclic AMP) occurring in a normal dog infused with tolbutamide. Note that the peak insulin response in the portal blood occurred 25-40 minutes after infusion and that no significant alterations in hepatic cyclic AMP were caused acutely by the tolbutamide itself. (By permission of *Surgery, Gynecology and Obstetrics,* 137:179, 1973.)

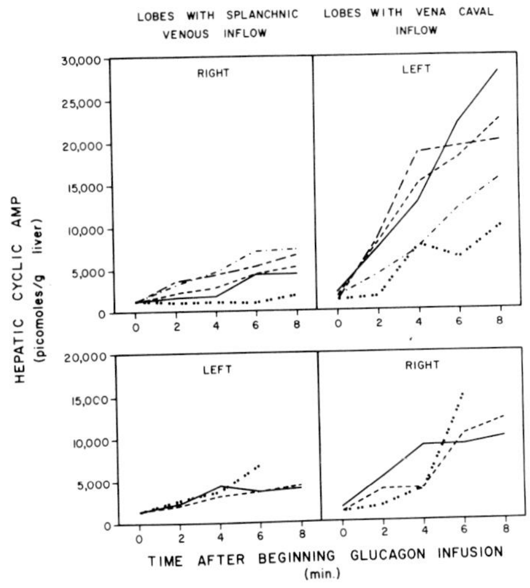

FIG. 8. Results of tolbutamide-glucagon tests in eight dogs with partial portacaval transposition, demonstrating the effect of endogenous insulin in the lobes receiving splanchnic venous blood. These insulin-controlled lobes had a restrained cyclic AMP response to the exogenous glucagon whereas the response in the other lobes was uninhibited. (By permission of *Surgery, Gynecology and Obstetrics,* 137:179, 1973.)

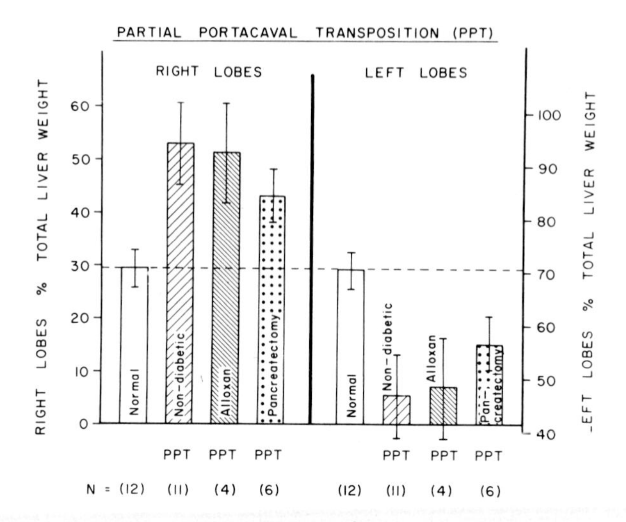

FIG. 9. Right and left liver lobe weights expressed as percentages of total liver mass in normal dogs and in dogs undergoing partial portacaval transposition (Fig. 5) with the splanchnic flow to the right lobes. About half of the operated animals were rendered diabetic, either by the prior administration of alloxan (four dogs) or by total pancreatectomy (six dogs). Note that the right lobes underwent remarkable hypertrophy and the left lobes atrophy after the transposition. This effect was only partially blunted by producing diabetes, less so by alloxan than by total pancreatectomy. N = Number of dogs in each experimental group.

eliminate all or even most of the hepatotrophic effect of splanchnic venous blood, at least as revealed by this model. In the absence of endogenous insulin or of the whole pancreas, nutrient-rich intestinal blood was better for the liver than was systemic blood from the vena cava. Histopathologically, this conclusion was even more striking. The left or so-called *vena caval lobes* contained hepatocytes that were fat laden. Although these were not particularly different in size than on the other side where perfusion was with splanchnic blood minus the pancreas, the tissue looked "sicker" on the vena caval side. Even the side receiving splanchnic flow had many abnormalities.

When the diabetes was induced with alloxan instead of total pancreatectomy, the degree of injury to both liver sides was reduced. The hepatocytes on the side receiving vena caval blood still had increased fat but not so much as after total pancreatectomy. The hepatocytes on the side receiving splanchnic blood minus insulin were in even better condition, although again not normal.

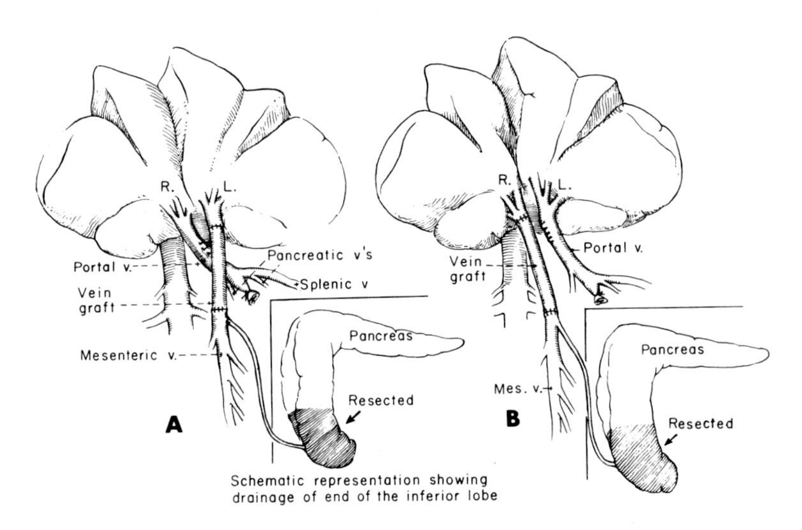

FIG. 10. Technique of division of splanchnic venous flow into a pancreatico-gastroduodenal-splenic compartment and an intestinal compartment. Blood from these respective sources is directed into the right or left lobes. The tail of the inferior lobe of the pancreas was resected since it drains separately into the mesenteric vein. (By permission of *Surgery, Gynecology and Obstetrics,* 137:179, 1973.)

Splanchnic Division Experiments

All the experiments I have just shown are consistent with the interpretation that the splanchnic blood contains hepatotrophic factors. They also indicated that no single hormone or even single organ represented the sole hepatotrophic effect. To get some idea of the relative hepatotrophic effects of the different organs or hormones, surgical techniques were developed that partitioned the splanchnic flow into its upper and lower components [22]. In some of these partitioning experiments (Fig. 10A), the right lobes of the liver were fed by a low volume of hormone-rich pancreatico-duodeno-splenic blood. By using a graft connecting the mesenteric vein to the left hepatic lobes, these left lobes were submitted to the somewhat greater volume of nutrition-rich blood returning from the intestine. In the dog, the tail of the inferior lobe of the pancreas drains separately into the mesenteric vein, for which reason it had to be resected in all such experiments. In other experiments (Fig. 10B), the lobar distribution of the different kinds of blood was just the opposite. The left lobes were now receiving the pancreatico-gastro-duodeno-splenic blood, and the right lobes were receiving intestinal blood.

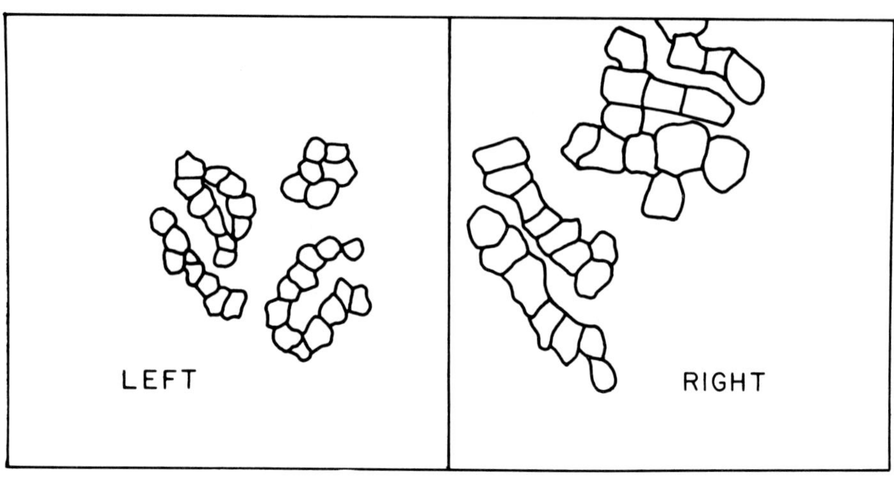

FIG. 11. Hepatocyte shadows traced during histopathologic examination. These were later cut out on standard paper and weighed as an index of hepatocyte size. The specimens depicted were from the experiment shown in Figure 2A. The right lobes with the large hepatic cells received venous blood from the pancreas, stomach, duodenum and spleen. The relatively shrunken left lobes with the small hepatocytes received intestinal blood. (By permission of *Surgery, Gynecology and Obstetrics,* 137:179, 1973.)

The effect of this kind of splanchnic division operation could be displayed dramatically on histopathologic and other morphologic grounds within 30 to 60 days. The lobules receiving pancreatico-duodenal venous effluent were big compared to the lobular atrophy and reticulin collapse in tissue given intestinal blood. With H and E stain, the individual hepatocytes on the side getting pancreatico-duodenal blood were obviously bigger and, in addition, there was evidence of hyperplasia. With a PAS stain, the same big hepatocytes contained much glycogen compared with the cells receiving nutrient-rich blood.

To obtain a quantitative estimation of the hepatocyte size in these liver fragments, a tracing device was attached to the light microscope and large numbers of hepatocytes in each experiment were drawn on a standard thickness paper and weighed. In the experiment shown on Figure 11, the hepatocytes on the left were from the liver side being perfused with intestinal blood. The right-sided and obviously much larger hepatocytes had their portal supply from the pancreatico-duodeno-splenic sources. The cell size data could then be summarized graphically as in Figure 12.

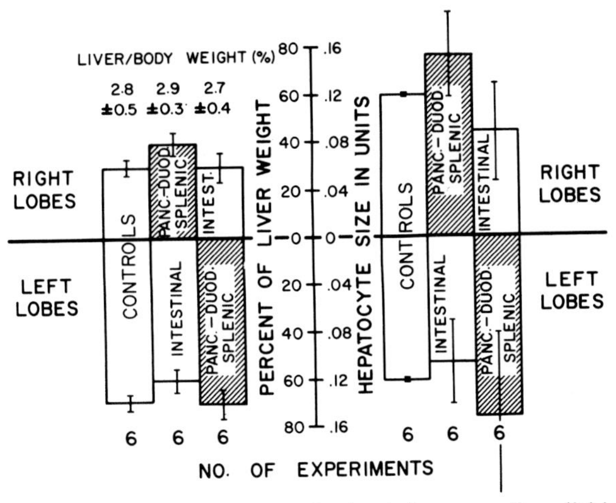

FIG. 12. The morphologic consequences of splanchnic venous flow division in the dogs shown in Figure 10 compared with normal dogs after 28 to 173 days, average 73. The liver fractions which were perfused with venous blood from the pancreatic, gastroduodenal and splenic areas are shaded. Note that these portions gained weight and underwent an increase in hepatocyte size relative to the other side while the total liver weight to body weight ratios were little altered. One standard deviation is depicted graphically on the bar graphs and written out for the weight percentages. (By permission of *Surgery, Gynecology and Obstetrics,* 137:179, 1973.)

The key data of Figure 12 are on the right, in which the size units of these hepatocytes are indicated. In normal control animals the hepatocytes were of essentially equal size with very small standard deviation in the right as opposed to the left lobes. However, when pancreatico-duodeno-splenic blood was diverted to the left hepatic lobes, the hepatocytes in this portion of the liver now became large in comparison to the hepatocytes in other liver fragments receiving intestinal blood. The same change occurred whether the pancreatico-duodeno-splenic blood was passed to the left or to the right side.

In these splanchnic division experiments, the side receiving pancreatic blood underwent glycogen storage. Also, the various other biochemical studies including glucokinase, cyclic AMP and phosphorylase determinations tended once more to show biochemical dissociation between the co-existing liver fragments. However, the results were far less predictable than with the originally employed split transposition. Because of this and because of the results I gave you a moment ago with split transposition animals made diabetic, we concluded that the hepatotrophic factors are mainly *interrelationships* of hormones rather than any single hormone, that the master anabolic hormone was probably insulin with a highly significant interplay with glucagon and probably other catabolic hormones including epinephrine. We further concluded that nutritional factors probably played a significant but secondary role. The complexity, changeability, interdependence and importance of these hormone-substrate relationships can be appreciated by perusing summary papers by Professors Hans Krebs, George Weber and others in the 1971 and 1972 issues of *Advances in Enzyme Regulation* or by reading the brilliant summary of the implications of the hepatotrophic concept by Hans Popper, which is being published in this month's issue of *Gastroenterology* [23].

Diabetes and Splanchnic Division

Although the results I just cited with the splanchnic division experiments were consistent with the conclusion that insulin was a hepatotrophic substance, the relative importance of insulin could still be debated. This question of the importance of insulin was examined in the splanchnic division model (Fig. 10) by the superimposition of alloxan diabetes and by total pancreatectomy. This was done in five and six

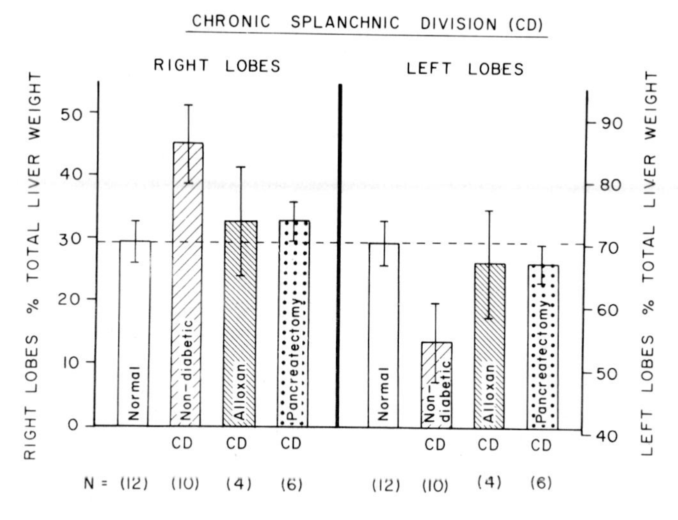

FIG. 13. Right and left liver lobe weights, expressed as percentages of total liver mass, in normal dogs and in dogs undergoing chronic splanchnic division (Fig. 10A). Half of the latter animals were rendered diabetic, either with alloxan (four dogs) or by total pancreatectomy (six dogs). Note that the hypertrophy of the right lobes produced by the surgical procedure was nearly abolished by the creation of diabetes. N = Number of dogs in each experimental group.

animals, respectively, and the results compared with 12 nondiabetic controls as well as with a dozen nonoperated normal animals. The diabetic dogs were treated with 15 to 20 units per day of NPH insulin for two months.

The results were extremely clear cut. The right lobes of completely normal dogs weighed the expected 30% of total liver mass. In nondiabetic animals, the splanchnic division operation caused a great increase in the right lobes which were receiving the hormone-rich pancreatico-duodeno-splenic blood, and striking atrophy of the left lobes which were receiving the nutritionally rich intestinal blood. This right lobar advantage was almost completely eliminated in the five animals which had alloxan diabetes established before the splanchnic division operation (Fig. 13). Almost exactly the same thing occurred in the animals with total pancreatectomy (Fig. 13). Bear in mind that these diabetic animals had to be treated with insulin which would eventually have been delivered in about the same proportions to both hepatic sides.

Another fascinating aspect of this study was that DNA synthesis as measured by the tritiated thymidine technique was much greater on the hormone-fed right side in otherwise unaltered (nondiabetic) animals (Fig.

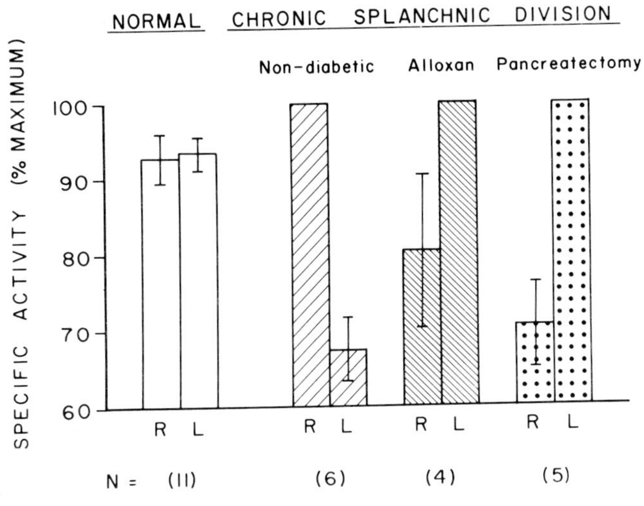

FIG. 14. DNA replication as measured by tritiated thymide uptake. The specific activity is expressed in percentages, the side with maximum uptake being assigned an arbitrary 100%. In normal dogs, there was no significant difference between the two sides. In the nondiabetic animals with chronic splanchnic division (Fig. 13A), the right lobes always had the greater activity. Note that the induction of diabetes reversed this pattern so that now the left lobes had the greater specific activity. N = Number of dogs in each experimental group.

14). The imposition of alloxan diabetes or the performance of total pancreatectomy completely reversed this situation. Now, the left, or nutritionally enriched liver lobes were predominant, thereby indicating that the dominant cell multiplication had shifted sides by the removal of endogenous insulin.

I emphasized at the beginning and do so again that our main preoccupation for more than a decade has been with the chronic animal and not with acute experiments on regeneration. Nevertheless, I have already stated that we observed long ago that liver tissue undergoing glycogen storage and hypertrophy under favorable hepatotrophic conditions also had evidence from old-fashioned mitotic indices of having relative hyperplasia. Consequently, it has been our tacit assumption that hepatotrophic factors are important to a full understanding of regeneration, a position which is supported by the data on DNA synthesis I just gave you and by much more of our work which I do not have time to go into. Recently, many authorities have supported this contention, including Lee [18], Chandler [19], Sgro and Orloff [24] of San Diego and by the more recent publications of Fisher to which I referred earlier [21]. It is only fair to say that Bucher of Harvard has been skeptical about any central role of hepatotrophic factors in regeneration [25]. Price et al of Columbia have even claimed that hypertrophy and hyperplasia as affected by splanchnic hepatotrophic factors bear an inverse relationship to each other [26].

To summarize to this point, I have reviewed work carried out mainly during the past decade which indicates that substances in the splanchnic venous blood are influential in the maintenance of hepatic structure and function. These substances appear to be predominantly, although not necessarily exclusively, trace quantities of interreacting hormones of which insulin is thought to be the major anabolic hormone, balanced by the converse effects of glucagon and presumably other hormones as well. The *interrelationship* of the hepatotrophic factors rather than any single hormone or other substance is thought to be responsible for the changes in chemical composition, hepatocyte size and the capacity for regeneration which the presence or absence of these hepatotrophic factors can markedly influence.

Clinical Application

What are some of the clinical implications of this work? One could start with auxiliary liver transplantation or with regeneration but these topics have been discussed already. In addition, there are direct connections of the hepatotrophic concept in the selection of portacaval shunt procedures. In patients who still have hepatopetal portal flow, the Warren shunt operation preserves, for liver perfusion, the hormone-rich pancreatic effluent, to say nothing of the intestinal venous drainage, while at the same time decompressing the gastro-esophageal varices. Because it retains maximally the perfusion of the liver by hepatotrophic portal factors, we believe in spite of its technical difficulties, that the Warren shunt is physiologically the most ideal shunt available today [27].

Glycogen Storage Disease

With the Warren shunt, the objective is to preserve normal hepatic physiology insofar as possible. But it is becoming increasingly obvious that the deliberate diversion of hepatotrophic factors *away* from the liver may be of significant therapeutic benefit in certain inborn errors of metabolism, of which I would like to mention two.

Table 2. Children with Glycogen Storage Disease Treated at the University of Colorado by Portal Diversion

Case No.	*Age at Operation*	*Type*	*Symptoms*		
			Hypoglycemia	*Acidosis*	*Growth Retardation*
1* (1963)	8½	III B	X	X	X
2* (1968)	7	I	X	X	X
3 (1972)	7	I	X	X	X
4 (1972)	11	I	X	X	X
5 (1972)	10	VI			X
6 (1972)	5	III	X	X	X
7 (1972)	3	III	X	X	X
8 (1973)	8	I	X	X	X
9 (1973)	13	I	X	X	X

*These two patients had portacaval transposition. All others had end-to-side portacaval shunt.

The first is glycogen storage disease, a disorder for which we recommended and first performed portal diversion more than ten years ago [7]. We have now treated a total of nine patients (Table 2). The second patient died of a technical surgical accident following the unnecessarily complicated procedure of portacaval transposition, but the other eight are still alive after six months to more than a decade. The glycogen storage diseases have been Type I, in which the enzyme deficiency responsible for hepatic glycogen accumulation is glucose-6-phosphatase, Type III (or amylo-1-6-glucosidase deficiency) and Type VI in which the deficient enzyme is phosphorylase. Stunting of growth was present in *all* the cases (Table 2). The patients with Types I and III all had metabolic acidosis and episodic hypoglycemia that required frequent night feedings (Table 2).

After portal diversion, the peripheral blood sugar response to a glucose meal was only a little prolonged in comparison to the preoperative study [28]. Thus, it would be a mistake in many of these cases, such as the child with Type I disease shown in Figure 15, to try to discontinue dietary management or to eliminate night feedings. Perhaps the reason that portacaval shunt did not produce a more dramatic glucose response what

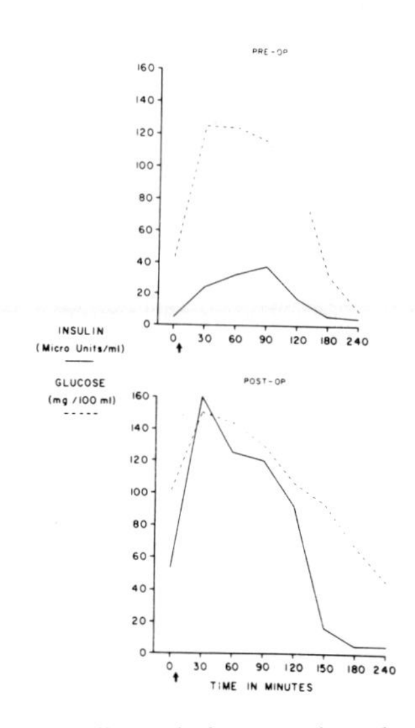

FIG. 15. Peripheral venous insulin and glucose values during oral glucose tolerance tests preoperatively (*top*) and two weeks after portacaval shunt (*bottom*). The arrow indicates the time of glucose ingestion. Note that the glucose curve is only slightly prolonged by the shunt, but that peripheral insulin levels have increased tremendously.

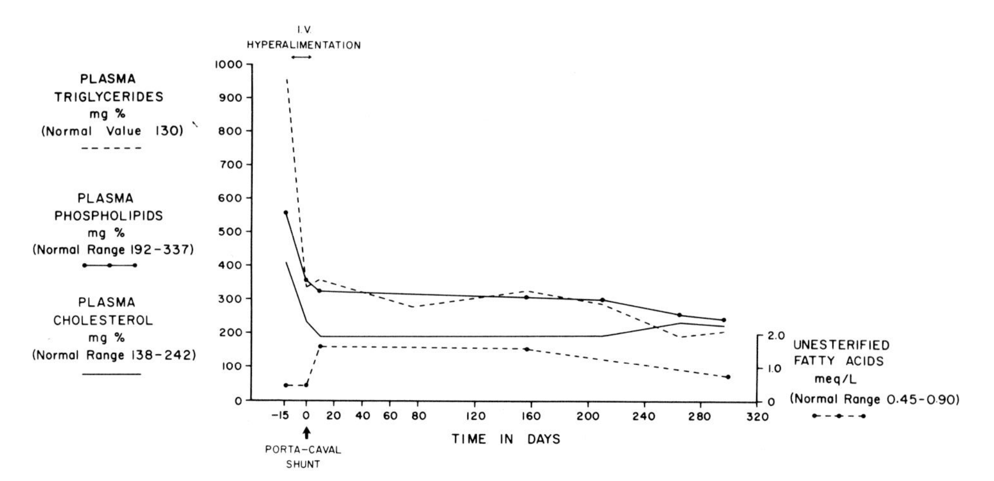

FIG. 16. Effect of parenteral hyperalimentation and end-to-side portacaval shunt on the plasma lipids of a patient whose diagnosis was Type I glycogen storage disease (glucose-6-phosphatase deficiency). Note the rapid and relatively complete reversal of all abnormalities. (By permission of *Annals of Surgery*, 178:525, 1973.)

that nutritional diversion was accompanied by a concomitant increase in circulating insulin (Fig. 15). It is well known [29] that patients with glycogen storage disease have low venous insulins, as in the preoperative study shown in Figure 15. Presumably, bypassing the liver, which normally extracts more than half of the portal venous insulin content, accounts for the augmentation of peripheral insulin which, in turn, we believe is responsible for many of the beneficial effects of portacaval shunt in these patients.

In contrast to the incomplete relief of hypoglycemia, all components of the hyperlipidemia which is characteristic of Type I disease are rapidly relieved by the procedure. In addition, there has been correction of other metabolic defects, including abnormal bleeding uric acid elevations and deranged calcium metabolism as we have described fully in an article [28].

One of the most interesting findings in these patients has been the effect of portal diversion on body growth. In our original case, a remarkable growth spurt was noted which ended ten years later in a "super-sized" teenager. Accelerated height increases have been seen in all of our patients followed for longer times. After operation, these previously dwarfed children have grown at a rate of 5/10 to one full centimeter every month (Table 3).

Table 3.

Case No.	Chronologic Age at Operation (Years)	Time of Follow-up (Months)	Postoperative Height Increase (cm)
1*	8½	113	47½
3	7	11½	11½
4	11	11	5½
5	10	8½	5¼

*These data have been published [28].

Comparison of the wrist and hand films before and 11½ months after operation show the effects of doubling the bone age in the child shown in Figure 17. The bracket shown was 5 cm in length. In addition to the size change, note that mineralization has occurred and that new bones have appeared in the wrists. Circulating somatrophins were normal. The growth spurts may have been at least partially attributable to the increased distribution of insulin to the periphery, as I discussed earlier. In recent years, insulin has been recognized to be a major growth hormone comparable in potency to somatotrophin [29].

Earlier, I provided some data from dog experiments which I have summarized in Figure 18 in terms of human anatomy. This work, which permitted the delineation of nutritional from hormonal effects in portal blood, has indicated that the hormonal influences are the more profound. Of course, in the children we have been discussing, nutritional as well as hormonal bypass was achieved and both factors may have contributed to the outcome.

In the dog experiments, there was shrinkage of the individual hepatocytes deprived of *pancreatic* blood. In the liver biopsies of our glycogen storage patients taken before and after portal diversion, there was a similar diminution in hepatocyte and lobular size. This observation explains, at least in part, why portal diversion has resulted in relief of hepatomegaly without, at the same time, resulting in a change in actual hepatic glycogen concentration.

Idiopathic Hyperlipidemia

Another example of the profound metabolic effects of portal diversion is its truly astonishing amelioration of homozygous Type II hyperlipidemia, a disease for which available therapy, including the ileal bypass of Buchwald and Varco [30], has not been very satisfactory. Sixteen

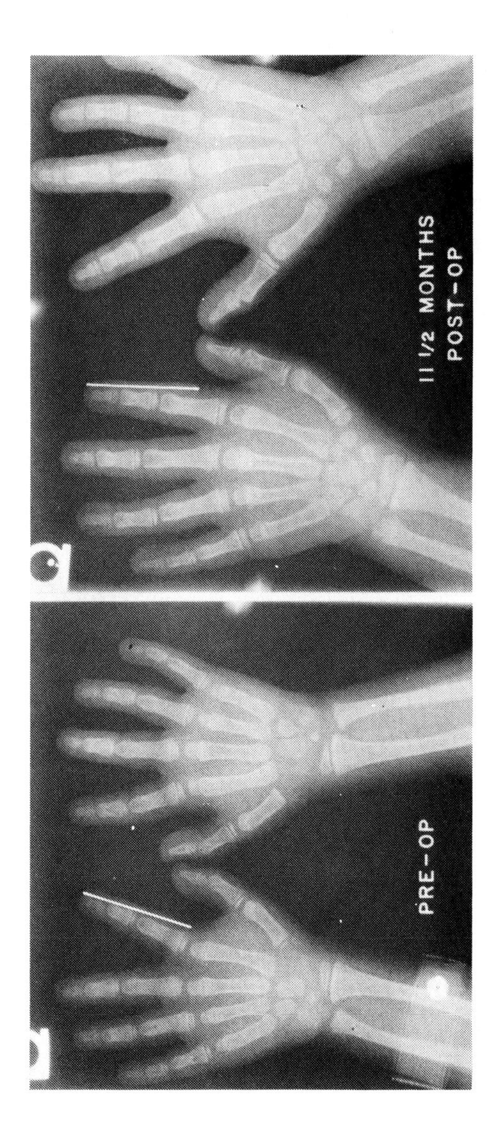

FIG. 17. The dramatic wrist and hand bone growth in a patient with Type I glycogen storage disease during the first 11½ postoperative months after portacaval shunt. The bracket on the left index finger is 5 cm in length. In addition to the size change, note the mineralization that has occurred, as well as the appearance of new bones, particularly of the wrist.

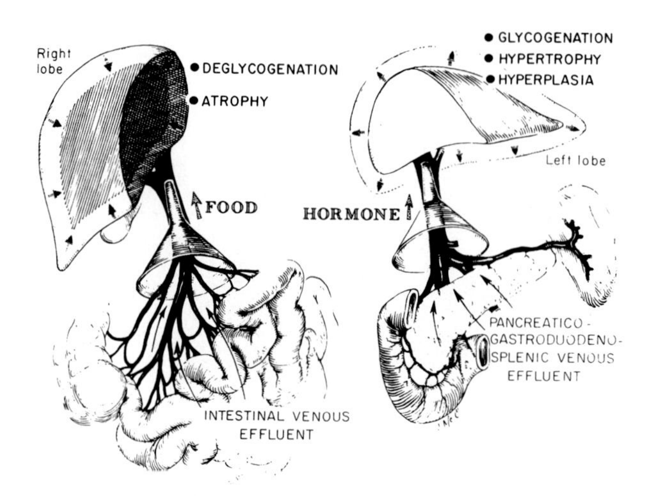

FIG. 18. Summary of the experimental results in the canine experiments in which one portion of the liver received portal venous inflow from the pancreas and the other portion received inflow from the intestine (prototype experiment as in Figure 10). The "food dominated" hepatic fragment underwent atrophy and deglycogenation whereas the "hormone dominated" fragment had hypertrophy, hyperplasia and glycogen storage. These experiments which permitted dissociation of nutritional and hormonal influences indicated that the latter were more influential than the former in affecting liver structure and function. (By permission of *Annals of Surgery,* 178:525, 1973.)

months ago we performed a portacaval shunt on a 12-year-old girl who had suffered a major myocardial infarction and who had significant aortic stenosis (60 mm Hg gradient), both presumably due to the deposition of xanthomas in her coronary arteries and aortic valve, despite therapy with diet, cholestramine, dextrothyroxin, chlofibrate and nicotinic acid.

After the portacaval shunt there was prompt regression of the hyperlipoproteinemia and hypercholesterolemia coupled with a remarkable subjective and objective clinical improvement [31]. The fall of the cholesterol values was from about 800 mg% preoperatively to just above the normal range six months later (Fig. 19).

The visible xanthomas decreased in size and it is clear that a similar reversal is occurring in her coronary arterial and aortic valvular lesions. The therapeutic effect in this case may have been due to a relative turning off of lipoprotein synthesis in the liver. At her original biopsy the hepatocytes were full of rough endoplasmic reticulum. After operation, the hepatocytes shrank and glycogen granules were scarce. Rough endoplasmic

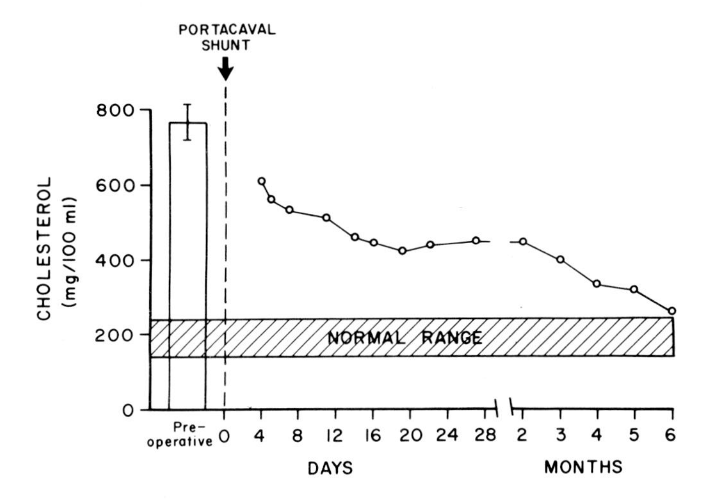

FIG. 19. Cholesterol concentrations before and for six months after portal diversion. The preoperative value represents the mean of nine determinations ± standard deviation.

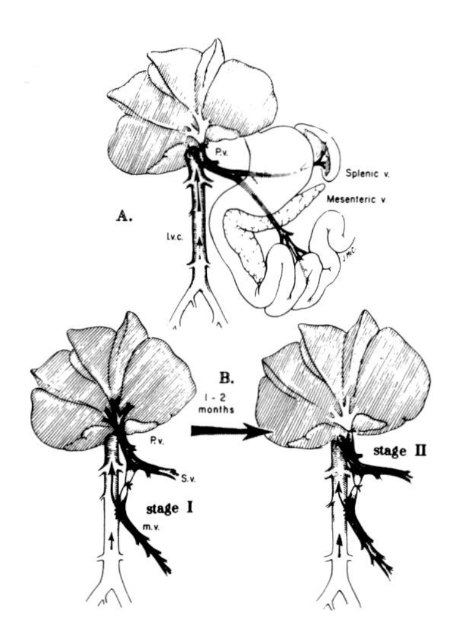

FIG. 20. (*A*) Complete portacaval shunt by which all nonhepatic splanchnic blood is diverted around the liver. In dogs, this procedure always lowers the serum concentration of cholesterol. (*B*) Selective diversion of the splanchnic blood. At the first stage the nutrient-rich intestinal blood is bypassed and subsequently the hormone-rich blood from upper splanchnic organs is rerouted.

reticulum was greatly decreased, to one-fourth or one-third of its original amount, as judged by a quantitative technique. Since rough endoplasmic reticulum is involved in lipoprotein synthesis, curtailment of this synthesis could be at least partly responsible for the improvement.

The role of hepatotrophic factors in this antilipidemia effect is suggested by the very simple experiment shown in Figure 20 which diverts intestinal nutrients around the liver by mesenteric-vena caval shunt. Later, hormone diversion can be added by a central portacaval shunt. Thus, in two stages the same thing is achieved as with a one-stage portal diversion. The same kind of result is almost always obtained in dogs and we think also in baboons. The mesenteric venous bypass has no effect on serum cholesterol concentrations, whereas when the pancreatic hormones are shunted at a second stage, the cholesterol starts down. Thus, we think the lipid lowering effect of portacaval shunt is from the shunting around the liver of hormones, particularly insulin.

The remarkable effects of portal diversion on lipid metabolism have implications far beyond the treatment of a few children with inborn errors of metabolism. At stake may be the chance to treat many adults with premature atherosclerosis.

Summary

The conclusion from these experiments and observations of the last 15 years is that hepatotrophic factors previously reported from our laboratories and by other investigators to be in splanchnic venous blood are, in fact, mainly trace quantities of hormones and, probably most importantly, insulin. However, it is the *interrelationship* of these hormones to each other and to nutritional substrate which is of key importance in the moment-to-moment regulation of nutrient and hepatic homeostasis. These interrelationships and their profound effects constitute a central and previously undefined fact of liver physiology that should reconcile a number of previously divergent opinions about portoprival syndromes, mechanisms of hepatic atrophy and hyperplasia, control of liver regeneration, and the effects of portal diversion for glycogen storage disease and idiopathic hyperlipidemia to mention only a few random examples.

References

1. Eck, N. V.: Ligature of the portal vein. Voen. Med. J., St. Petersburg 130 (2): 1-2, 1877. (Translated and discussed by Child, C. G., III: Eck's fistula. Surg. Gynec. Obstet., 96:375, 1953.)

2. Hahn, M., Massen, O., Nenchi, M. et al: Die Eck'sche Fistel zwischen der unteren Hohlvene und der Pfortader und ihre Folgen für den Organismus. Arch. Exp. Path. Pharmakol., 32:161, 1893.
3. Rous, P. and Larimore, L. D.: Relation of the portal blood to liver maintenance; a demonstration of liver atrophy conditional on compensation. J. Exp. Med., 31:609, 1920.
4. Mann, F. C.: Restoration and pathological reactions of the liver. J. Mount Sinai Hosp. N.Y., 11:65, 1944.
5. Child, C. G., Barr, D., Holswade, G. R. et al: Liver regeneration following portacaval transposition in dogs. Ann. Surg., 138:600, 1953.
6. Fisher, B., Russ, C., Updegraff, H. et al: Effect of increased hepatic blood flow upon liver regeneration. Arch. Surg., 69:263, 1954.
7. Starzl, T. E., Marchioro, T. L., Sexton, A. W. et al: The effect of portacaval transposition upon carbohydrate metabolism: Experimental and clinical observations. Surgery, 57:687, 1965.
8. Welch, C. S.: A note on transplantation of the whole liver in dogs. Transplantation Bull., 2:54, 1955.
9. Starzl, T. E., Marchioro, T. L., Rowlands, D. T., Jr. et al: Immunosuppression after experimental and clinical homotransplantation of the liver. Ann. Surg., 160:411, 1964.
10. Daloze, P. M., Huguet, C., Groth, C. G. et al: Blood flow in auxiliary canine liver homografts. J. Surg. Res., 9:10, 1969.
11. Marchioro, T. L., Porter, K. A., Dickinson, T. C. et al: Physiologic requirements for auxiliary liver homotransplantation. Surg. Gynec. Obstet., 121:17, 1965.
12. Halgrimson, C. G., Marchioro, T. L., Faris, T. D. et al: Auxiliary liver homotransplantation: Effect of host portacaval shunt. Arch. Surg., 93:107, 1966.
13. Faris, T. D., Dickhaus, A. J., Marchioro, T. L. et al: Liver radioisotope scanning in auxiliary hepatic homografts. Surg. Gynec. Obstet., 123:1261, 1966.
14. Thomford, N. R., Shorter, R. G. and Hallenbeck, G. A.: Homotransplantation of the canine liver. Arch. Surg., 90:527, 1965.
15. Tretbar, L. L., Beven, E. G. and Hermann, R. E.: The effects of portacaval shunt and portal flow occlusion on canine auxiliary liver homotransplants. Surgery, 61:733, 1967.
16. Marchioro, T. L., Porter, K. A., Illingworth, B. I. et al: The specific influence of nonhepatic splanchnic venous blood flow upon the liver. Surg. Forum, 16:280, 1965.
17. Price, J. B., Jr., Voorhees, A. B., Jr. and Britton, R. C.: The role of portal blood in regeneration and function of completely revascularized partial hepatic autografts. Surgery, 62:195, 1967.
18. Lee, S., Keiter, J. E., Rosen, H. et al: Influence of blood supply on regeneration of liver transplants. Surg. Forum, 20:369, 1969.
19. Chandler, J. G., Lee, S., Krubel, R. et al: The roles of inter-liver competition and portal blood in regeneration of auxiliary liver transplants. Surg. Forum, 22:341, 1971.
20. Fisher, B., Fisher, E. R. and Lee, S.: Experimental evaluation of liver atrophy and portacaval shunt. Surg. Gynec. Obstet., 125:1253, 1967.
21. Fisher, B., Fisher, E. R. and Saffer, E.: Investigations concerning the role of a

humoral factor in liver regeneration. Cancer Res., 23:914, 1963.
22. Starzl, T. E., Francavilla, A., Halgrimson, C. G. et al: The origin, hormonal nature and action of portal venous hepatotrophic substances. Surg. Gynec. Obstet., 137:179, 1973.
23. Popper, H.: Panel on portal hepatotrophic factors: Implications in hepatology. Gastroenterology. (In press.)
24. Sgro, J.-C., Charters, A. C., Chandler, J. G. et al: Site of origin of the hepatotrophic portal blood factor involved in liver regeneration. Surg. Forum, 24:377, 1973.
25. Bucher, N. L. R. and Swaffield, M. N.: Regeneration of liver in rats in the absence of portal splanchnic organs and a portal blood supply. Cancer Res., 33:3189, 1973.
26. Price, J. B., Jr., Takeshige, K., Max, M. H. et al: Glucagon as the portal factor modifying hepatic regeneration. Surgery, 72:74, 1972.
27. Warren, W. D., Zeppa, R. and Fomon, J. J.: Selective trans-splenic decompression of gastroesophageal varices by distal splenorenal shunt. Ann. Surg., 166:437, 1967.
28. Starzl, T. E., Putnam, C. W., Porter, K. A. et al: Portal diversion for the treatment of glycogen storage disease in humans. Ann. Surg., 178:525, 1973.
29. Lockwood, D. H., Merimee, T. J., Edgar, P. J. et al: Insulin secretion in Type I glycogen storage disease. Diabetes, 18:755, 1969.
30. Moore, R. B., Varco, R. L. and Buchwald, H.: Metabolic surgery in the hyperlipoproteinemias. Amer. J. Cardiol., 31:148, 1973.
31. Starzl, T. E., Chase, H. P., Putnam, C. W. et al: Portacaval shunt in hyperlipoproteinemia. Lancet, 2:940, 1973.

The work was supported by research grants from the Veterans Administration; by grants AI-AM-08898 and AM-07772 from the National Institutes of Health; by grants RR-00051 and RR-00069 from the General Clinical Research Centers Program of the Division of Research Resources, National Institutes of Health.

Liver Transplantation

Thomas E. Starzl, M.D., Ph.D. and Charles W. Putnam, M.D.

What I would like to do in this first paper is to give a general survey of liver transplantation but omit the overriding issue of liver sepsis, as this relates to biliary duct reconstruction. I will focus specifically on this problem of liver sepsis in a second report.

Varieties of Liver Transplantation

There are two fundamentally different kinds of hepatic transplantation procedures. In one, a second organ is placed in some abnormal location such as the paravertebral gutter, the splenic fossa or the pelvis. If an auxiliary graft is to succeed, I believe it should be revascularized according to the principles I discussed in connection with the hepatotrophic factors in my Judd Lecture (Fig. 1). Note in Figure 1 that the splanchnic blood perfuses the auxiliary liver through a mesenteric-portal anastomosis, that the hepatic artery is attached to the aorta and that the outflow is to the vena cava.

The results with auxiliary transplantation in patients (and for that matter in animals) have been so discouraging that I have not done one for about six years. However, Dr. Joseph Fortner of New York has an auxiliary graft recipient going now more than a year after the exact operation shown in Figure 1 for the indication of biliary atresia. This is a very important case which will certainly bear watching.

Incidentally, some of the most interesting possibilities for auxiliary transplantation are certain inborn errors of metabolism, of which I will mention just two. One is the Crigler-Najjar syndrome in which the function of the native liver is quite normal except for the inability to conjugate bilirubin due to the absence of glucuronyl transferase. The

Thomas E. Starzl, M.D., Ph.D. and Charles W. Putnam, M.D., Department of Surgery, University of Colorado Medical Center and the Veterans Administration Hospital, Denver.

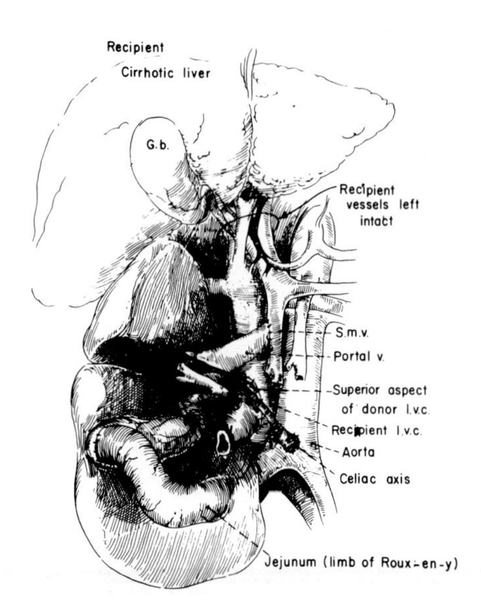

FIG. 1. Auxiliary liver transplantation as carried out clinically. Note that transplant was given a double blood supply and that the venous component was from nonhepatic splanchnic bed. Technique was almost identical to that developed in dogs. Biliary drainage should be with a Roux-en-Y cholecystojejunostomy. (By permission of W. B. Saunders Company, 1969.)

second possibility is juvenile Gaucher's disease. Here the missing enzyme is Beta glucosidase. The resulting cramming of the reticuloendothelial system may actually lead to liver failure. With either of these disorders, an auxiliary liver should be curative; in the Crigler-Najjar syndrome simply by clearing bilirubin and in the Gaucher's patient by providing the enzyme which would probably reverse the hepatic lesion and cause removal of the deposits of glucosyl ceramide elsewhere.

Orthotopic Transplantation

The rest of my remarks will deal with orthotopic liver transplantation, that is, about liver replacement. The diseased native liver is removed and revascularization of the graft is performed in as anatomically normal a way as possible – anastomosing the portal vein and hepatic artery end-to-end and reconstructing the vena cava above and below the liver. In most of our early cases, we have anastomosed the gallbladder to the duodenum after ligating the distal common duct (Fig. 2). I will be outlining the hazards of this approach in my second report.

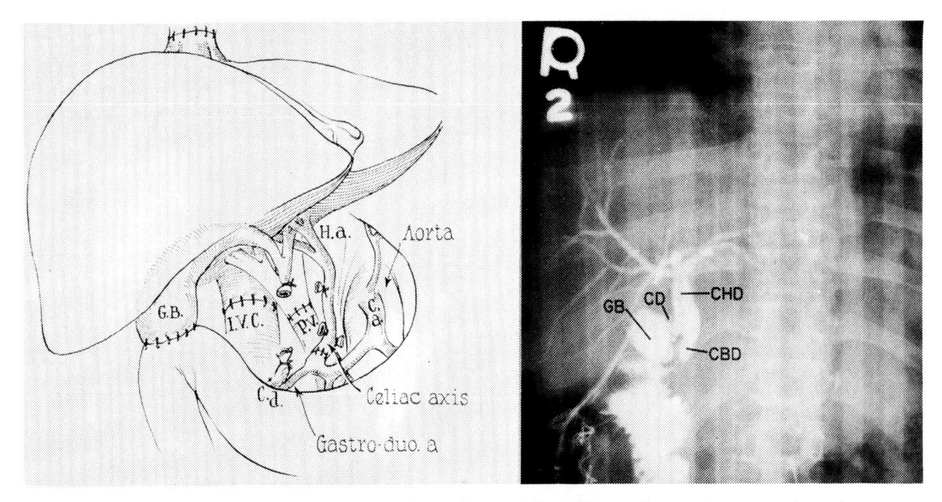

FIG. 2. Orthotopic liver transplantation with biliary duct reconstruction by cholecystoduodenostomy. The cholangiogram on right was obtained at reoperation by inserting a Foley catheter into gallbladder. There was no evidence of obstruction. CBD – common bile duct; CD – cystic duct; CHD – common hepatic duct; GB – gallbladder. (By permission of *Surgery*, 72:604, 1972.)

Indications for Operation

With these preliminary remarks I will now turn to the question about the indications for operation. At the beginning, we thought that the ideal reason for liver replacement would be primary hepatic malignancies, including hepatoma. Our enthusiasm was quickly dampened by the kind of experience which I will illustrate for you with a single case.

In Figure 3 are chest x-rays of a 15-year-old boy. A few weeks after "successful" orthotopic liver transplantation for a gigantic hepatoma, there was already a small pulmonary metastasis. He died 143 days after operation with his lungs almost replaced by metastases.

During the same interval, his new liver was similarly invaded as could be followed with serial scans (Fig. 4). There was evidence of metastases at all times after three months. He finally died of combined hepatic and pulmonary insufficiency. At autopsy, his lungs were a mass of tumor (Fig. 5). The same was true of his liver to an extent that only a tiny remnant of normal hepatic tissue remained (Fig. 6).

We have had a half a dozen other so-called successful liver transplantations with subsequent widespread metastases of hepatomas and one similar experience with a hemangioendotheliosarcoma. Three of the patients died beyond one year posttransplantation of tumor spread.

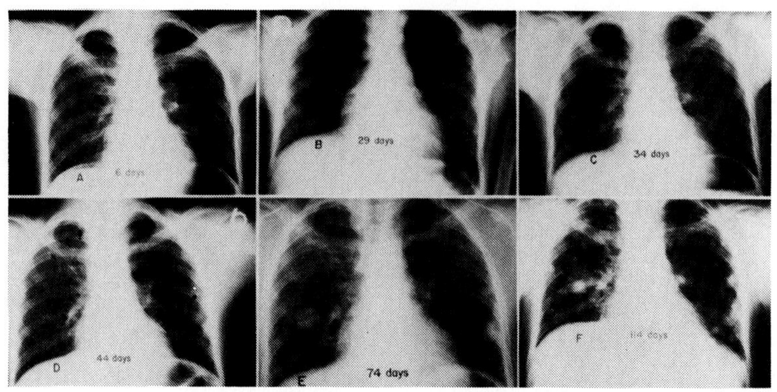

FIG. 3. The extremely rapid development of pulmonary metastases. (*A*) The chest is clear 6 days after liver replacement for indication of hepatoma; (*B*) 29 days postoperative. Two metastases are visible in left lower lung field (*arrows*); (*C*) 5 days later the tumor deposits previously seen have grown in size (*horizontal arrows*) and a third focus is now present in right upper lobe (*vertical arrow*); (*D*) 44 days. Only ten days have elapsed since last examination. Metastatic growths are scattered throughout lungs (*arrows*); (*E*) 74 days postoperative; (*F*) four months after operation. Transient dyspnea was first noticed a few days later. Patient died of pulmonary and hepatic insufficiency 143 days after transplantation. (By permission of W. B. Saunders Company, 1969.)

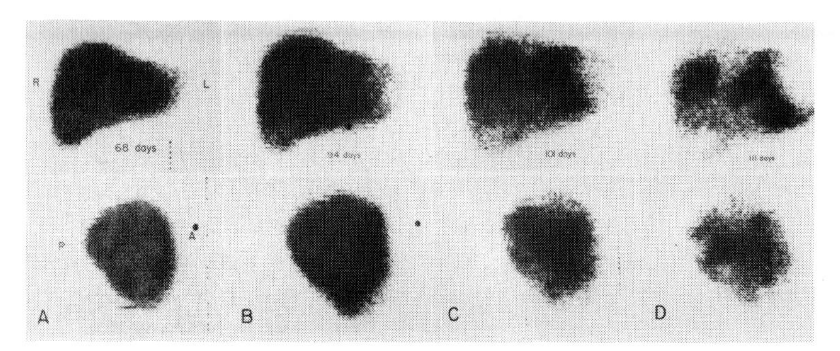

FIG. 4. Destruction of the homograft in the same patient as Figure 3 by tumor recurrence. Postero-anterior and lateral liver scans were obtained with 99m technetium. (*A*) 68 days; (*B*) 94 days: patient had become jaundiced; hepatomegaly is evident; (*C*) 101 days: multiple areas of poor isotope concentration are now visible; (*D*) 111 days: process has continued its rapid progression. By the time of death one month later, the homograft was almost completely replaced with carcinoma. (By permission of W. B. Saunders Company, 1969.)

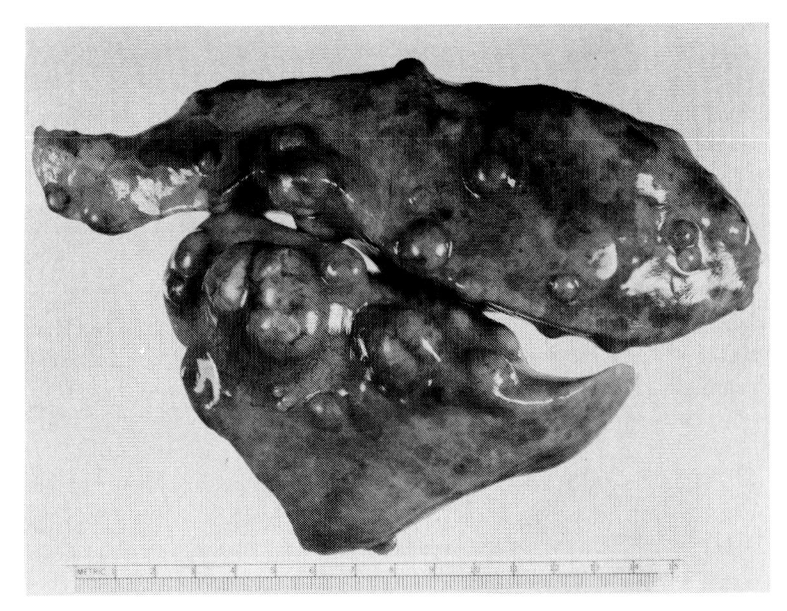

FIG. 5. Extensive pulmonary metastases in same patient as in Figures 3, 4 and 6.

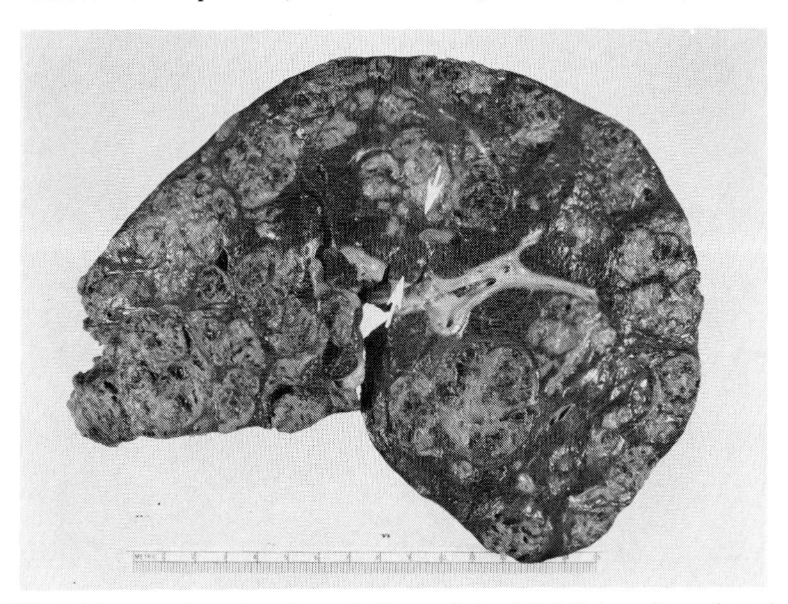

FIG. 6. Metastases in patient shown in Figures 3, 4 and 5. 143 days after orthotopic liver transplantation, liver homograft has been replaced by tumor except for a very small residual area of hepatic parenchyma (*arrows*). (By permission of W. B. Saunders Company, 1969.)

It would be inaccurate to say that liver transplantation can never be used to cure hepatoma, as can also be illustrated by another case. In Figure 7 is the liver of a child with biliary atresia in which was found a 2 cm hepatoma as an incidental pathologic feature. The alpha-fetoprotein that was present in her serum disappeared (Fig. 8) and has never returned. The child has a perfect result without evidence of tumor recurrence 4½ years later. Long survival after liver replacement for hepatoma has also been reported by Calne and Williams of Cambridge and a former fellow of ours, Daloze of Montreal. Nevertheless, I personally would prefer not to do more hepatomas at this time since the high incidence of metastases (exceeding 80% in our hands) has beclouded the kind of conclusions that must be reached in evaluating any new procedure.

It has seemed possible that the outlook might be less gloomy if the malignant tumor were some kind other than a hepatoma. For example, some of the slow growing proximal duct cell carcinomas might be worth treating. This is an example, which was diagnosed with transhepatic cholangiography, by Alan Redeker of Los Angeles (Fig. 9). Liver replacement was carried out in early February with a perfect result. The small tumor was not seen until after its removal.

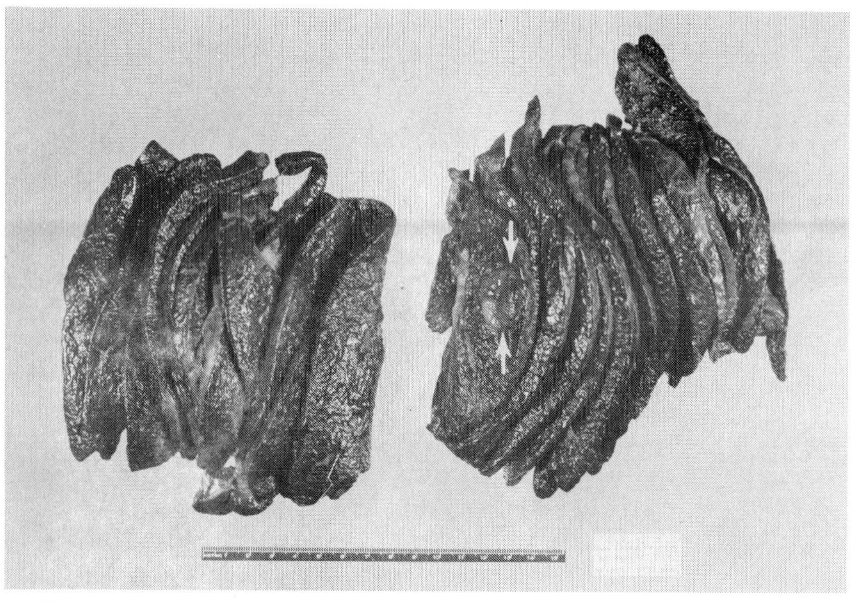

FIG. 7. Two centimeter hepatoma (*arrows*) in the liver of a 4-year-old child whose primary diagnosis was biliary atresia.

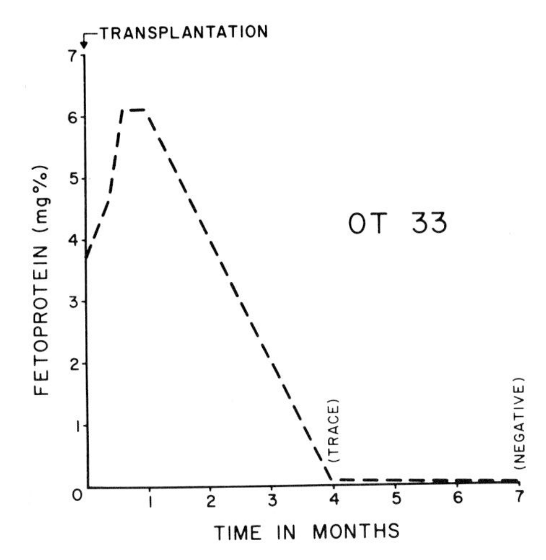

FIG. 8. Alpha-feto protein posttransplantation in child whose native liver is shown in Figure 7. (By permission of *Gastroenterology*, 61:144-148, 1971.)

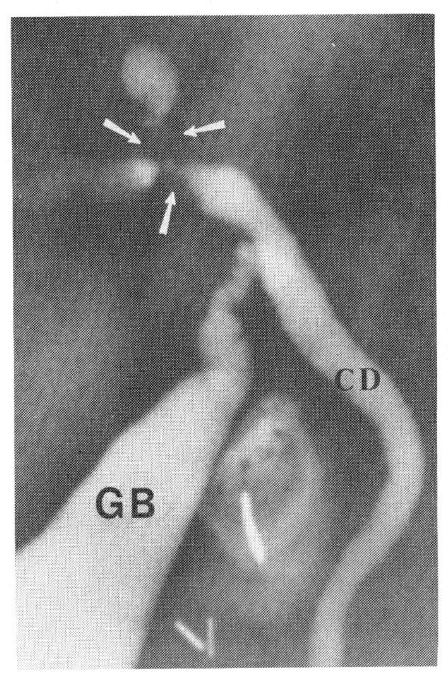

FIG. 9. The diagnosis of an intrahepatic duct carcinoma by preoperative transhepatic cholangiography. Procedure performed by Dr. Alan Redeker of Los Angeles.

Table 1. Criteria for Selection for Liver Transplantation

1. Are less than 40
2. Have a hopeless prognosis*
3. Do not have cancer
4. Do not have infection

*How is this known?

In any event, the important future of hepatic transplantation is for the treatment of *benign* hepatic disease. The most common diagnoses would be chronic aggressive hepatitis, biliary atresia and alcoholic cirrhosis. In all these situations, we would like to meet the criteria shown in Table 1. Of these criteria, the second one is the most difficult since the determination of "hopelessness" may be impossible until a few hours before death. Yet, if one waits this long, there will be no transplantations.

If liver transplantation is to be prosecuted successfully, case selection must be carried out by different doctors in widely separated cities on a national basis. In doing this, the dominating role of donor availability has to be recognized. Another key condition is a trustworthy system of prior evaluation *by experts* of any prospective patient. Then if a suitable donor is found, say in Denver, a recipient who has been judged otherwise hopeless can be transported to Colorado.

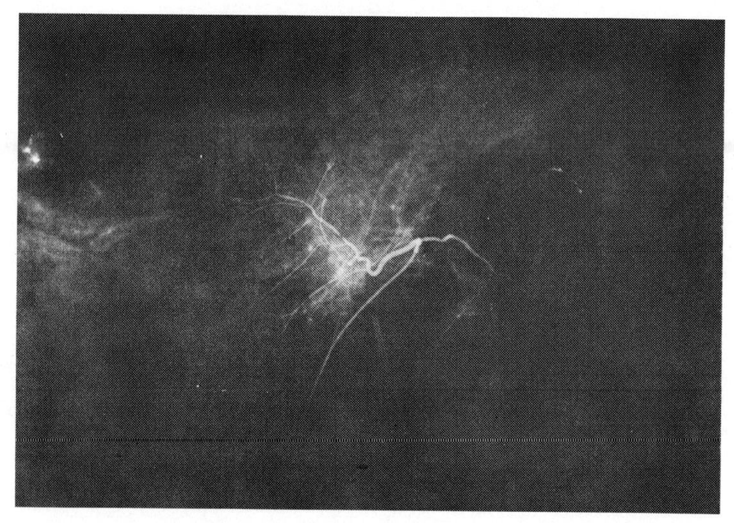

FIG. 10. Postmortem arteriogram of a liver homograft that had supported life for 3½ years. Note narrowed areas in some of the smaller vessels. (By permission of the *New England Journal of Medicine*, 289:82-84, 1973.)

The indication of biliary atresia for liver transplantation is perhaps the clearest one of all, since these children require a blind-end social input with no prospect of their getting better or of growing up. With successful transplantation they can become quite normal. The little girl, whose liver was shown in Figure 7, is now 4½ years posttransplantation and attending public school in Illinois. The boy, Jimmy Grund, who was well known to the Minnesota faculty, was well for 3½ years until his sudden death was precipitated by a *Hemophilus* septicemia. Incidentally, the arterial supply of his liver homograft was patent although it contained constrictions (Fig. 10) which were apparently due to the same kind of obliterative lesions which are so familiar in kidney transplants.

We have had two patients who underwent liver replacement for Wilson's disease, a disorder in which copper deposition in the tissues leads to neurologic, hepatic and other manifestations. The first patient had profound liver failure. The second patient recipient was treated because of uncontrolled neurologic manifestations despite conventional penicillamine therapy. Both of these patients are alive and very well after 5 and 3½ years, respectively. After operation, they underwent a massive cupriuresis (Fig. 11). As the copper was being mobilized, the Kayser-Fleischer (or copper) rings and the neurologic manifestations regressed. Repeated

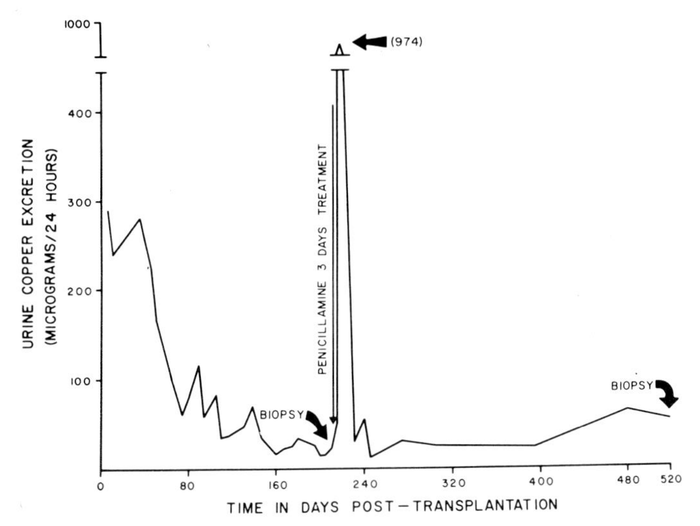

FIG. 11. Postoperative cupriuresis after liver replacement in a child who had Wilson's disease. Even after six months, note striking response to penicillamine. Child is still alive five years postoperative. (By permission of *Lancet*, March 13, 1971, pp. 505-508.)

biopsies of these livers have shown little or no reaccumulation of hepatic copper. The preoperative serum ceruloplasmin of the second child was zero. It promptly rose to normal.

Clinical Results

By showing you these pictures of healthy looking postoperative patients, I do not wish to give a false impression of the results that have been obtained. According to the April 1974 American College of Surgeons report on liver transplantation, about 200 patients have had liver replacement throughout the world. Since 1963, we have contributed 82 to this total, at a rate since 1967 ranging from 6% to 13% per year (Table 2). We have had 18 and 9 recipients, respectively, who have lived for more than one and two years. Thirteen recipients are still alive from eight weeks to almost five years postoperative. The four longest survivors are four years, 11 months; four years, 5 months; four years; and three years, 4 months.

There have been ten late deaths from 12 to 41 months postoperatively, and for the reasons listed in Table 3. The latest mortality at three years, five months was Jimmy Grund, the Minnesota child whom I mentioned previously.

With only 18 one-year survivors, it is obvious that the operation is presently unsafe. The single most important factor in the high acute failure rate has been a multiplicity of technical misadventures of which complications of biliary duct reconstruction usually with lethal sepsis lead the list. I will be devoting all of my later talk to this topic. It is surprising

Table 2. Cases of Orthotopic Liver Transplantation Treated in Denver

		Lived		
	Number	*1 year*	*2 years*	*Alive Now*
1963-1966	6	0	0	0
1967	6	1	0	0
1968	12	5	2	0
1969	6	2	1	1
1970	10	2	1	1
1971	11	2	2	2
1972	11	5	3	3
1973	13	1	0	3
1974 (To April 1)	7	0	0	3
	82	18	9	13

Table 3. The Present Status of 18 One-Year Survivors After Orthotopic Liver Transplantation. Eight are Still Alive From 14 to 58 Months. The Other 10 Eventually Died From the Causes Listed Below.

OT Number	*Time of Death (Months)*	*Causes of Death*
15	12	Recurrent cancer
29	12	Serum hepatitis and liver failure
8	13	Recurrent cancer
58	13½	? Chronic rejection ? Recurrent hepatitis
16	13½	Rejection and liver failure
14	14	Recurrent cancer
54	19	Multiple liver abscesses necessitating retransplantation
36	20	Systemic *Nocardia* infection and chronic aggressive hepatitis
13	30	Rejection and liver failure following retransplantation
19	41	*Hemophilus* septicemia and secondary liver and renal failure

how uncommonly failure to control rejection has been responsible for death.

One of the great unanswered questions about liver transplantation is whether chronic alcoholics are suitable candidates. First, cirrhotic patients have a predictably higher operative risk, in part due to the frequency of pulmonary and other infectious complications. Second, for all but those patients with clearly terminal esophageal variceal hemorrhage, hepatic coma or advanced secondary renal failure uncertainty about the natural course of the disease usually leads to a decision against transplantation until such time as the patient's condition becomes patently hopeless. Many then expire before a suitable liver becomes available; the few who are transplanted enter the operating room in a moribund state.

In Table 4, our experience with alcoholics has been separated out. Of the 82 consecutive recipients of hepatic homografts, one was treated for alcoholic hepatitis and nine carried the diagnosis of Laennec's cirrhosis without concurrent hepatoma. Nine of the ten patients have died, from 3 to 121 (mean 29) days posttransplantation; the only surviving recipient is in good condition six weeks postoperative. In contrast, 12 of the 72 patients transplanted for nonalcoholic liver disease are still alive from a few weeks to nearly five years later. The mean survival of the patients in the nonalcoholic group who have died is more than four times that of the

Table 4. Alcoholic vs. Nonalcoholic Liver Disease Treated by Orthotopic Hepatic Transplantation

	Alcoholic	*Nonalcoholic*	*Total*
No. of patients	10	72	82
Alive	1*	12	13
Dead	9	60	69
Mean survival of those who died	29 days	136 days	122 days

*Six weeks posttransplantation

alcoholic recipients. The causes of death among the alcoholics are shown in Table 5. If liver transplantation is to succeed in patients with alcoholic cirrhosis, potential recipients must be selected earlier, treated aggressively to prevent or correct infectious, pulmonary and other complications and transplanted before their condition has markedly deteriorated to the extent of coma, hepatorenal syndrome and other similar end points. In fact, no matter what the indication, I believe that operation needs to be considered earlier than we or our medical colleagues have been willing to recommend.

Table 5. Duration of Survival and Cause of Death in Ten Alcoholic Recipients of Hepatic Homografts

OT Number	*Age (Years)*	*Survival (Days)*	*Cause of Death*
22	33	10	Biliary obstruction
28	39	13	Disruption of choledochoduodenostomy; bile peritonitis
32	46	3	Unexplained coma
39	47	26	Unrelieved pre-existing coma
40	44	32	Rejection; pneumonitis; petechial hemorrhages of CNS
62	44	121	Rejection and liver failure; pulmonary emboli
70	40	34	Pneumonitis
75	48	8	Rejection and liver failure
81	47	15	*Aspergillus* pneumonitis with dissemination
82	37	Alive (6 weeks)	–

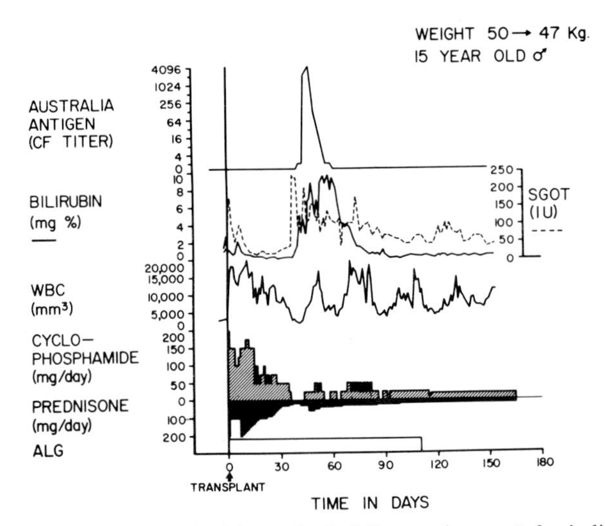

FIG. 12. The course of a teenaged boy who had liver replacement for indication of Wilson's disease. Acute derangements of liver function in second postoperative month were associated with development of Australia antigenemia. Thus, diagnosis was probably serum hepatitis, rather than rejection. After transplantation, the serum ceruloplasmin rose from zero to normal values.

The Question of Hepatitis

A few final thoughts may be in order. We still believe that under propitious circumstances, people with Australia antigenemia need not be arbitrarily eliminated from candidacy. We treated a former heroin addict under these circumstances who lived for almost two subsequent years, most of it with her family, although eventually she recapitulated her original disease.

I already mentioned (Table 3) that in patients who are Australia antigen *negative,* we have seen posttransplantation hepatitis. In Figure 12 is an example. During this flare-up of hepatic malfunction, the Australia antigen tests had turned positive. Then, the differential diagnosis of serum hepatitis versus rejection may be practically impossible.

Incidentally, I have said very little about the details of immunosuppressive treatment, since this is such a highly specialized area. We start out treating our patients with cyclophosphamide, steroids and ALG, later changing to azathioprine.

Summary

I would like to summarize now by making three brief statements. First, the prime indication for liver replacement is non-neoplastic hepatic disease. Second, it has been proved that patients can be restored to good health with liver transplantation, as evidenced by survival for as long as half a decade. Third, the greatest deterrent to improved results and, therefore, wider application is biliary duct reconstruction and hepatic sepsis, a combined subject which I will discuss later.

The work was supported by research grants from the Veterans Administration; by grants AI-AM-08898 and AM-07772 of the National Institutes of Health; by grants RR-00051 and RR-00069 from the General Clinical Research Centers Program of the Division of Research Resources, National Institutes of Health.

Hepatic Sepsis: Generally Applicable Lessons Learned from Liver Transplantation

Thomas E. Starzl, M.D., Ph.D. and Charles W. Putnam, M.D.

This paper should not be entitled "liver abscesses." There is no way I could possibly discuss liver abscesses briefly and I very much doubt if you would want me to try.

Instead, I will be talking about liver sepsis, using mainly our experience with liver transplantation as a model with which we think we have learned a lot about infections of the liver that can and should be applied to the understanding and treatment of abscesses, cholangitis and other conditions. In addition, the problems I will relate will have to be solved before the procedure of liver transplantation can become widely practical.

The most widely used method of bile duct reconstruction is the cholecystoduodenostomy that is shown in Figure 1A. With this operation, the distal common duct is ligated or sewn shut so that the bile passes through the cystic duct and gallbladder, to be delivered into the duodenum. The other biliary reconstruction we used early in our experience was a standard choledochocholedochostomy placing the T-tube through a stab wound in the recipient common duct (Fig. 2).

With liver transplantation and cholecystoduodenostomy, a series of terrible complications were encountered in several of our early cases in which prolonged survival was obtained. We called this complication "septic hepatic infarction" and its consequences were characteristic and resulted in three distinctive clinical and laboratory findings, of which two are shown in Figure 3. The components of the triad were gram negative septicemia and evidence from transaminase determinations of massive liver necrosis. The bacteremia and transaminasemia were relatively isolated

Thomas E. Starzl, M.D., Ph.D. and Charles W. Putnam, M.D., Department of Surgery, University of Colorado Medical Center and the Veterans Administration Hospital, Denver.

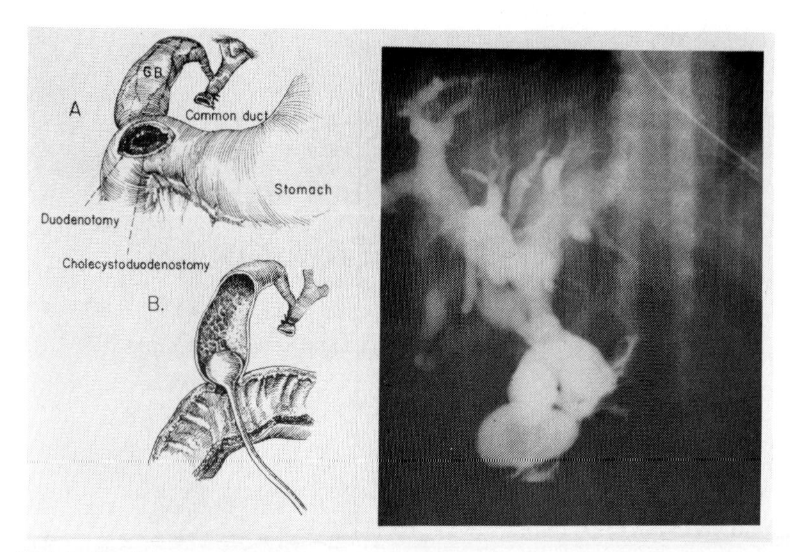

FIG. 1. The intra-operative diagnosis of a complication of cholecystoduodenostomy. On the left, cholecystoduodenostomy anastomosis was visualized through an anterior duodenotomy. Through an inflated Foley catheter, dye was introduced. Dilatation of the intrahepatic ducts was apparently due to partial obstruction of cystic duct. (By permission of *Surgery,* 72:604-610, 1972.)

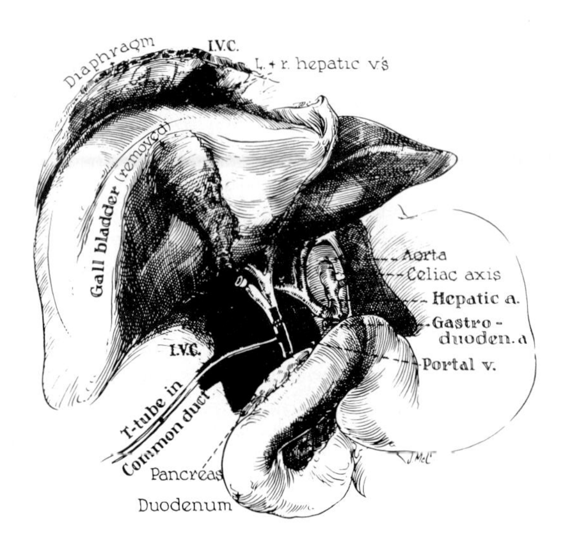

FIG. 2. Choledochocholedochostomy with T-tube drainage. This procedure has had a high incidence of biliary fistula. (By permission of W. B. Saunders Company, 1969.)

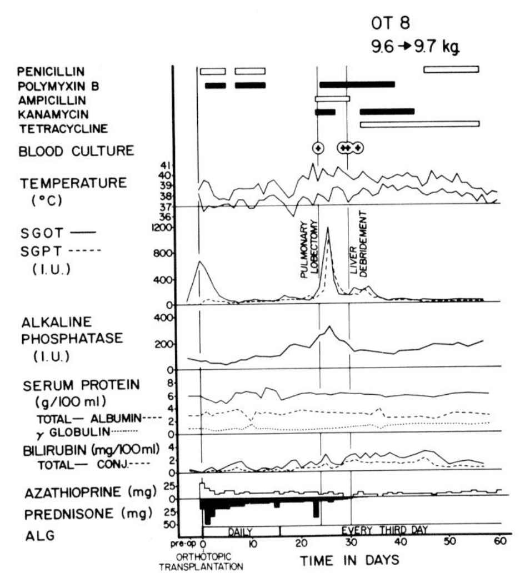

FIG. 3. The first 60 posttransplantation days in a patient after liver replacement. During third postoperative week there was evidence of an "anicteric" rejection, but significance of function changes was not appreciated at the time. Lung resection was carried out because right upper lobe was collapsed and it was suspected that this was the source of the unexplained fever. In retrospect, pulmonary lobectomy was probably not indicated. One day later, definitive evidence of septic hepatic infarction and abscess formation had appeared. All the positive blood cultures were of *Aerobacter-Klebsiella.* This patient was the first to survive for a prolonged period after human liver transplantation. Indication for operation was hepatoma. (By permission of W. B. Saunders Company, 1969.)

findings in the orthotopic liver recipient, shown in Figure 3. Protein synthesis, level of bilirubin and other liver functions were not particularly suggestive of a rejection.

The third component of the triad is seen in Figure 4, namely, the development on serial liver scans of persistently absent isotope concentration in the homograft. When these areas were explored, they were found to consist of gangrene with or without pus. In caring for these patients, who were usually children, we learned a lot about how to drain liver abscesses or to debride necrotic or infected hepatic tissue. Our approaches were subcostal, posterior extraperitoneal below the 12th rib and most commonly (Fig. 5) by the lateral route, sometimes using the two-stage procedure which was designed by Adams of the Leahy Clinic to avoid entering the pleural cavity.

Eventually, however, it was concluded that the combination of too little immunosuppression and inadequate antibiotic coverage made this

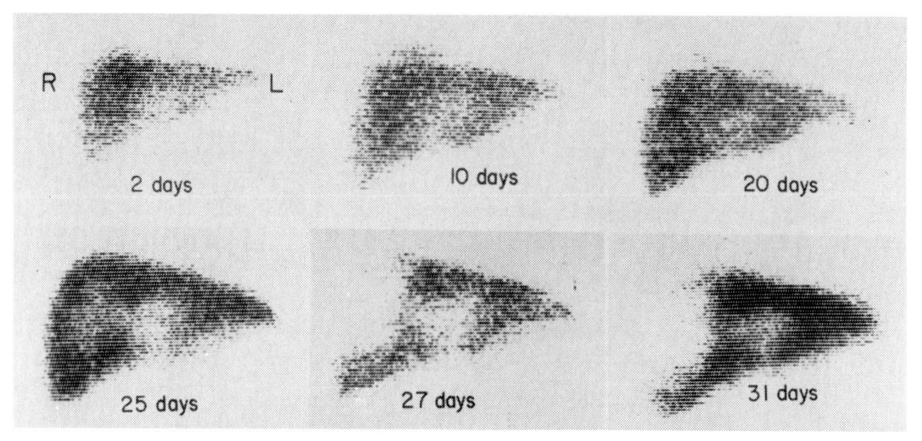

FIG. 4. Postoperative technetium scans of an orthotopic liver transplant – 2 days: small homograft is normal; 10 days: an increase in size is evident although the general configuration of the organ is still normal; 20 days: no further change is noted; 25 days: examination conducted as an emergency when child developed gram negative septicemia and very high increases in the transaminases. Areas of decreased isotope uptake are obvious in right lobe and central part of liver; 27 days: a striking extension of the process can be seen less than 48 hours later. A debridement procedure was carried out the same evening; 31 days: four days after debridement the radiographic appearance was improved. (By permission of W. B. Saunders Company, 1969.)

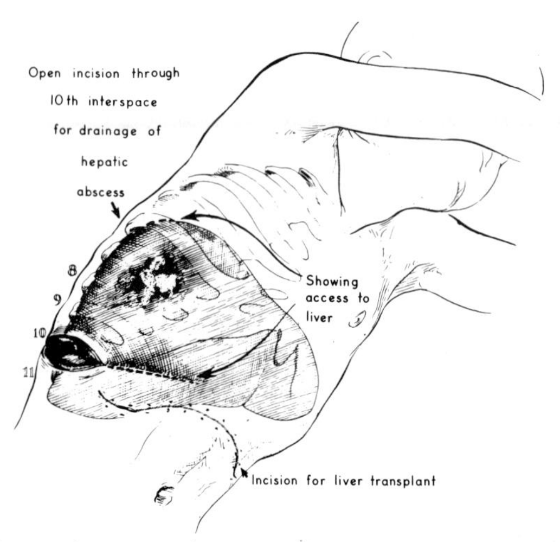

FIG. 5. Lateral operative approach to septic liver infarctions or abscesses of the right lobe through the tenth intercostal space. Neither pleural nor peritoneal cavities were entered. (By permission of *Annals of Surgery*, 168:392, 1968.)

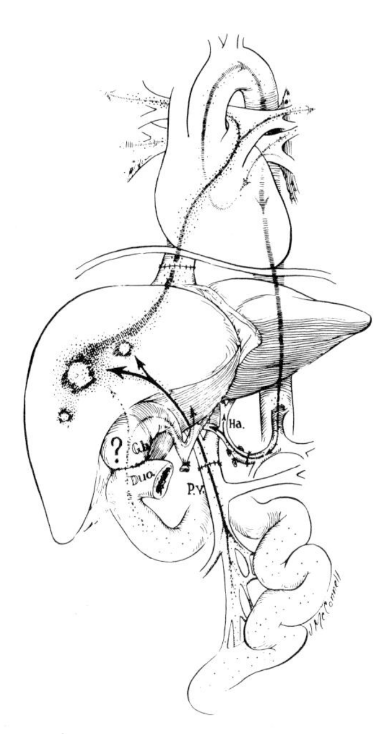

FIG. 6. An explanation of the predisposition of the liver to bacterial sepsis. Presumably, invading microorganisms enter via portal vein or through reconstructed biliary tract. (By permission of *Annals of Surgery,* 168:392, 1968.)

peculiar kind of septic infarction or abscess formation possible. The pathogenesis was envisioned as shown in Figure 6. An initiating event would be injury to the liver parenchyma whether caused by ischemic damage during the preservation, rejection (most commonly), vascular accidents or other factors. In any event, the liver, interposed as it is between the intestines and the heart, would be sure to become infected in its devitalized parts. Bacteremia, spreading infection within the liver itself, and toxicity followed. In those days which were in 1967 and 1968, our belief was that the portal of bacterial entry into the liver was almost surely hematogenous from the portal vein and that entry through the duct reconstruction was uncommon. We now believe that this was a foolish conclusion, as I will emphasize again later.

In time, it was learned how to more effectively prevent this lethal sequence of events leading to septic hepatic infarction. More intensive immunosuppression was given to avoid the necrosis of graft rejection. With the slightest impression of sepsis, intensive antibiotics were instituted.

Although septic hepatic infarction was thereby avoided, the liver transplant recipient has been at a very real risk from what we now recognize as liver sepsis long after operation. Periodic blood cultures at a time when these recipients have no symptoms may grow out *Proteus, Clostridium perfringens, E. coli* and other microorganisms at different times. Then, sudden death from overwhelming sepsis may follow. We now believe that these bacteremias are from this duct portal of entry (Fig. 7A).

The exposed relation of the duct system of the orthotopic liver to gastrointestinal flora is probably the first step in bacterial "leak" through a homograft which may well be bacteriologically porous *without* the presence of biliary duct obstruction or of histopathologically significant cholangitis. This special porosity would derive from the fact that all such patients are receiving immunosuppression and would not require a duct complication of the usual mechanical variety. This is not to say that the mechanical aspects of duct reconstruction have been satisfactorily handled. Indeed, the Achilles' heel of liver transplantation has been consistent flaws in biliary duct reconstruction. The different techniques we have tried to restore bile drainage include choledochocholedochostomy with or without a T-tube (Fig. 2), cholecystoduodenostomy after ligation of the graft common duct (Fig. 1) and choledochoduodenostomy. Because of continuing dissatisfaction with all of the aforementioned techniques of duct reconstruction, we have recently embarked on a trial of Roux-en-Y cholecystojejunostomy (Fig. 7B). The obvious biliary duct problems have been obstruction (Fig. 1) and biliary fistula from anastomotic leaks. In our 82 cases of orthotopic liver transplantation, the initial biliary reconstruction was eventually shown to be unsatisfactory and either led to death or early reoperation in these 25 cases for the staggering incidence of 30%; the true frequency was undoubtedly even higher, since many patients died so early postoperatively that an incipient duct problem would not yet be manifest.

Because of our profound conviction that the biliary duct reconstruction is the main reason, either for mechanical or the bacteriologic reasons I mentioned earlier, why liver transplantation has failed to become a practical clinical pursuit, we are now attempting to evolve a workable strategy based on five guiding principles. The principles are: (1) avoidance of stents or drains; (2) preservation of maximum extrahepatic biliary duct tissue; (3) intensification of diagnostic efforts to differentiate between duct obstruction and rejection, including performance of cholangiography in all homografts prior to transplantation; (4) early reoperation for suspicion of obstruction; and (5) placement of the liver in a relatively bacteria-free relation to the mainstream gastrointestinal continuity. None of the presently available operations completely meet all of these objectives, so that considerable individualization of care is necessary.

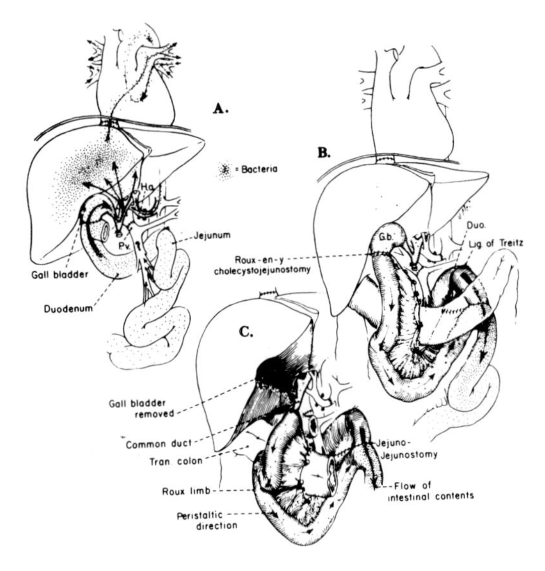

FIG. 7. Schematic representation of the bacterial contamination or lack thereof in three different kinds of biliary reconstruction. (*A*) Cholecystoduodenostomy. This extremely simple operation probably carries the greatest risk of graft infection. (*B*) Roux-en-Y cholecystojejunostomy. This operation protects from hepatic sepsis by placing the new liver outside the main gastrointestinal stream. Isoperistaltic limb is made at least 18 inches long. (*C*) Roux-en-Y choledochojejunostomy. The end-to-end duct to bowel anastomosis is simple if the duct is dilated as would be the case if a conversion became necessary from (*B*) to (*C*).

A Roux-en-Y cholecystojejunostomy (Fig. 7B), our present procedure of choice, permits all the above listed objectives to be partly met. If postoperative biliary obstruction later develops, the Roux limb can be detached, the gallbladder removed and an anastomosis performed to the now dilated common duct (Fig. 7C).

No matter what the initial procedure, an intense suspicion about the cause for postoperative jaundice is a necessary condition of postoperative management. The simplest precaution is to perform routine intravenous cholangiography in the early postoperative period. The intravenous cholangiogram of a cholecystojejunostomy, shown in Figure 8, was considered suspicious with slight dilatation of the ducts which contained air. However, the function was so perfect that reoperation has not been performed.

In almost all of our patients who develop jaundice, transhepatic cholangiography and percutaneous needle biopsy are now performed (Fig. 9). Cholangiography has been greatly expedited by our use of the Chiba needle introduced in Japan and now being used in several American

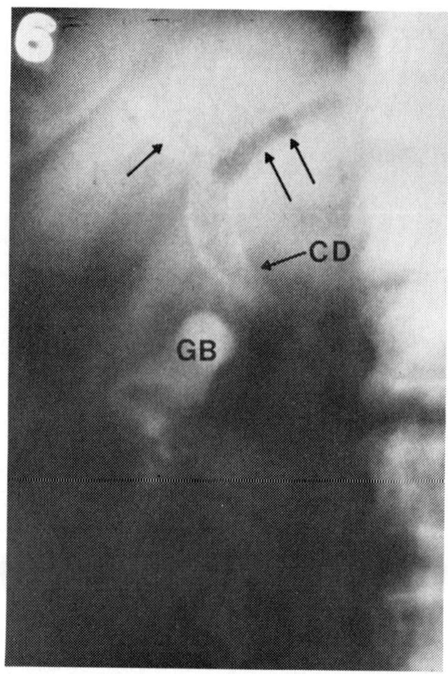

FIG. 8. Posttransplantation cholangiographic studies. Intravenous cholangiogram in a 47-year-old recipient of a hepatic homograft, the biliary drainage for which was with Roux-en-Y cholecystojejunostomy. Patient's liver function studies were normal at time of examination. However, findings of a very slightly dilated common duct and air in the biliary system (*arrows*) are suspicious for low grade obstruction.

centers. These thin-walled small caliber needles have great flexibility that permits the diagnostic studies to be done with an improvement in safety. The obstruction in Figure 9 after Roux-en-Y cholecystojejunostomy was relieved by conversion to a choledochojejunostomy using the same jejunal limb. The bilirubin, which had been about 10 mg%, fell immediately to normal.

In summary, I have used our experience in liver transplantation for two purposes. First, I wanted to show you how the pathogenesis of intrahepatic sepsis, including abscess formation, is probably almost always due to some combination of contamination from the intestines through either the portal vein or duct system, and that injury to the liver itself could very easily make the infectious foothold possible. These lessons so well learned in liver recipients surely have wide applicability. Second, I wanted to indicate to you that I believe contamination through the ducts is the main portal of bacterial entry, at least in the liver recipient. This probability has led to the evolution of a strategy for bile duct

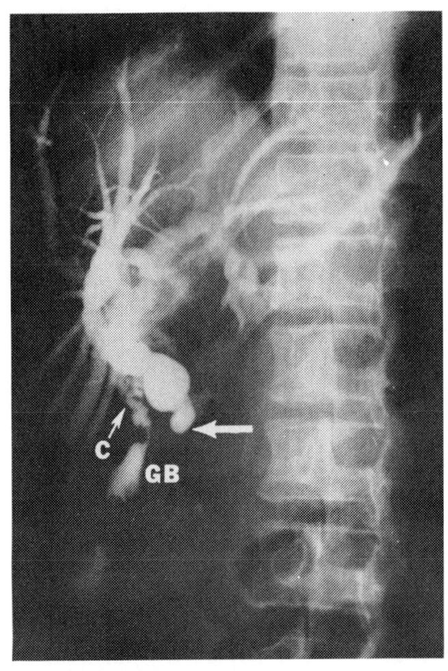

FIG. 9. A percutaneous transhepatic cholangiogram performed four weeks posttransplantation because of persistent elevations of the serum bilirubin (8-10 mg%). At time of transplantation, biliary drainage had been established with a Roux-en-Y cholecystojejunostomy (Fig. 7). After obtaining this study, patient was re-explored, gallbladder removed and Roux limb anastomosed to the dilated common duct (*large arrow*), as shown in Figure 7C. Patient's jaundice rapidly cleared and he now has normal liver function four months posttransplantation. GB – gallbladder; → – common bile duct; C – cystic duct.

reconstruction of liver homografts that puts the new liver as far away from the mainstream gastrointestinal tract as possible and which encourages reoperation for the slightest indication of duct obstruction or of cholangitis.

Bibliography

Starzl, T. E. (with the assistance of Putnam, C.W.): Experience in Hepatic Transplantation. Philadelphia:W. B. Saunders Company, 1969.

The work was supported by research grants from the Veterans Administration; by grants AI-AM-08898 and AM-07772 of the National Institutes of Health; by grants RR-00051 and RR-00069 from the General Clinical Research Centers Program of the Division of Research Resources, National Institutes of Health.

Surgical Treatment of Primary and Secondary Tumors of the Liver

Rodney Smith, M.S.

There is nothing new in the idea that a tumor of the liver, benign or malignant, may well be resected with profit. In the late 1930s I was a First Assistant to Sir Gordon Gordon-Taylor and he had several patients at that time who had undergone a hepatic resection. However, the technique at that time was a crude wedge excision and it may be said today that the whole character of resection as applied to liver tumors has become altered by a more detailed study of the hepatic architecture and also that, as regards malignancy, there are various methods other than resection for dealing with such a situation.

I intend only to make passing reference to the different varieties of hepatectomy, the method of choice in dealing with a benign tumor or, in most instances, in dealing with a single malignant tumor. Where malignancy is confirmed, the two other main varieties of treatment that should be considered are chemotherapy and arterial ligation. In addition, these two methods may sometimes be combined.

Cytotoxic drugs have been used now for a number of years in cases of hepatic malignancy. Although an occasional successful case is reported, drugs of this kind given by the oral, the intravenous or the intramuscular route are not likely to be successful and for this reason during the last few years surgeons have, in the main, sought to employ chemotherapy delivered by the intra-arterial route. If at operation the liver is found to contain a malignancy unsuitable for resection, it is often technically not difficult to insert a fine catheter into the hepatic artery for subsequent perfusion. Alternatively, in some cases where there has been an unequivocal demonstration of widespread involvement of the liver by malignancy, an operation can be avoided altogether by inserting a catheter into the celiac or hepatic artery using the Seldinger technique. This allows a short

---

Rodney Smith, M.S., F.R.C.S., Senior Surgeon, St. George's Hospital, London, England.

course, five to seven days, of chemotherapy to be given and if this is successful the patient can be readmitted for further courses of treatment at four to six month intervals. At St. George's Hospital in London, we had a relatively small series of patients treated by arterial perfusion alone, using a variety of techniques, before we became rather more interested in the possibilities of arterial ligation. In the cases treated by infusion alone, we had fewer successes with liver tumors than with pancreatic tumors and the results in neither of these lesions were particularly impressive. At the present time, however, even though the ultimate aim may be to perform a hepatic artery ligation, we would usually begin with a selective celiac

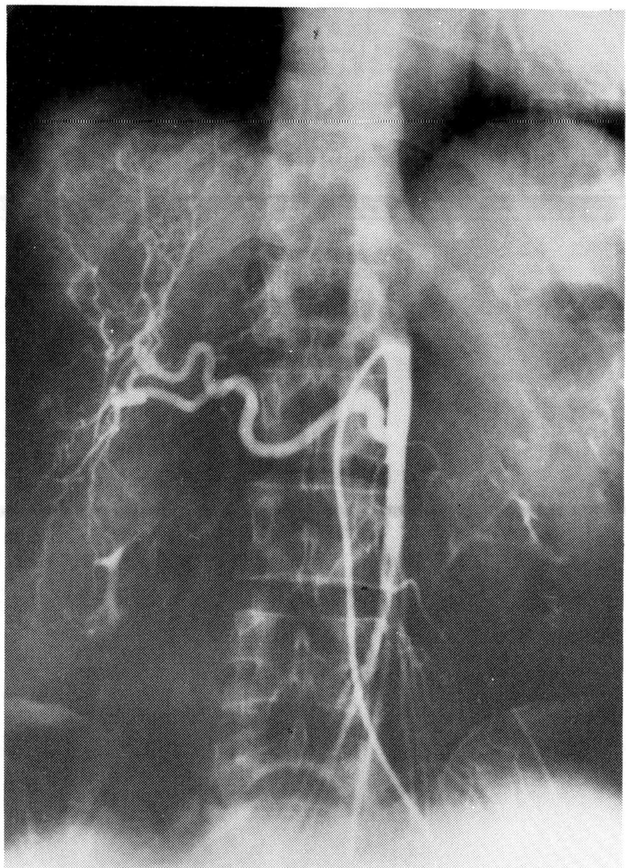

FIG. 1. The importance of preliminary angiography is shown well by this superior mesenteric arteriogram showing that this vessel gives off the right hepatic artery, a not uncommon finding.

artery angiogram first as a diagnostic measure; second, to display the precise anatomy of the hepatic artery and its branches (Fig. 1); and third, having a catheter in situ, with the intent of giving one course of arterial cytotoxic infusion as a preliminary to surgery.

Arterial Ligation

Arterial ligation is a relative newcomer on the scene. The basis is a reasonable one. In many cases of malignancy in the liver, it can be observed by angiography that the blood supply of the malignant tumor or tumors is predominantly arterial and that the portal vein contributes little (Figs. 2 and 3). If this is considered together with the amply demonstrated facts that the liver itself can survive perfectly well on the portal venous input with the main hepatic artery ligated just below the liver, it is not unreasonable to feel that arterial ligation might well result in necrosis of the tumor or tumors without any adverse effects upon the liver. In practice it does appear that this is sometimes achieved. A relatively small number of patients have been operated upon at St. George's Hospital in

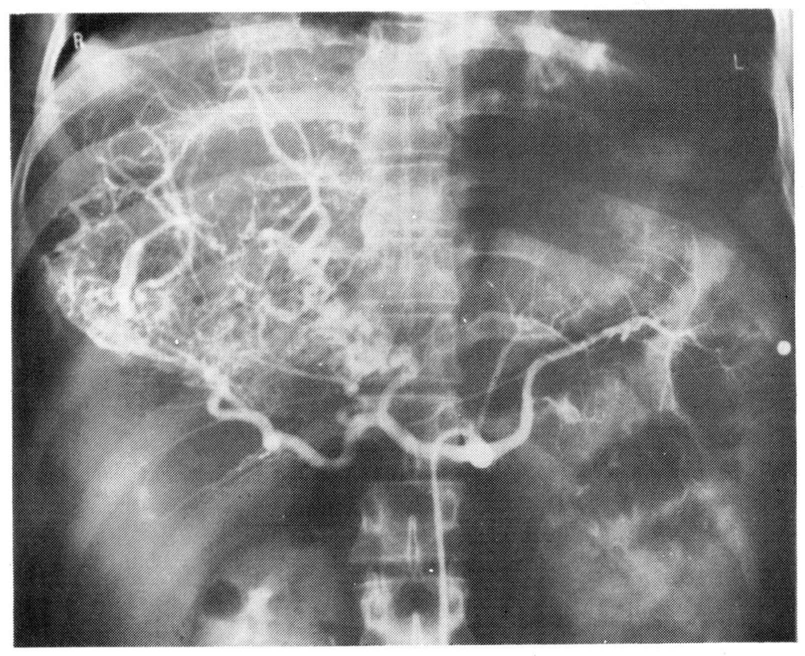

FIG. 2. Celiac angiogram showing the abnormal vascular pattern in a typical hepatoma in the upper part of the right lobe of the liver.

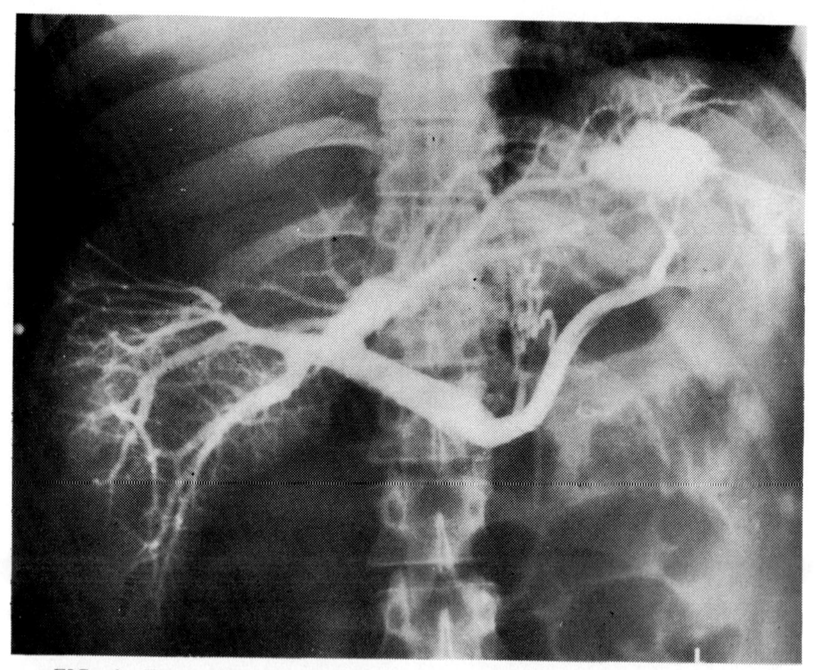

FIG. 3. From the same patient, a portal venogram shows the same area apparently not deriving any blood supply via the portal vein.

this way, but we have now moved on to treating most of these patients by an arterial ligation plus a fine catheter left in the hepatic end of the artery so that later perfusion can be added. In these patients the back-up chemotherapy has been intermittent, a five to seven day course of treatment being repeated at four to six month intervals. Between these, the fine catheter is filled with heparin solution and sealed off underneath the skin, where it can be recovered for the next perfusion.

As yet, of course, there is no means of determining whether arterial ligation alone or arterial ligation plus subsequent arterial chemotherapy is the better. Considerable study over a period of time must be allowed in order to investigate this problem. One way in which we are hoping to gain some information, in those cases where the liver is diffusely involved, both right and left halves, is the combination of arterial ligation plus the insertion of a catheter into one of the two terminal branches of the hepatic artery only. In this way each patient is, as it were, his own control. Here again, though, a number of years must elapse before any conclusion can be drawn.

Only a very preliminary assessment of results can be given. The operation is not dangerous unless it is performed upon the wrong patient. It could not, for instance, be performed if the patient has portal hypertension or malignant ascites. It can, however, be performed perfectly safely in cases of hepatoma in a cirrhotic liver, provided there is no portal hypertension in addition. To date, 30 patients have been treated in this way with one death. The interference with liver function has been transitory. It has been unusual to observe no improvement in the patient afterwards; some three quarters of the patients provide clear evidence of clinical improvement. Several patients in this small series have improved to a quite spectacular degree (Fig. 4). In one patient with an immense hepatoma filling practically the whole abdomen, the tumor rapidly diminished in size and eventually could no longer be felt. The patient remained asymptomatic for more than one year but the tumor did eventually recur after 18 months and then became widely disseminated

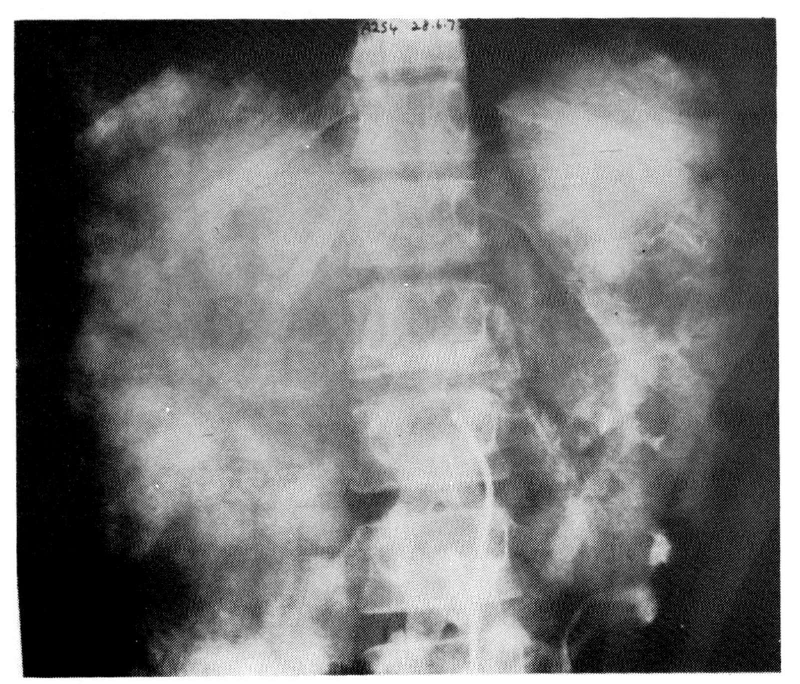

FIG. 4. Celiac angiogram in the capillary phase. Massive involvement of the whole liver by hepatoma. Survival in good health for more than 18 months followed arterial ligation.

and caused rapid death. In another patient, totally incapacitated by a liver full of functioning malignant insulinoma, with severe hyperinsulinism, arterial ligation alone (without chemotherapy) resulted in a total disappearance of the hypoglycemic symptoms, the patient returning to work for more than two years postoperatively.

It is, as yet, far too early to assess the possible results of arterial ligation, particularly with chemotherapy added, and a number of years must elapse before the place in surgery of procedures of this kind can be defined.

Finally, I think it should be said that for the benign and the single malignant tumor in the liver, however large this may be, the best treatment is a partial, or even subtotal, hepatic resection.

Intra-Arterial Hepatic Infusion Chemotherapy and Ligation of the Hepatic Artery in the Treatment of Metastatic Tumors to the Liver

Theodor B. Grage, M.D. and Charles L. Barbee, M.D.

Introduction

Colorectal carcinomas are the most common neoplasms seen in the adult population and approximately 50,000 deaths occur each year in the United States from this disease [1]. It is estimated that in more than half of the deaths from colorectal carcinoma, hepatic metastases constitute the major lethal route of spread. Although colorectal carcinomas are relatively slow-growing lesions, by the time hepatic metastases have occurred the average survival time is estimated to be about six months.

In a major study by Jaffee and co-workers, the lethality of hepatic metastases was well demonstrated [2]. The median survival time of 390 patients was 75 days from the date the diagnosis of hepatic metastases was made. This included all malignancies with hepatic metastases, and only 7% of the patients survived for more than one year. The survival rate of 177 patients with metastatic carcinoma of the colon was considerably better than that of metastatic gastric or pancreatic carcinoma. Nevertheless, the median survival time of 177 patients with metastatic carcinoma of the colon was about five months; at the end of one year, 80% of the patients had died from their disease. Similar observations have been made by others [3-5].

Cady reviewed the survival of 269 patients after colonic resection for carcinoma with simultaneous liver metastases seen at the Lahey Clinic and found a mean survival time of 13 months [6]. Factors adversely affecting

---

Theodor B. Grage, M.D., Associate Professor of Surgery, and Charles L. Barbee, M.D., Medical Fellow in Surgery, University of Minnesota Hospital, Minneapolis.
Supported by USPHS Grant #08832.

survival were weight loss, intestinal symptoms, ascites, peritoneal seeding and extension of the primary carcinoma to other viscera. What role selection of the patient population may play is indicated by Watkins et al, from the same institution [7]. In their study on intra-arterial infusion an untreated control group of 80 patients with colorectal carcinoma metastatic to the liver had a median survival time of 4.2 months.

From the foregoing data it is abundantly clear that the long-term prognosis of patients with metastatic cancer in the liver is poor. It is also apparent that the composition of the patients under study, the extent of the involvement of the liver by tumor, the extent of tumor involvement of other organs and many other factors influence the prognosis. Without randomization of the patients the difficulties in showing that a particular form of therapy has added a given number of months to survival time are enormous. It is easily understood why many of the reports of the literature indicating an improvement in survival or response to systemic chemotherapy or intra-arterial infusion or hepatic artery ligation have met considerable skepticism from the profession.

In an individual patient the response to a given therapy such as systemic chemotherapy may be quite dramatic and easily demonstrable by such clinical parameters as return of the liver to normal size, disappearance of a metastasis as demonstrated by a liver scan, improvement in liver function studies, improvement in performance status and nutritional intake, sense of well-being and ability to return to work. All too often, however, the ability to demonstrate response or lack of response is most difficult. The correlation between the abnormalities in liver function studies and the extent of involvement of the liver by tumor is frequently not very good. Consistent objective criteria for a response in patients with hepatic metastases are lacking.

Systemic Chemotherapy

The treatment of metastatic colorectal carcinoma with systemic intravenous 5-FU has been disappointing. Jacobs summarized nine reports from the literature and noted a 25% response rate in 674 patients [8]. The mean duration of response was approximately three months. When neoplasms other than from the colon and rectum are the source of the hepatic metastases, the response rate to systemic chemotherapy has been even lower. A number of other chemotherapeutic agents have been used, either singly or in combinations, including BCNU, cytosine arabinoside, mitomycin C, vinblastin, vincristine, methotrexate, cyclophosphamide and other alkylating agents. None of the drugs used alone have produced a response rate as great as that achieved with 5-Fluorouracil and combinations of these agents with 5-FU appear to be no more effective than 5-FU alone in the treatment of gastrointestinal neoplasms [9-13].

Intra-Arterial Infusion Chemotherapy

In 1965 Sullivan and Zurek [14] reported an objective response rate of 60% in patients with advanced liver metastases treated by a protracted, ambulatory intra-arterial hepatic infusion using FUDR. In a more recent report by Watkins et al from the same institution, their total experience in the treatment of 184 patients was summarized, including 108 patients with adenocarcinoma of the colon and rectum metastatic to the liver [7]. Of 108 patients, 82 had a satisfactory infusion; of these, 60 showed evidence of a favorable response to therapy. The patients with liver metastases from primary disease in the colon and rectum are believed to have had significant prolongation of survival after satisfactory infusion treatment. Measured from the onset of symptoms, the median survival time in the responders was 15 months. In 80 patients of a matched control group, not treated by intra-arterial hepatic infusion, the median survival time was 4.2 months.

Other reports of intra-arterial infusion include the report by Ansfield et al who treated 200 patients with intrahepatic arterial infusion with 5-FU [15]. Many of these patients had failed on systemic 5-FU. The median survival of the entire group was six months. The median survival of the 62% of the responders was 8.7 months compared to 2.5 months for the 38% who did not respond.

University of Minnesota Hospitals Experience

At the University of Minnesota Hospitals, 64 patients underwent 80 intra-arterial hepatic infusions with 5-FU for metastatic disease to the liver (Table 1). Thirty-four of these patients had adenocarcinoma of the colon and rectum. The remainder of the patients had primary disease originating in the breast, biliary tract, stomach, pancreas, unknown primary, carcinoid and miscellaneous tumors.

Preoperative Evaluation and Eligibility Criteria

In general, only those patients were subjected to an intra-arterial hepatic infusion whose primary clinical problem was due to hepatic involvement. In the majority, the primary tumor had been resected previously. A significant number of patients with colorectal carcinoma

Table 1. Intra-Arterial Hepatic Infusions

64 Patients
80 Infusions

Colo-rectum	34
Breast	4
Biliary tract	6
Hepatoma	4
Stomach	5
Pancreas	3
Carcinoid	3
Miscellaneous	5
Total	64

underwent simultaneous resection of the primary tumor and placement of an hepatic artery catheter at the same operation. Moribund patients, patients with impending hepatic failure and patients with significant infectious disease were excluded from the study. Nearly all of the patients had extensive involvement of the liver by metastatic tumor with significant symptoms from their disease.

Preoperative evaluation included a clinical evaluation of the extent of extrahepatic disease. Laboratory studies included hematological, liver function and renal function studies. Liver scans were usually obtained and occasionally were quite useful in assessing the response to therapy. However, in the majority of patients liver scans were of dubious value in determining the extent of the disease or in determining the degree of response to therapy.

Infusion Therapy

In 58 of the patients the catheter was placed percutaneously by way of the femoral artery, and in 22 patients the catheter was placed at the time of a laparotomy by threading a catheter into the hepatic artery via the gastroduodenal artery. The advantages of exploratory laparotomy and direct placement of a catheter are considerable. Recently, this method has been increasingly used to place the catheter. It permits removal of the primary tumor if this has not been resected, and exploration of the abdomen gives an accurate assessment of the extent of extrahepatic as well as hepatic involvement. Furthermore, direct placement of a catheter minimizes catheter problems and results in a more accurate placement in the hepatic artery. With the transfemoral route the catheter can usually be placed only in the common hepatic artery with consequent infusion of the drug into the bed of the gastroduodenal and left gastric vessels, at times resulting in gastritis and sloughing of the gastric mucosa. Also, the problems of thrombosis of the femoral artery and bleeding at the catheter entrance site are avoided. The disadvantage of direct placement is that it subjects the patient to a major operative procedure.

For details of the operative placement of the catheter the excellent paper by Watkins should be consulted [7]. A few technical points deserve emphasis. After the catheter has been secured in the gastroduodenal artery, this vessel is divided and the entire intra-abdominal course of the catheter is carefully covered with omentum to minimize problems of hemorrhage from the gastroduodenal artery at the time of removal. After the catheter has been placed, a small amount of fluorescin dye is injected to insure good distribution of the infusate to both the right and left lobes of the liver. The catheter is brought out through a separate stab wound on the abdominal wall and immediately hooked up to a pressure infusion set.

The Fenwal closed system was used to administer 1000 cc of 5% dextrose in water, with 1000 units of heparin added every 24 hours. Position of the catheter was checked radiographically at weekly intervals. Liver function studies were obtained weekly and the leukocyte and platelet counts were determined every other day.

Chemotherapy in this group of patients consisted of the administration of 5-FU. In the early part of this trial, 25 patients received 5-FU at a dose approximately equal to that given by the systemic route, consisting of 10 mg/kg given by continuous 24-hour daily infusion for a period of ten days. The average total dose of 5-FU given was 100 mg/kg and ranged between 50 and 150 mg. Once it became known that a significant amount of 5-FU is taken up by the liver and does not get into the systemic circulation, thereby increasing the tolerance to the drug, the next 39 patients were treated with much higher doses of 5-FU, receiving 20 mg/kg intravenously daily for a period of two weeks, followed by 10 mg daily for a period of from one to seven additional days. The average total dose of 5-FU given in these patients was 350 mg/kg and ranged from as low as 150 mg/kg to as high as 600 mg/kg.

Toxicity and Complications

Significant drug toxicity was seen only with the higher doses of 5-FU. Nine of 39 patients had significant bone marrow toxicity, as indicated by a drop in the white count to below 2000 or thrombocytopenia with a platelet count below 50,000. Three of these patients developed severe sepsis, one of whom died from necrotizing enterocolitis, undoubtedly related to drug toxicity.

Table 2. Intra-Arterial Hepatic Infusions Problems in 64 Patients

I.	Catheter problems		14
	Positional	6	
	Clotted	2	
	Broke	3	
	Bleeding	2	
	Thrombosis	1	
II.	Drug toxicity		
	Bone marrow		9
	G.I.		22
III.	Complications		
	Sepsis		3
	Myocardial infarct		1
	Pulmonary embolus		1
	Deaths		3

Catheter problems occurred in 14 patients, usually involving those patients in whom the catheter had been placed transfemorally (Table 2). It consisted of dislodgement of the catheter in six patients and clotting of the catheter in two patients. In three patients the catheter broke; bleeding from the femoral artery at the entrance site of the catheter occurred in two patients. Thrombosis of the femoral artery necessitated thrombectomy in one patient.

There were three deaths in this entire group. One patient died from a myocardial infarct five days after exploratory laparotomy and placement of the catheter. One patient died from a pulmonary embolus and one patient died from necrotizing enterocolitis.

With the high dosage of 5-FU currently being used, it is important to immediately stop infusion therapy at the earliest sign of toxicity such as a drop in the white count to below 3000, a drop in the platelet count below 100,000, evidence of diarrhea or ulceration of the oral mucosa.

After completion of the intra-arterial infusion the catheter was removed. As soon as the patients had fully recovered from the therapy, usually requiring one to two weeks, weekly doses of 5-FU were begun at a dose level of 12 to 15 mg/kg given by the intravenous route.

Results of Intra-Arterial Infusion

The criteria of response in patients who underwent hepatic artery infusion included decrease of hepatomegaly by more than 5 cm, decrease in the size of a measurable metastasis by 50%, return of liver function

Table 3. Clinical Result of Intrahepatic Arterial Infusion Chemotherapy

Primary Tumor	*Number Improved**	*Number Not Improved*	*Total*	*Survival in Months Range*	*Survival in Months Average*
Colon and rectum:					
Low dose 5-FU	5	7	12	0-19	5.0
High dose 5-FU	17	5	22	0-27	11.5†
Breast	2	2	4	1-16	6.5
Biliary tract	4	2	6	1- 9	4.5
Hepatoma	1	3	4	2- 9	5.0
Stomach	4	1	5	1-24	7.0
Pancreas	2	1	3	2-11	5.0
Carcinoid	3	0	3	1-96	–
Miscellaneous	1	4	5	1- 7	3.5
TOTAL	37	27	64	0-27	6.0‡

*See text for criteria of clinical improvement.
†Three of these patients are still alive.
‡Does not include the eight year survivor with carcinoid tumor.

studies to normal or decrease of abnormal liver function tests by 50% and improvement in the performance status of the patient. Evidence of clinical response in one or more of these parameters was noted in two out of four patients with carcinoma of the breast, three out of three patients with carcinoid tumors, two out of three patients with carcinoma of the pancreas, four out of six patients with carcinoma of the biliary tract and four out of five patients with carcinoma of the stomach (Table 3).

Of major interest and significance is the group of 34 patients with colorectal carcinomas, since it is the only group with sufficiently large numbers to permit an estimate of the increment in survival. Twelve patients with metastatic colorectal carcinoma were treated with a low dose infusion, receiving an average of 100 mg/kg of 5-FU. Five of these 12 showed evidence of clinical response and the survival time for the entire group of patients was five months. Twenty-two patients received a high dose infusion with 5-FU, averaging 340 mg/kg. Seventeen of these 22 showed evidence of a response. The average survival time for this group was 11.5 months and three of these patients are still living, indicating that the average survival of this group is significantly prolonged over that seen when a lower dose of 5-FU was in use.

Comment

There continues to be substantial controversy surrounding the use of intra-arterial hepatic infusion for the treatment of metastatic carcinoma to the liver. Many surgeons are convinced that intra-arterial infusion of 5-FU into the liver is far superior, in terms of response rate and prolongation of survival, to systemic chemotherapy. Other individuals feel that systemic chemotherapy is as good and certainly has less complications and is less troublesome to the patient.

To resolve this issue, the Central Oncology Group has embarked upon a program of prospectively studying this problem in a randomized fashion to compare the effectiveness of sustained systemic chemotherapy with 5-FU vs. hepatic artery infusion of 5-FU followed by systemic 5-FU in selected patients with hepatic metastases from adenocarcinoma of the colon and rectum [16]. The study is on-going and the number of patients so far admitted is still small. Preliminary data in 22 patients studied indicate that the survival and response rate in those patients receiving intra-arterial infusion is significantly better than in those patients who receive the systemic chemotherapy. With sufficient patient accrual to this study, a more precise estimate should be available to what extent patients benefit from intra-arterial infusion in terms of response rate and prolongation of survival.

Hepatic Artery Ligation for Metastatic Carcinoma to the Liver

Ligation of the hepatic artery and hepatic dearterialization in the treatment of primary and secondary carcinoma of the liver has recently received increasing attention [17-22]. The rationale for this procedure is based upon the observation that these tumors receive their blood supply entirely or predominantly from the hepatic artery and that ligation induces selective tumor necrosis [23, 24]. Because the normal liver parenchyma receives its blood supply from both the arterial and portal systems the normal liver has tolerated ligation of the hepatic artery remarkably well.

The postoperative mortality of hepatic artery ligation has ranged from 8% to 40% with the average reported to be 20% (Table 4). The mortality appears to be highest in those patients with the most extensive involvement of the liver; hepatic artery ligation is not tolerated at all in a patient whose portal vein is thrombosed. Few authors believe that hepatic artery ligation alone has had a significant effect upon prolongation of the survival, although most investigators feel that some of their patients have distinctly benefited from the procedure.

Collateral arterial flow developing after hepatic artery ligation has been well documented [25]. This collateral flow may be the reason that hepatic

Table 4. Postoperative Mortality After Hepatic Artery Ligation

Author	*Number of Patients*	*Deaths*	
		Number	*Percent*
Almersjo [18]	44	10	23
Nilsson [22]	7	1	14
Koudahl [19]	20	8	40
Fortner [21]	23	4	17
Balasegaram [17]	26	4	12
Total	120	27	22.5

artery ligation alone has not improved survival as much as might be expected from the necrosis seen in postoperative biopsies of the tumors. In some centers the hepatic artery is simply divided and ligated whereas in others complete arterial devascularization is performed by taking down the round ligament, the falciform ligament, the triangular ligament and ligating the phrenic arteries. At the present time, there are no solid data to determine what effect total devascularization of the liver vs. simple ligation of the hepatic artery has upon the extent of morbidity, the mortality rate, the response rate and the survival time of the patients.

A case report will illustrate some of the problems associated with hepatic artery ligation.

Case report: A 50-year-old man was seen at the University of Minnesota Hospitals in June 1971 with a carcinoma of the transverse colon. At the time of the resection of the transverse colon, he was found to have extensive metastatic disease to both lobes of the liver. A catheter was placed into the hepatic artery and he received a course of intra-arterial infusion with a total of 350 mg/kg of 5-FU given over a 20-day period. The patient had an excellent regression of his tumor with return of liver function studies to normal and a massively enlarged liver returned back to normal size. He was treated with weekly doses of 5-FU and for an entire year was essentially asymptomatic and was able to return to full time work.

Within two months thereafter he had substantial progression of his disease with increasing hepatomegaly and was admitted in a coma. A fasting blood sugar level was 25 mg%. It was readily apparent that he was one of the rare examples of severe hypoglycemia secondary to colonic carcinoma. Despite the administration of intravenous glucose, as much as 1000 gm of glucose given by intravenous infusion daily, we were unable to maintain his blood sugar about 100 mg%. Because of the increasingly desperate situation, he was taken to the operating room and the abdomen was explored.

Intra-operative venogram of the portal vein indicated a patent portal vein; the hepatic artery was ligated and divided just beyond the takeoff of the pancreatico-duodenal artery. The clinical response was dramatic. The hypoglycemia promptly disappeared. The immediate postoperative period was characterized by worsening of liver function studies with a rise in the alkaline phosphatase to 2800 I.U., SGOT reached a peak of 410 milliunits and LDH reached a peak of 1100 units. However, the clinical benefits of hepatic artery ligation were short-lived. Within six weeks after the hepatic artery ligation, he again showed signs of increasing hypoglycemia and despite increasing amounts of intravenous glucose his condition rapidly deteriorated and he expired two months after the hepatic artery ligation.

Autopsy examination revealed a massively enlarged liver with numerous necrotic nodules scattered throughout. The liver volume was about three times normal size due to extensive replacement by tumor.

Summary and Conclusion

Intra-arterial hepatic infusion chemotherapy appears to be a worthwhile procedure in patients with metastatic malignancies to the liver. The response rate to intra-arterial infusion chemotherapy is substantially higher than that seen by the systemic route and there is increasing evidence to suggest a distinct prolongation of survival. A prospectively randomized study will be needed to identify more clearly the extent of improvement and the extent of increase in survival in patients thus treated.

Ligation of the hepatic artery appears to have a dramatic effect with tumor necrosis; however, the morbidity and mortality with the procedure continue to remain high and the benefits to the patient appear to be dubious. At the moment sufficient data are not available to recommend hepatic artery ligation.

References

1. Silverberg, E. and Holleb, A. I.: Cancer Statistics, 1974 – Worldwide Epidemiology. CA, 24:2, 1974.
2. Jaffee, B. M., Donegan, W. L., Watson, F. et al: An investigation of the factors which influence the survival in patients with untreated hepatic metastases. Surg. Gynec. Obstet., 127:1, 1968.
3. Bengmark, S. and Hafstrom, L.: The natural history of primary and secondary malignant tumors of the liver. Cancer, 23:198, 1969.
4. Flanagan, L., Jr. and Foster, J. H.: Hepatic resection for metastatic cancer. Amer. J. Surg., 113:551, 1967.
5. Pestana, C., Reitemeier, R. J., Moertel, C. G. et al: The natural history of carcinoma of the colon and rectum. Amer. J. Surg., 108:826, 1964.

6. Cady, B., Monson, D. O. and Swinton, N. W.: Survival of patients after colonic resection for carcinoma with simultaneous liver metastases. Surg. Gynec. Obstet., 131:697, 1970.
7. Watkins, E., Jr., Khazei, A. M. and Nahra, K. S.: Surgical basis for arterial infusion chemotherapy of disseminated carcinoma of the liver. Surg. Gynec. Obstet., 130:581, 1970.
8. Jacobs, E. M., Luce, J. K. and Wood, D. A.: Treatment of cancer with weekly intravenous 5-Fluorouracil. Cancer, 22:1233, 1968.
9. Reitemeier, R. J., Moertel, C. G. and Hahn, R. G.: Combination chemotherapy in gastrointestinal cancer. Cancer Res., 30:1425, 1970.
10. Kaufman, S.: 5-Fluorouracil in the treatment of gastrointestinal neoplasia. New Eng. J. Med., 288:199, 1973.
11. Gailani, S., Holland, J. F., Falkson, G. et al: Comparison of treatment of metastatic gastrointestinal cancer with 5-Fluorouracil (5-FU) to a combination of 5-FU with cytosine arabinoside. Cancer, 29:1308, 1972.
12. Krakoff, I. H.: Chemotherapy of gastrointestinal cancer. Cancer, 30:1600, 1972.
13. Horton, J., Olson, K. B., Gehrt, P. et al: Combination therapy with 5-fluorouracil (NSC-19893), mitomycin C (NSC 26980), vincristine (NSC 67574) and thiotepa (NSC 6396) for advanced cancer. Cancer Chemother. Rep., 4:59, 1965.
14. Sullivan, R. D. and Zurek, W. Z.: Chemotherapy for liver cancer by protracted ambulatory infusion. JAMA, 194:481, 1965.
15. Ansfield, F. J., Ramirez, G., Skibba, J. L. et al: Intrahepatic arterial infusion with 5-Fluorouracil. Cancer, 28:1147, 1971.
16. Shingleton, W. W. and Grage, T. B.: Central Oncology Group Protocol 7032. A study of the chemotherapy of carcinoma of the colon and rectum, metastatic to the liver.
17. Balasegaram, M.: Complete dearterialization for primary carcinoma of the liver. Amer. J. Surg., 124:340, 1972.
18. Almersjö, O., Bengmark, S., Rudenstam, C. S. et al: Evaluation of hepatic dearterialization in primary and secondary cancer of the liver. Amer. J. Surg., 124:5, 1972.
19. Koudahl, G. and Funding, J.: Hepatic artery ligation in primary and secondary hepatic cancer. Acta Chir. Scand., 138:289, 1972.
20. Plengvanit, U., Limwonges, K., Viranuvatti, V. et al: Treatment of primary carcinoma of the liver by hepatic artery ligation. Preliminary report of 40 cases. Liver Research, Kyoto, 1967 p. 490.
21. Fortner, J. G., Mulcare, R. J., Solis, A. et al: Treatment of primary and secondary liver cancer by hepatic artery ligation and infusion chemotherapy. Ann. Surg., 178:162, 1973.
22. Nilsson, L. A.: Therapeutic hepatic artery ligation in patients with secondary liver tumors. Rev. Surg., 23:374, 1966.
23. Segall, H. N.: An experimental anatomical investigation of the blood and bile channels of the liver. Surg. Gynec. Obstet., 37:152, 1923.
24. Healey, J. E.: Vascular patterns in human metastatic liver tumors. Surg. Gynec. Obstet., 120:1187, 1965.
25. Bengmark, S. and Rosengren, K.: Angiographic study of the collateral circulation to the liver after ligation of the hepatic artery in man. Amer. J. Surg., 119:620, 1970.

Panel Discussion

Moderator: C. McKhann, M.D.

Panelists: T. E. Starzl, M.D. S. Sherlock, M.D.
S. Schwartz, M.D. T. Grage, M.D.

Dr. McKhann: I have several questions for Dr. Sherlock. First, is there any cross immunity between hepatitis-A and hepatitis-B?

Dr. Sherlock: No, there is no cross immunity between hepatitis-A and hepatitis-B, as far as we know. If one has had one type, then one can get the other. The best evidence for this comes from the Willowbrook studies, where M.S.-1 was a short incubation type and M.S.-2 was a long incubation type. And there turned out to be no cross immunity.

Dr. McKhann: Do you isolate hospitalized cases of hepatitis and, if so, for how long?

Dr. Sherlock: No, we are not really that strict. We usually take care with disposal of excreta and with the washing of bed linen and night clothes. We do not have isolation facilities for this type of patient. I don't think it is necessary. In all honesty, I think hepatitis is rather a noninfectious disease. It has had a lot of publicity in the last few years. But most hepatologists will tell you that there is virtually never any cross infection from one patient to another, on a ward, with hepatitis.

Dr. McKhann: Should the otherwise healthy surgeon avoid doing surgery, if he is hepatitis-B antigen-positive? In other words, can he give it to his patients?

Dr. Sherlock: The evidence at the moment is that he does not give it to his patients. I think that he would be unwise to work in an area where there are particularly susceptible patients, such as the transplant service, a renal unit, an oncology service. But if he takes normal precautions, I think he can lead a normal surgical life. This is the view adopted at the present time by such authorities as Dr. Thomas Chalmers.

Dr. McKhann: Dr. Schwartz, I have quite a few questions and some editorials on your and Dr. Lin's technique. One from Dr. William Halstead. He is appalled! What incision do you use in doing your hepatectomy?

Dr. Schwartz: I have to defend myself because I do regard Dr. Starzl and Mr. Rodney Smith very highly as my surgical confreres. I guess that I should begin with a confession. I think that it is an ecclesiastic aphorism that the convert is always the most zealous enthusiast. And I am a convert, having watched Professor Lin work. Before I answer your question regarding the incision I think that the reason why I have converted to using this technique for the elective hepatic resections is the one that we usually employ for the more common indication for hepatic resection, namely, the massively traumatized liver. If you are going to apply the anatomic dissection technic to a massively traumatized liver requiring a 50% hepatic resection, you are going to be in a terrific mess. So we have really extrapolated from early experience with trama. Most of our liver resections are related to the New York Thruway and the automobile accident rather than to gunshot wounds. These are massive traumas to the dome of the liver. Others, who have had more experience with trauma than we, the group at San Francisco General Hospital, and Dr. Thomas Shires group at Parkland Hospital in Dallas, have also employed this technic for trauma. If it is employable for a circumstance which is more difficult, then why not use it when you have a clean field? I have been pleased with it, despite the fact that it does look artistic. Before making the incision, even in the trauma patients, if they are not in intense shock, we do an angiogram. We think that this is extremely important and use it in all elective resections. In the trauma patient, there is an added bonus of differentiating between splenic rupture and hepatic rupture with the celiac angiogram. By slipping the catheter down into the superior mesenteric artery, you can determine whether you have one of the hepatic arteries emanating from the superior mesenteric vein as is the case in 25%. For a left lobectomy, or for a left lateral segmentectomy, the operation is readily accomplishable through a midline incision, occasionally taking the xiphoid, without any extension into the thorax. For lesions of the dome and for massive trauma, I usually do extend the incision up into the right pleural space. This particularly in the trauma patients because I anticipate the possibility of using a Cable catheter as a stent, if there is hepatic vein disruption. Despite the fact that I enjoy and appreciate the criticism, made by Mr. Rodney Smith and by Dr. Starzl, the next one that I do at the hospital will still be by this technic.

Dr. McKhann: The next question is from Professor Lin in Taiwan, and it is for Dr. Starzl. He says "Confucius says that fingers were made before forks." Don't you agree?

Dr. Starzl: That stops me. I'll even accept my colleague Dr. Schwartz's classification of where we should be sitting. I agree with almost everything that he has said and I accept almost everything that was in his presentation. But I do think that the technique shown in the movie is a poor way to do a major hepatic resection for tumors. Dr. Schwartz graciously referred to Dr. Lin's publication, which appeared in *The Annals of Surgery*, April 1973. At about that time, I was reviewing trisegmentectomies, since most hepatic resections that I do are trisegmentectomies. I had done a resection about a year before which I thought was 90+%. I was trying to find out how many of these resections or resections of this magnitude had actually been carried out. The answer was surprisingly few. But it occurred to me that there must be a large experience in the Far East with trisegmentectomy, so I looked at Dr. Lin's article with considerable interest. There were none. His cases were all bisegmentectomies or less. It is my judgment that a true trisegmentectomy, which is necessary to get an adequate margin in many hepatic tumors, is not possible, using that method. I think that a very clean Halsteadian dissection and ligation of the right and left hepatic ducts is the first step in a trisegmentectomy. There is a very important piece of anatomy that Mr. Rodney Smith and I were discussing, which I think should be passed on because it is always misrepresented in drawings of the anatomy of the human hilum. I noticed that there was an error, even in Dr. Schwartz's picture of the anatomy of the hilum. The anatomy as it is actually encountered is that the left portal structures come over and don't enter the liver until they reach about the level of the falciform ligament. Then the blood supply of the medial segment turns back. If one is to do a trisegmentectomy, it becomes very necessary to get that whole complex of structures moved off the undersurface of the liver and then to separately ligate and divide the blood supply and the ducts going back to the medial segment. I have seen now on several occasions people who have tried trisegmentectomies and, having failed to do the maneuver that I have just described, end up with a lateral segment that doesn't have anything going to it, or, at least, anything worthwhile, that is, no blood vessels or ducts. There are several other tricks that I think are important in carrying out carefully controlled hepatic resections. One of them is that if you want to ligate a right portal branch and are having trouble because of overhanging tumor, one of the slickest tricks that I know is to lift the whole right lobe up and to approach the right portal branch from posteriorly, rather than from what would be the standard way, coming at it from the front. Another is that as you dissect the ducts and vessels, going to the right and left lobes of liver, it is almost invariable that the ducts bifurcate surprisingly high. The duct bifurcation will be the last structure that you encounter, as you do this dissection. I think that Dr. Schwartz and his great success with the Lin technic merely represents a tribute to one of the world's great surgeons, Dr. Schwartz himself. For residents who are being brought up and who are doing their first hepatic resections, or in anybody's hands, if you are looking at an 85% or greater percent resection, this really has to be done by the more traditional technic that Mr. Rodney Smith described.

Dr. Schwartz: Dr. Starzl, how would you approach a patient who required a 50%-60% resection, due to a massive traumatic injury of the dome of the liver?

Dr. Starzl: I would go into a scramble pattern, which is what I think the Lin procedure is.

Dr. Schwartz: You would do it that way, then?

Dr. Starzl: Yes, I think that that would be reasonable. If you have massive trauma to the liver, very often the site of transection has already been defined for you. It is only a matter of completing the lobectomy.

Dr. McKhann: One topic about which many questions were asked is the indications for liver resection versus repair in trauma.

Dr. Schwartz: I think all of us interested in liver surgery have done a disservice in the first phase of discussion of hepatic resection for trauma, by using that nomenclature. What we are doing, in most instances, is a nonanatomic debridement. It is a debridement and not an anatomic resection. I am guilty as are others, early in the phase of hepatic trauma discussions, of using the term, anatomic resection. As Dr. Starzl indicates, your plane or at least the initiation of your plane, if it is going to require resection, has been established by the trauma and you debride so that you leave no avascular tissue. In most of the large series, the successful results that you see relate to knife wounds and occasionally to gunshot wounds, which are entirely dissimilar from vehicular trauma, which is much more profound. None of us have good results with vehicular trauma. I think that the overall mortality rate is in the range of 50%, with massive resection subsequent to vehicular trauma. We surgeons relate this to associated injuries which, more often than not, are present; nevertheless, we are looking at a poor mortality statistic. So I think that regarding the traumatized liver, one should be more conservative than we have thought in the past and do essentially a resectional debridement.

Dr. McKhann: What about hepatic artery ligation for trauma?

Dr. Schwartz: I think that the question alludes to an experience reported by Truman Mays, of Louisville, who had good results with it. I have had no personal experience with hepatic artery ligation for trauma. But I am somewhat dubious because the type of bleeding that I see in the extensively traumatized liver is venous bleeding, frequently related to the hepatic veins, and I don't see how ligating an artery is going to satisfy that circumstance.

Dr. McKhann: Dr. Grage, several people would like to know how oral 5-FU compares with systemic administration and infusion.

Dr. Grage: There are several articles now in the literature that clearly indicate that 5-FU is as effective, if given orally, as by the intravenous route. There is no oral preparation. You must use the preparation that comes for intravenous use. It is usually mixed with fruit juice. The GI complications tend to be slightly higher; the nausea and vomiting are a little more frequent with oral administration. In terms of effectiveness, the two appear to be about equivalent. Intravenous infusion enjoyed a trial for awhile, but there doesn't seem to be any advantage to that over the single IV push technic. I think that the main thing in either the oral or the IV method is that you treat a patient to slight toxicity. This usually entails a weekly administration of 15 mg/kg, even as high as 20 mg/kg. It is better to titrate the patient to toxicity rather than rigidly stick to a certain dose that the textbook may advise. There are times when the patient will tolerate higher doses than others. In general, I think that you ought to titrate to slight toxicity.

Dr. McKhann: Dr. Grage, if the hepatic arteries are shown by angiography to come from separate origins, do you try to infuse these patients and, if so, how do you go about it?

Dr. Grage: The most common deviation that I see is the hepatic artery coming directly from the superior mesenteric. The radiologist is usually able to put a catheter transfemorally out to the superior mesenteric artery and from there up into the hepatic. But it is a little tricky. Every so often one might tip the catheter over backwards, because it is very easy to occlude the superior mesenteric artery which would be absolutely disastrous. But, if at all possible, you try to determine the vascular abnormalities preoperatively and, if necessary, put two catheters in.

Dr. McKhann: If there are two separate hepatic arteries, one to the right lobe and one to the left lobe with different origins, do you cannulate both of them with catheters?

Dr. Grage: Yes, we do.

Dr. McKhann: Dr. Schwartz and Dr. Starzl, how about T-tubes after hepatic resection?

Dr. Schwartz: I no longer employ the T-tube after hepatic resection and rarely, if ever, after an elective hepatic resection with a normal sized duct and very rarely in patients with trauma because of the experience of Lucas and Walt in Detroit, which I think was a fairly definitive study.

Dr. McKhann: How about the rest of your drainage; do you drain the chest and the subhepatic space?

Dr. Schwartz: Yes, I drain the chest, if I am in the chest. If not, I always drain the subhepatic space, what is now the subphrenic space, quite extensively, because I think drainage is imperative whenever there is liver trauma.

Dr. McKhann: Do you ever use large compressive suture ligatures on "liver" needles for the control of bleeding in hepatectomy?

Dr. Schwartz: Rarely, now. Since we have had the use of the clamp and have been able to apply it, take it off and apply it again, we have relied mainly on ligature and suture ligature of the major vessels as they pass across. There has been a rare circumstance, anteriorly, in which we have used the chromic catgut on the liver needle. Posteriorly, they are hard to place and I really never can get a compressive force, using that technique. I try to avoid it, if at all possible.

Dr. McKhann: Do you use oxygen and high concentrations of glucose, postoperatively?

Dr. Schwartz: Yes, we use 10% glucose in our patients. We do not alter the postoperative course, as far as oxygen is concerned. Concerning the use of hypothermia, we do not employ hypothermia and we do not employ hypotensive anesthesia, in the elective cases.

Dr. McKhann: Dr. Starzl, do you agree with Dr. Schwartz?

Dr. Starzl: Yes, I think that the critical thing is really broad drainage because if you don't have perfect drainage after a large hepatic resection, you are certain to have an infection. So I agree with Dr. Schwartz completely. I have never really used a T-tube. There is one detail: If you do a big resection, anything over 75%, and use those large "liver" needles and have a continuous suture in the raw surface, you can imperil your venous drainage, particularly if you are down to one or almost your last hepatic vein.

Dr. McKhann: Liver resections showed a mortality rate in at least one slide of about 11% or more. What have been the causes of these deaths?

Dr. Schwartz: First, you want to describe which patients you are talking about. One point has to be emphasized, one made by Mr. Rodney Smith. We don't regard liver resection as appropriate in a patient who has a hepatoma superimposed upon cirrhosis. Some of the nice, early work by Professor Lin showed that these livers do not regenerate, albumin is not synthesized and the patients get into a great deal of trouble. The mortality rate, the black beast in our menagerie, is infection, overwhelmingly so. We have had very little trouble with coagulation problems. We anticipate hyperbilirubinemia for a period of time; all of the enzymes do change for a period of time. But the real problem in our hands has been infection. Most of our resections, of course, have been related to trauma. But, even in elective cases, infection has been a major problem. Secondary hemorrhage has occurred in some. This requires early exploration rather than implicating coagulation factors. I think that the biggest error the surgeon can make, after doing a partial resection of the liver, is to indict coagulation factors as causing a continuous ooze. It is usually due to something that you must go back in and remedy in a technical fashion.

Dr. Starzl: There is a very special problem with children. In the last decade or so, I have had one death after removing a tumor from the liver. It was not with a formal hepatic resection. A little child came out to Denver with a huge lesion, called a cystic hamartoma. The patient had been at Baltimore, operated upon and was sent to me from Emory University Hospital for a liver transplant. I explored the child. The boy had the cystic hamartoma, a perfectly benign lesion. I peeled it out of the surface of the liver and the child died on the operating table. It wasn't a formal hepatic resection. I didn't look up what I had done in the last 10 to 12 years – I would think that probably 30 trisegmentectomies – and I have had no deaths nor any deaths from any hepatic resection. So I consider an 11% mortality for an elective hepatic resection to be an unacceptable figure. I will say, to get back to the situation with the child with the cystic hamartoma who died, that was such a disquieting experience that we looked into the literature of deaths from hepatic resection in pediatric recipients and there was plenty of reason for us to have anticipated trouble because the mortality has been said to be about 25%, that is, intra-operative deaths in pediatric recipients undergoing major hepatic resections. And for three reasons: (1) hemorrhage, which was just mentioned; (2) hypothermia, which has not been properly controlled in these children; and (3) air embolus. Apparently this last is a peculiar risk in the pediatric patient because it is unnecessary to go into the chest in these children to do a hepatic resection; they have such a nice, pliable chest cage. So there is a great temptation to stay out of the chest. But, if you do this, and the anesthesiologist does the natural thing during the dangerous part of the procedure, which is to have the children light, and if you get into your vena cava, or the hepatic veins, near the vena cava, and the children are struggling to breathe, they can easily suck up air. Of course, if you have a thoraco-abdominal incision, this will not happen. But, if you have an intact bellows, you can have that complication. So, I think that knowing these things, with children, where your great operative risk is to be expected, you can avoid all three of those hazards that I mentioned.

V

Portal Hypertension

The Pathology of Portal Hypertension

Hans Popper, M.D., Ph.D.

Portal hypertension may be best defined as a gradient greater than 5 mm Hg between portal venous pressure and systemic venous pressure below the diaphragm. Increased portal pressure, therefore, as result of an elevated systemic venous pressure is excluded by this conventional definition. Portal hypertension as now defined may be the result of (1) increased resistance of venous flow to, within and from the liver, (2) augmented splanchnic blood flow and (3) though to a lesser degree, increased pressure in the inferior vena cava [1]. The pathology of portal hypertension [2] encompasses thus a discussion of (a) the mechanism of portal hypertension and the sites where it is produced with disease processes serving as examples of the functional derangement, (b) the consequences of portal hypertension, (c) the enumeration of main diseases in which the various forms of portal hypertension are key manifestations with separation of those in which one mechanism from those in which several ones are involved. The knowledge of the thus defined pathology of portal hypertension influences the medical and surgical management of the diseases.

Mechanism of Portal Hypertension

Resistance to the venous flow may take place either below, within or above the liver:

Infrahepatic causes of portal hypertension are obstruction of the lumen of the portal vein produced by thrombosis or its compression by tumors, abscesses or malformations. By definition, interference below the confluence of the tributaries of the portal veins is not designated portal hypertension but rather splenic or mesenteric vein hypertension, depending upon the vein involved.

Hans Popper, M.D., Ph.D., The Stratton Laboratory for the Study of Liver Diseases, Mount Sinai School of Medicine of The City University of New York. At present Fogarty Scholar-in-Residence, Fogarty International Center, National Institutes of Health, Bethesda, Md.

Portal vein thrombosis is more frequent in infants and children in whom it is usually caused by preceding infections such as from umbilical postnatal sepsis or other often suppurative processes in the abdomen. In adults the thrombosis may also be produced by infections but more frequently by increased coagulability as in polycythemia or as a result of tumor thrombi as in primary hepatic carcinoma.

Intrahepatic interference with the venous flow may be presinusoidal which means before the blood enters the sinusoidal labyrinth; it may be sinusoidal within the lobules or postsinusoidal involving the hepatic vein tributaries.

Presinusoidal portal hypertension may result from lesions of the intrahepatic branches of the portal vein such as thrombosis, frequently an extension of the processes discussed under infrahepatic portal hypertension, or vein involvement from schistosomiasis. Further, it may be caused by compression of the portal tracts as also produced by schistosomiasis and by various inflammatory and granulomatous conditions such as rarely by sarcoidosis [3] as well as by malformations and particularly by most types of cirrhosis including the precirrhotic stage of primary biliary cirrhosis [4]. The compression of the portal vein tributaries by scarring in the portal tract is recognized in a christmas tree-like appearance in portovenograms, which is considered characteristic of cirrhosis [5]. Phlebosclerosis of the portal vein branches, either idiopathic or secondary to portal hypertension, must also be listed.

Sinusoidal portal hypertension may be produced by increase of the intralobular connective tissue framework as result of various types of chronic hepatitis in that active fibroplasia occurs either around damaged hepatocytes which are frequently arranged in rosette-like fashion, around proliferated bile ductules, and sometimes around intralobular granulomas or other accumulations of macrophages [6]. Moreover, alterations of the hepatocytes raise transiently the portal pressure, as observed in the conspicuous steatosis of nutritional disorders or following alcohol abuse and with augmented smooth endoplasmic reticulum induced by drug treatment [7]. Necrosis of the hepatocytes causes areas of collapse in which the blood flow may be compromised. Finally, in various forms of hepatitis, eg, acute viral hepatitis, sinusoidal cells including macrophages and lymphocytes are sufficiently proliferated to at least transiently raise portal pressure. Carcinoma metastases may compromise the portal flow by thrombosis or compression.

Postsinusoidal portal hypertension is induced by processes which act upon the tributaries of the hepatic veins or by diseases of these veins.

Regenerative nodules in cirrhosis, also occasionally in other conditions, compress the hepatic vein tributaries, as is well demonstrated after injection of the hepatic venous tree by synthetic resins followed by digestion of the soft tissue: the flattened hepatic veins are arranged in basket form around the nodules [8, 9]. The slit-like shape of their lumen is also readily seen on the cut surface of autopsy specimens where the nodules seem to compress the veins. Scarring around the hepatic vein tributaries particularly characterizes the initial stage of alcoholic liver injury: the central hyaline sclerosis [10]. In contrast to previous belief that alcoholic liver injury is a portal process reflected in the now rejected term "portal cirrhosis," chronic and recurrent alcoholic hepatitis is characterized by ballooned hepatocytes, accumulation of leukocytes, as well as deposition of alcoholic hyaline in the centrolobular zone. This induces presinusoidal accumulation of fibrous tissue but hemodynamically far more important perivenous scarring which compromises the lumen of the central veins and other hepatic vein tributaries and thus produces an outflow block similar to that produced by a regenerative nodule. Eventually, the lesion extends to the portal tract to produce a pull resulting in approximation of central and portal fields as first step of transformation to cirrhosis [11].

Diseases of the smaller branches of the hepatic vein tributaries may be the result of exposure to seneccio and crotalaria alkaloids in bush tea, primarily in malnourished children in the Caribbean areas, but is also seen in other parts of the world and designated as veno-occlusive disease [12]. This disorder of children between 6 and 10 years of age slowly leads to death. Similar occluding lesions may be the result of thrombosis and recanalization, eg, in polycythemia or occasionally after administration of contraceptive drugs [13]. The latter two processes may also involve larger tributaries of the hepatic veins.

Suprahepatic portal hypertension is created in the main tributaries of the hepatic veins and in the inferior vena cava by compression by tumors or abscesses, by thrombosis occasionally extending from the smaller vessels, particularly with increased blood coagulability, or by developmental changes.

Portal hypertension may also result from *increased blood flow to the venous bed* in the liver, in comparison to the size of the bed. This mechanism is hard to prove except by blood flow measurements. Splenomegaly, particularly extensive enlargement, is associated with increased blood flow to the liver. This has been assumed to be the cause of portal hypertension in myeloid metaplasia [14, 15] rather than increased resistance in the liver from portal infiltration [16]. However, not all studies have demonstrated increased hepatic blood flow [17]. Moreover, severe splenomegaly in Africa on presumably infectious basis, including malaria, is not accompanied by portal hypertension. Also after portacaval shunt the total splenic flow increases although the portal venous pressure is reduced, indicating the limited role of increased splenic flow in the portal hypertension [15].

Other factors increasing portal flow or pressure are arterial/venous anastomoses as they may occur as traumatic extrahepatic fistulas between portal vein and hepatic artery. Such fistulas have been postulated in the intestine and radiologically demonstrated in the spleen [18]. In cirrhosis, vascular anastomoses between the artery and both portal vein branches and hepatic vein tributaries develop in the connective tissue septa as seen in injection preparations [9]. However, the fact that hepatic arterial ligation in cirrhosis does not significantly reduce the portal hypertension shows them to be only a minor contributing factor.

There is a large group of conditions of primary or idiopathic portal hypertension in which a cause cannot be readily established. In some of these instances, application of special techniques may demonstrate an overlooked etiology, eg, organized thrombi in the intrahepatic portal veins, as visualized at postmortem injection techniques [19]. Humoral factors have been incriminated, but are not proven. In a group of cases, hepatic fibrosis is found intralobular, subcapsular and portal, but not of sufficient degree to account mechanically for a significant portal hypertension with prominent splenomegaly and bleeding esophageal varices. This lesion has been previously designated as Banti's syndrome, to be distinguished from cirrhosis with splenomegaly [20]. Such cases have been found sporadically in the Western world, usually without obvious etiology [21, 22]. Such inconspicuous hepatic fibrosis and bleeding esophageal varices associated with portal hypertension and splenomegaly have been also observed following prolonged administration of anorganic arsenicals, eg, in treatment of psoriasis [23] or recently after prolonged exposure to vinyl chloride of workers engaged in its polymerization [24]. In both of these circumstances the changes have been followed in some instances by development of hepatic angiosarcoma [25, 26]. Other instances of so-called Banti's syndrome of unknown etiology may have an unrecognized toxic basis. Such cases have been reported with greater frequency in India [27] and Uganda [28] than in the Western world; particularly thorough examinations in India have not elucidated the hemodynamic reason for the lesion [29]. Some have incriminated primary alterations of the intrahepatic portal vein branches [30].

Consequences of Portal Hypertension

The presented topographic classification of portal hypertension requires modification, particularly in evaluating the consequences. Infrahepatic and presinusoidal hypertension have to be separated from sinusoidal, postsinusoidal and suprahepatic hypertension. Most cases of hypertension resulting from increased portal blood flow and the idiopathic forms mainly belong to the group of infrahepatic and presinusoidal portal hypertension. In the first group the hepatic parenchyma itself is not under increased pressure and only the portal pressure is elevated as measured either during operation in the mesenteric vein or by splenoportal or umbilical manometry, while the wedged hepatic vein pressure is normal. By contrast, in the form represented by the postsinusoidal, sinusoidal and suprahepatic forms the increased pressure makes itself felt on the hepatic parenchyma. Here not only the portal blood flow but also the wedge hepatic blood pressure is increased and both pressures are about equal and the portal pressure even higher. It therefore may be justified to designate the first group as nonparenchymal and the other parenchymal portal hypertension.

This separation has major practical significance in that the increased pressure in parenchymal hypertension impairs hepatocellular function. It also alters the structure of the hepatic sinusoids. While they normally differ from capillaries by a lack of a basement membrane, such a membrane forms in the perisinusoidal tissue space in chronic liver injury, particularly that associated with portal hypertension. This leads to an interference with the exchange between hepatocytes and blood and thus reduces the effective hepatic blood flow. Increased sinusoidal pressure favors ascites formation, in contrast to the nonparenchymal group, in which it only develops in the presence of complicating hepatocellular injury or of hypoproteinemia. Similarly, nonparenchymal portal hypertension if not associated with liver cell injury tolerates further reduction of portal flow, eg, brought on by shunt operations, much better than the parenchymal hypertension, in which shunt operations may more readily lead to hepatic failure in the short run and hepatic encephalopathy in the long run. Furthermore, coagulation defects after gastrointestinal hemorrhage in portal hypertension are much better tolerated in the nonparenchymal form because, in the parenchymal form impaired formation of clotting factors interferes with the control of the hemorrhage. Increased formation of hepatic lymph leads to increased lymph pressure and dilatation of the thoracic duct [31] and of the lymphatics in the portal tract [32].

Other sequelae of portal hypertension are found equally in both forms, however, they are the more conspicuous the closer the obstruction is to the target. Therefore, in nonparenchymal portal hypertension the consequences are usually more conspicuous with equal pressure, particularly since the sinusoidal bed of the liver acts as a buffer reducing somewhat the effects of postsinusoidal and suprahepatic hypertension.

Dilatation of collaterals between splanchnic and systemic circulation and enlargement of the spleen are the two major consequences of portal hypertension in general. The collaterals are found in the posterior abdominal wall when they are only recognized at operation or at laparoscopy, in the anterior abdominal wall when they may be detected by dilated subcutaneous veins especially conspicuous in the Cruveilhier-Baumgarten syndrome and, particularly important, at the upper and lower border of the gland-bearing portion of the gastrointestinal tract. The hemorrhoidal veins drain both toward the inferior mesenteric vein as well as to the pudendal veins and dilatation of these hemorrhoidal veins has previously been considered as typical hemorrhoids. The common anal hemorrhoids, however, which often contain arterial blood, do not result from portal hypertension which causes submucosal varices in the rectum above the anus. Bleeding from the latter yields only venous blood. The dilated veins in the gastric portion of the stomach and particularly the submucosal veins of the esophagus are communications from the short gastric and coronary veins to the vena hemiazygous. This intensive collateral network is well illustrated by various angiographic methods in which the dilatation of the coronary vein is particularly characteristic. Erosion of the esophageal varices is one of the main causes of death in patients with portal hypertension. However, esophageal varices are not necessarily an indication of portal hypertension since they may be found without it, particularly in older people. Esophageal varices, therefore, do not correlate with the degree of portal hypertension and are not effective collaterals; for instance, their presence is not reflected in increased arterial ammonia levels.

Splenomegaly in patients with portal hypertension need not only be the result of a mechanical factor. Increased intrasplenal pressure causes fibrosis of the pulp cords which closes the previously open circulation [33, 34] as well as atrophy of the lymph follicles frequently associated with intrafollicular or perifollicular sclerotic areas containing both iron and calcium deposits (Gamna-Gander bodies) as indication of preceding follicular hemorrhage. However, the size of the spleen is not a measure of portal hypertension since in addition to hemodynamic factors a hyperplasia of splenic reticuloendothelial and lymphoid cells contributes. The latter is stimulated by either the liver injury or by immunologic processes. Pressure and cellular hyperplasia as factors in portal hypertension were separated in studies on rats chronically intoxicated by ethionine in which the spleen was enlarged six times. After discontinuation of ethionine feeding, the spleen size reduced to three times the normal simultaneously with a drop of the previously elevated serum gamma globulin. The persisting three times enlargement in the scar stage reflects the effects of pressure [35]. The nature of the inflammatory or immunologic insult which is responsible for the lack of correlation between the degree of portal hypertension and the splenic enlargement is not fully established. There is little, if any, evidence that circulating antibodies to liver tissue cause liver injury, although the possibility of autoaggression by cell-bound immunity is not excluded. However, the immune state is altered in many diseases with portal hypertension [36], for instance the frequent excess of immune gamma globulin is not directed against hepatic structures but rather against antigens from intestinal bacteria [37] and some persisting viral antigens [38] which both reach the lymphatic tissue including the spleen in chronic liver diseases because of bypass of blood from the liver and of the inability of the Kupffer cells to take up these antigens. This discrepancy between increased portal pressure and the size of the spleen is conspicuous in alcoholic liver disease, in which the spleen is usually smaller than would be expected from the liver disorder because of nutritional deficiency of cofactors which inhibits the splenic cellular reaction.

Increased renal vascular resistance has been associated with portal hypertension and might play a role in renal failure in cirrhosis [39, 40]. The claim that portal hypertension causes peptic ulceration has not been substantiated by statistical studies. Hepatocellular dysfunction may play a greater role than pressure. Most of the other consequences associated with portal hypertension are also not its direct result but rather produced by the associated hepatic functional defect and particularly by the vascular shunts which divert blood from the liver.

Diseases in Which Portal Hypertension Is Prominent

In some diseases, one site of portal hypertension is present while in others several factors play a role to different degrees. Similarly, the same factor may act on several sites. Increased blood coagulability for instance, as in polycythemia vera, may cause thrombosis in infrahepatic, presinusoidal, postsinusoidal, as well as in suprahepatic location. Tumors, extrahepatic, metastatic and primary hepatic carcinomas, may also exert their effects in any of these locations. Table 1 lists the diseases in which blockage in a specific location is prominent. The identification of the

Table 1. Localizations of Origin of Portal Hypertension Produced by Resistance

A. Infrahepatic
  1. Thrombosis of portal vein
  2. Obstruction of portal vein by tumor or abscess
  3. Malformations of portal veins

B. Intrahepatic
  1. Postsinusoidal
  2. Schistosomiasis
  3. Congenital hepatic fibrosis and occasionally microhamartomas
  4. Syphilitic hepar lobatum
  5. Chronic nonsuppurative destructive cholangitis
  6. Chronic suppurative cholangitis (E. coli)
  7. Neoplastic processes
  8. Diffuse nodular hyperplasia
  9. Partial nodular transformation
  10. Sarcoidosis

C. Sinusoidal
  1. Toxic agents
  2. Hypervitaminosis A
  3. Steatosis
  4. Hepatitis

D. Postsinusoidal
  1. Alcoholic sclerosing hyaline necrosis
  2. Veno-occlusive disease (in malnourished children in the Caribbean area)
  3. Radiation hepatitis
  4. Anticancer therapy
  5. Intrahepatic Budd-Chiari syndrome (thrombosis with recanalization)

E. Suprahepatic
  1. Congenital web in vena cava inferior and at entrance of hepatic veins
  2. Thrombosis
  3. Compression of hepatic veins by tumor

cause is essential in surgical management with radiographic, manometric and biopsy methods – important diagnostic tools. If biopsy demonstrates hepatitis, particularly alcoholic, surgery is being delayed just as detection of cancerous growths alters indications.

Prolonged thrombotic obstruction of the portal vein may cause infrahepatic portal hypertension followed by the recanalization of its original lumen. Collaterals may bring blood from the tributaries of the portal vein to the hilus bypassing the obstructive area. This lesion has been designated as cavernomatous transformation of the portal vein and has been wrongly considered as a malformation. Acute portal vein thrombosis usually causes an abdominal catastrophy with hemorrhagic ascites and infarction of the intestine. The lack of return of blood from the splanchnic system is the cause of the "drowning of the patient in his own ascites fluid." By contrast, surgical ligation of the portal vein above the origin of the coronary vein fails to lead to serious consequences since the latter vein drains the splanchnic blood through collaterals to the systemic circulation.

Schistosomiasis is the most important presinusoidal form [41] because it is the most widespread variety of portal hypertension; it has been estimated that more than 100 million people suffer from this condition. Recent studies [42] indicate that it is not a simple mechanical reaction to the deposition of schistosoma ova but rather a complex immunologic process in which cell-bound immunity to schistosoma antigens causes the scarring around the veins, as well as intravenous processes. Schistosomiasis usually produces nonparenchymal portal hypertension; the parenchymal form occurring particularly in Brazil and Egypt is caused by complicating cirrhosis [43]. Congenital hepatic fibrosis [44, 45] which differs morphologically from cirrhosis by the lack of displacement of the hepatic vein tributaries to the septa is associated with presinusoidal portal hypertension and sometimes with cholangitis, which may be the predominant feature. Related to it is the polycystic liver which does not lead to portal hypertension. Microhamartomas (Meyenburg complexes) [46], which usually are innocent incidental findings, sometimes may cause portal hypertension in adolescents for reasons not clear. Portal scarring may obstruct the portal vein branches, they may be underdeveloped; moreover, a frequent excess of hepatic arterial branches in the portal tracts implicates arterial/venous anastomoses in the hemodynamic alteration as is assumed for the Osler-Rendu-Weber syndrome [47]. Diffuse nodular hyperplasia seldom causes portal hypertension, though parenchymal nodules in the caudal lobe (partial nodular transformation) [48] may do it although portal vein thrombosis is often encountered in this later condition.

Sometimes presinusoidal and sinusoidal are combined, eg, in the mentioned examples of hepatic fibrosis. The Budd-Chiari syndrome is designated as narrowing and occluding disorders of the hepatic vein tree [49, 50]. The syndrome may involve the intrahepatic smaller tributaries, but mainly the large trunks or the vena cava inferior compromising the ostia of the hepatic veins. Obstruction of larger vessels leads frequently to secondary thrombosis in smaller ones. In acute Budd-Chiari syndrome, the clinical manifestations are dramatic with jaundice, rapidly developing ascities and hepatic failure, while in chronic disease they may be insidious. The disease should be suspected when liver biopsy performed on the enlarged liver shows passive congestion in the absence of systemic cardiac insufficiency. With obstruction of larger veins, the caudate lobe may be enlarged since its drainage is independent of the major hepatic veins. This is sometimes recognized as opacity on hepatic scintigraphy. Chemical and radiation therapy against cancer may cause edema, thrombosis and fibrosis of the walls of the intrahepatic branches of the hepatic veins associated with hepatomegaly, ascites and jaundice. This may occur even in the absence of hepatic metastases [51].

According to recent, mainly Japanese studies, congenital webs covering the ostia of the main hepatic veins or located in the inferior vena cava produce the Budd-Chiari syndrome. This may be in the form of thin diaphragms or of thick fibrotic bands which almost create a stricture [52, 53]. Peculiarly enough, clinical manifestations may appear only in the second or third decade of life; this has been explained by kinking of the veins resulting from changes in position of the growing liver. It is important to distinguish the form involving the large veins from the other, since if demonstrated by angiographic methods it can be corrected by either abdominal or thoracic surgery [54].

Among conditions with multifactorial portal hypertension, cirrhosis is the single most important example. The main factor is the compression of the hepatic vein tributaries by the regenerative nodules, the more effective the smaller the nodules. Second, portal scarring associated with inflammation plays a role which is dominant in the precirrhotic precursor stage of primary and secondary biliary cirrhosis when nodule formation has not yet set in. Third, the anastomoses between hepatic artery and the portal and hepatic vein system [9, 55] bring hepatic arterial pressure to bear on the portal vein. The hepatic artery carries smaller amounts of blood under high pressure while in the portal vein much blood flows under low pressure, a situation often compared with the relation of a torrent to a river. The anastomoses cause visible pulsations in the upper limb of the portal vein during end-to-side portal caval shunt. They also disturb the circulation as visualized on X-ray cinematography by the movement of a radiopaque bolus injected into the liver. It sometimes moves retrograde to the portal vein and more frequently to the hepatic veins [56, 57]. With progression of cirrhosis the arterial blood flow assumes quantitatively more significance because the regenerative nodules become gradually separated from the portal flow. A fourth factor is perisinusoidal fibrosis, the significance of which is not established. A fifth contributing factor to portal hypertension is splenomegaly since the addition of blood flowing to the enlarged spleen, though the result of cirrhosis, has to be accommodated in the hepatic bed with splenic vascular resistance usually reduced in cirrhosis because of general vasodilatation. Finally, the scarring of the liver prevents an expansion of the vascular bed in cirrhosis which also increases the pressure. However, parenchymal portal hypertension is the most important cause of hypertension in cirrhosis and this disease is its most frequent cause. The portal scarring accounts for the enlargement of the spleen and less for the overall pressure.

Finally, a vicious circle is often established in that in any type of portal hypertension the trunk and branches of the portal vein show secondary changes of phlebosclerosis with thickening of the intima, as already mentioned. This so-called hepatoportal [21] sclerosis was also considered a primary lesion in some forms of portal hypertension, eg, in India [30]. Anyway, wherever the process starts, the portal sclerosis increases portal pressure and portal hypertension in turn augments portal sclerosis.

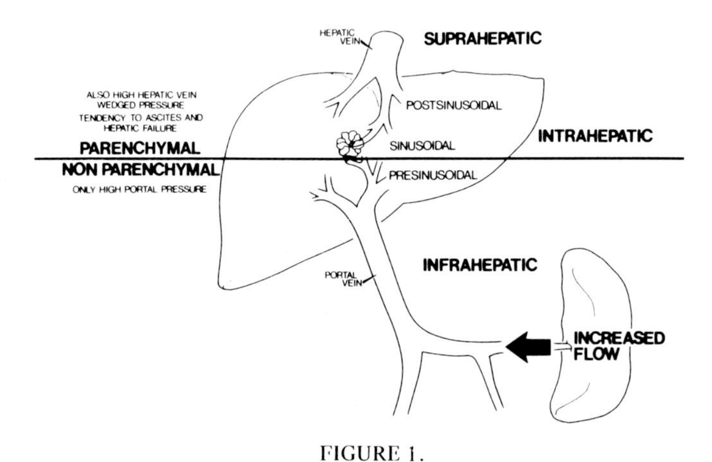

FIGURE 1.

Summary

Portal hypertension has been classified as to localization of its origin, namely, below the liver, within the liver and above the liver. But functionally more important is the separation of the conditions in which the hepatic parenchyma is under increased pressure from those in which it is not (Fig. 1). Infrahepatic and presinusoidal locations, as well as the conditions resulting from increased blood flow, represent nonparenchymal hypertension in which only the portal pressure is elevated, but not the wedged hepatic vein pressure. By contrast, sinusoidal, postsinusoidal and suprahepatic locations cause parenchymal portal hypertension in which both pressures are equally raised and hepatic function is impaired or at least threatened. This is significant in prognosis and in the sequelae of shunt surgery and particularly in the probability of portasystemic encephalopathy. Some forms of portal hypertension are created in one location, eg, portal vein thrombosis and schistosomiasis result in nonparenchymal hypertension and Budd-Chiari syndrome in the parenchymal form. Portal hypertension in cirrhosis results from a variety of factors in which postsinusoidal compression by regenerative nodules usually is the most important. But other mechanisms may play a significant role which accounts for the variations of hemodynamic conditions in cirrhosis and indicates hemodynamic evaluation of each patient before surgical intervention.

References

1. Sherlock, S.: Classification and functional aspects of portal hypertension. Amer. J. Surg., 127:121-128, 1974.
2. Popper, H.: Pathology of portal hypertension. The therapy of portal hypertension. Proceedings from International Symposium, Oct. 29-31, 1967, Bad Ragaz, Switzerland, pp. 58-63.
3. Porter, G. H.: Hepatic sarcoidosis. A cause of portal hypertension and liver failure; review. Arch. Intern. Med., 108:483, 1961.
4. Kew, M. C., Varma, R. R., Dos Santos, H. A. et al: Portal hypertension in primary biliary cirrhosis. Gut, 12:830, 1971.
5. Viamonte, M., Warren, D., Foman, J. et al: Angiographic investigations in portal hypertension. Surg. Gynec. Obstet., 130:37-53, 1970.
6. Popper, H. and Udenfriend, S.: Hepatic fibrosis – Correlation of biochemical and morphologic investigations. Amer. J. Med., 49:707-721, 1970.
7. Leevy, C.L., Ten Hove, W., Opper, A. et al: Influence of ethanol and microsomal drugs on hepatic hemodynamics. Amer. NY Acad., 178:315-331, 1970.
8. Kelty, R. H., Baggenstoss, A. H. and Butt, H. R.: The relation of the regenerated liver nodule to the vascular bed in cirrhosis. Gastroenterology, 15:285, 1950.

9. Popper, H., Elias, H. and Petty, D.E.: Vascular pattern of the cirrhotic liver. Amer. J. Clin. Path., 22:717, 1952.
10. Reynolds, T. B., Ito, S. and Iwatsuki, S.: Measurement of portal pressure and its clinical applications. Amer. J. Med., 49:649, 1970.
11. Gerber, M. A. and Popper, H.: Relation between central canals and portal tracts in alcoholic hepatitis. A contribution to the pathogenesis of cirrhosis in alcoholics. Hum. Path., 3:199-207, 1972.
12. Stuart, K. L. and Bras, G.: Veno-occlusive disease of the liver. Quart. J. Med., 26:291, 1957.
13. Hoyumpa, A. M., Jr., Schiff, L. and Helfman, E. L.: Budd-Chiari syndrome in women taking oral contraceptives. Amer. J. Med., 50:137-140, 1971.
14. Shaldon, S. and Sherlock, S.: Portal hypertension in the myeloproliferative syndrome and the reticuloses. Amer. J. Med., 32:758, 1962.
15. Sullivan, A., Rheinlander, H. and Weintraub, L. R.: Esophageal varices in agnogenic myeloid metaplasia: Disappearance after splenectomy. Gastroenterology, 66:429-432, 1974.
16. Ward, H. R. and Block, M. H.: The natural history of agnogenic myeloid metaplasia (AMM) and a critical evaluation of its relationship with the myeloproliferative syndrome. Medicine, 50:357-420, 1971.
17. Kew, M. C., Lumbrick, C. and Varma, R. R.: Renal and intrarenal blood flow in non-cirrhotic portal hypertension. Gut, 13:763, 1972.
18. Stone, H. H., Jordan, W. D., Acker, J. J. et al: Portal arteriovenous fistulae. Review and case report. Amer. J. Surg., 109:191, 1965.
19. Boyer, J. L., Hales, M. r. and Klatskin, G.: "Idiopathic" portal hypertension due to occlusion of intrahepatic portal veins by organized thrombi. Medicine, 53:77, 1974.
20. Sato, T., Koyama, K. and Yamauchi, H.: Developmental mechanism of splenomegaly and portal hypertension in noncirrhotic periportal fibrosis with splenomegaly (so-called Banti's syndrome). Jap. Soc. Gastroent., 8:115-130, 1973.
21. Mikkelsen, W. P., Edmondson, H. A., Peters, R. L. et al: Extra- and intrahepatic portal hypertension without cirrhosis (hepatoportal sclerosis). Ann. Surg., 162:602, 1965.
22. Benhamou, J. P., Guillemot, R., Tricot, R. et al: Hypertension portale essentielle. Presse Med., 70:2397, 1962.
23. Morris, J. S., Schmid, M., Newman, S. et al: Arsenic and noncirrhotic portal hypertension. Gastroenterology, 64:86, 1974.
24. Popper, H. and Thomas, L. B.: Alterations of liver and spleen among workers exposed to vinyl chloride. Ann. NY Acad. Sci. (In press.)
25. Roth, F.: Arsen-Leber-Tumoren (Haemangioendothelium). Z. Krebsforsch. 61:468, 1957.
26. Thomas, L. B. and Popper, H.: Pathology of angiosarcoma of the liver among vinyl chloride polyvinyl chloride workers. Amer. NY Acad. Sci. (In press.)
27. Basu, A. K. and Aikat, B. K.: Tropical splenomegaly. London:Publ. Butterworths, 1963.
28. Williams, R., Parsonson, A., Somers, K. et al: Portal hypertension in idiopathic tropical splenomegaly. Lancet, 1:329, 1966.

29. Boyer, J. L., Gupta, K.P.S., Biswas, S. K. et al: Idiopathic portal hypertension. Comparison with the portal hypertension of cirrhosis and extrahepatic portal vein obstruction. Ann. Intern. Med., 66:41, 1967.
30. Ramalingaswami, V. and Nayak, N. C.: Liver disease in India. *In* Popper, H. and Schaffner, F. (eds.): Progress in Liver Diseases, Vol. 111. New York:Grune & Stratton, 1970, pp. 222-235.
31. Dumont, A. E. and Mulholland, J. H.: Hepatic lymph in cirrhosis. *In* Popper, H. and Schaffner, F., (eds.): Progress in Liver Diseases Vol 11. New York:Grune & Stratton, 1965, pp. 427-441.
32. Baggenstoss, A. H.: The relationship of the hepatic hilar lymph vessels of man to ascites. Arch. De Vecchi Anat. Pat., 31:11, 1960.
33. Moschcowitz, E.: The pathogenesis of splenomegaly in hypertension of the portal circulation; "congestive splenomegaly." Medicine, 27:187, 1948.
34. Wennberg, E. and Weiss, L.: The structure of the spleen and hemolysis. Amer. Rev. Med., 20:29-40, 1969.
35. Kent, G., Popper, H., Dubin, A. et al: The spleen in ethionine-induced cirrhosis. Its role in gamma globulin elevation. AMA Arch. Path., 64:398, 1957.
36. Popper, H., Gerber, M. A. and Vernace, S.: Immunologic factors in liver disease. Israel J. Med. Sci., 9:103-113, 1973.
37. Bjorneboe, M., Prytz, H. and Orskov, F.: Antibodies to intestinal microbes in serum of patients with cirrhosis of the liver. Lancet, 1:58, 1972.
38. Triger, D. R., Kurtz, J. B., Maccallum, F. O. et al: Raised antibody titer to measles and rubella viruses in chronic active hepatitis. Lancet, 1:665, 1972.
39. Kew, M. C., Brunt, P. W., Varma, R. R. et al: Renal and internal blood-flow in cirrhosis of the liver. Lancet, 2:504, 1971.
40. Kew, M. C., Limbrick, C., Varma, R. R. et al: Renal and intrarenal blood flow in noncirrhotic portal hypertension. Gut, 13:763, 1972.
41. Aufses, A. H., Jr., Schaffner, F., Rosenthal, W. S. et al: Portal venous pressure in "pipestem" fibrosis of the liver due to schistosomiasis. Amer. J. Med., 27:807, 1959.
42. Warren, S., Domingo, E. O. and Cowan, R. B. T.: Granuloma formation around schistosoma eggs as manifestation of delayed hypersensitivity. Amer. J. Path., 51:735, 1967.
43. Andrade, Z. A.: Hepatic schistosomiasis. *In* Popper, H., and Schaffner, F., (eds.): Progress in Liver Diseases, Vol. 11. New York:Grune & Stratton, 1965, p. 228.
44. Kerr, D. N. S., Harrison, C. V., Sherlock, S. et al: Congenital hepatic fibrosis. Quart. J. Med., 30:91, 1961.
45. Fauvert, R., and Benhamou, J. P.: Congenital hepatic fibrosis. *In* Schaffner, F., Sherlock, S. and Leevy, C. M. (eds.): The Liver and Its Diseases. New York:Intercontinental Medical Book Corporation, 1974, p. 283.
46. Popper, H. and Schaffner, F.: Liver: Structure and Function. New York:The Blakiston Division, McGraw-Hill Book Company, Inc., 1957.
47. Martini, G. A.: Lebercirrhose bei Morbus Osler, Cirrhosis hepatic telangiectatica. Gastroenterologia, 83:157, 1955.
48. Sherlock, S., Feldman, C. A., Muran, B. et al: Partial nodular transformation of the liver with portal hypertension. Amer. J. Med., 40:195, 1966.
49. Parker, R. G. F.: Occlusion of the hepatic veins in man. Medicine, 38:369, 1959.
50. Westcott, J. L.: The Budd-Chiari syndrome. Amer. J. Gastroent. 60:625, 1973.

51. Scott, R. B., Budinger, J. M., Prendergast, R. A. M. et al: Hepatic veno-occlusive syndrome in American adult. Gastroenterology, 42:631, 1962.
52. Takeuchi, J., Takada, A., Hasumura, Y. et al: Budd-Chiari syndrome associated with obstruction of the inferior vena cava. Amer. J. Med., 51:11, 1971.
53. Kimura, C., Shirotani, H. and Kirooka, H.: Membranous obliteration of the inferior vena cava in the hepatic portion. J. Cariovasc. Surg., 4:87, 1963.
54. Schaffner, F., Gadboys, H. L., Safran, A. P. et al: Budd-Chiari syndrome caused by a web in the inferior vena cava. Amer. J. Med., 42:838, 1967.
55. Hales, M. r., Allan, J. S. and Hall, E. M.: Injection-corrosion studies of normal and cirrhotic livers. Amer. J. Path., 53:909-941, 1959.
56. Kessler, R. E., Tice, D. A. and Zimmon, D. S.: Retrograde flow of portal vein blood in patients with cirrhosis. Radiology, 92:1038, 1969.
57. Okuda, K., Moriyama, M., Yasumoto, M. et al: Roentgenologic demonstration of spontaneous reversal of portal blood flow in cirrhosis and primary carcinoma of the liver. Amer. J. Roentgen., 99:419-428, 1973.

The "H" Shunt for Portal Decompression

Marvin L. Gliedman, M.D. and Barry Driscoll, M.D.

Introduction

The "H" graft mesocaval shunt is an evolutionary extension of the classic mesocaval shunt (Fig. 1) described by Marion [1] and Clatworthy [2]. From July 1962 to 1967 the side-to-end superior mesenteric vein to inferior vena cava shunt for portal decompression was our standard decompressive procedure. In June 1967 we attempted a mesocaval shunt in a patient who had previous gastric and biliary surgery and a lysis of adhesions. Eventually we were able to free the superior mesenteric vein; however, it appeared impossible to get the abdomen sufficiently dissected to allow for the routine mesocaval shunt. On this basis we simply dissected through the posterior peritoneum below the duodenum and freed the anterior portion of the cava and by use of a 20 mm Dacron graft accomplished a side-to-side shunt between the "cava" and superior mesenteric vein. Since that time we have used the technic in 27 patients. Of the 27 early patients, ten were in desperate circumstances and two other procedures were presumed preludes to liver transplantation.

Technic

The technic is based on our previous description for the mesocaval shunt, which has changed little since the description in 1965 [3, 4]. In the "H" graft procedure the routine dissection of the superior mesenteric vein is carried out, but the inferior vena cava is freed directly through the retroperitoneum below the transverse portion of the duodenum. The

Marvin L. Gliedman, M.D., Professor and Chairman, Department of Surgery, Albert Einstein College of Medicine (MHMC); Chief of Surgery, Montefiore Hospital and Medical Center and Barry Driscoll, M.D., Instructor in Surgery, Albert Einstein College of Medicine; Assistant Attending, Montefiore Hospital and Medical Center, Bronx, N.Y.

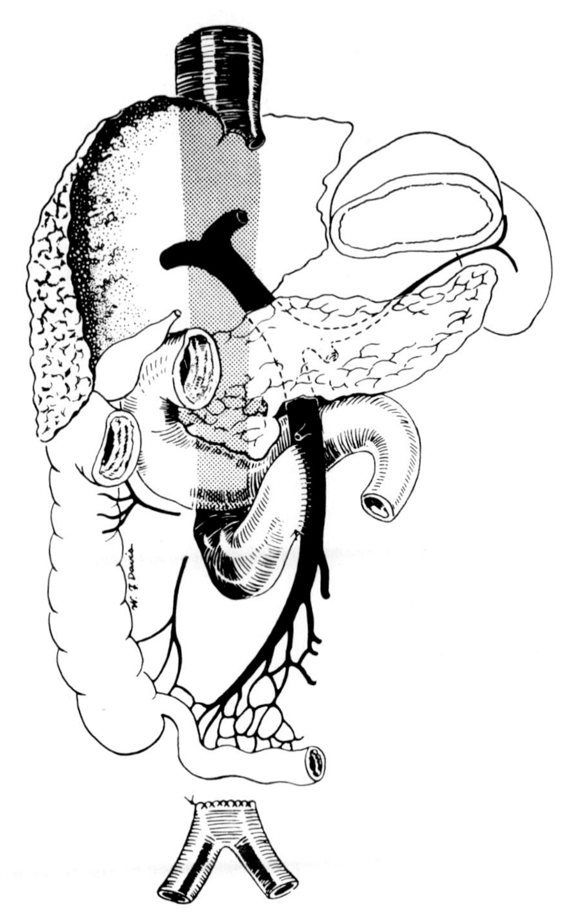

FIG. 1. The side-to-end ("J") mesocaval shunt.

inferior vena cava is freed anteriorly and laterally only enough to allow the placement of a Satinsky vascular clamp. Usually, no lumbar veins are divided. The technic is described in more detail in Figures 2-4.

Results

From 1967 to 1970 there were three survivors in the so-called disaster cases. These patients were not candidates for a surgical procedure except perhaps for a rapid and blood sparing one. For example, one patient was immediately postoperative from a double cardiac valve replacement procedure, one patient was not typable for any blood in the city and the

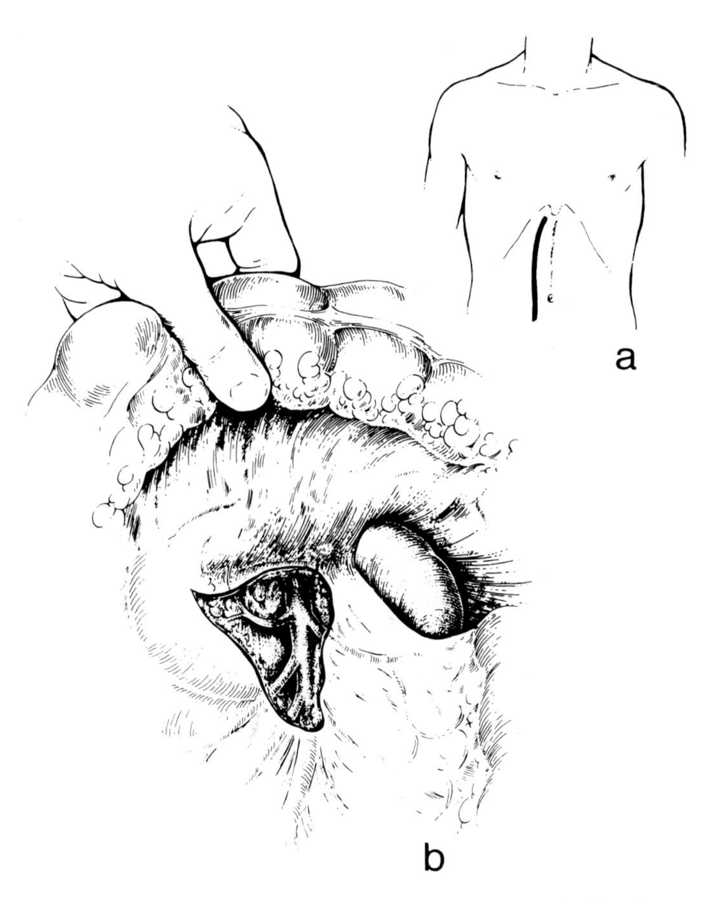

FIG. 2. (a) A mid-line or right paramedian incision is used. (b) The superior mesenteric vein is immediately behind the posterior peritoneum, running parallel to the right vertebral body border, where the under surface of the mesocolon turns upon the posterior peritoneum.

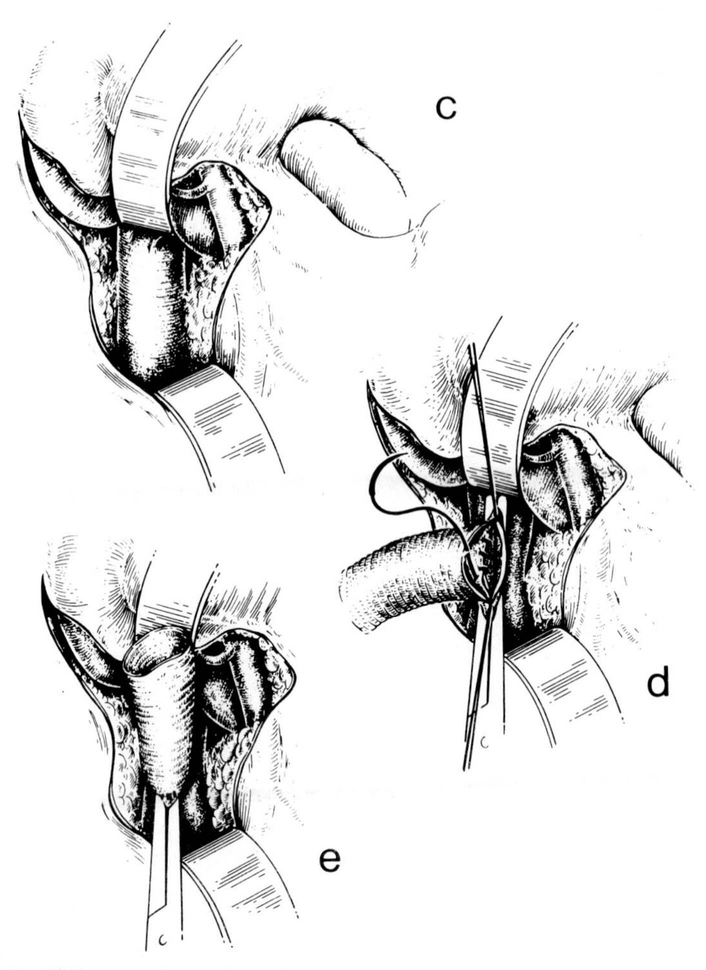

FIG. 3. (c) The posterior peritoneal incision is widened, the duodenum is freed and elevated to expose the inferior vena cava. (d) An 18 or 20 mm woven Dacron tube is sutured to the inferior vena cava with a continuous 4-0 Tevdek suture, interrupted at the superior and inferior pole of the anastomosis. (e) The Dacron tube is then anastomosed to the superior mesenteric vein which lies anterior and medial to the cava.

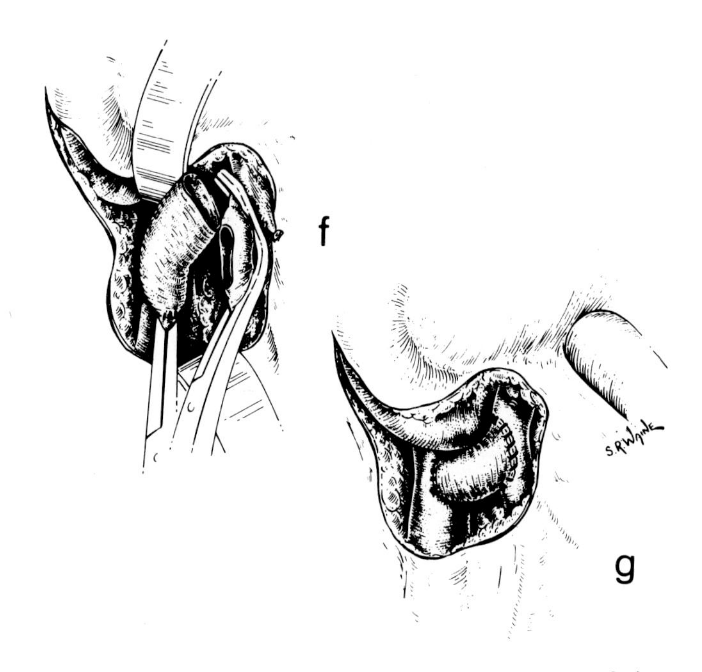

FIG. 4. (f) The 4-6 cm graft is anastomosed to the long axis of the superior mesenteric vein usually with 5-0 Tevdek. (g) The graft, with the duodenum freed and elevated, extends from the normally retroduodenal inferior vena cava to the superior mesenteric vein above the confluence with the iliocolic vein, anterior to the duodenum.

others represented the category of jaundice, ascitic, comatose, cirrhotic that are not salvaged by us. However, three did leave the hospital following the shunting procedure. One succumbed 18 months later from a cerebral vascular accident with a patent shunt; the others continue.

From 1970 to the present we did 17 more cases with 13 patients leaving the hospital. One of the latter, a 72-year-old man, died 13 months later after hemorrhaging from a duodenal ulcer. Two patients who appeared to be candidates for liver transplants succumbed from liver failure after the shunting procedure. One patient died in the postoperative period from massive hemolysis after a blood transfusion and one died as a result of technical errors at surgery.

Discussion

In the recent literature Lord [5], Read [6] as well as our own group [7-9] have commented on the clinical use of this type of shunt. The

17 PATIENTS HAD

68 BLEEDING EPISODES

No. of Episodes	1	2-3	4-5	6-10	17
No. of Patients	1	9	4	2	1

FIG. 5. The incidence of bleeding in the last 17 patients undergoing "H" shunt portal decompression for variceal bleeding.

fall in portal pressure, shunt patency and freedom from subsequent variceal bleeding appear to support its continued use. There is little evidence that there is a significant "metabolic" advantage over other shunts. While it does avoid the caval division of the "J" mesocaval shunt and the edema problem in the lower extremities, its greatest advantages are technical ease and rapidity of accomplishment. Most recently, Drapanas [10] has discovered the technic and reported an enviable record of its successful use.

In an attempt to decrease the magnitude of the portosystemic shunt, we now tend to use a somewhat longer (6-8 cm) 18 mm Dacron tube in the older patients. Hopefully, the greater resistance of the longer, narrow conduit will reduce the sequelae of the shunting procedure by decreasing portal diversion.

Because of our relative disenchantment with shunting procedures we have noted a tendency to operate upon our patients later than we did previously. In the later group of 17 patients we have had 68 episodes of bleeding (Fig. 5). While these patients were not matched or statistically related to another group, our previous policy was to operate after the first massive variceal hemorrhage. Though there has been an emphasis on selective shunting [11], we have not yet seen apparent advantages in our small group of so treated patients.

For the occasional "shunt-surgeon" we believe the simplicity of the "H" graft has much to offer.

Summary

The technic of the "H" superior mesenteric to inferior vena cava shunt is described. Early attitudes on 27 experiences are reported.

References

1. Marion, P.: Les obstructions portales. Sem. Hop. Paris, 29:2781, 1953.
2. Clatworthy, H. W., Wall, T. and Watman, R. W.: A new type of portal-to-systemic venous shunt for portal hypertension. Arch. Surg., 71:588, 1955.
3. Gliedman, M. L. and Margulies, M.: The side-to-end superior mesenteric vein-inferior vena cava shunt for portal decompression. Surgery, 56:473, 1964.
4. Gliedman, M. L.: The technique of the side-to-end superior mesenteric vein to inferior vena cava shunt for portal hypertension. Surg. Gynec. Obstet., 121:1101, 1965.
5. Lord, J. W., Jr., Rossi, G., Daliana, M. et al: Mesocaval shunt modified by the use of a teflon prosthesis. Surg. Gynec. Obstet., 130, 1970.
6. Read, R. C., Thompson, B. W., Wise, W. S. et al: Mesocaval H venous homografts. Arch. Surg., 101:785, 1970.
7. Gliedman, M. L.: Discussion of Read, R. C., Thompson, B. W., Wise, W. S. et al: Mesocaval H venous homografts. Arch. Surg., 101:785, 1970.
8. Gliedman, M. L. and Margulies, M.: The mesocaval shunt for portal decompression. In Haimovici, H. (ed.): The Surgical Management of Vascular Diseases. Philadelphia: J. P. Lippincott Co., 1970.
9. Gliedman, M. L.: The mesocaval shunt for portal hypertension. Amer. J. Gastroent., 56:323, 1971.
10. Drapanas, T.: Interposition mesocaval shunt for treatment of portal hypertension. Ann. Surg., 176:435, 1972.
11. Warren, W. D., Zeppa, R., Fomon, J. J.: Selective transplenic decompression of gastroesophageal varices by distal splenorenal shunt. Ann. Surg., 166:437, 1967.

Portacaval and Splenorenal Shunts

Frank G. Moody, M.D.

It is a pleasure for me to defend the "little guy" who by chance treats patients with portal hypertension; by that I mean the individual who is doing five or less portal decompressive operations per year. Those who do five or less shunts a year may represent the majority of surgeons who do shunt surgery. Therefore, we must provide a good operation that is standardized and has predictable results. I would like to consider several operations for portal hypertension which fit these criteria.

Over the past decade, we have had to defend the use of the portacaval shunt against medical therapy. It has taken much effort to establish the fact that such a shunt is efficacious. That esophageal bleeding can be reduced to almost nil by a portacaval shunt has been known for a long time. But we have been constantly plagued by the problem of whether, in fact, the procedure increases survival time of these patients.

I currently perform an end-to-side anastomosis between the splanchnic end of the divided portal vein and the inferior vena cava in the majority of patients who have bled from esophageal varices. On occasion, in the type of patient that Dr. Warren has described, who has demonstrable outflow block (usually, this is the patient who has ascites which is difficult to manage), I do the anastomosis in side-to-side fashion. I see no value in placing a prosthesis between the inferior vena cava and the superior mesenteric vein or the portal vein. A unique operation described by Dr. Warren and his colleagues offers a very attractive alternative to a portacaval shunt [1]. He describes how blood can be selectively drained away from esophageal varices and maintain flow through the mesenteric-portal systems.

At this point in time, I feel that Dr. Warren's argument is much more persuasive than his results. We have to take what Dr. Warren says and what I say against the background of what happens to the alcoholic cirrhotic as he filters down through this hopper offered by the Michigan group [2].

Frank G. Moody, M.D., Professor and Chairman, Department of Surgery, University of Utah School of Medicine, Salt Lake City.

We have 100 patients with cirrhosis. Half of them develop varices. One third or more of them bleed from the varices and come to our attention. About two thirds of the patients survive their bleeds and become candidates for shunt. Then, depending upon the philosophy of your institution and yourself, some of them are shunted. We end up at the bottom no matter what we do, with 10 patients out of 100 that began with cirrhosis. There are those who believe that if a shunt is done prior to the time a patient bleeds, survival will be increased by salvage of patients who would die on their first or subsequent bleeds, the so-called prophylactic shunt. Randomized trials have conclusively shown that prophylactic portacaval shunts do not prolong survival [3]. You merely change the way the patient dies. He now succumbs to progressive hepatic failure or infection, but not of variceal hemorrhage.

The Veterans Administration randomized control trial of the therapeutic shunt (a shunt done after the patient has one or more bleeds from esophageal varices) has been carried on for a long enough period of time to show that the shunted patient appears to have a small advantage over the nonshunted patient [4]. There are two other randomized control trials that show the same thing. None of these studies have reached a level of statistical significance as of one year ago. The three studies together, however, do establish statistical significance. I am convinced that the portacaval shunt does provide the patient who has bled from varices a small edge over his medically-treated counterpart.

Dr. Child [5] has emphasized the potential role of liver function tests in identifying the degree of hepatic compromise in cirrhosis. Unfortunately, they are not quantitative. There are patients with very advanced cirrhosis who have relatively normal liver function, at least as measured by usual parameters such as bilirubin, alkaline phosphatase, albumin or transaminase. Dr. Child has popularized the use of serum albumin and bilirubin levels, as well as ascites, wasting and encephalopathy, as being parameters that categorize the patient in terms of risk of operation. Figure 1 shows the results of the Michigan group, in terms of mortality, with the patient who has almost normal liver function versus the patient who has severely compromised hepatic function. You will note that mortality significantly increases with worsening hepatic function. An interesting thing is that the survival curve, seen by the slope of this line as a function of time, appears to be the same in the three groups. In other words, the use of hepatic function tests predict early survival but apparently do not predict the long-term outcome for these patients. I think that most people would agree with that statement.

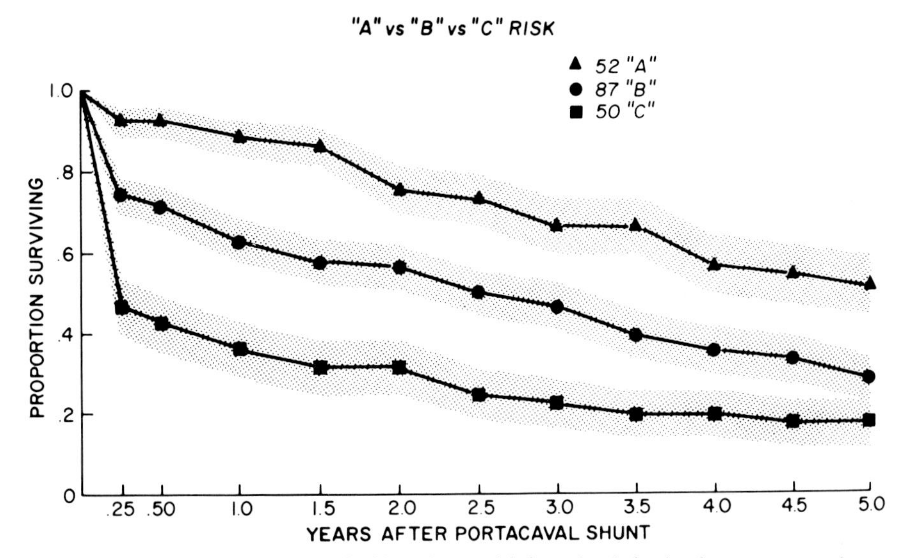

FIG. 1. Cumulative survival of 189 patients with hepatic cirrhosis after a portacaval shunt. The portacaval shunts were performed consecutively between 1959 and 1972. Risk refers to Child's criteria to estimate hepatic reserve. The shaded areas represent one standard error of the proportion surviving at each interval. (From Turcotte [2].)

The measurement of portal pressure at the time of surgery has become a popular way to try to identify patients who might gain benefit from a shunt [6]. I have not found such a measurement useful in helping to determine what operation to perform in the usual case of portal hypertension. I have tried to use pressures to identify the patient who, indeed, does have the portal vein as an outflow tract, but have not been successful even in this regard. The idea is that one can get an indication of perfusion by measuring pressures on either side of the cross-clamped portal vein. But one is doing this under anesthesia, in an operative situation, and I would seriously question whether these are very reliable measurements upon which to make judgments. I was pleased to hear Dr. Warren state, rather emphatically, that we cannot quantitate liver blood flow at this point in time. Dr. Warren, in 1963 [7], was certainly on the right track. He put a great deal of effort into the measurement of hepatic blood flow, but now has come to recognize that these tests are just beyond our technical expertise. So I shall not say anything further about blood flow.

The old saw as to whether one should do an end-to-side or a side-to-side shunt was played for about ten years. The Michigan group has kept it alive by their observation that patients who have side-to-side

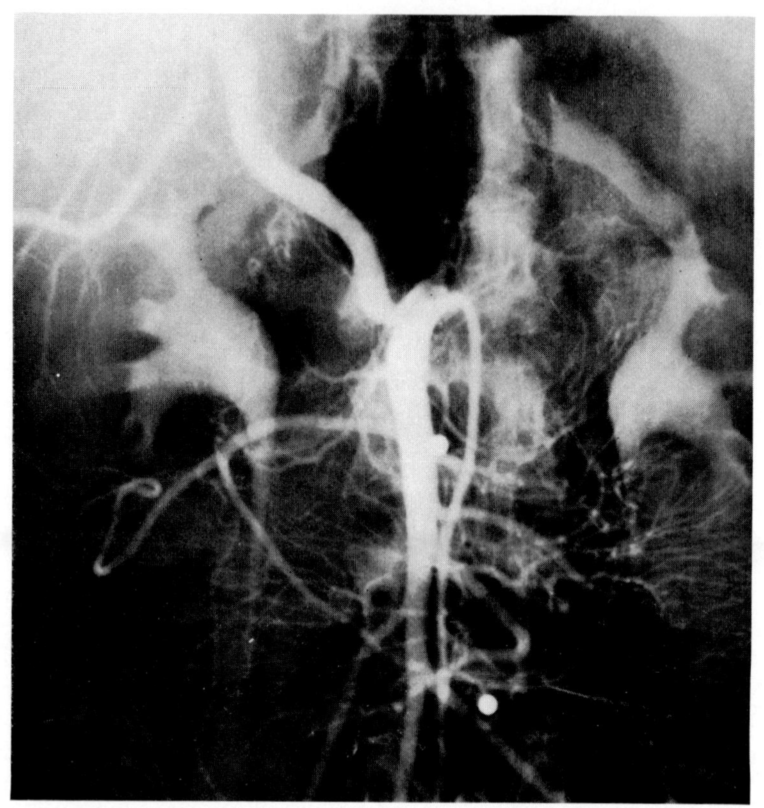

FIG. 2. Superior mesenteric arteriogram demonstrating a right dominant hepatic artery in a patient being prepared for portacaval shunt.

shunts, with advanced liver disease, appear to have a slight edge over the patient who has an end-to-side shunt [2]. I tend to agree with Dr. Mikkelsen and his group [8] as shown in their randomized prospective study, looking at all comers, not putting them into groups, that the end-to-side and side-to-side shunts appear to give about the same survival rate.

I prefer to use arteriographic as well as splenophotographic assessment of shunt candidates. Figure 2 demonstrates the value of mesenteric arteriography, where a dominant right hepatic artery is seen to arise from the superior mesenteric artery. It is very important to recognize this variation prior to performing a portacaval shunt. Once identified, the artery can be mobilized to give access to the portal vein. Splenoportograms are also quite helpful in terms of looking at the anatomy of the portal system. I have yet to encounter a case in which we weren't able to visualize the portal vein when it was patent. But, certainly, in patients who have huge collaterals with the coronary azygous systems siphoning blood away, visualization of the main portal system may be suboptimal. Poor visualization of the portal vein by splenoportography offers three possibilities: (1) occlusion, (2) dilution or (3) retrograde flow.

Dr. Aldrete and I embarked upon a series of portasystemic shunts about seven years ago [9]. To date, 50 have had portacaval and 10 splenorenal anastomoses (personal communication – Aldrete). Our indications for splenorenal shunt included the presence of a large splenic vein, a large spleen and hypersplenism in patients with mild bleeds. We felt patients with profound depression in the formed elements of the blood might indeed benefit from a prophylactic shunt. Seven patients underwent portacaval shunt for bleeding varices secondary to postnecrotic cirrhosis. These patients as a group were older than the alcoholic cirrhotics, the oldest being 65. Age did not appear to influence the operative mortality, or the morbidity of encephalopathy.

The majority of patients in our series are alcoholic cirrhotics. They had all bled, so their operation would be termed an elective shunt. Thirty-one had ascites at some point in their hospital course. Our approach was to make every effort to improve the patient's nutritional status, utilizing two or three months if necessary. This has the inherent risk that they might start to drink and rebleed. But, by and large, most of these patients, if you maintain a good relationship and close follow-up, will be motivated toward being prepared for operation. But even with this conservative approach, most only attained a Child's Class B state, reflecting a moderate depression in hepatic function. We had to operate on five because we could not remove the Sengstaken tube without recurrent hemorrhage. Five others were weaned from tube tamponade but rebled in the hospital, so we operated on a semi-urgent basis; 40 underwent elective portacaval shunts. There were six operative deaths, four of those occurring in the emergency or semi-emergency group. Therefore, we had two deaths in the 40 elective portacaval shunts, which yields a mortality of 5% in that population. Twelve patients died within the next three years from progressive hepatic failure; three patients died from causes not related to liver disease. We have not pursued life survival analysis since the numbers are too few. But, 11 patients are alive for more than three years. Encephalopathy has not been a problem in this group. Only one patient in this series has required hospitalization for encephalopathy on a single occasion during a six year follow-up and continues to survive. Twelve patients who died of

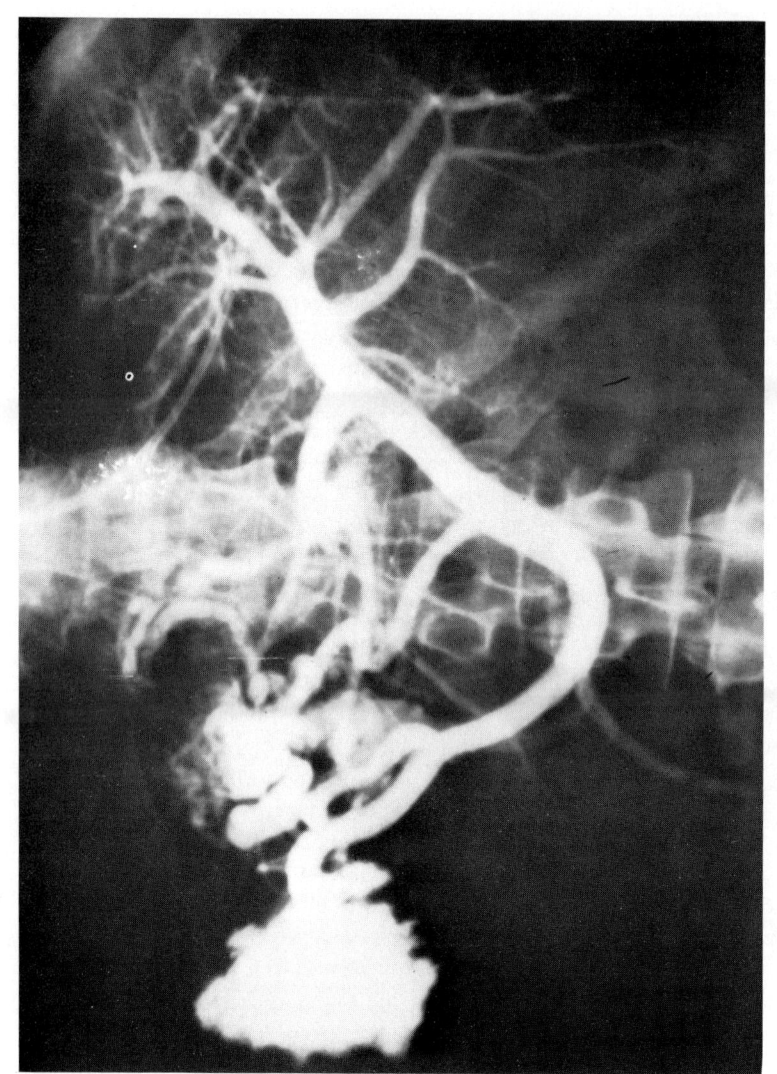

FIG. 3. Splenoportogram in a patient with cirrhosis and esophageal varices. This study was performed on the morning prior to portacaval shunt.

progressive hepatic failure had encephalopathy when they came back into the hospital; possibly we are weeding out patients who would have gone on to develop chronic episodes of encephalopathy. We have three other patients who have had mild episodes of encephalopathy who are easily controlled with diet. For some reason or other, encephalopathy does not seem to be a problem in the South. I would remind you that these patients were done in Birmingham, Alabama, which is not very far from Atlanta. Dr. Drapanas in New Orleans has also had a very low incidence of encephalopathy in a large number of patients who received a side-to-side shunt. There are other parts of the country where encephalopathy is not a major problem. For example, it is a rare complication in Salt Lake City. Encephalopathy postshunt seems to have a geographic type of distribution. Perhaps Dr. Warren could tell us about the incidence of encephalopathy in Miami and Atlanta which, of course, are becoming Yankee towns.

In closing, I would like to again consider how we should proceed as the Warren shunt sweeps the country and becomes the "in" thing. Even with this innovative approach, we are going to have a large number of patients who are not going to survive for a very long time because of the advanced nature of their liver disease. The question as to whether the Warren shunt offers an improved survival over conventional shunts has not as yet been answered. Dr. Zeppa has reported that in the Miami selective shunt series, there does not appear to be an increased survival over that reported for portacaval shunts (personal communication). So it appears that we are not doing much better in this regard, but there is no doubt that encephalopathy is reduced by a reversed splenorenal shunt.

We have attempted to approach this general problem by studying hepatic functional mass in the cirrhotic before and after portal decompression. Indocyanine green has been used for this purpose, since it is removed from the bloodstream exclusively by the liver. It, therefore, represents an ideal molecule for the study of hepatic function since its rate of disappearance from the bloodstream reflects its rate of uptake by the liver. We found that the maximal uptake of ICG correlates with the dry weight of rat liver following two-thirds hepatectomy and during subsequent regeneration [10]. Functional hepatic mass can also be assessed in this way in dog [11] and man [12]. We have found ICG to be a safe substance to use in human beings. The test consists of studying the removal rate of three different doses of ICG (0.5, 1.0 and 5.0 mg/kg). The disappearance curves are plotted employing classical enzyme kinetics. Alcoholic cirrhotics show a tenfold decrease in the maximum removal rate of the dye. We believe that this population of patients have a tenfold decrease in functioning hepatocytes and more specifically a marked decrease in protein-receptor-mass on the sinusoidal side of the hepatocytes. If this is true, then the alcoholic cirrhotic has a fantastic compromise of his functional hepatic mass. Therefore, it is no wonder that their survival is decreased following portal decompression.

We have also studied patients with noncirrhotic liver disease and they are not too different from controls. The biliary cirrhotics fall somewhere in between controls and alcoholic cirrhotics. An interesting thing is that a portacaval shunt does not appear to affect this parameter. We have done it serially in eight patients, before portacaval shunt, at three weeks and three months following the shunt. Other patients have been studied anywhere from three months to five years postoperatively. We haven't studied enough patients to predict which are going to do poorly after portacaval shunt; we believe that with further work and refinement of this technique, we might identify a number that will tell us which patient will or won't survive portacaval shunt.

Does portal decompression prevent variceal bleeding? Absolutely, yes. Do prophylactic portacaval shunts prolong survival? No. Maybe the Warren shunt, done prophylactically, will be efficacious in this regard. Will a therapeutic shunt prolong survival? Probably. What factors will predict operative mortality? The Child's Classification and modifications of it? Certainly, if you use the Child's Classification retrospectively, it does; the patients with advanced liver disease seem to have the highest mortality. What about predicting long-term survival? Which shunt is preferable? I don't think I have to comment on this, since I shall not have the last word.

References

1. Warren, W. D., Zeppa, R. and Fomon, J. T.: Selective trans-splenic decompression of gastroesophageal varices by distal splenorenal shunt. Ann. Surg., 166:437, 1967.
2. Turcotte, J. G.: Portal hypertension as I see it. Portal Hypertension, Major Problems in Clinical Surgery XIV, Philadelphia:W. B. Saunders, 1974.
3. Callow, A. D., Resnick, R. H., Chalmers, T. C. et al: Conclusions from a controlled trial of the prophylactic portacaval shunt. Surgery, 67:97, 1970.
4. Jackson, F. C., Perrin, E. B., Felix, W. R. et al: A clinical investigation of the portacaval shunt. V. Survival analysis of the therapeutic operation. Ann. Surg., 174:672, 1971.
5. Child, C. G. and Turcotte, J. G.: Surgery and portal hypertension. The Liver and Portal Hypertension, Major Problems in Clinical Surgery I, 1964.

6. McDermott, W. V. Jr.: Evaluation of the hemodynamics of portal hypertension in the selection of patients for shunt surgery. Ann. Surg., 176:449, 1972.
7. Warren, W. D., Restreppo, J. E., Respess, J. E. et al: The importance of hemodynamic studies in the management of portal hypertension. Ann. Surg., 158:387, 1963.
8. Reynolds, T. B., Hudson, N. M., Mikkelsen, W. P. et al: Clinical comparison of end-to-side and side-to-side portacaval shunt. New Eng. J. Med., 274:706, 1966.
9. Moody, F. G. and Aldrete, J. S.: Current status of surgically created portasystemic shunts in the management of portal hypertension. Amer. Surgeon, 37:605, 1971.
10. Rikkers, L. F. and Moody, F. G.: Estimation of hepatic mass in rat liver. Gastroenterology, 67:691, 1974.
11. Rikkers, L. F. and Moody, F. G.: Estimation of functional reserve of normal and regenerating dog livers. Surgery, 75:421,1974.
12. Moody, F. G., Rikkers, L. F. and Aldrete, J. S.: Estimation of the functional reserve of human liver. Ann. Surg., 180:592, 1974.

Emergency Shunts for Patients With Esophageal Bleeding and Portal Hypertension

Seymour I. Schwartz, M.D.

Consideration of the applicability of emergency portal decompressive operations for bleeding esophagogastric varices evolves around three simple questions: (1) Is an operation indicated? (2) Is there need for selectivity? (3) What operation should be performed? I shall confine my comments to the problem of the cirrhotic patient with bleeding varices and dispense with the patient whose varices are secondary to portal vein thrombosis and who has no associated hepatic dysfunction. The axiom in reference to these latter patients is that emergency surgery is rarely required. In fact, they are generally best managed by bed rest and transfusion and rarely require either balloon tamponade or vasopressin. We prefer to wait for elective surgery until the patients are older and have larger vessels for shunts; however, if repeated bleeding episodes necessitate an elective shunting procedure, then obviously a choice is made between a mesocaval and a splenorenal shunt.

In presenting data regarding the applicability of emergency portal decompression in the cirrhotic bleeding patient, it is hardly necessary for me to indicate that at present there is no randomized series which will satisfy either the scientist or the sceptic. Evaluation of the problem is clouded by a definition of the term "emergency shunt." Some have considered this as a shunt performed while the patient was still actively bleeding, while others have included in this nomenclature procedures performed on patients either during the bleeding episode or shortly after the bleeding episode has subsided, either spontaneously or having been controlled with tamponade or vasopressin. Although we have considered emergency shunts only as procedures performed while the patient was

Seymour I. Schwartz, M.D., Department of Surgery, University of Rochester School of Medicine, N. Y.

actively and massively bleeding, perhaps the more inclusive definition is appropriate since control of bleeding can be effected in a temporary fashion in a great majority of patients.

The base figure which serves as a frame of reference and comparison is the mortality for patients with bleeding varices not subjected to emergency portacaval shunts. As pointed out by Conn, a mortality rate of approximately 66% is generally to be expected from a variceal hemorrhage. Orloff's compilation from many sources indicated that 73% of cirrhotics died during hospitalization for a first hemorrhage from esophageal varices. In the nonoperated group, death is generally related to continuance of bleeding. There is little question that an effective portal-systemic decompressive procedure almost always interrupts bleeding, and therefore evaluation of the shunts centers around the comparison of mortality. Review of reported experiences indicates that the so-called emergency shunts are associated with survival for immediate hospitalization in 50% to 71% (Fig. 1) of the cases. This figure pertains despite a more liberal attitude toward acceptability of patients in reference to their liver profile.

To indicate the experience in the past ten years, we have reviewed the literature and would like to present the only reported series. In 1964, Peskin reported that three of their 13 patients, subjected to emergency portacaval shunts, died within 30 days for an operative mortality of 23%, or as the surgeon would perhaps prefer to put it, for a survival of 77%. In every instance, the hematemesis had been severe, with a fall in arterial blood pressure and a significant lowering of the hematocrit. In this article

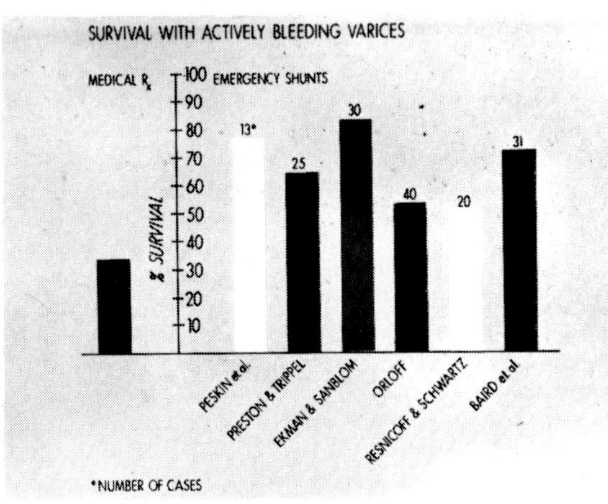

FIGURE 1.

the authors reviewed the previously reported results of emergency portacaval shunts in cirrhotic patients with bleeding varices. The operative mortalities range from 20% to 46%.

In 1965, Preston and Trippel reported on 25 alcoholics, 36% of whom had ascites, 24% had preoperative coma and 32% had jaundice. The survival rate in this group was 64%. Interestingly, in six of the nine patients who died, the shunts apparently did not control the hemorrhage. In the 15 survivors, ten were alive 3 to 40 months, with an average of 20 months at the time of their report. In 1964, Ekman and Sandblom in Sweden reported an 83% survival in 30 patients shunted because of continued bleeding and at the time of their report, 54% were still alive.

In 1967, Orloff compared three groups of cirrhotic patients with massive bleeding. Forty were subjected to an emergency shunt with a 30 day survival of 53% and a four year survival of 43%. The patients subjected to emergency transesophageal ligation had a 30 day survival of 57%, quite comparable. But this dropped off rapidly and the four year survival was 22%. In the medical group, the three year survival was 18% with the four year survival of 3%.

In 1968, we reported our own experience with 20 emergency shunts performed over a two year period. As mentioned earlier, the term emergency was applied only to those patients in whom active and massive bleeding was continuing at the time the patient was taken to the operating room. The overall survival was 50%.

There were 15 Laennec cirrhotics, and nine of these died within 30 days of surgery, while there were five non-Laennec cirrhotics, four of whom survived. We compared our experience with emergency shunts during the same period for patients in whom an elective shunt was performed with an operative mortality rate of 5%. In our experience with emergency shunts, the 30 day mortality was related to thrombosis of the shunt in two cases, infection in six cases and the presence of florid cirrhosis in two. Our experience agrees totally with the report of Ekman and Sandblom which demonstrates reduced mortality for patients operated on two to seven days after the hemorrhage had ceased, as compared with the mortality for procedures carried out while the patients continued to bleed. Included in our group of elective shunts are those patients in whom the bleeding was controlled by vasopressin who were taken to the operating room perhaps 24 hours after their hemorrhage.

The final and most encouraging report appeared in 1971 when Baird and his associates in Canada reported on 31 consecutive patients operated on within 48 hours of massive bleeding episode including 18 nutritional and 13 postnecrotic cirrhotics with a hospital survival rate of 71%. In the follow-up of these patients, there were no recurrent hemorrhages and only two late deaths from hepatic failure.

In an article which appeared just two months ago, a prospective evaluation of emergency portacaval shunts, conducted over a ten year period in 115 unselective consecutive patients with alcoholic cirrhosis and bleeding varices, was reported by Orloff and his associates. Surgery was generally performed within eight hours of admission. The operative survival rate was 48% with an actual seven year survival rate of 42.5%. Thus the data seem to indicate at least an improvement in immediate survival figures for patients subjected to shunts as compared to those treated nonoperatively. In addition, shunted patients almost always stop bleeding while the nonshunted patients frequently continue to bleed and exhaust blood banks and the time of hospital personnel, therefore crediting the shunting procedure with improving the logistics of medical care. These two factors, improved survival and improved logistics, lead us to answer the nuclear question: yes, portacaval shunts are indicated on an emergency basis for cirrhotic patients.

We come then to the second question regarding patient selection. In our experience with emergency shunts, we did not have the good fortune of managing patients with excellent liver functions, and there is really little statistically significant difference in the so-called Child's B and Child's C category in our series. We have gradually liberalized our indications and presently are willing to shunt patients who are actively bleeding if the serum albumin is greater than 2, the prothrombin time greater than 25% and the bilirubin less than 4. We have adhered to the dictum that the patient in coma who cannot be improved by catharsis should be excluded from consideration for surgery since we have had no salvage in this group. However, this is not a uniform conclusion in the literature.

In Peskin's series, the results could not be correlated with the liver index but one patient with hepatic coma died four days after injury. In the experience of Preston and Trippel, hepatic function was a most important factor in determining postoperative survival. Among six patients in whom the BSP retention was less than 29%, there were no postoperative deaths, while in ten patients with BSP retention in the 30%-39% range, there were two postoperative deaths; of five patients with retention greater than 40%, three died. In their series, among the 14 patients who had a total bilirubin of 4 mg% or less, there were two postoperative deaths while there were five deaths among the group with bilirubin levels greater than 4. Ascites which did not respond to medical management had a poor prognosis and seven of 13 patients shunted on an emergency basis with ascites died. In their series, the survival statistics in patients with preoperative coma were approximately the same as those without coma. Orloff's findings were quite similar. He evaluated factors which might have influenced survival, and he could attribute no significance to the presence or absence of jaundice, to the presence or absence of encephalopathy, or to any individual liver function test. However, ascites, when present, was associated with a survival rate of 24% in contrast to the survival rate of 74% in the nonascitic patient. Thus, there are essentially no valid data to offer guidance in selection of patients although my conversations revealing visceral reactions of surgeons throughout the country lead me to believe that frank coma should preclude serious consideration.

The remaining question is what shunt should be performed. Functionally, portal-systemic shunts can be categorized as either totally or partially diverting portal venous flow away from the liver and also either decompressing or failing to decompress intrahepatic venous hypertension. The end-to-side portacaval shunt prevents blood from reaching the liver by providing complete drainage of the splanchnic venous circulation into the inferior vena cava. The argument that this shunt deprives the liver of an important source of blood has been refuted by some studies. The alteration of hepatic blood flow associated with end-to-side shunt is extremely variable, ranging from an increase of 34% to a decrease of 53%. The end-to-side shunt certainly also prevents the portal vein from serving as an efferent conduit from the liver. However studies have shown that following an end-to-side shunt, the wedge hepatic venous pressure which reflects the hepatosinusoidal pressure declines in most patients. In reference to the point at issue, namely, decompressing the splanchnic venous circulation and therefore the esophageal varices, both the end-to-side and side-to-side shunts will effect equal reduction in portal pressure and equal decreases in hepatic flow, since the simple laws of hydrodynamics apply.

Briefly summarizing the hemodynamic effects, portal pressure reduction should be equivalent with equivalently constructed stomas. The sinusoidal pressure may be reduced equivalently by either an end-to-side or a side-to-side shunt. The afferent portal blood flow and the efferent portal blood flow are obviated by the end-to-side shunt. However, the side-to-side shunt allows little liver blood flow. If blood flow away from the liver occurs, the question as to whether this is salutary or detrimental, ie, is there a siphoning effect away from the liver cell, has not been resolved.

Because of the great confusion and the lack of scientific data regarding the efficacies of the shunting procedure in the patient who is bleeding significantly and is frequently suffering from major hepatic dysfunction, the type of shunt to be selected, in my mind, is based on ease and accessibility. When a readily accessible and shuntable portal vein is present, an end-to-side portacaval shunt is generally performed, since we feel it is the easiest procedure. It is associated with the lowest incidence of thrombosis, and in the presence of a large caudad lobe is frequently the only procedure which can be performed. Interestingly, when Mikkelsen and his associates compared equal numbers of patients subjected to end-to-side and side-to-side shunts, he concluded that the end-to-side shunts were associated with the lowest operative mortality, and in addition, with the lowest incidence of postoperative encephalopathy. If the portal vein is thrombosed, or if the patient has undergone multiple procedures in the right upper quadrant, suggesting a difficult, prolonged procedure, then the H graft with interposition of a Dacron prosthesis between the mesenteric vein and the inferior vena cava can be used.

In summary, in the absence of control randomized trials, it is felt that emergency portacaval anastomosis does offer greater survival potential than more conservative forms of therapy. Interestingly, there is no series in the literature which presents data refuting this concept. In addition, the operative approach provides improvement in the logistical management of patients. One can make a case for liberalization of criteria of patient selection and presently we exclude only patients with significant icterus, ie, a bilirubin greater than 4, frank hepatic coma and tense ascites or active florid cirrhosis. The operation which should be performed is one which the individual surgeon feels that he can carry out with the greatest dispatch in order to effect a permanent reduction of the portal hypertension.

Bibliography

Orloff, M. J.: An appraisal of progress in the treatment of portal hypertension. Arch. Surg., Vol. 108, March 1974.

Resnicoff, S. A. and Schwartz, S. I.: Portal decompressive surgery: Comparative evaluation of patients with Laennec's cirrhosis and other causes. Arch. Surg., 97:371, 1968.

Barker, C. F., Nance, F. C. and Peskin, G. W.: Regional hypothermia for massive bleeding. Surgery, Vol. 56, No. 4, 1964.

Baird, R. J., Tutassaura, H. and Miyagishima, R.: Emergency portal decompression. Arch. Surg., 103:73, 1971.

Mikkelsen, W. P.: Emergency portacaval shunt. Rev. Surg., Vol. 19, No. 3, 1962.

Conn, H. O.: Progress in management of bleeding esophageal varices, hepatic circulation and portal hypertension. Ann. N. Y. Acad. Sci., 170:345, 1970.

The Management of Extrahepatic Portal Venous Obstruction in Children

Stacy A. Roback, M.D. and Arnold S. Leonard, M.D., Ph.D.

Extrahepatic portal venous obstruction in childhood is an uncommon problem, which can challenge the skill of the most experienced surgeon. Although unusual lesions such as intravenous webs, valves, or actual congenital stenoses of the portal vein have been described in the literature, the vast majority of children with extrahepatic portal venous obstruction and resultant varices have thrombosis of the portal vein as the primary cause. This is most often due to omphalitis, often unrecognized, at birth with extension of the thrombotic process originating in the umbilical vein to the portal vein and its major branches. This discussion will be limited to a consideration of this entity and, in particular, the management of the child with bleeding esophageal varices. However, it should not be forgotten that ascites, nutritional deficiency, protein losing enteropathy, diarrhea and secondary hypersplenism constitute important features of the clinical syndrome.

Diagnosis

The child who enters the hospital with upper gastrointestinal bleeding presumed to be due to esophageal varices must be subjected to immediate diagnostic evaluation, lest another cause of bleeding be overlooked. At least 25% of these children will be found to be bleeding from other sites in the upper gastrointestinal tract. We employ diagnostic endoscopy, with an infant endoscope if indicated by the size of the child, as the initial procedure in all patients who enter the University of Minnesota Hospitals with upper gastrointestinal hemorrhage, despite previous documentation of esophageal varices. Often, the cause of bleeding can be ascribed to other lesions or to the ingestion of aspirin for upper respiratory tract infections.

Stacy A. Roback, M.D., Medical Fellow in Surgery and Arnold S. Leonard, M.D., Ph.D., Professor of Surgery, Head, Pediatric Surgery, University of Minnesota Hospitals, Minneapolis.

The direct erosive action of aspirin on the distal esophagus, stomach or duodenum can cause alarming bleeding in the child with or without known varices. Indeed, 80% of our recent cases of bleeding varices in children were preceded by aspirin ingestion for respiratory tract infection, gastroenteritis or other types of common pediatric febrile illnesses. If endoscopy is equivocal or nondiagnostic, upper gastrointestinal x-ray studies are also employed to exclude other causes of bleeding.

If acute bleeding has not been responsible for admission or if conservative therapy has been successful in arresting hemorrhage, it is our belief that these children should undergo limited laparotomy for portal venograms, portal venous pressure measurements and liver biopsy. This surgical procedure is best deferred, if possible, until the child reaches at least 6 or 7 years of age so that a reliable estimate of splenic vein size can be made in anticipation of a possible portal systemic shunt. This procedure also identifies children with an intrahepatic etiology for portal hypertension in whom additional or alternative modes of therapy may be critical. This category includes children with biliary atresia, cystic fibrosis, postnecrotic cirrhosis, viral or toxic hepatitis, as well as those with cirrhosis secondary to alpha 1 antitrypsin deficiency.

Treatment

Essential to the treatment of children with esophageal varices are measures directed at prevention of a bleeding episode. Parents should be instructed in the avoidance of aspirin either orally or rectally for any febrile episodes. A diet free of roughage and spicy foods should be prescribed. The role of antacid therapy in such a patient is not established and at the present time probably is not helpful on a prophylactic basis.

In the acutely bleeding patient, after diagnosis has been established, therapy should be conservative; success in the high percentage of cases can be anticipated. The child is put to bed and sedated. A nasogastric tube is passed, confirmed to be in proper position by x-ray and the stomach is emptied. Hourly antacids are given and fresh whole blood administered as dictated by the rate of bleeding. If bleeding is persistent in spite of these measures, intra-arterial Pitressin is infused via the superior mesenteric artery to decrease portal pressure. We have virtually abandoned the use of the Sengstaken tube in the treatment of children with bleeding esophageal varices unless all other measures fail to stop bleeding. This has occurred only twice in the last seven years at our institution.

Children tolerate bleeding esophageal varices remarkably well and a nonoperative approach in extrahepatic portal vein obstruction is not only quite successful but results in a low mortality rate. At the Columbus

Children's Hospital, 68 patients bleeding from esophageal varices were treated nonoperatively, with a mortality rate of zero [1]. In Dr. Voorhees' series of 129 patients with multiple bleeding episodes, observed over a 30-year period, the mortality was 7% [2]. This pattern is true in our patients as well, suggesting that emergency portosystemic shunts in children are unwarranted and shunting should be planned during non-bleeding intervals in the optimally prepared patient.

Surgical Treatment

In the child with a history of multiple and/or massive bleeding episodes, portosystemic shunting becomes the primary mode of therapy. The type of shunt (splenorenal or mesocaval) to be used is dependent upon the cross-sectional diameter of the mesenteric vein. The diameter must be equal to or greater than 1 cm if adequate decompression is to be achieved and long-term patency expected. This will eliminate occasionally the splenorenal shunt from consideration. If the vein is of adequate caliber, we favor a splenorenal shunt with the anastomosis carried out as close to the junction of the inferior mesenteric vein as is technically possible. This provides a vein of adequate caliber and obviates dissection of the entire splenic vein on the posterior pancreatic surface. In addition, the kidney requires no mobilization and there is no angulation of either vein. Fine suture of 5-0 or 6-0 proline insures a hemostatic anastomosis.

Collective experience indicates that if this procedure is performed in a technically satisfactory manner, rebleeding is almost always attributable to inadequate size of the splenic vein.

Summary

Extrahepatic portal venous obstruction in children demands precise early diagnosis and reconfirmation with each bleeding episode. Non-operative therapy for the acute hemorrhagic episode will yield high success and low mortality. Portosystemic shunts are successful in a large majority of children if the vein used is of adequate caliber.

References

1. Voorhees, A. B., Jr. and Price, J. B.: Extrahepatic portal hypertension. Arch. Surg., 108:338-341, 1974.
2. Boles, E. T., Jr.: Centrally placed splenorenal shunt. Reprinted from Cooper (ed.): The Craft of Surgery. Boston:Little, Brown and Company, Inc., 1964. Also personal communication from Dr. Boles to Dr. Leonard on April 25, 1974.

Complications of Portacaval Shunts

Seymour I. Schwartz, M.D.

The successful management of patients undergoing portal decompressive procedures definitely necessitates an appreciation and anticipation of the many complications which may ensue. The fact that recently there has been an introduction of several new procedures, ostensibly to reduce the incidence of complication, is evidence that at present the perfect solution is not in hand.

The complications uniquely associated with portal systemic shunting procedures may be divided into those which are encountered intraoperatively and those which are postoperative. The intraoperative complications include bleeding and a non-shuntable situation, while the postoperative complications include rebleeding, hepatic failure, changes in the cardiorespiratory dynamics, and the so-called hepatorenal syndrome. Late postoperative complications include hemosiderosis, peptic ulceration and encephalopathy.

Diffuse bleeding during the operative procedure may be related to technical factors, coagulation defects which frequently accompany cirrhosis, or a combination of the two. We have found that the most important preoperative assessment is a platelet count. It is generally felt that below the level of 70,000/cu mm, one is in a critical situation. This can be corrected by administering 20 frozen platelet packs and then repeating the platelet count to determine the effect. If there is little change, then removal of the spleen, which acts as a platelet sequestering or destructive organ, may be required. Following splenectomy, additional platelet packs may then be effective. Deficiency in specific coagulation factors, usually prothrombin, can be corrected by administering the deficient factors, generally with fresh frozen plasma. In this regard fresh blood is generally preferable to banked blood for the cirrhotic patient, since it does contain platelets and coagulation factors and does not have the increased ammonia levels noted in banked blood. Ammonia increases

---

Seymour I. Schwartz, M.D., Department of Surgery, University of Rochester School of Medicine, N. Y.

from a baseline of 5μg to 580μg during 21 days of storage. Although some have reported that a large portion of surgical patients with cirrhosis have increased fibrinolytic activity, which could be reversed with epsilon aminocaproic acid, we have been hesitant to use this drug because of its potential for causing diffuse clotting and embolization.

Mechanical control of the bleeding site is most important. The recent addition to the armamentarium of continued infusion of vasopressin, which has been initiated preoperatively and continued during the operation, has reduced the amount of bleeding from the veins of Retzius. The other approach to this significant ooze is performance of the shunting procedure with relative dispatch, since once the pressure within the portal system is reduced, bleeding stops most dramatically.

The second intraoperative complication occurs when the surgeon encounters an anatomic or pathologic situation which precludes the creation of a portal systemic shunt. The most common circumstance is the patient with cavernomatous transformation of the portal vein, in whom the process extends to involve the superior mesenteric and splenic veins. We have seen three such patients during the last year and a half. A so-called make-shift shunt, using large collaterals, is doomed to failure. The operative approach to this problem is the immediate employment of an esophagogastrectomy with interposition. All of our patients in this category have done well with this procedure. The immediate bleeding has ceased, and there has been no rebleeding during a short period of follow-up.

Perhaps the most unusual difficulty is caval hypertension, generally caused by hypertrophy or nodularity of the caudate lobe, but occasionally due to extensive thrombosis of the suprahepatic inferior vena cava. In the usual circumstance of the Budd-Chiari syndrome, there is no hypertension in the inferior vena cava, since the process is confined to the hepatic veins. However, if the process does extend to the cava, hypertension may occur. In the Japanese, the extraordinarily rare situation of web formation in the suprahepatic inferior vena cava has been described and may account for this syndrome. An inferior vena cavagram reveals membraneous obstruction of the vena cava, readily corrected by rupture of the membrane with a transcardiac approach.

When hypertension is related to encroachment by a caudate lobe, partial resection of this lobe may reduce pressure within the cava, but usually this is not the case. The situation may preclude a conventional portal decompressive procedure. Fonkalsrud successfully decompressed the portal system in such a circumstance by anastomosing the splenic vein to the isolated left pulmonary artery but the patient eventually died of a massive bleed eight years after the procedure. We have recently been confronted with such a situation in a child with cystic fibrosis and bleeding varices, in whom the portal pressure was 510 mm of saline, and the caval pressure was an elevated 330 mm of saline. Despite the caval hypertension, since a gradient existed, we elected to perform a portacaval shunt. The bleeding stopped, and the patient has done well during the short period of follow-up.

This then brings us to a consideration of the early postoperative complications. In the patient who continues to bleed from varices following an operation, or who rebleeds having ceased bleeding prior to the procedure, a differential diagnosis must be established between thrombosis of the shunt, and acute gastric erosions, or peptic ulceration. In the great majority of cases, rebleeding is due to thrombosis of the shunt. In order to avoid this situation, we have routinely, subsequent to the establishment of the usual end-to-side portacaval shunt, measured pressures with a simple spinal manometer in the vein and in the cava, and insist on the absence of a significant gradient. If a significant gradient does exist, the anterior aspect of the shunt is taken down. On such occasions, a clot has been noted at the suture line. In a relatively large personal experience, in which an insignificant gradient was demonstrated at the end of the procedure, we have had no instance of rebleeding from varices related to shunt thrombosis. It is to be emphasized that duodenal ulcers infrequently cause bleeding in the early postoperative phase, and when peptic ulcer is indicted, it is usually the stress variety. The only way of establishing the site of bleeding is by esophagogastroscopy. In our hands, the yield of angiographic studies to determine the bleeding site in these patients has been extremely poor.

In the patient with recurrent bleeding, and also in the patient with rapidly progressive ascites, attempts should be made to determine whether the shunt is patent or has become occluded. Intrasplenic pulp manometry provides a reliable estimate of portal hypertension. We have employed isotopic evaluation of circulation and splenoportography in this regard. Injection of 0.5 ml of radioactive material directly into the spleen, and counting simultaneously over the liver and esophagus, shows a classic tracing with a patent portacaval shunt. A splenoportogram will show a patent portacaval shunt and, more important, the absence of collaterals, as an index of adequate decompression of the portal system. If the shunt is shown to be occluded, one can re-explore the patient within several days, perform a thrombectomy and reestablish the shunt. We have done such a procedure 2½ days following the initial operation with success. Or one can perform a second decompressive procedure such as a mesocaval or splenorenal, if a portacaval shunt had been the initial operation. If the shunt is found to be patent, then therapy is directed at stress ulceration.

The appearance or persistence of ascites following a portacaval shunt is due to either insufficient reduction of hepatic sinusoidal pressure or the impairment of hepatocellular function. The formation or accentuation of ascites has been thought to be related to the type of shunting procedure, but several authors could find no correlation between the procedure and, in fact, no correlation between the intrahepatic venous pressure and the development of ascites. It has also been noted that the end-to-side shunt may significantly reduce hepatic sinusoidal pressure. The management of patients is based on a regimen of low sodium intake, accompanied by fluid restriction; potassium supplements are given; albumin is generally not required; and a variety of diuretic agents can be used. Repeated abdominal paracenteses are to be condemned.

Hepatic function may deteriorate after shunting procedures, and the incidence of hepatic failure is significantly higher in patients with advanced impairment of hepatic function prior to surgery. When coma occurs in the early postoperative period, a mortality rate of over 66% can be anticipated. If the coma is associated with continued postoperative variceal bleeding, the mortality rate is well over 90%. The various treatments for fulminant hepatic failure are generally not applicable to patients with hepatic failure following shunting procedures, since the yield approaches zero.

In reference to the alterations in cardiorespiratory dynamics and the hepatorenal syndrome, the shunting of a patient with normodynamic circulation may place him in a hyperdynamic situation with an increased cardiac output, an increased venous return and a fall of peripheral resistance. In general, the shunt will not improve the patient's systemic circulatory status and, in fact, increases the risk of eventual high output heart failure. Renal failure, following a portal systemic decompressive procedure, is not predictable, but is quite uncommon in patients without ascites. There is dilutional hyponatremia, which may reverse spontaneously, but the prognosis is related primarily to the degree of the reversibility of the hepatic disease. The treatment directed at renal failure generally consists of supportive measures. Recently the use of essential amino acids and hyperalimentation for chronic renal disease has added another treatment possibility. Although beneficial effects on this syndrome have been reported by administering metaraminol, this is not generally substantiated.

Progressing to the late postoperative complications, considering first, hemosiderosis. This is reported more frequently in the shunted patient. Conn recorded an incidence of hemosiderin accumulation of 27% in shunted patients. This increase in hepatic hemosiderin may be more apparent than real. Dr. Sherlock has indicated that treatment, including chelating agents or phlebotomy, is rarely required, but it should be emphasized that about one half of the cases in one series did develop congestive heart failure and diabetes.

The whole chapter regarding postshunt peptic ulceration has been rewritten. It is now appreciated that the incidence of peptic ulcer in the nonshunted patient is not significantly increased and that the cirrhotic patient is, in fact, a hyposecretor. Although an overall incidence of peptic ulceration of 27% has been reported following portacaval shunts, the overwhelming majority of these are superficial erosions and not true peptic ulcer. In the Veteran's Administration review there was no increase in ulcer incidence in patients subjected to therapeutic shunts.

We come then to perhaps the most significant complication in the long-term management of patients after portal decompressive procedures, the neuropsychiatric manifestations, or the so-called portal systemic encephalopathy. The syndrome is unusual in patients with portal hypertension secondary to obstruction of the portal vein and is rarely seen before the age of 12. The question of whether shunting of blood per se is a critical factor is now open, since recent experience with portacaval shunts in nonhypertensive patients operated on for glycogen storage disease was not associated with any encephalopathy. The incidence of encephalopathy in the cirrhotic has varied markedly. I imagine that this discrepancy is based on the criteria used for establishing the diagnosis. Dr. Sherlock and her associates reported that about 42% of surviving patients developed encephalopathy during the first five years, and more than 72% had neuropsychiatric manifestations after five years. Significant encephalopathy was noted in about 20% of these patients, and a similar percentage was noted in McDermott's series. But only half of McDermott's patients found the symptoms truly incapacitating. In our own experience, somewhat less than 10% have had significant encephalopathy requiring active medical interference. In our own experience, the etiology of cirrhosis did not influence the incidence of encephalopathy, but more severe encephalopathy develops in the older patients and in those who resume drinking.

Supportive therapy is directed at restriction of protein, the use of nonabsorbable antibiotics, and the administration of potassium if hypokalemia is present. The results of lactulose therapy have been encouraging in our hands and in a double-blind study conducted by Conn and his associates. In contrast, the use of L-Dopa has been singularly ineffective. Since the colon is the site of bacterial degradation, and there most of the ammonia is absorbed into the portal circulation, resection of the colon has been carried out in some cases of severe intractable encephalopathy. A matched group of 38 has been studied in randomized fashion. The longevity of the two groups was identical, and the dietary protein tolerance. Encephalopathy control only slightly and not significantly favored the colon bypass group.

The problem of portal systemic encephalopathy has been the major stimulus for the introduction of new approaches to treatment of bleeding varices, which leads to a brief discussion of the relative merits of the various new shunting procedures with reference to the intent, a reduced incidence of encephalopathy. When one compares an end-to-side shunt with a side-to-side shunt, most figures show less encephalopathy is present in those patients shunted in end-to-side fashion. The question raised in performing a side-to-side portacaval shunt is, does the portal vein, acting as an outflow tract from the liver, have a beneficial or harmful effect, a siphoning effect, reducing the blood available to the hepatic cell?

The first of the new shunts to be considered is the "H" graft, introduced years ago by Lord and associates, and popularized recently by Drapanas, in which a conduit is placed between the superior mesenteric vein and the inferior vena cava. This is, in essence, a side-to-side shunt and does not enhance blood flow going to the liver. By the laws of hydrodynamics, one would not expect any flow to course up the mesenteric vein to the portal vein with fluid flowing from high pressure sinusoidal system to the low pressure systemic system. In addition, it was shown many years ago that the classic mesocaval shunt, as described by Clatworthy and Marion, is associated with as high, if not higher, incidence of encephalopathy, when compared to the end-to-side shunt. Therefore, one would not expect a reduction in encephalopathy with "H" graft interposition.

The next procedure is one described initially by Maillard, in France, and championed in our country by Adamson and his associates. It consists of an end-to-side portacaval shunt, coupled with a method of arterializing the liver, either constructing a conduit directly from the aorta or using the gastroduodenal artery to arterialize the end of the portal vein. As the authors indicate, the procedure is not directed at improving liver function, but at delaying or eliminating functional deterioration due to reduction in hepatic blood flow. When a classic end-to-side portacaval shunt is carried out, the hepatic circulation is entirely arterialized; there is a 30% increase in hepatic arterial flow; polarographic studies show that the oxygen tension of the liver increases markedly. If one believes, as several studies have shown, that there is something special in splanchnic venous blood as far as liver regeneration and function is concerned, this operation does not address itself to that problem. There are no data regarding the incidence of encephalopathy which can be considered meaningful in this regard.

The final, so-called new procedure is the one popularized by Dr. Warren. It does have the theoretical advantage that blood will continue to course to the liver, through the portal vein, while supposedly the esophageal varices are decompressed. At present there is a suggestion that this procedure is associated with a reduced incidence of postshunt encephalopathy, with the greatest enthusiasm coming from countries such as Brazil where they have bilharzial disease and the patients have a high incidence of postshunt encephalopathy. This procedure is not generally applied to poorest risk patients and is contraindicated in patients with ascites who certainly fall in the poor risk category. For these reasons, at this time, we feel that the end-to-side portacaval shunt is to be continued as a standard reference by which all new procedures are judged, and we eagerly await the randomized, control studies by Dr. Warren and his group.

It is appropriate to close with a quote from a recent article which appeared in the *Annals of Surgery* by Bismuth and associates who evaluated a variety of portacaval shunts. In their study was a highly laudable postoperative mortality of 1.6% and a five year survival of 66%, with a very low incidence of hemorrhage and encephalopathy. Their concluding sentence is: "Efforts to devise shunting procedures which may appear in theory to be more effective hemodynamically, should not divert attention from these other auxiliary influences."

Bibliography

Bismuth, H., Franco, D. and Hepp, J.: Portal-systemic shunt in hepatic cirrhosis: Does the type of shunt decisively influence the clinical result? Ann. Surg., Vol. 179, No. 2, Feb. 1974.

Schwartz, S. I.: Complications of portal-systemic shunting procedures. *In* Complications in Vascular Surgery. Lippincott, 1973.

Preoperative Assessment and Choice of Operative Procedure for Portal Hypertension

W. Dean Warren, M.D.

A surgeon who does the same operation for every patient with portal hypertension does not perform optimally no matter which operation he chooses. In the preoperative assessment of potential shunt patients, we try to determine the immediate operative risk and we try to establish what operation may be most useful in a particular patient. In recent years we have developed techniques which are beginning to give us a handle on the risk of encephalopathy following a shunt.

The first thing to estimate is the risk to a particular patient of going through an operation. I mean any operation, whether it be nonshunting, distal shunt, or total shunt. What is the risk of a major operative procedure for a particular patient? The evaluation of operative risk depends mainly upon conventional liver function tests.

Table 1 shows Child's classification and Table 2 illustrates McDermott's criteria for defining risk factors. By empiric observation certain aspects of hepatic function have been correlated with the patient's ability to survive a major operative procedure. They are serum albumin, bilirubin and prothrombin time. Another very important evaluative test is the serum transaminase to look for the possibility of acute cell necrosis. Another factor, which should be stressed, is the presence of ascites, particularly if of recent onset. If there is loss of appetite and loss of weight and the clinical evaluation indicates active liver disease, then the patient is a much worse risk than liver function tests suggest. You must evaluate the patient clinically as well as by means of laboratory tests.

We disagree strongly with Orloff [1], who has suggested that every patient should be shunted immediately upon admission following the

---

W. Dean Warren, M.D., Joseph B. Whitehead Professor and Chairman, Department of Surgery, Emory University School of Medicine, Atlanta, Ga.

Table 1. Clinical and Laboratory Classification of Patients With Cirrhosis in Terms of Hepatic Functional Reserve

Group Designation	*"A" Minimal*	*"B" Moderate*	*"C" Advanced*
Serum bilirubin* (mg%)	Below 2.0	2.0-3.0	Over 3.0
Serum albumin (gm%)	Over 3.5	3.0-3.5	Under 3.0
Ascites	None	Easily controlled	Poorly controlled
Neurological disorder	None	Minimal	Advanced, "coma"
Nutrition	Excellent	Good	Poor, "wasting"

*Equivocal in biliary cirrhosis.

occurrence of an esophageal variceal hemorrhage. During the bleeding episode, these patients are usually poor risks and face a high operative mortality. There is not enough time to prepare for an optimal surgical procedure. We believe that the best interests of the patient are served by controlling the bleeding nonoperatively, by careful preoperative study and then by operating at a later date. I will admit that we may be dealing with a different population than Dr. Orloff. Perhaps in his setting, the safest thing is to operate on an emergency basis, but the mortality is tremendously high.

An example to illustrate this point was a lady who came into our hospital in 1971 with a serum albumin of 3.3, which isn't bad, but the bilirubin was markedly elevated. She was a class 4 patient, or Child's classification C. The prothrombin time was acceptable, but she had massive ascites and severely compromised nutrition. Of great importance, in this case, was the liver biopsy. Histologic sections showed this patient to have cirrhosis with active alcoholic hepatitis. Such individuals carry a tremendous operative mortality. In the series done by Mikkelsen [2] at Southern California, patients with this finding on liver biopsy had an

Table 2.

Rating for liver index	0	1	2	3	4
Bromsulphalein % retention	<4	<10	<20	<30	<30
Albumin (gm%)	>3.9	<4.0	<3.5	<3.0	<2.5
Van den Bergh (mg%)	<1.0	<1.5	<3.0	<6.0	>5.9
Alkaline phosphatase (Bodansky units)	<4.0	<6.0	<15	<30	<29
Cephalin flocculation (48 hours)	0	1	2	3	4
Prothrombin time (% of normal)	>80	<80	<60	<40	<20

operative morality of 70%. That is simply too high, unless the bleeding won't stop without operation. The hemorrhage did stop in this particular lady. She returned some months later with a good serum albumin; the bilirubin was down to normal and the ascites had cleared completely. She had gained weight in terms of lean body mass. There was no evidence of cell necrosis on repeat liver biopsy. At this time she was a Class A candidate and was put into our randomized series. She has done extremely well since the shunt procedure. Her chance of survival with an early operation would have been poor.

We now rely heavily upon endoscopy and angiography for establishing varices, but the barium swallow is also still a good method. When a patient with cirrhosis has bled, one of the critical questions is whether the bleeding comes from varices. Frequently, it may be from other sources, such as a Mallory-Weiss tear, ulcer or gastritis. Proof of the presence of varices is extremely important, but only direct endoscopic visualization will prove that the bleeding actually arises from the varices.

Certain physiologic features are important in terms of selecting patients for operation. These factors have become even more important, since we have demonstrated the value of the selective shunt, which is unique in permitting continued portal venous flow to the liver. We want to know the intrahepatic and portal vein pressures not because they, in themselves, are of great help, but because the diagnosis is sometimes not cirrhosis. For example, in a patient with schistosomiasis, the intrahepatic pressure (wedge hepatic vein pressure) is low, but the portal venous pressure is very high, as measured by splenic manometry. If the intrahepatic pressure is high, indicating cirrhosis, then splenic manometry is unnecessary.

Hepatic blood flow is of great importance but, unfortunately, cannot be measured. There are presently no practical techniques that can assess this parameter except cannulation of the portal vein and the xenon washout technique. Such cannulation is hazardous because it may lead to portal vein thrombosis. Hemodynamically, what we really want to quantitate is (1) hepatic arterial compensation for the diminished portal vein flow and (2) portal venous perfusion of the liver. At present we try to estimate by angiography the probability of maintaining venous flow to the liver. An important observation in angiographic study is the location and size of collateral vessels. In the selective shunt operation, one deliberately ligates the collaterals that take blood away from the liver. Of course, in doing a portacaval shunt, you like to know where the coronary vein is and the angiogram provides this information.

Splenoportography, one of the oldest angiographic techniques, will show patency of the portal vein but cannot definitely establish occlusion. Failure to visualize the vein may be due to reverse flow rather than occlusion. The splenoportogram demonstrates the size and location of venous collaterals, knowledge which is of real importance in the selective shunt and of moderate importance in other shunting procedures. Splenoportography is currently the best available practical assessment of portal venous flow to the liver. We do not do direct portal vein studies because of the reported occurrence of portal vein thrombosis following cannulation. For a mesocaval shunt, portal vein thrombosis doesn't make much difference, but it makes a tremendous difference if you hope to preserve portal venous perfusion of the liver. A patient who shows large portal vein flow to the liver and very little collateral is an excellent candidate for selective distal splenorenal shunt.

When the splenoportogram shows no portal flow to the liver, a conventional portacaval shunt does not induce any severe change in the hepatic hemodynamic status. We do not consider such patients candidates for a distal splenorenal shunt but rather for some type of side-to-side procedure, for example, mesocaval interposition.

In the late stages of hemodynamic block in the liver, manometry shows that there is inflow block, there is trans-sinus block and, most significantly, an outflow block from the sinusoids. The intrahepatic pressure becomes so high that it exceeds the pressure in the portal vein, which is decompressed by big collaterals. On the splenic angiogram the portal vein may look as if it is clotted.

Many surgeons do not perform portal-systemic shunting procedures but all are involved in treating upper gastrointestinal hemorrhage. Splenic vein thrombosis is an important although unusual cause of such bleeding. This condition shows an absolutely characteristic x-ray feature, a hugely dilated gastroepiploic vein (Fig. 1). Why isn't that vein dilated in portal vein thrombosis or in cirrhosis? The reason is that the portal vein pressure is high, so there is no pressure gradient to utilize the gastroepiploic vein as a collateral from spleen to portal vein. In splenic vein thrombosis, there is high pressure distally and a normal pressure centrally. Because of the pressure difference, the gastroepiploic vein becomes grossly dilated. In our series of eight such patients, three underwent gastrectomy. In each case the surgeon commented on an enormous gastroepiploic vein but did not remove the spleen, which is the curative procedure. Every patient bled again. When operating upon a bleeding patient who has a normal looking liver and a huge spleen, think of splenic vein thrombosis. These factors help to think of the diagnosis: Is there pancreatic disease? Has there been

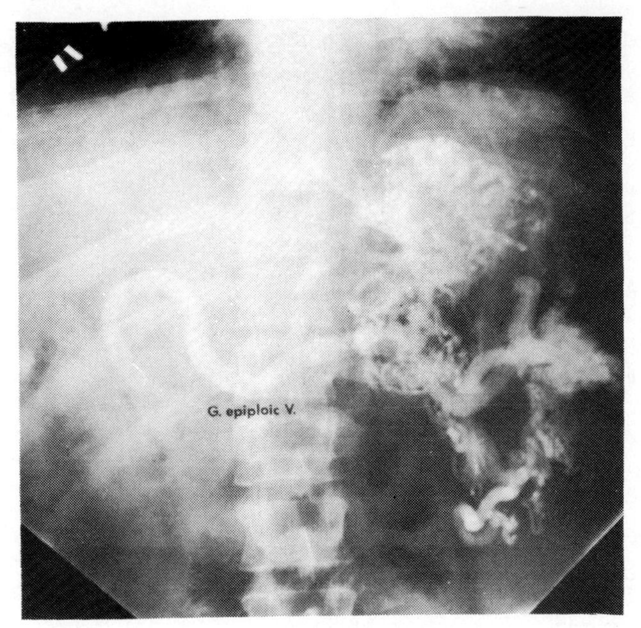

FIGURE 1.

pancreatic trauma? Is there a lymphoma that could obstruct the splenic vein? When in doubt, you can measure splenic pulp pressure, which will be very high, while the portal vein pressure is normal. If, in addition to splenic vein thrombosis, you suspect portal vein thrombosis, inject radiographic media into one of the mesenteric veins to determine its patency or occlusion.

We utilize hepatic vein catheterization frequently. It is essentially risk free and serves to establish the level of portal hypertension under basal conditions. It will separate out the schistosomiasis patient, the portal vein thrombosis patient and the idiopathic portal hypertension patient, which conditions are always accompanied by a low intrahepatic pressure. Hepatic vein wedge pressure and wedge hepatic venography are very useful in establishing the cause of the portal hypertension. Hepatic vein angiography can show spontaneous retrograde portal flow and thus separate this circumstance from that of a thrombosed portal vein. Splenic or portal venography will not do so.

We correlate hepatic vein wedge pressure with hepatic venography. Together they are extremely reliable in demonstrating the degree of portal flow. With significant portal flow to the liver the picture is the sinusoidal bed full of dye with no retrograde filling into the portal system following

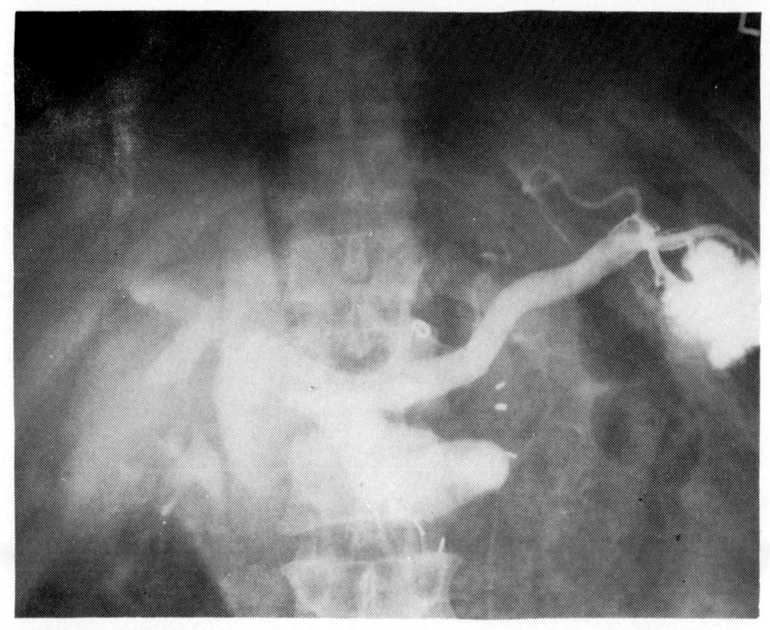

FIGURE 2.

wedge hepatic vein injection. With moderate portal flow, the sinusoidogram shows some dye entering the portal vein to continue out toward the periphery. With severe reduction in portal flow to the liver, the portal vein clearly fills in a retrograde fashion.

Figure 2 shows a splenoportogram after a mesocaval interposition H-graft. The portal vein fills with dye which exits via the shunt. Every one of our H-graft subjects shows the picture of retrograde portal flow out of the liver.

Indirect portography by superior mesenteric arteriogram is comparatively risk-free. It is the only method for the postsplenectomy patient. You obtain additional helpful information from arteriography, particularly as relates to anatomy of the hepatic artery. The very common hepatic artery anomalies can lead to technical problems during a shunting procedure.

A study that we have begun to employ in the last three or four years is renal vein angiography to locate the left renal vein with respect to the splenic vein. This is helpful in planning a selective splenorenal shunt.

A new test from our lab will not find immediate general use but is of tremendous ultimate importance in the field of portal hypertension surgery in the cirrhotic [3]. Figure 3 outlines the Krebs-Henseleit cycle,

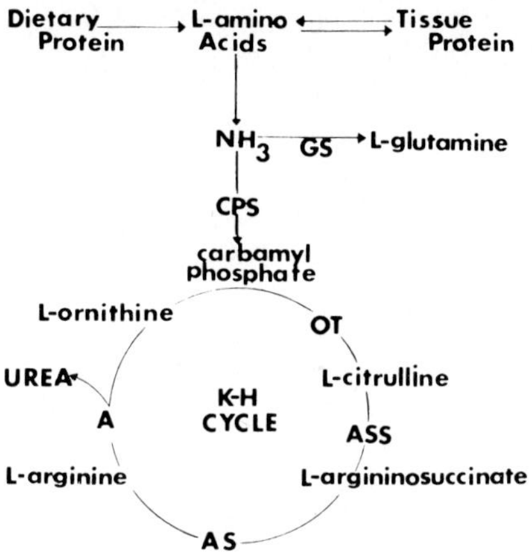

FIGURE 3.

which is a major pathway for protein catabolism. If encephalopathy is related to ammonia, then it must be related to the ability of the liver to carry out the functions of the Krebs-Henseleit cycle. In cirrhosis, there is marked reduction in the enzymes involved in this cycle and a quantitative depression of the liver's ability to handle ammonia and amino acid metabolism. I was always taught that the last thing to fall in liver disease was urea metabolism, this only shortly before death. That is not true! Amino acids are broken down by specific enzymes to ammonia. The ammonia may go through carbamyl synthetase and then into the Krebs-Henseleit cycle and out as urea. The name of the test we have developed is the Maximal Rate of Urea Synthesis (M.R.U.S.). The test is based on giving an excess of protein to make the Krebs-Henseleit cycle function maximally. Urine urea nitrogen is measured. After a protein load, a peak is reached and urea excretion no longer climbs but continues level for a considerable time without any additional protein input and then later falls. This determines the maximal rate of urea excretion, but does not necessarily represent urea synthesis, because urea may be stored or may be destroyed in the gut. To convert from the maximal rate of urea excretion to the maximal rate of urea synthesis we calculate for urea synthesized but not excreted. This is accomplished by noting the change in the BUN during the test period and by measuring total body water. Values are calculated in milligrams of urea nitrogen per hour per body weight to the three-quarters power. This is a complicated metabolic test that has been shown to relate very closely to encephalopathy. We feel that it will be possible in the relatively near future to categorize a patient with regard to how much hepatic reserve he has before he enters a metabolic insufficiency state and, therefore, encephalopathy.

Summary

1. Careful study allows prediction of the immediate operative mortality risk of a particular patient.

2. Objective hemodynamic measurements help to select which operative procedure is best for each patient.

3. The risk of severe morbidity from portal systemic encephalopathy, which heretofore has so blunted the effects of our surgical endeavors, may soon be predictable by metabolic testing.

References

1. Orloff, M. J.: Emergency portacaval shunt. A comparative study of shunt, varix ligation and nonsurgical treatment of bleeding esophageal varices in unselected patients with cirrhosis. Ann. Surg., 166:456-478, 1967.
2. Mikkelsen, W., Turril, F. and Kern, W.: Acute hyealine necrosis of the liver. Amer. J. Surg., 116:266-272, 1968.
3. Warren, W. D., Rudman, D., Millikan, W. et al: The metabolic basis of portasystemic encephalopathy and the effect of selective versus nonselective shunts. Ann. Surg., 180:573-579, 1974.

Physiology and Results of the Selective Distal Splenorenal Shunt

W. Dean Warren, M.D.

It would be a mistake to think that the type of portal systemic shunt makes no difference. Some surgeons propose to do the one technically easiest and that's all there is to it. The hard facts are that that is not all there is to it. I want to present some scientific data, something which you are not accustomed to seeing on this subject.

The prophylactic shunt prospective series [1, 2] have clearly shown that a portacaval shunt will not prolong the life of a cirrhotic patient who has not bled. Other current data indicate that a portacaval shunt probably prolongs life slightly for a patient who has bled; but this has not been established at a level of statistical significance. The prophylactic series came out with a very acceptable 7% operative mortality. Yet, the shunted patients died slightly sooner than the control patients who did not have an operation.

The fact that the major cause of death was hemorrhage in the control or nonoperative group is of extreme importance. There were also a significant number of patients in the control group who did not bleed but who developed progressive, fatal hepatic failure. In the shunt group, there was excellent control of bleeding. Shunting, however, led to an accelerated rate of hepatic failure, as has been noted in every study ever conducted on total portal systemic shunt procedures. There is invariably an acceleration of the rate of hepatic failure and death. Only the mechanism of death changes from the frightening rush to the emergency room with exsanguinating hemorrhage to one of quiet somnolence in hepatic failure. Total diversion of portal flow unquestionably leads to hepatic atrophy and death at a far more rapid rate than seen in the group of patients on medical therapy who do not bleed.

The surgeons at the University of North Carolina became disenchanted with shunt operations and turned to nonshunting procedures,

---

W. Dean Warren, M.D., Joseph B. Whitehead Professor and Chairman, Department of Surgery, Emory University School of Medicine, Atlanta, Ga.

ligation of varices, splenectomy, pyloroplasty and vagotomy [3]. They had a high immediate postoperative mortality but then a less rapid rate of death. With respect to overall survival, these patients ended up about the same as groups of patients with shunts. Two important facts emerged from the North Carolina study:

1. The major cause of continuing mortality was hemorrhage, as with every nonshunting procedure that has been studied thus far.
2. Encephalopathy was not a significant problem.

I simply do not understand surgeons who claim that they do not see encephalopathy. Every objective study directed at the question has shown a tremendous incidence of encephalopathy following portacaval shunts. Virtually all patients go through a stage of encephalopathy before they die of hepatic failure.

The original portacaval shunt series from New York Presbyterian Hospital was followed up by Voorhees [4]. In the patients surviving for five years or longer, over two thirds had moderate to marked encephalopathy. At the end of five years, less than 15% of the patients could be said to be functioning in a normal socioeconomic fashion. There are two associated problems, hepatic failure and portal-systemic encephalopathy, as sequelae to the total portal-systemic shunting procedures.

We once did many side-to-side portacaval shunts and have studied them for years. Because our own data indicated that this operation precipitated an increased rate of hepatic failure, we felt the need for a new procedure. Total portal-systemic shunting led to increased rates of death from hepatic failure and encephalopathy. Nonshunt procedures failed to control bleeding and had a high operative mortality. At the outset, we established these criteria for an acceptable operation:

1. Effective decompression of gastroesophageal veins, not by ligation but by shunting.
2. Preservation of hepatopetal portal flow, that is, portal flow to the liver. The reasons for this criterion are two: (a) Encephalopathy is related to nitrogen metabolism. Sustaining portal blood flow through the liver should at least modify the patient's tendency to develop encephalopathy following protein ingestion. (b) Equally important is avoidance of progressive hepatic atrophy and liver failure, which frequently develops after total portal diversion. We were later supported in this opinion by the work of Starzl and others who showed the great importance of hepatotrophic factors in the portal blood [5].

Our operation for selective decompression of gastroesophageal varices is shown in Figure 1. Ninety-six percent of all fatal hemorrhages from

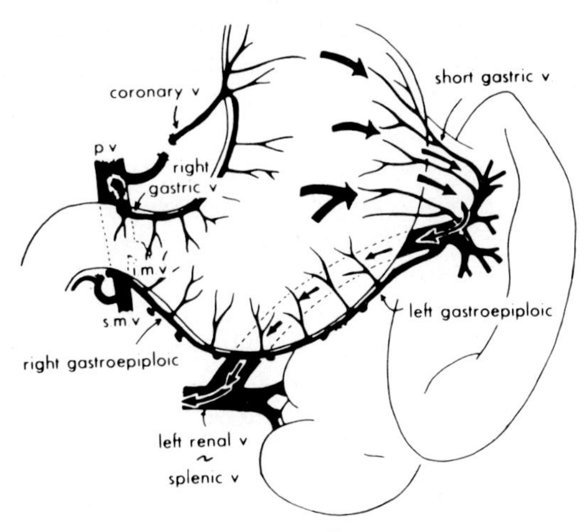

FIGURE 1.

varices in portal hypertension come from a 2 inch segment in the region of the esophagogastric junction. Our aim is to decompress that region while maintaining high portal pressure so that mesenteric and pancreatic effluent blood perfuse the liver. The operation includes disconnection of portal-mesenteric from gastrosplenic veins so that portal blood will not overload the splenic collaterals, nor will mesenteric blood be diverted away from the liver. With the procedure depicted, the pressure in the spleen falls to normal.

We have routinely studied shunt patency following the selective operation by observing the venous phase in splenic arteriography. Patency has been determined in every patient, either by angiography or at autopsy. There has been over a 95% patency rate of these distal splenorenal shunts in our series. The apparent reason for success is that the anastomosis is made at the point of maximal splenic vein circumference and enters in line with the flow of the renal vein to minimize turbulence. The splenic vein enters the renal like a tributary and not against the stream as do conventional splenorenal shunts, which have a 30%-40% occlusion rate in most series. Without question, the patency of the splenorenal anastomosis is maintained after our operation.

A second major issue is whether the operation prevents bleeding. In the last seven years we have had one patient readmitted for bleeding esophageal varices. This individual had a thrombosed shunt and ultimately died from hemorrhage.

A third important question is maintenance of portal perfusion to the liver. Superior mesenteric arteriography has demonstrated clearly that superior mesenteric vein blood perfuses the liver after the selective shunt. We can tell, angiographically, that portal vein blood reaches the liver but cannot do so at autopsy. Of the patients studied angiographically, over 95% showed portal perfusion of the liver, a figure similar to that of shunt patency.

One reason we are conducting a randomized study of selective splenorenal shunts versus mesocaval or mesorenal H-grafts is that Drapanas, who popularized the procedure, has claimed continued portal perfusion of the liver and has contended that these patients do not get encephalopathy [6]. We have been unable to demonstrate portal perfusion of the liver in a single patient in the H-graft series. Conversely, wedge hepatic vein catheterization with hepatic venography shows blood refluxing into the liver, passing back down the portal vein and out through the shunt into the vena cava. Portal blood does not perfuse the liver following a mesorenal or a mesocaval shunt.

Study of the maximum ability of the liver to synthesize urea has been a helpful tool with which to evaluate these operative procedures. The postoperative cases studied for this function show two things:

1. The H-graft shunt group is significantly diminished from the normal in its ability to synthesize urea.
2. The encephalopathic group is lower (.001 significance) than the total group of postoperative patients. We have clearly correlated the presence of encephalopathy with marked restriction in ability to remove and metabolize ammonia and amino acids from the circulation.

Only one patient in the selective group has developed encephalopathy. We later learned that she had been to a dentist, who had administered Demerol and Seconal. After these medications, the patient became confused. She is included in our results as an example of encephalopathy even though she was not nitrogen-intolerant and has not showed further signs of encephalopathy in the subsequent three years.

In comparing ability to synthesize urea for the nonselective H-graft group versus the selective shunt before and after operation statistical analyses show several things:

1. The preoperative values in the two groups were equal.
2. The postoperative values in the selective shunt group were unchanged. There has been no demonstrable injury to these patients with regard to ability to metabolize ammonia to urea. In marked contrast are the H-graft patients. The nonselective shunt patients show a decrease in ability to synthesize urea significant at the .025 confidence level. Urea synthesis is unequivocally

depressed following total diversion of portal flow from the liver.

3. The frequency of encephalopathy in those patients who were not encephalopathic before surgery is also highly significant in the H-graft group.

These data show that the nonselective H-graft shunt results in significant metabolic impairment of the liver and that this impairment is correlated, virtually 1 to 1, with the development of encephalopathy. In the next few years, we anticipate that we will be able to show that patients who start off with low urea synthesizing capacity are going to be more prone to encephalopathy because even a little liver injury will be intolerable. A good preoperative maximal urea synthesis will not, of itself, insure freedom from encephalopathy but a poor one indicates an increased danger. On the other hand, starting out with a good urea synthesizing ability does not assure that it will be maintained after total portal diversion.

We are developing an ammonium chloride tolerance test which will soon be available to hospitals around the country [7]. Using this test in the selective shunt group, only two patients out of seven changed. In the nonselective or H-graft group all showed diminished ammonium chloride tolerance and encephalopathy correlated with this fall. The difference between these two groups is highly significant. This test provides objective, unequivocal metabolic evidence that there is major hepatic impairment following a total portacaval shunt.

In our prospective clinical series all patients are studied to decide whether they are good risks for operation. If so, they are randomized by drawing a sealed envelope. Among selective shunt patients one has been hospitalized for encephalopathy – the patient who took the Demerol and Seconal following a dental extraction. Five patients have been readmitted for encephalopathy in the nonselective H-graft group. Two more developed encephalopathy before leaving the hospital and were, therefore, placed on markedly restricted protein intake and on oral neomycin. In the selective shunt group there has been one death, a lady who actually never left the hospital after shunt thrombosis. She developed ascites, recurrent infections, and finally died with bleeding as the terminal episode. This patient is counted as a recurrent hemorrhage.

There is no question that the difference between a selective shunt, which maintains portal perfusion of the liver, and a total shunt, which diverts portal blood from the liver, is highly significant. It does make a great deal of difference which shunt is done. You are fooling yourself, and I think that you are subjecting the patient to severe hazards, if you take the attitude that any shunt is equally satisfactory. It should be mentioned that all these data refer to elective surgery. In an emergency situation you must do the best you can to get a live patient.

In our early experience with the selective shunt, we had a high operative mortality [8]. At first only the very sick patients were operated on because we knew that no other procedure would permit survival. More recently, operating on good risk patients, now about 70 in number, the operative mortality is around 5%, the hospital mortality about 7%.

Summary

1. The selective splenorenal shunt operation is unequivocally effective in the control of variceal hemorrhage, as effective as a conventional portacaval shunt.

2. There are major demonstrable metabolic differences between total and selective shunts. We have already established a statistically significant advantage for the selective distal splenorenal shunt in the ability to synthesize urea and in the prevention of encephalopathy. The only thing that remains to be demonstrated, and these patients are not yet three years into the randomized study, is that increased survival will follow this shunt compared to a total shunt, as epitomized by an H-graft interposition.

References

1. Conn, H. O. and Lindenmuth, W. W.: Prophylactic portacaval anastomosis in cirrhotic patients with esophageal varices. New Eng. J. Med., 279:725-732, 1968.
2. Garceau, A. J., Donaldson, R. M., O'Hara, E. T. et al: A controlled trial of prophylactic portacaval-shunt surgery. New Eng. J. Med., 270:496-500, 1964.
3. Peters, R. M. and Womack, N. A.: Surgery of vascular distortions in cirrhosis of the liver. Ann. Surg., 154:432-445, 1961.
4. Voorhees, A. B., Jr., Price, J. B., Jr. and Britton, R. C.: Portasystemic shunting procedure for portal hypertension. Amer. J. Surg., 119:501-505, 1970.
5. Starzl, T. E., Francavilla, A., Halgrimson, C. G. et al: The origin, hormonal nature and action of hepatrophic substances in portal venous blood. Surg. Gynec. Obstet., 137:179-199, 1973.
6. Drapanas, T.: Interposition mesocaval shunt for treatment of portal hypertension. Ann. Surg., 176:435-448, 1972.
7. Warren, W. D., Rudman, D., Millikan, W. et al: The metabolic basis of portasystemic encephalopathy and the effect of selective venous nonselective shunts. Ann. Surg., 180:573-579, 1974.
8. Warren, W. D., Zeppa, R. and Fomon, J. J.: Selective transplenic decompression of gastroesophageal varices by distal splenorenal shunt. Ann. Surg., 166:437-455, 1967.

Panel Discussion

Moderator:	R. L. Varco, M.D.	
Panelists:	H. Popper, M.D.	W. D. Warren, M.D.
	F. G. Moody, M.D.	S. Schwartz, M.D.
	M. L. Gliedman, M.D.	A. S. Leonard, M.D.

Dr. Varco: Dr. Gliedman, do you make any particular efforts to try to protect the duodenum against the adjacent rigidity of the graft when you create the cavo-mesenteric grafts?

Dr. Gliedman: A long time ago, when we started to do the mesocaval shunts, we were impressed with the way the duodenum hung on the graft. We are still impressed with the way it hangs on the dacron prosthesis. But, aside from thinking about it and talking about it, we really don't do anything except completely free up the duodenum so that it is not really pressed against the graft but is simply resting against it. It is a commonly thought of concern. It has not, apparently, in anyone's series been a significant problem.

Dr. Varco: Questions have been raised about differences in the length of the graft material used. Drs. Gliedman, Schwartz and Warren, please comment about your prejudices or cite the facts determining the length of the graft that you prefer. Obviously, it must reach between the two places, but is there any appropriate point of emphasis on short versus long?

Dr. Gliedman: In the H-graft, our initial attitude was to make it as short and wide as possible to get the greatest decompression. We did that, largely, in our young adult males. As time has passed, we have gone on occasion to a longer, narrower graft. As the patient gets older, we tend to use a smaller diameter, 18 mm longer length graft. Therefore, we are, in some way, decompressing the liver less. Whether or not that is correct, I cannot say because it is a small group of patients. We don't decompress as well. We sacrifice decompression for what we think is sustained perfusion.

Dr. Varco: Dr. Schwartz, do you have any comments?

Dr. Schwartz: We use as short a graft as possible when we do the H-graft. I am interested to hear Dr. Gliedman's comments that he does have a differential between the long and the short grafts. I would not anticipate much of a pressure drop in that system, over an additional 12 inches, when you are dealing with that large a conduit. The one case in which we did use a long graft – because of the circumstance which he described, of having difficulty with the duodenum – did thrombose. But we have not had a short graft thrombose now for longer than two years.

Dr. Warren: In contrast to my confreres, we have actually measured the length of these things that have been put in, in the mesocaval side. Dr. Atef Salam, of our group at Emory University Hospital, has measured them, and they average 7 cm in length in the typical mesocaval position. In contrast with the mesorenal shunt, you have a direct shot from the superior mesenteric to renal, there is 4 cm. So there is significantly less length in using the mesorenal approach. Whether or not this is important, I don't know. But I would say that the argument of "I would use the H-graft if it would stay patent" is no longer viable. They will stay patent in the vast majority of instances.

Dr. Varco: Dr. Warren, a number of people raise questions about residual hypersplenism in an individual who has had that problem and in whom you do your type of anastomosis. Has this been a difficulty? Have they all responded?

Dr. Warren: That is an interesting question because the same people who ask that question will do an H-graft, which does not relieve the hypersplenism any more than anything else, but they don't think anything about it. This shunt is just like an end-to-side portacaval shunt, a side-to-side portacaval shunt, or an H-graft shunt. It decompresses the spleen to normal pressure. One third stay the same; one third will get a little better; one third get significantly better. But we have not had to operate upon any patient for severe hypersplenism, either in the selective shunt group or in the portacaval shunt group. I would say that the theoretic disadvantage of severe hypersplenism is what Dr. Schwartz said – you have a markedly depressed platelet count and you might have interoperative bleeding. In two instances, we have ligated the splenic artery, as a result of concern about this; although we don't have the data, the shunt stayed open and that is all we can say.

Dr. Varco: Is it concern about the shunt staying open that guides you in not doing it more frequently?

Dr. Warren: Yes, that is correct. As soon as we get the scientific data, which we are fairly sure will be within the next two or three years, this will be the conclusive period, then we are going to make several technical changes, which we don't want to introduce at this time. One would be ligation of the splenic artery in patients with a huge spleen and severe hypersplenism. I believe that they will continue to stay patent because of the large arterial collateral flow that enters the spleen. The others are related to the use of an H-graft between the splenic vein and the renal vein and then ligation of the splenic vein. Dr. Schwartz had a mistake on one of his slides. But I have learned to live with Dr. Schwartz's mistakes over the years. A side-to-side splenorenal shunt does not perfuse the liver. We wrote a classic paper on this. Dr. Schwartz, on one of your drawings you said, "Question perfusion of the liver." Would you take that question out?

Dr. Gliedman: I must take issue with one of Dr. Warren's comments about hypersplenism. I think that that was well answered by a monograph many years ago by Dr. Carl Axel Eckmann; he measured the splenic size, the white count change, the platelet count and the hematocrit in control and postshunt patients. It has been duplicated many times by many people. In our experience, people who have secondary hypersplenism, that is, congestive splenomegaly with decompression, will lose their congestive splenomegaly. I am not talking about the H-graft, particularly; I am just talking about successful shunting procedures. I have no information at all on the patients on whom we have done the reverse splenorenal shunt. But good "first line" decompressive procedures for the portal system will take care of hypersplenism in nine out of ten patients.

Dr. Warren: Dr. Gliedman, do you mean return to normal? If you do, that is absolutely wrong. Dr. Sheila Sherlock has studied this most carefully, with Roger Williams, measuring splenic blood flow before and after shunt. The splenic blood flow actually increases significantly after shunt. If they have had a platelet count of 50,000 or lower, they rarely return to normal.

Dr. Gliedman: I was very cautious about what I said. I said, congestive splenomegaly and hypersplenism. There was an article in *The Quarterly Review of Medicine* some years ago that reviews all of this. There are three or four good reasons why these cirrhotics have hematologic disorders. And there are other reasons why they have some deficiencies in the postshunt period: measuring stasis within the spleen, spleen size, and the things that appear to relate to secondary hypersplenism will revert after a successful decompressive procedure in about nine out of ten patients.

Dr. Varco: Dr. Popper, what are your thoughts about this problem?

Dr. Popper: I have already discussed in my presentation at least two reasons for splenic enlargement: one is a mechanical process and its correction will depend upon the hemodynamic change. The second is far more mysterious, namely, reticuloendothelial as well as lymphoid cell hyperplasia, which, by some mechanism, is related to liver injury. These two have been separated. I am not quite clear about what these latter irritation factors are. But we have known for many years that splenomegalic cirrhosis, with spleens the size of 1,550 gm, is not simply mechanically explained. The mechanical factor may or may not be corrected by plumbing, such as portacaval shunts, whereas the irritative factor is not changed.

Dr. Varco: Dr. Moody, some of our audience is questioning the point you raised about the apparent difference in the attack rate of encephalopathy in certain geographic areas. Do you have any additional information that you can give us in elaboration of this seeming difference?

Dr. Moody: I can only say that our follow-up, in the Birmingham series, is very short; we have only been seven years in this study. We have tried very carefully to document changes in mentation of these patients. But the follow-up in the ones who continue to drink is most difficult. I wonder if Dr. Warren would tell us how he is able to keep this group together so he can follow them so carefully. I think that it is extremely important to bring these people back at intervals, talk to them and find out how they are doing. Before Dr. Warren answers that question, may I ask Dr. Warren another question? I must say that I hope that his operation works out, because it will be a marvelous thing for people who need to have portal hypertension. Was the mortality in the control group 24%? For some reason or other, this doesn't quite fit in with what I think it should be for an end-to-side portacaval shunt. So will you spell out in a little clearer way what has happened to the people in the control group.

Dr. Warren: There was no operative mortality in either group. I would like to ask you if you could improve on that? Second, the figures that you quoted were those who required actual rehospitalization for encephalopathy. There were five out of 17 in the total shunt group, one out of 17 in the selective shunt group.

Dr. Moody: No one has died, Dr. Warren?

Dr. Warren: They have died postoperatively, after they have gone home. These are all after they go home.

Dr. Moody: Do they go home in seven days?

Dr. Warren: They do, if there is no available bed in the Metabolic Research Unit.

Dr. Varco: Dr. Schwartz, a few questions on Pitressin, with particular regard to details. Given a patient whom you have decided to treat with intra-arterial Pitressin, please tell us the regimen and what you use for end points.

Dr. Schwartz: The catheter is inserted, with the Seldinger technique, into the superior mesenteric artery. We use a lambda pump but any type of infusion pump can be used. After an angiogram is done by the radiologist, we start the Pitressin, and we see if there is an effect on the vasculature. Not all people are doing that. But we are interested to see, directly, what the vasoconstrictive effect is. We infuse 0.2 units of Pitressin per milliliter, 1 ml/min, into the catheter. We follow the patients with x-rays daily. By merely looking at the curve of the tip, you can tell whether it is still in the superior mesenteric artery. We generally maintain the Pitressin, if bleeding stops, for a period of about 12 hours after the cessation of bleeding and then switch to a non-Pitressin infusion, leaving the catheter in place. More frequently than not we operate on the reasonable risk patients and so prior to going to the operating room, reinstitute the Pitressin to decrease the bleeding from the veins of Retzius. There have been problems reported with the use of vasopressin. We have seen one unusual one. There are two reported cases, as far as I know, of intestinal necrosis related to the drug. We have not seen this. One inadvertent positioning of the catheter in the hepatic artery, causing hepatic necrosis, has been reported. The complication that we saw was an unusual one in a patient who was a poor risk, whom we did not think would be suitable for surgery; the Pitressin therapy was maintained for 17 days! He was bleeding intermittently. When he stopped bleeding, we decreased the Pitressin, and he had the most enormous diuresis I have ever seen! We had to reinstitute the Pitressin and then taper him off again. What is necessary for this technic is a cadre of radiologists willing to get up in the middle of the night. Although we were initially enthusiastic about the intravenous technic, we rarely use it now. Only when all of the angiologists are out of town will we go back to the intravenous technic. We rely solely on the intra-arterial infusion.

Dr. Moody: Dr. Schwartz, do you use the intravenous technic in the emergency room to get them to the x-ray suite?

Dr. Schwartz: No, we have not been doing that. The only ones who have had the intravenous Pitressin have been those cases when the radiologists have been out of town. We have had two such patients in the past 1½ years.

Dr. Gliedman: We have had an experience with over 150 of these cannulations now. You must do an angiogram before you start the infusion. Not infrequently you will see a large flow to the liver. The catheter should be beyond an aberrant hepatic artery or large inferior pancreatic duodenal branch. If you are flushing that Pitressin into the liver, you can get significant liver dysfunction. We have used the usual dosage, which Dr. Schwartz has described. Recently, where we have not been able to stop the bleeding, we have doubled it to 0.4 units of Pitressin per minute. Interestingly enough, we have seen no side effects, other than a somewhat greater increase in the systemic blood pressure. It is an extremely important addition, I think, to our capability. I warn against the intravenous infusion of Pitressin. By that route the greatest effect of Pitressin is on the heart. If the patient has just come into the emergency room, he is hypovolemic and depleted. If you start the patient on intravenous Pitressin with a low cardiac output, you may have an abrupt, unexpected cardiac arrest.

Dr. Varco: Dr. Leonard, given a child under age 4 whom you have decided to operate upon and do a splenorenal shunt, describe those technical aspects which you think are most helpful in obtaining the best result, granted that you have evidence a vein adequate in size.

Dr. Leonard: As shown in my slide presentation, the central splenorenal shunt for us has been the best shunt. One does not have to dissect the distal portion of the splenic vein. I think that this is one of the only places where you really get into trouble because of the myriad of small veins that come off into the pancreas. If one then identifies the large splenic vein, centrally cuts it off at that point and brings that vein down onto the renal vein, one should get an adequate shunt and a much easier dissection. I agree, also, with Dr. Warren that it is important to know where that left renal vein is. One should have an IVP to be sure that you have a good kidney; occasionally, you will have a very small fibrotic kidney on that side. Moreover, a large spleen makes the dissection easier in that the splenic vein migrates inferior to the fixed portion of the renal vein.

Dr. Varco: Dr. Popper, is there any help for us through use of serial biopsies of the liver in hopefully comparable cases, following a variety of shunts, for chronicling what happens to the liver after a given shunt versus what happens after another type of shunt?

Dr. Popper: It really depends upon what you are expecting from the liver biopsy. If you expect information which deals with the cirrhotic status of the liver, a serial biopsy is misleading. We know that fibrotic nodular and other similar changes vary throughout the organ while liver cell injury usually does not. The liver biopsy picture is therefore not representative of what you are interested in and serial biopsy may confuse you. If you are dealing with macronodular cirrhosis, the various nodules may show quite different changes and you may not even obtain fibrous tissue. It has been used in a large series which I, myself, examined. It took some 10 to 12 years in doing the follow-up study and I had to report that the correlation between what was seen in the liver biopsy and the final outcome was miserable.

Dr. Varco: For all panel members who operate on the alcoholic cirrhotic, this question is the final one for them: At this time, on the basis of all the therapies that are available to you and assuming for purposes of discussion the comparability between the cases that you are looking at, do you think that you are doing the same number of shunts, more shunts or less shunts as you view your case load profile of patients in 1974. For Dr. Warren, while the other panel members are thinking, please answer this question: Have you included in this prospective study of the randomized patients undergoing two different types of shunts any attempt at what might be called early or intra-operative morphology studies, followed by subsequent morphology studies, as a bulwark to the biochemical data that you are accumulating? And the second part of the question: Can you give us any help with technical details so that we can avoid some unfortunate dissections in attempting to free up this splenic vein?

Dr. Warren: In answer to the first part of the question, the only morphologic studies that we do are liver biopsies. We follow those periodically, as we follow these people and readmit them to the Metabolic Unit. So we do have data of that sort. As Dr. Popper has said, it has not been very helpful in predicting prognosis, except as it predicts immediate mortality. We have been able to identify when some people came back in with a real fatty liver that they had reinstituted alcoholic drinking. I would like to take this opportunity to discuss something which I apparently did not do during my presentation, that this shunt is contraindicated if there is intense ascites. That means that in about three-quarters of the emergency shunts that you do, the patients will not be candidates for the distal shunt. We have done a good number of emergency shunts in patients who did not have ascites. The big mortality which we originally had was operating on people with ascites. That is the one thing that you should avoid. I apparently overlooked mentioning that in my presentation.

Dr. Varco: Dr. Warren, that concept isn't to extend to include persons with ascities who have been treated and have had the situation corrected?

Dr. Warren: No, we will operate upon these patients during the same hospital admission, if they clear the ascites. The other part of the question, about technic, is one that is, of course, extremely important. You can do all of the physiology, you can do all of the pathology. But, in operating upon this group of patients, I am convinced that much of the nature of your results is going to be related to the technical finesse with which the operation is performed. We had a diagrammatic demonstration of this operation. Dr. Varco showed one of the slides in his presentation, from *Hospital Practice,* and I think that it was about the best operative description of this procedure, yet published. I think that between the two institutions, Miami, where this was started, and Atlanta, where I am now located, we have done over 50 consecutive elective cases without a mortality in either institution. So it can be done! It is not an operation which requires a genius to perform. I personally have trained six people, some of whom do it better than I. You should not leave this symposium thinking that it is all right for me but that no one else can do it. That isn't so. In fact, I trained a man whom Dr. Schwartz once told me could not operate, to do this technic.

Dr. Moody: Dr. Warren, what procedure do you do if the patient has ascites? The last time you and I were on a panel I think you replied that the procedure you would do would be a side-to-side splenorenal shunt?

Dr. Warren: I think that you have to do some variety of a side-to-side procedure. If we can get to the splenic vein easily, without a major operation, it is simply a little sort of zip, zip, and it is up, and you put in an H-graft between the two of them. That will decompress the ascites and control the bleeding. You will have a candidate for encephalopathy and accelerated hepatic failure. If you have that situation, you go back in and simply ligate the splenic vein between the shunt and the superior mesenteric, and then devascularize the stomach, converting it to a selective shunt. But with massive ascites, jaundice, hemorrhage, I think it would be absolutely contraindicated to try to do a distal shunt. If I were you, I think I would do a mesocaval and just say, "The hell with it! We just have to do the best we can, under the circumstances!"

Dr. Varco: Please comment on the question I asked of the other surgeons on the panel.

Dr. Warren: We are doing more operations because we have less fear of encephalopathy. For instance, we have done a distal shunt on one patient, 74 years of age, who is not encephalopathic. Dr. Robert Zeppa brought her back four years postshunt and she is still not encephalopathic! So we feel much more confident about operating on the elderly than we did before. We have not decreased our surgical approach to this problem. But I know that, in general, the rest of the country has. Dr. Sherlock has encouraged us, and also the people in Miami, to look again at the problem of a prophylactic shunt. Theoretically, our operation is like a medical patient who won't bleed. In those circumstances, if they stop drinking, you can get 75%-80% five-year survival in those patients. So I think that in the next two or three years we are going to restudy the prophylactic shunt which with the total portal systemic shunt was shown to be not helpful but to be harmful.

Dr. Moody: My position does not change acutely by sitting on a panel or by reading the surgical literature. I stick with things that I have learned and then gradually modify them. When I moved from Birmingham to Salt Lake City I was in a population where there were very few patients who required shunting and the ones who did, by and large, were not alcoholics, so I have continued to employ the end-to-side portacaval shunt, as I have described it. If, indeed, I should become responsible for a regional center for portal hypertension, then I shall go to Dr. Warren's institution and learn how to do his operation and learn how to do it very well, so that I don't have to go through a period of trial and error. I believe that it is a shunt which should be applied when you are dealing with large numbers of patients who are alcoholics.

Dr. Schwartz: On direct questioning, just focusing on the one point of the alcoholic, the answer would be that we are doing fewer operations. We are doing an equivalent number of shunts. Of course, we are being referred more which are nonalcoholics. In the alcoholic patient, we are doing fewer, because, as I indicated, we will not accept a patient who is in a coma; we will not accept an intensely jaundiced patient, or one with intense ascites or other stigmata of advanced liver disease. In our hands, the alcoholic patients do not do well. Rarely, we have a patient who indicates that he will absolutely stop drinking. I am always astonished by Dr. Orloff's figures of his capability of getting 71% of his alcoholic patients to stop drinking. My figure would be closer to 5%.

Dr. Gliedman: As I started my presentation, I remarked that we do fewer shunts, one reason being the downhill course of the postshunt patient who drinks. If I were convinced about what Dr. Warren claims in terms of the ability of the prophylactic reverse splenorenal shunt to do no harm, I guess that I could be convinced to do more. I don't know why our experience is such, but the worst case of encephalopathy that I personally have seen was in a patient upon whom I had done the procedure Dr. Warren recommends specifically to avoid encephalopathy. I don't know what I did wrong. In any event, as things stand now, with the outlook for the postshunt patient, and with the difficulties that the general surgeon has, in doing shunt procedures and the rarity of the times that he does it, I suspect that most surgeons are going to be doing fewer shunts unless they are willing to do the procedure with which they are comfortable.

Subject Index